Drug Synthesis, Properties and Reactions

Drug Synthesis, Properties and Reactions

Edited by **Judith Baker**

SYRAWOOD
PUBLISHING HOUSE
New York

Published by Syrawood Publishing House,
750 Third Avenue, 9th Floor,
New York, NY 10017, USA
www.syrawoodpublishinghouse.com

Drug Synthesis, Properties and Reactions
Edited by Judith Baker

International Standard Book Number: 978-1-68286-347-3 (Hardback)

Printed in China.

Contents

Preface

Every book is a source of knowledge and this one is no exception. The idea that led to the conceptualization of this book was the fact that the world is advancing rapidly; which makes it crucial to document the progress in every field. I am aware that a lot of data is already available, yet, there is a lot more to learn. Hence, I accepted the responsibility of editing this book and contributing my knowledge to the community.

Pharmacology has become a very prominent field of study in the recent decades. It plays a crucial role in the development of therapeutic medicines and novel drugs that can be used for treatment of critical illnesses. The chapters included in this book provide significant information on the mechanism of drug action, methods of synthesis, adverse chemical reactions, evaluation of different drugs and chemical compounds, etc. Researches and case studies compiled herein aim to provide an overview of the latest advancements in this field. The important concepts that are discussed in the book will benefit students, researchers and professionals engaged in this field at various levels.

While editing this book, I had multiple visions for it. Then I finally narrowed down to make every chapter a sole standing text explaining a particular topic, so that they can be used independently. However, the umbrella subject sinews them into a common theme. This makes the book a unique platform of knowledge.

I would like to give the major credit of this book to the experts from every corner of the world, who took the time to share their expertise with us. Also, I owe the completion of this book to the never-ending support of my family, who supported me throughout the project.

Editor

1

Cytotoxicity and radiosensitising activity of synthesized dinitrophenyl derivatives of 5-fluorouracil

Khosrou Abdi[1,2], Ali Khalaj[1,2*], Syeed-Naser Ostad[3] and Mohammad Reza Khoshayand[4]

Abstract

Background and the purpose of the study: Dual functional agents in which nitroaromatic or nitroheterocyclic compounds are attached through a linker unit to mustards and aziridines have shown higher cytotoxicities than the corresponding counterparts to both aerobic and hypoxic cells and enhanced radiosensitizing activity. In the present investigation cytotoxicity and radiosensitizing activity of 2,4-dinitrobenzyl, 2,4-dinitrobenzoyl, and 2, 4-dinitrophenacetyl derivatives of 5-fluorouracil which was assumed to release cytotoxic active quinone methidide and 5-fluorouracil under hypoxic conditions on HT-29 cell line under both aerobic and hypoxic conditions was investigated.

Methods: 5-fluorouracil derivative X-XIII were prepared by the reaction of the corresponding di-nitro substituted benzyl, benzoyl and phenacetyl halides with 5-fluorouracil protected at N-1 with di-*t*-butoxydicarbonate (BOC) in dimethyl formamide (DMF) in the presence of the potassium carbonate followed by hydrolysis of the blocking group by potassium carbonate in methanol. Cytotoxicity of fluorouracil VIII and tested compounds X-XIII against HT-29 cell line under both aerobic and hypoxic conditions after 48 hrs incubation were measured by determination of the percent of the survival cells using 3-(4,5-Dimethylthiazol-2-yl)-2,5-diphenyltetrazolium bromide (MTT) assay and percent of the dead cells using propidium iodide(PI)-digitonine assay and results were used to calculate the corresponding IC_{50} values. Radiosensitization experiments were carried out by irradiation of the incubations with a ^{60}Co source and clonogenic assay was performed to determine the cell viabilities following treatment with the tested compounds and/or radiation. Sensitization Enhancement Ratio (SER) of each tested compound was obtained from the radiation survival curves in the absence and presence of each sensitizer for 37% survival respectively.

Results and major conclusion: Findings of the present study showed that alkylation or acylation of 5-fluorouracil result in compounds which have little or no cytotoxicity and radiosensitizing activity under aerobic conditions, but have high cytotoxicity and radiosensitizing effects under hypoxic conditions. Furthermore radiosensitizing activities of compounds under hypoxic conditions increased by increase in their concentrations and SER of the tested 5-FU derivatives at concentrations higher than 50 μmol were equal or higher than 1.6 which is the minimum effective SER of a radiosensitizer in an *in vitro* assay.

Keywords: Nitroaromatic compounds, HT-29 cell line, Radiosensitizing activity, Cytotoxicity, 5-FU

* Correspondence: khalaj@ams.ac.ir
[1]Department of Medicinal Chemistry, Tehran, Iran
[2]Department of Nuclear Pharmacy, Tehran, Iran
Full list of author information is available at the end of the article

Introduction

One of the most important reasoning for the resistance of solid tumors to chemotherapy and radiotherapy is the presence of hypoxic cells in these tumors due to insufficient blood supply. Oxygen as a radiosensitizer increases the effects of radiation by the formation of free radicals that damage DNA [1]. Nitroaromatic and nitroheterocyclic compounds known as electron affinic compounds act like oxygen in the hypoxic cells and increase the sensitivity of these cells to radiation by formation of radical anions through one electron reduction which is reversed by oxygen in aerobic cells [2]. In the absence of radiation, radiosensitizers are also toxic to hypoxic cells due to the formation of the nitro radical anion and suppressing intracellular sulfhydryl compounds which are radioprotectors [3]. In the normal oxygenated cells in which the initially reduced species can be readily re-oxidized by molecular oxygen, the cytotoxicity of the radiosensitizers has been attributed to the parent nitro compound or its bioactivation by NADPH:quinine oxidoreductase which can act as an oxygen insensitive reductase [4].

Several hybrid or dual functional agents have been described in which nitroaromatic or nitroheterocyclic compounds are attached through a linker unit to cytotoxic nitrogen mustards [2] and aziridine moieties [5] which act as a leaving group. These compounds have shown higher cytotoxicities and enhanced radiosensitizing activity on both aerobic and hypoxic cells than the corresponding counterparts [5]. In these compounds cellular reduction of the nitro group to more electron donating species activate the nitrogen of the cytotoxic group by the release of electron through the aromatic ring and generate reactive alkylating species[2]. Previously it was shown that 3[3-(2,4-dinitro-phenylamino)-propyl]-5-fluoro-1 H-pyrimidine-2,4-dione resulting from linkage of 2,4-dinitrophenylamine through three carbon atoms with 5-fluorouracil which is not a leaving group, under aerobic conditions is not cytotoxic but is radiosensitizer [6].

In the present study, the cytotoxicity and radiosensitizing activity of 2,4-dinitrobenzoyl, 2,4- and 3,5-dinitrobenzoyl and 2,4-dinitrophenylacetyl derivatives of 5-fluorouracil which was assumed to produce quinone methides and 5-fluorouracil [7] by increase in the electron density of the aromatic ring through reduction of the nitro to electron releasing groups under both aerobic and anaerobic conditions was investigated (Scheme 1).

Material and methods

Materials and instrumentation

5-Flourouracil, 2,4-dinitrobenzoic acid, 2,4-dinitrophenylacetic acid, 3,5-dinitrobenzoyl chloride, 2,4-dinitrobenzyl chloride, di-t-butoxydicarbonate $(Boc)_2O$, thionyl chloride, 4-Dimethyl aminopyridine (4-DMAP), digitonine, and other chemicals and solvents not listed here were from Merck Chemical Co. (Germany). HT-29 Cells (Human colon cancer cells) from Pasteur Institute (Iran), RPMI 1640 from Gibco (England), Fetal Bovine Serum (FBS), Penicillin/streptomycin 100X, Trypsin-EDTA 10X and Trypan blue from Biosera (England),MTT and PI from Sigma (USA) were used in this study. Thin layer chromatography was carried out using silica gel (Kieselgel 60, 230–400 mesh, Merck) to monitor the progress of reactions. Melting points were determined on a MEL-270 Sibata melting point apparatus and are uncorrected. ^{1}HNMR spectra were recorded on 500 MHz Bruker (Germany), using DMSO-d_6 or $CDCl_3$ as solvent. Chemical shifts (δ) are reported in ppm relative to TMS as internal standard. Mass spectra were obtained on a Finningan TSQ-70 instrument. Infrared spectra were recorded on a Nicolet Magna IR- 550 spectrometer (USA). All compounds were characterized by the analytical and spectral data. 3,5-dinitrobenzoyl chloride and 2,4-dinitrobenzyl chloride were commercially available and the known 2,4-dinitrobenzoyl, and 2,4-dinitrophenylacetyl chloride were prepared by the reported method [8] through the reaction of the corresponding acids with thionyl chloride. Analytical and spectroscopic data for the known compounds were consistent with the reported literature values and data only for new compounds are presented.

Chemistry

Preparation of compounds X-XIII

Synthesis of 3-(2,4-Dinitrobenzyl)-5-fluoropyrimidine-2,4(1 H,3 H)-dione X:

A solution of 5-Fu-Boc IX (2.30 g, 10 mmol) prepared by the reported method [9] in 30 ml of DMF, was treated with K_2CO_3 (1.38 g, 10 mmol), KI (0.41 g, 2.5 mmol), and 2,4-dinitrobezyl chloride (2.2 g, 10 mmol) and the mixture was heated at 78°C for 4 hrs. The mixture was then treated with water, acidified with HCl, and extracted with ethyl acetate (3 × 50 ml) and the organic layer was washed with cold water (5 × 30 ml). The organic phase was evaporated under reduced pressure and the residue was dissolved in MeOH (30 ml) and treated with K_2CO_3 (1.4 g, 5.1 mmol) and the reaction mixture was stirred for 2 hrs at room temperature. After evaporation of methanol under vacuum, the residue was diluted with EtOAc (30 ml) and washed with cold water (30 ml). The organic phase was dried over Na_2SO_4, evaporated under reduce pressure and the residue was purified by flash column chromatography (silica gel, hexane-EtOAc, 70:30) to give 1.74 g (56%) of the compound X as pale yellowish white color solid; mp: 252-254°C (EtOAc, hexane); IR (KBr) : 3129, 1736, 1659, 1541, 1347 cm^{-1}; ^{1}H NMR (500 MHz, DMSO-d_6): 5.33 (s, 2 H, CH2), 7.63 (d, J = 8.5 Hz, 1 H, H6 phenyl), 8.01. (d, J = 8.5,1 H, H-6 FU), 8.43 (dd, J = 8.5, 2.5 Hz, 1 H, H5 phenyl), 8.79 (d, J = 2.5 Hz 1 H, H3 phenyl); MS: 310

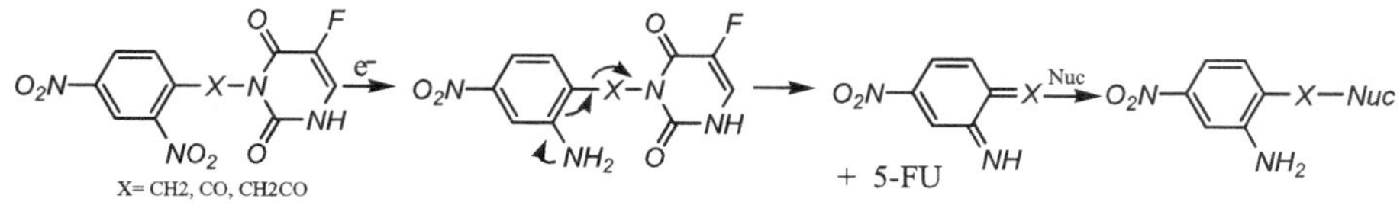

Scheme 1 Proposed metabolic reduction of compounds X-XIII on the basis of reference 7.

(7%), 264(43%), 181(100%), 167 (75%), 130 (70%), 91 (44%), 75 (76%).

Synthesis of 3-(2,4-dinitrobenzoyl)-5-fluoropyrimidine-2,4(1H,3H)-dione XI, 3-(2-(2,4-dinitrophenyl)acetyl)-5-fluoropyrimidine-2,4(1H,3H)-dione XII and 3-(3,5-dinitrobenzoyl)-5-fluoropyrimidine-2,4(1H,3H)-dione XIII:

A mixture of 5-Fu-Boc IX (2.30 g, 10 mmol) [9] and K_2CO_3 (1.3 g, 10 mmol) in 20 ml of CH_3CN were stirred for 30 min and the mixture then was added dropwise over 30 min to a well-stirred, ice-cold CH_3CN (25 ml) solution containing 10 mmol of the appropriate dinitrobenzene acid chloride. The mixture was stirred for another one hour at 0°C, filtered and washed with CH_3CN (30 ml). After evaporation of the solvent under reduced pressure, the residue was crystallized from an appropriate solvent to give pure compounds XI-XIII.

XI: As pale yellowish white color (73%); mp: 195-198°C (EtOAc, hexane); IR (KBr): 3131, 1734, 1656, 1536, 1349 cm^{-1}; ^1H NMR (500 MHz, DMSO-d_6): 8.01 (d, $J = 8.5$ Hz, 1 H, H-6 FU), 8.69 (d, $J = 6.5$ Hz, 1 H, H6 phenyl), 8.77 (dd, $J = 6.5$, 2.5 Hz, 1 H, H5 phenyl), 8.91 (d, $J = 2.5$ Hz 1 H, H3 phenyl); MS : 324 (5%), 278 (20%), 277 (45%), 195(100%), 167 (26%), 130 (72%), 91 (42%), 75 (78%).

XII: As pale yellowish white color solid (57%), mp: 222-225°C (EtOAc, hexane); IR (KBr): 3125, 1730, 1652, 1540, 1345 cm^{-1}; 1 H NMR (500 MHz, DMSO-d_6): 3.35 (s, 2 H, CH2), 8.03 (d, $J = 8.5$ Hz, 1 H, H6 phenyl), 8.69 (d, $J = 6.5$, 1 H, H-6 FU), 8.77 (dd, $J = 8.5$, 2.5 Hz, 1 H, H5 phenyl), 8.91 (d, $J = 2.5$ Hz 1 H, H3 phenyl); MS: 338 (8%), 292 (18%), 209 (100%), 181 (19%), 157(38%), 130 (70%), 91 (47%), 75 (74%).

XIII As pale yellowish white color solid, (67%), mp: 184-187°C (EtOAc, hexane); IR (KBr): 3133, 1738, 1656, 1547, 1350 cm^{-1}; ^1H NMR (500 MHz, DMSO-d_6): 7.76 (d, $J = 6.5$ Hz, 1 H, H-6 FU), 9.15 (d, $J = 3.1$ Hz, 2 H, H2, H6 phenyl), 9.25 (d, $J = 3.1$ Hz 1 H, H4 phenyl); MS : 324 (6%), 278 (23%), 277 (40%), 195(100%), 167 (28%), 130 (70%), 91 (43%), 75 (75%).

Biology

Cell culture

Studies were carried out with HT-29 cells, originally derived from human colorectal carcinoma, obtained from Pasteur Institute of Iran. Cells were grown as an attached monolayer in RPMI 1640 supplemented with 10% fetal bovine serum, penicillin (50 unit/ml), and streptomycin (50 µg/ml). Cells were routinely grown in tissue culture flasks and kept in a humidified atmosphere of 5% CO_2 and 95% air at 37°C.

Determination of the cytotoxicity

The experiments were carried out in 96-well culture dishes. HT-29 cells were seeded at the density of 10^4 cells/well. Compounds VIII and X- XIII were dissolved in DMSO to a stock concentration of 50 mmol and stored at -20°C. The stock solutions were diluted with culture media to final concentrations of 6.75-400 µmol and added to each well of dish. Culture mediums containing DMSO in concentration equal to those which were used in incubations treated with the tested compound served as control. Cell incubations were kept at 37°C for 48 hrs under air by purging with 95% nitrogen and 5% CO_2 or hypoxia in sealed GasPak jar by using Anoximat (Netherland) and an anaerobic chamber GasPak Jar (Merck, Germany) and GasPak pluss (Merck, Germany) [10]. After removal of the supernatant of the culture medium, wells were washed with phosphate buffer saline (PBS), and the numbers of live or dead cells were determined by MTT [11] and PI [12] assays respectively as follows:

MTT assay

To each well of a 96 well plate was added 25 µl of MTT (5 mg/ml in PBS) and incubated for 4 hrs at 37°C and then 100 µl of DMSO was added to dissolve the precipitated formazan and its absorbance was read in Elisa reader at 550 nm and a background wavelength of 690 nm.

Survival was scored by the ratio of the absorbance of the treated cells to untreated cells with the tested compounds (control) and is expressed as percentage of the cell survival. Cytotoxicity was assessed using cell survival curves in which the percentages of cells that survive were plotted as a function of concentration of tested compounds from which the corresponding IC_{50} values were determined [11].

PI-digitonine assay

To each well of a 96 well plate was added 20 µl of a 1.53 mmol solution of propidium iodide (PI) in PBS for a final concentration of 30 µmol. After 60 min

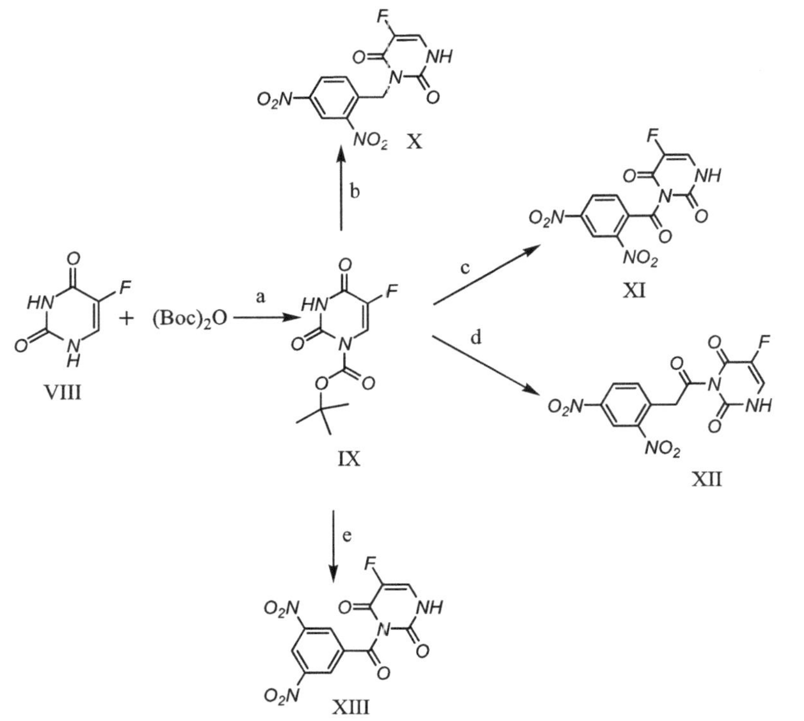

Scheme 2 (a) 4-DMAP/CH_3CN (b) 2,4-dinitrobenzyl chloride, K_2CO_3, KI, DMF (c) 2,4-dinitrobenzoyl chloride, K_2CO_3, CH_3CN (d) 2,4-dinitrophenylacetyl chloride, K_2CO_3, CH_3CN (e) 3,5-dinitrobenzoyl chloride, K_2CO_3, CH_3CN.

incubation at 37°C the initial fluorescence intensity from the dead cells was measured in a multi-well plate reader, (BioTek, Synergy HT, USA) with 530-nm excitation and 645-nm emission filters. Then digitonine (600 nmol) was added to each well to permeabilize all cells and label all nuclei with PI and after 30 min incubation, the fluorescence intensity was measured again to obtain a value corresponding to the total number of cells [12]. The percentage of dead cells was calculated as the proportion of the initial fluorescence intensity over that corresponding to the total number of cells [13]. Cytotoxicity was assessed using cell survival curves in which the percentages of cells that survive were plotted as a function of the concentration of the tested compounds from which the corresponding IC_{50} values were determined.

Radiosensitization experiments

Cell cultures were exposed to a range of concentrations (0, 25, 50, 100 and 200 μmol) of each compound which were lower than their corresponding IC_{50} values and incubated in air or hypoxic condition at 37°C for 3 hrs. Incubations were then irradiated with 5 different doses of radiation (2, 4, 6, 8 and 12 Gy) at room temperature at the dose rate of 1.67 Gy/min and Source Surface Distance (SSD) = 80 cm^2 by a ^{60}Co source (Theratron 780 MDS – Nordion).

Clonogenic forming assay and cell survival curves

The medium of the cell cultures after treatment with the tested compounds and/or irradiation were first separated to remove the tested compounds, and washed with PBS. Cells were seeded in 6-well plates at concentration of 5×10^3 cells per well and maintained at 37°C for 14 days. The cells were then fixed in methanol, colonies which

Table 1 The IC_{50} values for 5-Fluorouracil VIII and tested compounds X-XIII determined by MTT and PI assays on human colon cancer (HT-29) cells under aerobic and hypoxic conditions

		IC_{50}				
		VIII	X	XI	XII	XIII
*MTT	**Aerobic**	**93 ± 9**	**350 ± 15**	**372 ± 19**	**382 ± 12**	**386 ± 24**
	Hypoxic	**89 ± 7**	**308.9 ± 19**	**301 ± 16**	**302.1 ± 20**	**350 ± 17**
**PI	**Aerobic**	**88 ± 7**	**345 ± 14**	**380 ± 20**	**393 ± 18**	**379 ± 9**
	Hypoxic	**84 ± 5**	**301 ± 19**	**311 ± 12**	**317 ± 17**	**342 ± 21x**

Data points were obtained from three independent experiments, and the standard deviations are given for each point (Mean ± SD).
*: 3-(4,5-Dimethylthiazol-2-yl)-2,5-diphenyltetrazolium bromide.
**: Propidium Iodide.

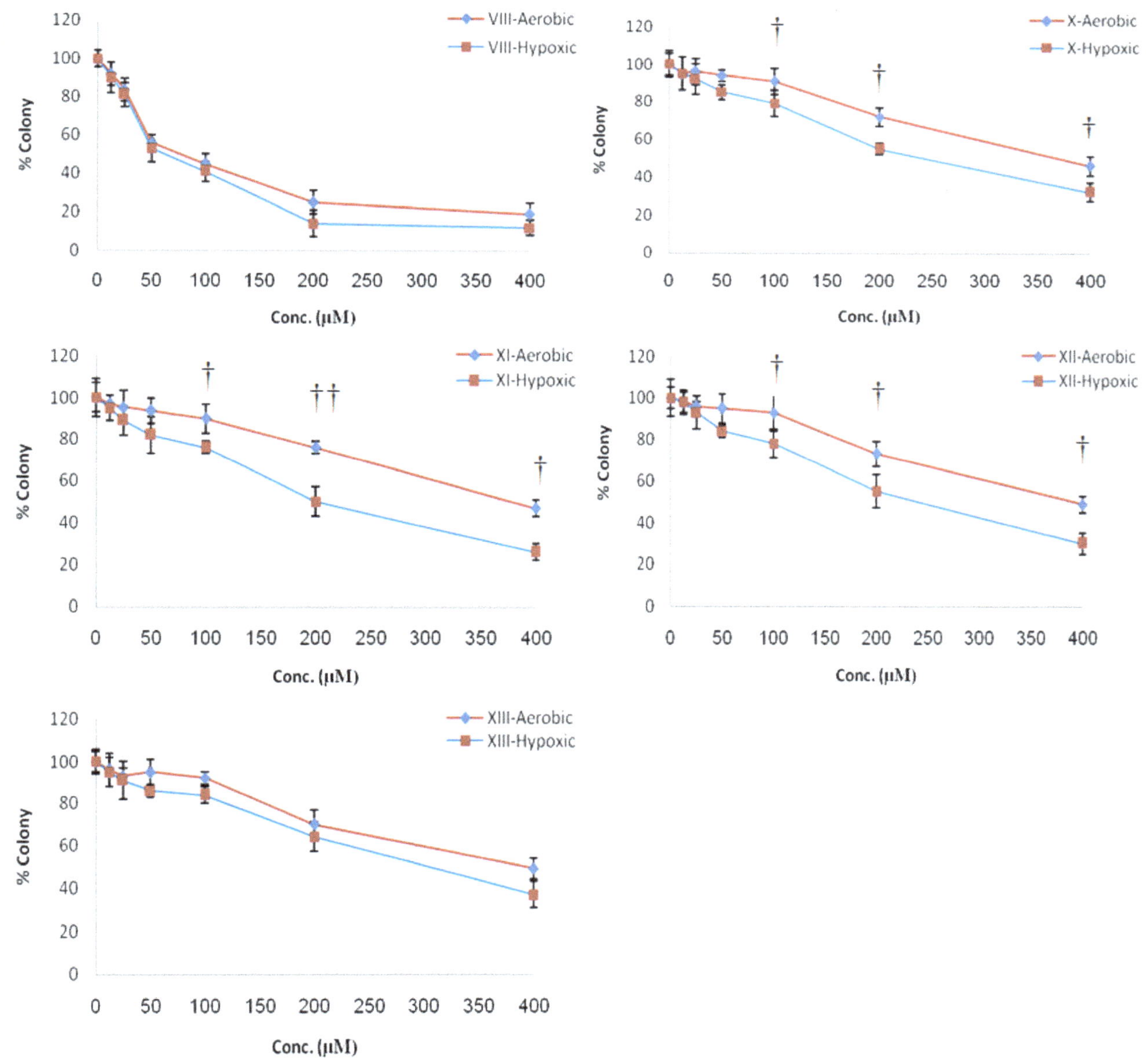

Figure 1 Clonogenic cell survival after 48 hrs incubation of HT-29 cell line with different concentration (6.25, 12.5, 25, 50, 100, 200, 400 μmol) of 5-Fluorouracil VIII and tested compounds X-XIII under Aerobic (♦) and Hypoxic (■) conditions (Mean ± SD), († = P < 0.05, †† = P < 0.01).

were formed stained with crystal violet and those containing more than 50 cells were scored. Sensitization Enhancement Ratio (SER) were obtained from the survival curves of irradiation in the presence and absence of the tested compounds from the equation SER = D_0 untreated cells/D_0 treated cells, where D_0 values represent radiation dose that leading to 37% cell survival [14].

Statistical analyses

For the cell survival and cell death assays each experiment was repeated three times and results are mean ± SD of three independent experiments. Statistical analysis was performed using SPSS11.0 for window (SPSS Inc, USA) and descriptive statistics are shown as arithmetic mean ± standard deviation. Independent samples' *t*-test was used to investigate the differences between irradiated and unirradiated cells treated with the tested compounds and for comparing more than two groups One Way Analysis of Variance were performed and p value smaller than 0.05 was considered statistically significant.

Results and discussion

Direct acylation or alkylation of 5-fluorouracil usually give a mixture of N-3, N-1, and N-1,3 substituted compounds

[15] and preparation of the N-3 derivatives by this approach result in low yield and require chromatographic separation. Therefore three-step sequences involving protection of the N-1 position, acylation or alkylation at N-3 and removal of the protecting group have been employed for the preparation of N-3 substituted 5-fluorouracils.

For the protection of N-1 position, the use of acyl [16], benzyl [17], benzyloxymethyl [18], tetrahydropyranyl [19], 2-(trimethylsilyl)ethoxymethyl (SEM) [20] and di- t-butoxydicarbonate [9] groups have been described. However introduction or removal of the most of these groups are associated with some difficulties and in this study BOC which is introduced and removed rapidly and its uses is practical and economical was employed for the protection of N-1 position of 5-FU [9]. Reaction of the resulting N-1 protected 5-fluorouracil with dinitro substituted benzyl, benzoyl and phenacetyl halides in DMF in the presence of the potassium carbonate resulted in the formation of the corresponding N-3 derivative which upon treatment with potassium carbonate in methanol for removal of the protecting group gave compounds X-XIII (Scheme 2).

Cytotoxicity of 5-Fu and tested compounds X-XIII against HT-29 cell line under both aerobic and hypoxic conditions after 48 hrs incubation, were determined by measurement of the percent of the cell survival using MTT assay [11] and the percent of the dead cell using PI-digitonine assay [12]. The results of these assays were used to obtain the IC_{50} values of the tested compounds as well as the dose of the tested compounds at which under aerobic conditions less than 10% growth inhibition occurred ($< IC_{10}$) as an appropriate dose for the radiosensitization experiments. The cytotoxicity of the compounds under both aerobic and hypoxic conditions were similar after 3 hrs and within this period of time there was no differential cytotoxicity at various concentrations. However after 48 hrs the cytotoxicity of the tested compounds were significantly different. Results of this study showed that IC_{50} values measured by PI-digitonine assay were not significantly different from those determined by MTT assay (Table 1). While the tested compounds under hypoxic conditions at different concentration reduced the cell viability significantly (Figure 1 and Table 1), these compounds were not cytotoxic under aerobic conditions and at concentrations up to 100 μmol reduced the cell viability only to less than 10%.

The cytotoxicity of 5-FU was not significantly different under both aerobic and hypoxic conditions which is in agreement with results of other investigations that N-acylation or alkylation of 5-Fu reduces its cytotoxicity [15].

In contrast to a number of (*O*- and *P*- Nitrobenzyloxycarbonyl)-5-fluorouracils which have shown [7] equal cell killings under both aerobic and hypoxic conditions, which has been attributed to the instability and decomposition of compounds, the cytotoxicity of the tested compounds of this study under hypoxic in comparison with aerobic conditions were higher indicating the possibility that under this condition one electron reduction of these compounds produce cytotoxic reactive intermediates. With exception of 5-FU which under both conditions and compound XIII which under hypoxic conditions showed highest and lowest IC_{50} values respectively, IC_{50} values of other tested compounds under either conditions were not significantly different from each other indicating that they have similar mechanism of action and might produce the same reactive species. The low cytotoxicity of compound XIII could be attributed to the presence of the nitro groups in the *meta* position which in contrast to *ortho* positions after one electron reduction does not produce reactive quinone methiodide species and 5-FU.

Radiosensitization experiments was carried out under conditions identical to the cytotoxicity measurement using MTT assays by incubating HT-29 cells with compounds under hypoxic and aerobic conditions at 37°C. After 3 hrs where none of the compounds had shown significant cytotoxicity, cells were irradiated with a ^{60}Co source.

Table 2 Sensitizing Enhancement Ratios (SER) of different concentrations (25, 50, 100, 200 μmol) of 5-Fluorouracil VIII and tested compounds X-XIII on human colon cancer (HT-29) cells upon exposure to different doses of radiation(0, 2, 4, 8 and 12 Gy) under aerobic and hypoxic conditions

Compound	Concentration (μmole)	SER	
		Hypoxic	Aerobic
VIII	25	1.04 ± 0.04	1.09 ± 0.06
	50	1.18 ± 0.11	1.12 ± 0.09
	100	1.20 ± 0.12	1.16 ± 0.10
	200	1.29 ± 0.10	1.21 ± 0.15
X	25	1.20 ± 0.12	1.10 ± 0.10
	50	1.51 ± 0.09	1.16 ± 0.11
	100	1.78 ± 0.15	1.24 ± 0.14
	200	2.23 ± 0.21	1.29 ± 0.12
XI	25	1.30 ± 0.18	1.11 ± 0.08
	50	1.57 ± 0.12	1.21 ± 0.16
	100	1.85 ± 0.16	1.23 ± 0.10
	200	2.39 ± 0.10	1.35 ± 0.17
XII	25	1.16 ± 0.14	1.10 ± 0.09
	50	1.37 ± 0.18	1.15 ± 0.10
	100	1.73 ± 0.11	1.26 ± 0.15
	200	2.28 ± 0.21	1.33 ± 0.13
XIII	25	1.14 ± 0.09	1.07 ± 0.10
	50	1.18 ± 0.14	1.13 ± 0.09
	100	1.22 ± 0.23	1.18 ± 0.14
	200	1.37 ± 0.15	1.25 ± 0.11

Means ± SD, each set of experiments was performed in triplicates.

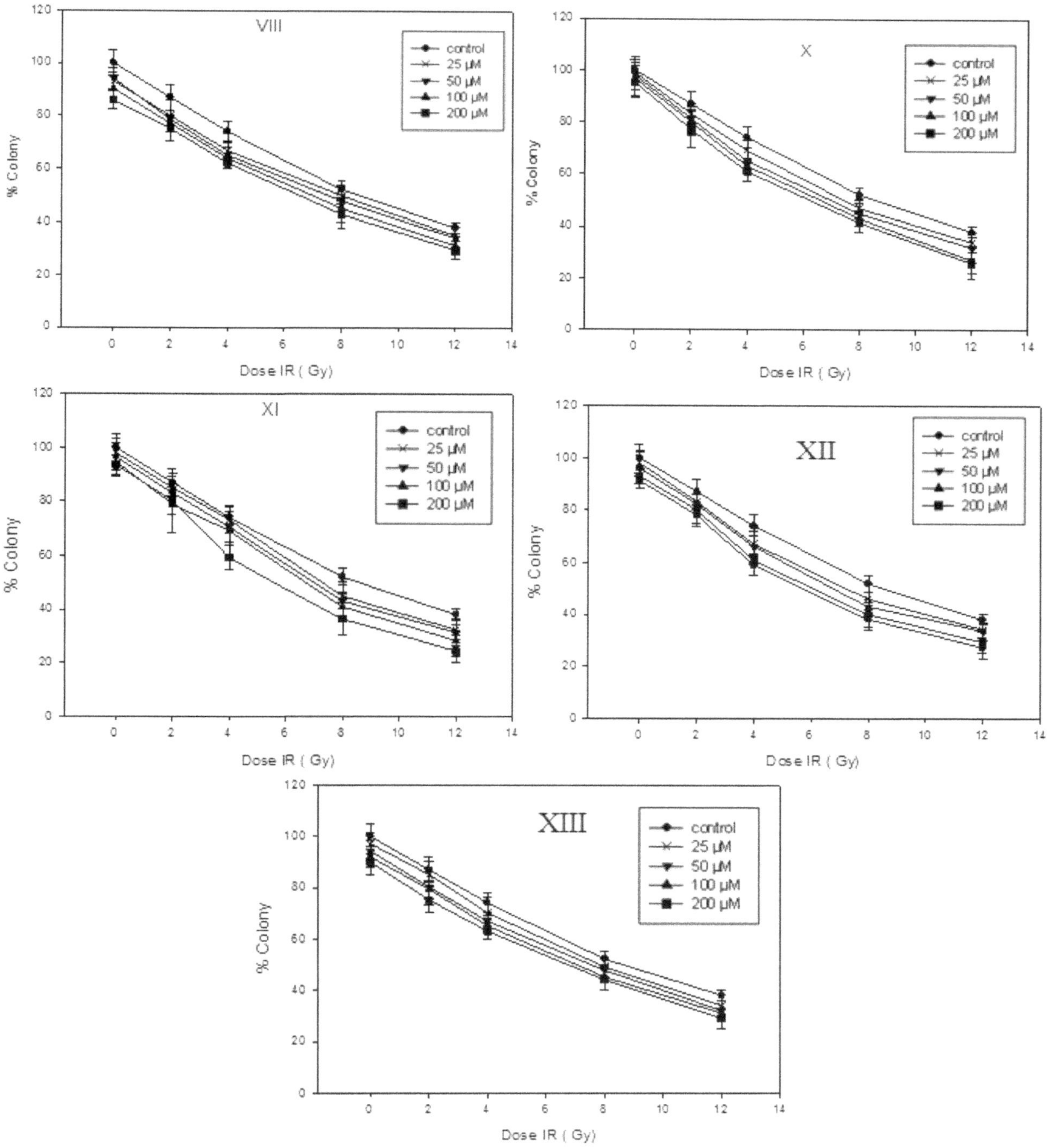

Figure 2 Clonogenic cell survival of HT-29 cells upon exposure to different dose of Gamma-radiation (2, 4, 6, 8 and 12 Gy) after incubation with different concentration (25, 50, 100 and 200 μmol) of 5-Fluorouracil VIII and tested compounds X-XIII under Aerobic condition. Data points were obtained from three independent experiments, and the standard deviations are given for each point. (Mean ± SD, each set of experiments was performed in triplicates).

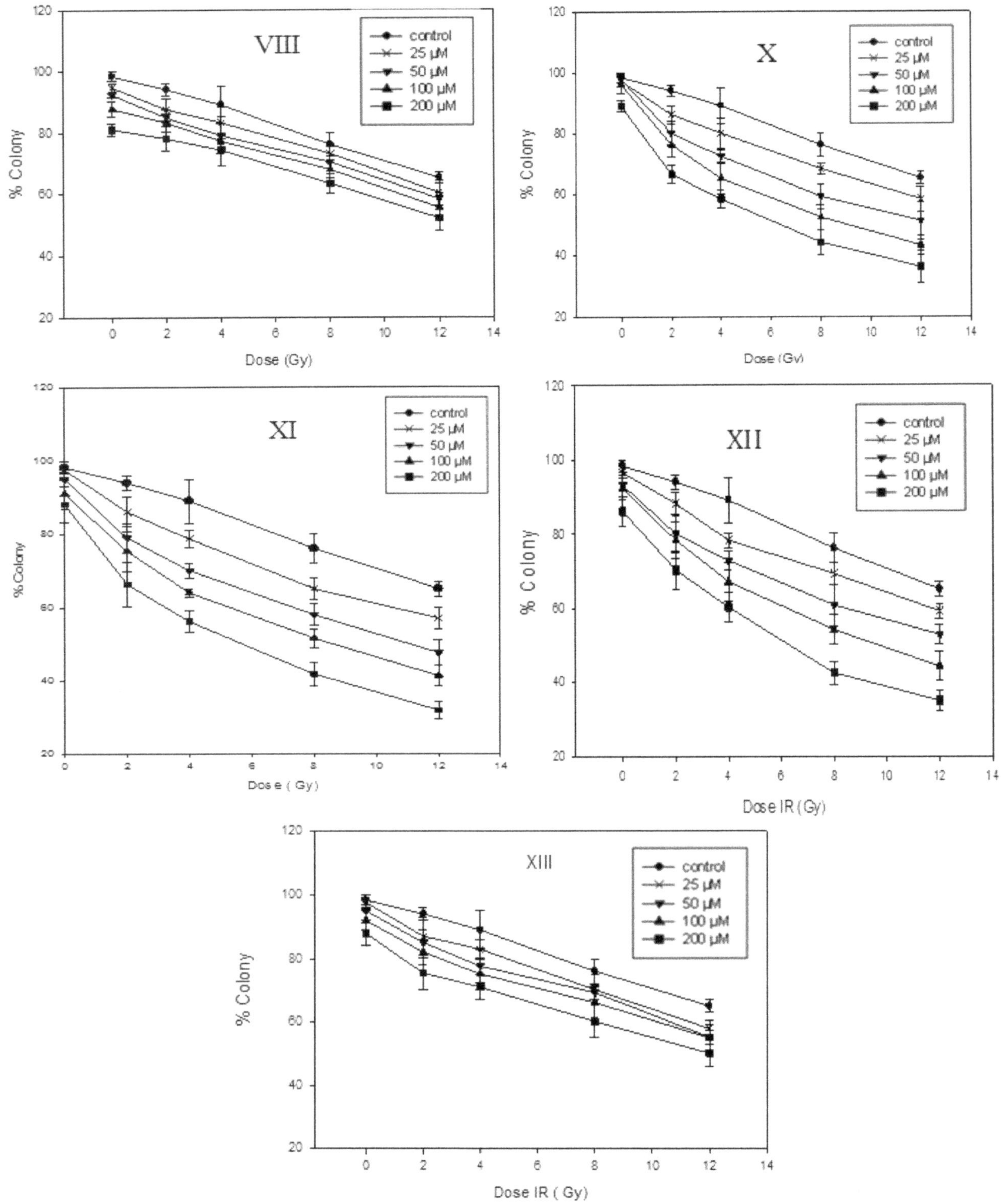

Figure 3 Clonogenic cell survival of HT-29 cells upon exposure to different dose of Gamma-radiation (2, 4, 6, 8 and 12 Gy) after incubation with different concentration (25, 50, 100 and 200 μmol) of 5-Fluorouracil VIII and tested compounds X-XIII under Hypoxic condition. Data points were obtained from three independent experiments, and the standard deviations are given for each point. (Mean ± SD, each set of experiments was performed in triplicates).

Radiosensitivity of the tested compounds were determined through measurement of the cell growth inhibition using colony formation [13] and the clonogenic cells was determined by staining with crystal violet and counting on Dissecting microscope. Results are presented in terms of Sensitization Enhancement Ratio (SER) which were obtained from the survival curves of irradiation in the presence and absence of the tested compounds from the equation SER = D_0 untreated cells/D_0 treated cells, where D_0 values represent radiation dose that leads to 37% cell survival [21].

A comparison of the sensitizer enhancement ratio values of the tested compounds (Table 2) revealed that under aerobic condition none of the compounds and under hypoxia 5-fluorouracil VIII and its 3,5-dinitrophenyl derivative XIII had no radiosensitizing activity.

As it is shown in Figures 2 and 3 cells viability was reduced dose dependently by irradiation which was significant in the presence of the compounds X-XII under hypoxic conditions. Radiosensitizing activities of these compounds increased by increase in their concentrations and at concentrations higher than 50 were equal or higher than 1.6 which is the minimum effective SER [22] of a radiosensitizer in an *in vitro* assay.

Conclusion

The present study showed that alkylation or acylation of 5-fluorouracil, results in compounds which have little or no cytotoxicity and radiosensitizing activity on aerobic cells but are toxic and radiosensitizer on hypoxic cells and their uses may be advantageous in adjunct cancer treatment by radiotherapy.

Competing interest

The authors declare that they have no competing interests

Author details

[1]Department of Medicinal Chemistry, Tehran, Iran. [2]Department of Nuclear Pharmacy, Tehran, Iran. [3]Department of Pharmacology & toxicology, Tehran, Iran. [4]Department of Drug and Food Control, Faculty of Pharmacy, Tehran University of Medical Sciences, Tehran, Iran.

Authors' contribution

AK: Synthesis and determination of cytotoxicity and radiosensitizing activity of the tested compounds. KA: Designer of the project, supervisor of the synthesis and corresponding author of the manuscript. OS-N: Supervisor for the determination of the cytotoxocity and radiosensitizing activity of the tested compounds. KMR: supervising statistical analyses. All authors read and approved the final manuscript.

References

1. Nagasawa H, Uto Y, Kirk KL, Hori H: **Design of hypoxia-targeting drugs as new cancer chemotherapeutics.** *Biol Pharm Bull* 2006, 29(12):2335–42.
2. Lee HH, Palmer BD, Wilson WR, Denny WA: **Synthesis and hypoxia-selective cytotoxicity of A 2-nitroimidazole mustard.** *Bioorg Med Chem Lett* 1998, **8**:1741–1744.
3. Tao C, Desai NP, Soon-Shiong P, Sandford PA: **Dual functional cytotoxic/radiosensitizer compounds and methods for the preparation thereof.** *Chem Abstr* 1996, **126**:131664n. PCT Int Appl WO 96 40,091.
4. Palmer BD, Wilson WR, Pullen SM, Denny WA: **Hypoxia-selective antitumor agents. 5. Synthesis of water-soluble nitroaniline mustards with selective cytotoxicity for hypoxic mammalian cells.** *J Med Chem* 1990, **35**:3214–3222.
5. Ahmed L, Jenkins TC, Walling JM, Stratford IJ, Sheldon PW, Adams GE, Fielden EM: **Analogues of RSU-1069: radiosensitization and toxicity in vitro and in vivo.** *Int J Radiat Oncol Biol Phys* 1986, **12**:1079–1081.
6. Khalaj A, Doroudi AR, Ostad SN, Khoshayand MR, Babai M, Adibpour N: **Synthesis, aerobic cytotoxicity, and radiosensitizing activity of novel 2,4-dinitrophenylamine tethered 5-fluorouracil and hydroxyurea.** *Bioorg Med Chem Lett* 2006, **16**(23):6034–6038.
7. Lin TS, Wang L, Antonini I, Cosby LA, Shiba DA, Kirkpatrick DL, Sartorelli AC: **(o- and p-nitrobenzyloxycarbonyl)-5-fluorouracil derivatives as potential conjugated bioreductive alkylating agents.** *J Med Chem* 1986, **29**:84–89.
8. Serebryakov EA, Kislitsin PG, Semenov VV, Zlotin SG: **Selective synthesis of 1,2-benzisothiazol-3-one-1-oxide nitro derivatives.** *Synthesis* 2001, **11**:1659–1664.
9. Jaime-Figueroa S, Zamilpa A, Guzman A, Morgans DJ: **N-3-Alkylation of uracil and derivatives via N-1-Boc protection.** *Synthetic Communications* 2001, **31**(24):3739–3746.
10. Mikihiko N, Chizuko H, Shigeki M, Takashi T: **Caspase-independent necrotic cell death induced by a radiosensitizer, 8-nitrocaffeine.** *Cancer Sci* 2004, **95**(4):361–366.
11. Mosmann T: **Rapid Colorimetric Assay for Cellular Growth and Survival: Application to Proliferation and Cytotoxicity Assays.** *J Immunol Methods* 1983, **65**:55–63.
12. Zhang L, Mizumoto K, Sato N, Ogawa T, Kusumoto M, Niiyama H, Tanaka M: **Quantitative determination of apoptotic death in cultured human pancreatic cancer cells by propodium iodide and digitonin.** *Cancer Lett* 1999, **142**:129–137.
13. Moore A, Donahue CJ, Bauer KD, Mather JP: **Simultaneous measurement of cell cycle and apoptotic cell death.** *Methods Cell Biol* 1998, **57**:265–78.
14. Franken NP, Rodermond HM, Stap J, Haveman J, van Bree C: **Clonogenic assay of cells in vitro.** *Nat Protoc* 2006, **1**:2315–2319.
15. Ozaki S, Watanabe Y, Hoshiko T, Nagase T, Ogasawara T, Furukawa H, Hemura A, Ishikawa K, Mori H, Hoshi A, Iigo M, Tokuzen R: **5-Fluorouracil derivatives. X. Synthesis and antitumor activity of α-alkoxyalkyl-5-fluorouracils.** *Chem Pharm Bull* 1986, **34**(1):150–157.
16. Pogolotti ALJr Failla, Santi DV: **A facile synthesis of 3-alkyluracils and thymines.** *J Hetrocycl Chem* 1972, **9**:1423–1428.
17. Ishikawa I, Itoh T, Takayanagi H, Oshima J, Kawahara N, Mizuno Y, Ogura H: **The Photocycloaddition Reactions of Uridine and Related Compounds with 2, 3-Dimethyl-2-butene.** *Chem Pharm Bull* 1991, **39**:1922–1927.
18. Kundu NG, Khatri SG: **Studies on Uracil Derivatives and Analogs VII. Synthesis of N1-Iodomethyl Derivatives of Uracil and Dihydrouracil.** *Synthesis* 1985, :323–327.
19. Manfredine S, Baraldi PG, Bazzanini R, Guarneri M, Simoni D: **A new direct glycosylation of pyrimidine, pyrazole, imidazole and purine heterocycles via their N-tetrahydropyranyl (THP) derivatives.** *J Chem Soc Chem Commun* 1994, :583–584.
20. Arias L, Guzman A, Jamie-Figuera S, Lopez FJ, Morgans DJ Jr, Padilla F, Perez-Medrano A, Quintero C, Romero M, Sandoval L: **Direct N3 Alkylation of Uracil and Derivatives via n1-[2-(trimethylsilyl) ethoxymethyl] Protection.** *Synlett* 1997, **11**:1233–1234.
21. Cariveau MJ, Stackhouse M, Cui X, Tiwari K, Waud W, Secrist JA, Xu B: **Clofarabine acts as radiosensitizer in vitro and in vivo by interfering with DNA damage response.** *Int J Radiation Oncology Biol Phys* 2008, **70**(1):213–220.
22. Nakae T, Uto Y, Tanaka M, Shibata H, Nakata E, Tominaga M, Maezawa H, Hashomoto T, Kirk KL, Nagasdawa H, Hori H: **Design, synthesis, and radiosensitizing activities of sugar-hybrid hypoxic cell radiosensitizers.** *Bioorg Med Chem Lett* 2008, **16**:675–682.

The role of prophylactic ibuprofen and N-acetylcysteine on the level of cytokines in periapical exudates and the post-treatment pain

Maryam Ehsani[1], Ali-Akbar Moghadamnia[2], Samir Zahedpasha[1*], Ghorban Maliji[3], Sina Haghanifar[4], Seyyed Mohsen Aghajanpour Mir[3] and Narges Mousavi Kani[3]

Abstract

Background: Periapical lesions are inflammatory diseases that result in periapical bone destruction because of host defensive–microbial disturbances.

Objective: To evaluate the role of prophylactic ibuprofen and N-acetylcysteine (NAC) on the levels of tumor necrosis factor alpha (TNF- α), interleukin- 6(IL-6) and IL-17 and post-treatment pain level in chronic periapical lesions.

Materials and methods: Eighty patients with chronic apical lesions less than 1 cm were randomly assigned to receive NAC tablets (400 mg), ibuprofen tablets (400 mg), NAC (400 mg)/ibuprofen (200 mg) combination and placebo 90 minutes prior to sampling. Periapical exudates were collected from root canals. TNF- α, IL-6 and IL-17 levels were determined by ELISA and post-treatment pain was assessed using a visual analog scale (VAS).

Results: There was a significant difference in IL-6 level between ibuprofen group and placebo ($p = 0.019$). Significant difference in IL-17 level was observed between NAC/ibuprofen combination group and placebo ($p = 0.043$). Four hours after treatment, a significant difference was observed in VAS pain score between ibuprofen group and placebo ($p = 0.017$). Eight hours post-treatment, VAS pain score for NAC group was statistically lower than placebo group ($p = 0.033$). After 12 hours VAS pain score showed a significant decrease in NAC group compared to placebo ($p = 0.049$).

Conclusion: The prophylactic ibuprofen and NAC failed to clearly reflect their effect on cytokines levels in exudates of chronic periapical lesions. On the other hand it seems that NAC can be a substitute for ibuprofen in the management of post endodontic pain.

Keywords: Periapical exudate, N-acetylcysteine, Ibuprofen, Cytokine, Pain

Introduction

Periapical lesions are inflammatory diseases that develop as result of root canal bacterial infections and may result in periapical bone destruction because of host defensive–microbial disturbances [1,2]. Neutrophil granulocytes, among infiltrating leukocytes, are the first line of defense which stimulate the migration of monocytes and lymphocytes [3]. Infiltrates of mononuclear cell, composed of antigen-presenting cells, T and B lymphocytes and their effectors are characteristic of chronic periapical processes [3]. Cytokines are low-weight messenger molecules between the host cells secreted by different immune cells and believed to have an important role in treatment and pathogenesis of many inflammatory diseases such as periradicular lesions [4,5]. Tumor necrosis factor alpha (TNF-α) has a wide range of pro-inflammatory and immunomodulatory effects on a number of different cell populations. It stimulates prostaglandin synthesis, bone resorption, and protease production by many cell types, including fibroblasts and osteoblasts. Extraproduction or inappropriate expression of TNF-α can lead to a variety

* Correspondence: Samirzahedpasha@gmail.com
[1]Department of Endodontics, Dental Material Research Center, Faculty of Dentistry, Babol University of Medical Sciences, Babol, Iran
Full list of author information is available at the end of the article

of pathological conditions [6]. Interleukin- 6 (IL-6) has been traditionally considered to be a pro-inflammatory cytokine that may have a part in inflammatory process of periapical lesions [7]. IL-6 may also release locally in inflamed pulp and periradicular lesions, especially of chronic types [8]. IL-17 is the first member of an emerging family of inflammatory cytokines whose biological activities remain incompletely defined. IL-17 is produced exclusively by activated memory T-cells. IL-17, derived from T-cells, may play an important role in the initiation and maintenance of pro-inflammatory responses, and has recently been found to stimulate osteoclastic resorption [9,10]. For tooth pain, none steroidal anti-inflammatory drugs (NSAIDs) are the most frequently administered analgesics. Many studies have shown ibuprofen to be very effective in control or reducing dental pain [11,12]. Ibuprofen blocks the cyclo-oxygenase-1 (COX-1) and - 2 (COX-2) enzymes both together, with a highly effective analgesic and anti-inflammatory action for post endodontic pain [11]. However, many NSAIDs have undesirable side effects like gastrointestinal (GI) irritation, ulcers and bleeding. NSAIDs exacerbate some inflammatory responses, such as in inflammatory bowel disease [13-15]. Tugendreich et al. offered an interesting explanation for the mechanism by which certain NSAIDS could increase the production of inflammatory mediators [16]. They showed that the administration of several NSAIDs to rats resulted in the stimulation of gene expression similar to that observed when rats were exposed to LPS. They concluded that NSAIDs cause injury to the gastrointestinal system and lead to leakage of commensal bacteria and/or LPS into the circulation provoking a systemic inflammatory response. N acetylcysteine (NAC) is a derivative of the amino acid L-cysteine and is currently indicated for acute paracetamol overdose [17]. Pharmacological functions include repletion of intracellular glutathione stores, scavenging of toxic oxygen free radicals (both directly and indirectly via increased glutathione concentrations) and suppression of TNF production [18]. NAC is well known as a mucolytic agent and exerts anti-inflammatory activity [19,20]. The anti-inflammatory activity of NAC takes place through its ability to inhibit the expression and release of a variety of pro-inflammatory cytokines [21] and it down-regulates cytokine-stimulated expression of leukocyte adhesion molecules [22,23]. Simultaneous administration of NAC and diclofenac potentiates the NSAID drug anti-inflammatory effect and helps obtaining the same effect at lower drug levels [24]. The aim of this randomized clinical trial mainly was to evaluate the role of prophylactic ibuprofen and NAC on the levels of TNF- α, IL-6, IL-17 in chronic periapical lesions and evaluation of the post treatment pain.

Methods

This double-blinded randomized clinical trial (Registration code of clinical trial: IRCT201008114547N1) was done on 80 subjects of different age and sex. Selection criteria included patients with good general health who had a recent panoramic radiograph. Exclusion criteria included: 1) systemic diseases such as diabetes, hepatitis, HIV infection, immunosuppressive chemotherapy, bleeding disorder, inflammatory or autoimmune diseases like Behçet's syndrome, arthritis, and AIDS; 2) history and/or presence of other infections; 3) specific physiological condition such as pregnancy or menstruation; 4) periodontal diseases; 5) oral ulcers; 6) current smoking; 7) GI problems, such as peptic ulcer; 8) treatment with any medication in the preceding week. Following recruitment all subjects were given verbal and written information concerning the study and gave their written consent prior to the clinical examination. The study was approved by ethics review board of Babol University of Medical Sciences and was performed in agreement with the declaration of Helsinki. For careful evaluation, a periapical radiographic examination with bisecting-angle technique was performed after detection of periapical lesion in panoramic radiographic view of involved tooth. Two examiners (an oral and maxillofacial radiologist and an endodontist) evaluated the radiographs and determined the size of periapical radiolucent area by a ruler. Subjects with radiolucent asymptomatic periapical lesions with a diameter of less than 1 centimeter were included in the study. All of the subjects in the case group were asymptomatic at the time of sample collection without any history of previous exacerbation of periapical lesions. The teeth studied could be as follows: All single rooted teeth, distal root of mandibular molars and palatal roots of maxillary molars. Further, groups, each containing 20 subjects, were randomly assigned to receive either NAC tablets (400 mg), ibuprofen tablets (400 mg), NAC (400 mg)/ibuprofen (200 mg) combination and placebo (starch), all were packaged in identical 500 mg capsules with the same color and size and then encoded by a third person unaware of the study protocol. Each participant received a package containing 2 capsules and consumed it 90 minutes before sampling. The teeth were anesthetized with 2 % lidocaine with 1/100000 epinephrine and access cavity was prepared using an end-cutting fissure bur (Dentsply Maillefer, Ballaigues, Switzerland). The involved teeth were isolated with a rubber dam. Following the measurement of the working length, the root canal was enlarged to size 40 using K-Flexofile (Dentsply Maillefer, Ballaigues, Switzerland). After the root canal was dried with sterilized paper points, two size 40 paper points (Absorbent paper points, Kerr Manufacturing Co., Romulus, MI, USA) were subsequently inserted into the root canal close to the established working length and held for 30 s. The actively draining teeth were supposed to be excluded from the study. If the paper point withdrawn from the canal was dry, a thin endodontic file was used carefully to penetrate through the apical foramen to bring exudates into the root canal from the periapical area. The tooth was excluded from the study when blood was visible along the paper point. The wetted length of paper points was measured immediately. The volume of the fluid was calculated from a standard curve as described before [25] and expressed as μL. Both paper points were immersed into sterile Ependorf vials containing 300 μL phosphate buffered saline (PBS), vortexed for 1 min and stored at −70 ° C until time of assay. Routine treatment of the patient was then continued.

Measurement of TNF- α, IL-6, and IL-17 levels

TNF- α, IL-6, and IL-17 were measured by ELISA. Assays were carried out in accordance with manufacturer's instructions (eBioscience, Vienna, Austria). The amount of TNF- α, IL-6, and IL-17 were determined by reference to standard curves (0–1000 $pg\,mL^{-1}$) constructed with each assay. The concentrations of IL-6, TNF- a, and IL-17 in each sample were calculated based on the dilutions and exudates volumes. The results were expressed as picograms per milliliter ($pg\,mL^{-1}$) for cytokine concentration. The detection limit for TNF-alpha was 2.3 $pg\,mL^{-1}$, 0.92 $pg\,mL^{-1}$ for IL-6, and 0.5 $pg\,mL^{-1}$ for IL-17 respectively.

Pain recordings

Following the endodontic treatment, the patients were asked to record the level of pain and discomfort using a standard VAS scale and complete the postoperative questionnaires at pre-defined time points according to the following schedule: at 4, 8, 12, and 24 h after treatment [26]. Pain was defined as the presence of any degree of discomfort and was scored from 0 (no pain) to 10 (worst pain). Escape medication was included in the patients' packets were (Darou Pakhsh Pharmaceutical Co., Tehran, Iran) for inadequate pain control from the trial medication.

Statistical analysis

Cytokine levels in the periapical exudates were compared between groups by using Mann–Whitney *U* test. VAS pain scores were compared using one-way ANOVA post hoc Tukey test. A value of $p < 0.05$ was required for statistical significance.

Results

Assessment of TNF- α level

TNF- α was detected in all periapical exudates samples. However the difference between groups was not statistically significant regarding TNF- α levels (Figure 1).

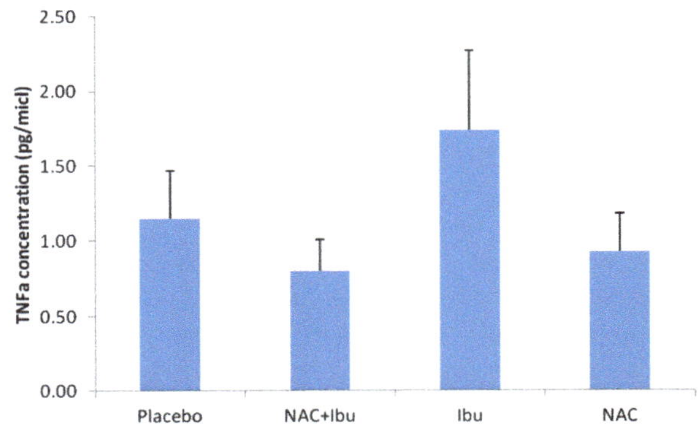

Figure 1 Mean ± SEM of TNF- α concentration ($pg\,ml^{-1}$) in the four study groups (n = 20). No significant differences were seen between treatment groups compared to placebo. NAC; N-acetyl cysteine, Ibu; ibuprofen.

Assessment of IL-6 level

IL-6 was not detected in all periapical exudates samples. There was a significant difference in IL-6 level between ibuprofen and placebo receiving groups ($p = 0.019$) (Figure 2).

Assessment of IL-17 level

Undetectable levels of IL-17 were more pronounced compared to the other two cytokines. There was a significant difference in IL-17 level between NAC/ibuprofen combination group and placebo ($p = 0.043$) (Figure 3). No significant difference detected for ibuprofen and NAC treatment group compared to placebo.

Assessment of pain level

No patients took any of the escape medication, which was provided in case of inadequate pain control. Figure 4 shows the mean VAS pain scores during 24 hours post treatment in four study groups. Considering VAS pain

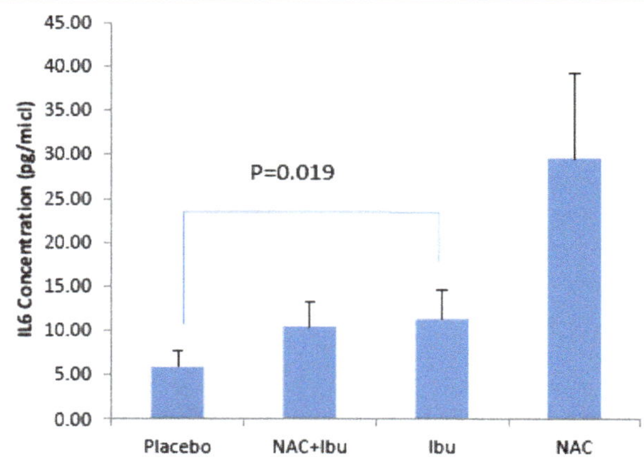

Figure 2 Mean ± SEM of IL-6 concentration ($pg\,ml^{-1}$) in the four study groups (with significant differerence between ibuprofen and placebo groups).

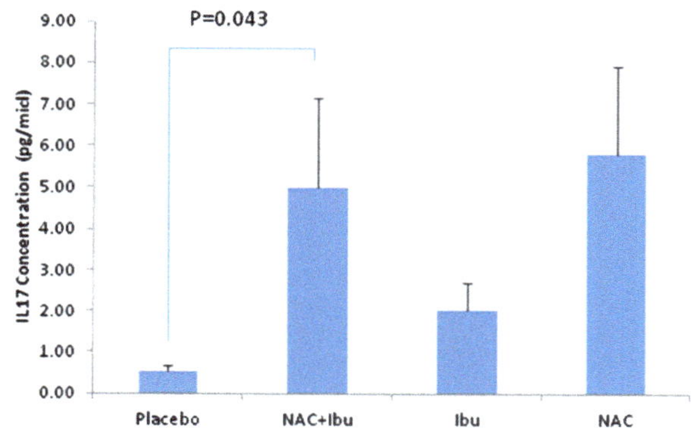

Figure 3 Mean ± SEM of IL-17 concentration (pg ml^{-1}) in the four study groups (with significant difference between NAC/Ibu and placebo groups).

score, 4 hours after treatment, a significant difference was observed between ibuprofen and placebo receiving subjects ($p = 0.017$). Eight hours post-treatment, VAS pain score was statistically different between NAC group and placebo ($p = 0.033$). After 12 hours VAS pain score showed significant difference between NAC group and placebo ($p = 0.049$). No significant difference was found in VAS pain score at 24 hours after treatment between study groups ($P > 0.05$). Based on assessment of VAS pain scores by time after treatment, there were both inter-groups ($p = 0.015$) and intra-groups ($p = 0.0001$) differences in four study groups.

Discussion

In this study we investigated the effect of prophylactic ibuprofen and NAC on the levels of TNF- α, IL-6 and IL-17 and post treatment pain level in chronic periapical lesions. Study drugs were given 90 minutes prior sampling. Ibuprofen is absorbed from the GI tract and its peak plasma concentrations are reached within about 1 to 2 hours after

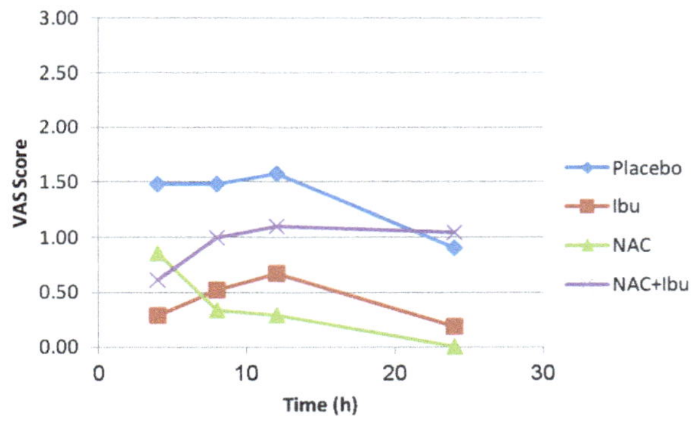

Figure 4 Mean of VAS score changes by time (h) in four study groups (n = 20). NAC; N-acetyl cysteine, Ibu; ibuprofen. The score for NAC group tends to zero after 24 hours post administration in comparison with other treatments.

ingestion [27,28]. NAC is a thiol, a mucolytic agent and a source of sulfhydryl groups in cells and scavenger of free radicals as it interacts with ROS such as OH· and H_2O_2 [29]. Uses of NAC in different diseases including cancer, cardiovascular diseases, human immunodeficiency virus (HIV) infections, acetaminophen-induced liver toxicity and metal toxicity have been reviewed previously [30]. After an oral dose of NAC 200 to 400 mg the peak plasma concentration of 0.35 to 4 mg/L is achieved within 1 to 2 hours [31]. We collected the exudates from the root canals using noninvasive methods. There were no actively draining teeth in this experiment and none of the cases showed blood along the paper point. TNF- α was detected in all samples of periapical exudates but there were no significant differences between four study groups. Our results demonstrate the presence of IL-6 in the majority of tissue samples, but analysis of the data revealed that there was significant difference in IL-6 level only between ibuprofen group and placebo. This means ibuprofen 400 mg could not augment TNF-a to levels beyond the other groups but on the other hand increased IL-6 to much a level that was statistically different to placebo, but not to the other groups. Shahriari et al. [32] studied the effect of ibuprofen on IL-1β, TNF-α and PGE2 levels in periapical exudates. Ibuprofen was prescribed one tablet every 6 hour for three days and in the fourth day second samples were taken. Their results showed that PGE2 levels were decreased significantly in the case group following ibuprofen treatment comparing with the pre-treatment and placebo group. But there were no significant differences in IL-1β and TNF-α level between the two groups and in each group before and after treatment. In a study done by Spinas et al. [33] plasma levels of TNF- α, IL-1, and IL-6 were monitored after intravenous administration of Escherichia coli endotoxin with or without ibuprofen pretreatment to healthy volunteers. Pretreatment with ibuprofen caused a significant augmentation and temporal shift in cytokine elaboration. In a study by Sironi et al.[34]the effect of dexamethasone and two NSAIDs, ibuprofen and indomethacin, on the production of serum IL-6 and TNF levels in mice treated with endotoxin was investigated. Pretreatment with indomethacin or ibuprofen potentiated the production of both IL-6 and TNF. In the case of IL-6, indomethacin and ibuprofen were able per se to induce significant levels of this cytokine even in the absence of lipopolysaccharide (LPS). These data indicate that prostaglandins can physiologically provide a negative feedback regulation of IL-6 and TNF synthesis. Peristeris et al. [18] in their study investigated the effect of NAC on TNF production and LPS lethality in mice. The results indicated that oral administration of NAC inhibits the increase in serum TNF levels in LPS-treated mice and protects against

LPS toxicity. The inhibition was not confined to the released form of TNF, since NAC also inhibited LPS-induced spleen-associated TNF. Hulten et al. [35] found that NAC attenuates TNF- α mRNA expression and secretion in macrophages from human lung transplant recipients and may be beneficial against transplant rejection. In a study carried out by Confalone et al.[36] NAC, a scavenger of reactive oxygen species, inhibited the activation of NF-κB and induction of IL-6 by TNF-α, being ineffective on IL- 1 β activity. It is apparent that the mentioned investigations are structurally different from our study and logically they cannot be compared. Our findings showed that undetectable levels of IL-17 were more pronounced compared to the other two cytokines. We found that NAC 400 mg/ibuprofen 200 mg combination increased the level of IL-17 to a level that a significant difference could be observed with control group. Data indicating the effect of these drugs on the level of cytokines in chronic periapical lesions are lacking in the literature. We measured post treatment pain level and discomfort using a standard VAS scale at pre-defined time points according to the following schedule: at 4, 8, 12, and 24 h after treatment. Four hours after treatment, a significant difference was observed in VAS pain score between ibuprofen group and placebo. Eight hours later, VAS pain score was statistically different between NAC group and placebo. After 12 hours VAS pain score showed significant difference between NAC group and placebo. No significant difference was found in VAS pain score at 24 hours after treatment between study groups. Hoffer et al. [24] found that LPS-induced prostaglandin E2 formation was significantly reduced by rofecoxib and by diclofenac, two NSAIDs. Adding NAC to each of these drugs enhanced the effect of the NSAIDs. They suggest the potentiation of the anti-inflammatory effect of COX inhibitors by their simultaneous administration with NAC, or obtaining the same anti-inflammatory effect at lower drug levels. In our investigation, no patients took any of the escape medication, which was provided in case of inadequate pain control; this could be due to the fact that in chronic periapical lesions pain is not a big issue following root canal therapy. From this study we can conclude that, the effect of ibuprofen and NAC on the periapical immunological events in chronic periapical lesions is still questionable, and more clinical trials are recommended to clarify these relationships. On the other hand, it seems that NAC can be a substitute for ibuprofen for post endodontic pain, but it is better to do more experiments especially in acute cases where an indication for analgesics seems more appropriate and rational.

Competing interests

The author(s) declare that they have no competing interests.

Authors' contribution

ME participated in the design and conception of the study and has given final approval of the version to be published. AAM participated in the design of the study, performed the statistical analysis, and approved the English structure of manuscript to be published. SZ participated in the design of the study, patient management, drug delivery, acquisition of the data, drafted and revised the manuscript. GM participated in the design and conception of the study, helped in the immunological process of the samples and lab procedures and has given final approval of the version to be published.SH participated in the design of the study, and controlled the radiographic aspect of the study and has given final approval of the version to be published. SMAM participated in the acquisition of the data, performed the lab procedures and coordinated the immunological processes. NMK participated in the acquisition of the data, performed the lab procedures and coordinated the immunological processes. All authors read and approved the final manuscript.

Acknowledgements

The authors would like to thank Maria Hashemi, for her technical assistance. This investigation has been financially supported by Babol University of Medical Sciences.

Author details

[1]Department of Endodontics, Dental Material Research Center, Faculty of Dentistry, Babol University of Medical Sciences, Babol, Iran. [2]Department of Pharmacology, Faculty of Medicine, Babol University of Medical Sciences, Babol, Iran. [3]Cellular and Molecular Biology Research Center, Babol University of Medical Sciences, Babol, Iran. [4]Department of Oral and Maxillofacial Radiology, Faculty of Dentistry, Babol University of Medical Sciences, Babol, Iran.

References

1. Colic M, Vasilijic S, Gazivoda D, Vucevic D, Marjanovic M, Lukic A: **Interleukin-17 plays a role in exacerbation of inflammation within chronic periapical lesions.** *Eur J Oral Sci* 2007, **115**:315–320.
2. Prso IB, Kocjan W, Simic H, Brumini G, Pezelj-Ribaric S, Borcic J, *et al*: **Tumor necrosis factor-alpha and interleukin 6 in human periapical lesions.** *Mediators Inflamm* 2007, **2007**:1–4.
3. Marton IJ, Kiss C: **Protective and destructive immune reactions in apical periodontitis.** *Oral Microbiol Immunol* 2000, **15**:139–150.
4. Danin J, Linder L, Lundqvist G, Wretlind B: **Cytokines in periradicular lesions: the effect of linezolid treatment.** *Oral Surg Oral Med Oral Pathol Oral Radiol Endod* 2003, **96**:492–498.
5. Mousavi-Jazi M, Aslroosta H, Moayer AR, Baeeri M, Abdollahi M: **Effects of Angipars on oxidative inflammatory indices in a murine model of periodontitis.** *DARU* 2010, **18**:260–264.
6. Girardin E, Roux-Lombard P, Grau GE, Suter P, Gallati H, Dayer JM: **Imbalance between tumour necrosis factor-alpha and soluble TNF receptor concentrations in severe meningococcaemia. The J5 Study Group.** *Immunology* 1992, **76**:20–23.
7. Balto K, Sasaki H, Stashenko P: **Interleukin-6 deficiency increases inflammatory bone destruction.** *Infect Immun* 2001, **69**:744–750.
8. Barkhordar RA, Hayashi C, Hussain MZ: **Detection of interleukin-6 in human dental pulp and periapical lesions.** *Endod Dent Traumatol* 1999, **15**:26–27.
9. Vernal R, Dutzan N, Chaparro A, Puente J, Antonieta VM, Gamonal J: **Levels of interleukin-17 in gingival crevicular fluid and in supernatants of cellular cultures of gingival tissue from patients with chronic periodontitis.** *J Clin Periodontol* 2005, **32**:383–389.
10. Van Bezooijen RL, Papapoulos SE, Lowik CW: **Effect of interleukin-17 on nitric oxide production and osteoclastic bone resorption: is there dependency on nuclear factor-kappaB and receptor activator of nuclear factor kappaB (RANK)/RANK ligand signaling?** *Bone* 2001, **28**:378–386.
11. Cooper SA: **Five studies on ibuprofen for postsurgical dental pain.** *Am J Med* 1984, **13**(77):70–77.
12. Dionne RA, Campbell RA, Cooper SA, Hall DL, Buckingham B: **Suppression of postoperative pain by preoperative administration of ibuprofen in**

comparison to placebo, acetaminophen, and acetaminophen plus codeine. *J Clin Pharmacol* 1983, **23**:37–43.
13. Tanaka K, Suemasu S, Ishihara T, Tasaka Y, Arai Y, Mizushima T: **Inhibition of both COX-1 and COX-2 and resulting decrease in the level of prostaglandins E2 is responsible for non-steroidal anti-inflammatory drug (NSAID)-dependent exacerbation of colitis.** *Eur J Pharmacol* 2009, **28**:120–132.
14. Endres S, Whitaker RE, Ghorbani R, Meydani SN, Dinarello CA: **Oral aspirin and ibuprofen increase cytokine-induced synthesis of IL-1 beta and of tumour necrosis factor-alpha ex vivo.** *Immunology* 1996, **87**:264–270.
15. Ertel W, Morrison MH, Ayala A, Perrin MM, Chaudry IH: **Blockade of prostaglandin production increases cachectin synthesis and prevents depression of macrophage functions after hemorrhagic shock.** *Ann Surg* 1991, **213**:265–271.
16. Tugendreich S, Pearson CI, Sagartz J, Jarnagin K, Kolaja K: **NSAID-induced acute phase response is due to increased intestinal permeability and characterized by early and consistent alterations in hepatic gene expression.** *Toxicol Pathol* 2006, **34**:168–179.
17. Brok J, Buckley N, Gluud C: **Interventions for paracetamol (acetaminophen) overdose.** *Cochrane Database Syst Rev* 2006, :CD003328.
18. Peristeris P, Clark BD, Gatti S, Faggioni R, Mantovani A, Mengozzi M, *et al*: **N-acetylcysteine and glutathione as inhibitors of tumor necrosis factor production.** *Cell Immunol* 1992, **140**:390–399.
19. Sadowska AM, Manuel YK, De Backer WA: **Antioxidant and anti-inflammatory efficacy of NAC in the treatment of COPD: discordant in vitro and in vivo dose-effects: a review.** *Pulm Pharmacol Ther* 2007, **20**:9–22.
20. Dekhuijzen PN: **Antioxidant properties of N-acetylcysteine: their relevance in relation to chronic obstructive pulmonary disease.** *Eur Respir J* 2004, **23**:629–636.
21. Lappas M, Permezel M, Rice GE: **N-Acetyl-cysteine inhibits phospholipid metabolism, proinflammatory cytokine release, protease activity, and nuclear factor-kappaB deoxyribonucleic acid-binding activity in human fetal membranes in vitro.** *J Clin Endocrinol Metab* 2003, **88**:1723–1729.
22. Paterson RL, Galley HF, Webster NR: **The effect of N-acetylcysteine on nuclear factor-kappa B activation, interleukin-6, interleukin-8, and intercellular adhesion molecule-1 expression in patients with sepsis.** *Crit Care Med* 2003, **31**:2574–2578.
23. Radomska-Lesniewska DM, Sadowska AM, Van Overveld FJ, Demkow U, Zielinski J, De Backer WA: **Influence of N-acetylcysteine on ICAM-1 expression and IL-8 release from endothelial and epithelial cells.** *J Physiol Pharmacol* 2006, **57**:325–334.
24. Hoffer E, Baum Y, Nahir AM: **N-Acetylcysteine enhances the action of anti-inflammatory drugs as suppressors of prostaglandin production in monocytes.** *Mediators Inflamm* 2002, **11**:321–323.
25. Shimauchi H, Miki Y, Takayama S, Imai T, Okada H: **Development of a quantitative sampling method for periapical exudates from human root canals.** *J Endod* 1996, **22**:612–615.
26. Gopikrishna V, Parameswaran A: **Effectiveness of prophylactic use of rofecoxib in comparison with ibuprofen on postendodontic pain.** *J Endod* 2003, **29**:62–64.
27. Bramlage P, Goldis A: **Bioequivalence study of three ibuprofen formulations after single dose administration in healthy volunteers.** *BMC Pharmacol* 2008, **8**:18.
28. Schultze-Mosgau S, Schmelzeisen R, Frolich JC, Schmele H: **Use of ibuprofen and methylprednisolone for the prevention of pain and swelling after removal of impacted third molars.** *J Oral Maxillofac Surg* 1995, **53**:2–7.
29. Aruoma OI, Halliwell B, Hoey BM, Butler J: **The antioxidant action of N-acetylcysteine: its reaction with hydrogen peroxide, hydroxyl radical, superoxide, and hypochlorous acid.** *Free Radic Biol Med* 1989, **6**:593–597.
30. Zafarullah M, Li WQ, Sylvester J, Ahmad M: **Molecular mechanisms of N-acetylcysteine actions.** *Cell Mol Life Sci* 2003, **60**:6–20.
31. Holdiness MR: **Clinical pharmacokinetics of N-acetylcysteine.** *Clin Pharmacokinet* 1991, **20**:123–134.
32. Shahriari S, Rezaei A, Jalalzadeh SM, Mani K, Zamani A: **Effect of Ibuprofen on IL-1beta, TNF-alpha and PGE2 levels in periapical exudates: a double blinded clinical trial.** *Iran J Immunol* 2011, **8**:176–182.
33. Spinas GA, Bloesch D, Keller U, Zimmerli W, Cammisuli S: **Pretreatment with ibuprofen augments circulating tumor necrosis factor-alpha, interleukin-6, and elastase during acute endotoxinemia.** *J Infect Dis* 1991, **163**:89–95.
34. Sironi M, Gadina M, Kankova M, Riganti F, Mantovani A, Zandalasini M, *et al*: **Differential sensitivity of in vivo TNF and IL-6 production to modulation by anti-inflammatory drugs in mice.** *Int J Immunopharmacol* 1992, **14**:1045–1050.
35. Hulten LM, Lindmark H, Schersten H, Wiklund O, Nilsson FN, Riise GC: **Butylated hydroxytoluene and N-acetylcysteine attenuates tumor necrosis factor-alpha (TNF-alpha) secretion and TNF-alpha mRNA expression in alveolar macrophages from human lung transplant recipients in vitro.** *Transplantation* 1998, **66**:364–369.
36. Confalone E, D'Alessio G, Furia A: **IL-6 Induction by TNFá and IL-1â in an Osteoblast-Like Cell Line.** *Int J Biomed Sci* 2010, **6**:135–140.

Positive effect of septimeb™ on mortality rate in severe sepsis: a novel non antibiotic strategy

Kaveh Eslami[1,2], Ata Mahmoodpoor[3], Arezoo Ahmadi[4], Mohammad Abdollahi[1], Koorosh Kamali[5], Sarah Mousavi[6], Atabak Najafi[4], Maryam Baeeri[1], Hadi Hamishehkar[7], Leila Kouti[2], Mohammad Reza Javadi[1] and Mojtaba Mojtahedzadeh[1,4*]

Abstract

Background: Septimeb is a new herbal-derived remedy, recently approved for its potential immunomodulatory effects. Regarding the key role of immune system in the pathogenesis of severe sepsis and lack of any standard treatment for improving survival of these patients; we evaluated the effect of Septimeb -as an adjutant to standard treatment-on inflammatory biomarkers and mortality rates in patients with severe sepsis.

Methods: In this multicenter, randomized, single-blind trial, we assigned patients with severe sepsis and Acute Physiology and Chronic Health Evaluation (APACHE II) score of more than 20 to receive standard treatment of severe sepsis (control group) or standard treatment plus Septimeb. This group was treated with Septimeb for 14 days then followed up for another14 days. APACHE score, Sequential Organ Failure Assessment (SOFA) and Simplified Acute Physiology Score (SAPS) were calculated daily. Blood samples were analyzed for interleukin 2 tumor necrosis factor-α, total antioxidant power, platelet growth factor and matrix metalloproteinase 2.

Results: A total of 29 patients underwent randomization (13 in control group and 16 in Septimeb group). There was significant difference between the Septimeb and control group in the 14 days mortality rate (18.8% vs. 53.85 respectively, P=0.048). Compared to control group, Septimeb was significantly effective in improving SAPS (P= 0.029), SOFA (P=0.003) and APACHE II (P=0.008) scores. Inflammatory biomarkers didn't change significantly between the two groups (P>0.05).

Conclusion: Septimeb reduces mortality rates among patients with severe sepsis and it could be added as a safe adjutant to standard treatment of sepsis.

Keywords: Severe sepsis, Immunomodulation, Septimeb, ICU

Introduction

Sepsis is one of the most prevalent and fatal diseases in Intensive Care Units (ICU) resulted in 30-60% mortality [1,2]. Sepsis is a systemic inflammatory response to an infection leading to endothelial dysfunction, impairment of microcirculation, tissue hypoxia, apoptosis and finally multiple organ failure and death [3]. Nowadays the role of inflammatory cytokines, oxidative stress and immune system in the pathogenesis of sepsis is obvious. Continuous elevated levels of various cytokines in severe sepsis could result in uncontrolled inflammation [4-7]. Breaking of inflammatory cascade may lead to improving of survival [8]. A significant association exists between inflammatory cytokine levels in the first 72 hours of severe sepsis and severity of tissue hypoxia, organ dysfunction and mortality [9]. IL-6 and Acute Physiology and Chronic Health Evaluation (APACHE) II score are used respectively in prediction of mortality and clinical evaluation of severe septic patients [10]. Therefore modulation of inflammation and immune system response could be one of the strategic plans to manage sepsis.

Several immunomodulatory therapies have been evaluated in sepsis. Corticosteroids [11,12], anti Tumor Necrosis Factor α (TNF α) antibodies [13,14], Anti Interleukin 1 antibodies [15], Platelet Aggregating Factor (PAF)

* Correspondence: mojtahed@tums.ac.ir
[1]Faculty of Pharmacy and Pharmaceutical Sciences Research Centre, Tehran University of Medical Sciences, Tehran, Iran
[4]Department of Anesthesiology and Critical Care Medicine, Sina Hospital, Faculty of Medicine, Tehran University of Medical Sciences, Tehran, Iran
Full list of author information is available at the end of the article

antagonist [16,17], antioxidants especially selenium [18,19], modulation of nutrition [20], modulation of coagulation [21] and complement pathway [22] are examples of immunotherapy in sepsis, but none of them were effective on survival of patients. Procedures such as plasmapheresis and hemofiltration slightly improve prognosis of sepsis by reducing circulating levels of inflammatory cytokines but couldn't decrease mortality rate [23].

Analysis of current immunomodulating strategies indicates that monovalent approaches in isolation are unlikely to restore immunostasis or attain status of complete therapy. It is likely that multiple immunomodulating strategies will be necessary to achieve clinical success owing to complex interplay between pathways. Botanical extracts provide cytoprotective, antiinflammatory, and antimicrobial activities in addition to immunoregulatory activity [24].

Septimeb (a more potent form of IMOD™) is a herbal extracts including Tanacetum vulgare (tansy), Rosa canina and Urtica dioica (nettle) in addition to selenium, flavonoids and carotenes. Tanacetum vulgare may relieve anti-inflammatory symptoms and Rosa canina defers blood glucose and cholesterol elevation. Extracts from Urtica dioica may prevent maturation of myeloid dendritic cells and reduce T cell responses [25]. Septimeb can regulate TNF-α, interferon-γ (IFN-γ) and IL-2 [26]. IMOD has been patented in Europe with code of WO/2007/087825 for its immunomodulator and anti-TNF-α capacities and improving CD4 in HIV positive patients [27,28]. The pre-clinical safety studies of IMOD in animals and phases I and II trials have been successfully conducted, showing optimistic results [29,30]. As sepsis is an immune mediated disease and modulating of immune system might be effective in improving prognosis and survival, we aim to evaluate Septimeb's effect on plasma levels of inflammatory biomarkers, and mortality rates of patients with severe sepsis.

Methods

Patient selection

In all cases, informed consents were received from patients or their legal guardian. The study procedure and protocol were approved by the ethical committee of Tehran University of Medical Sciences (TUMS). Our clinical trial was registered in Australian Newzeland Clinical Trial Organization with code number of (ACTRN012607000376448).

Study subjects

Between March 2009 and April 2011, 29 patients with severe sepsis and Acute Physiology and Chronic Health Evaluation (APACHE) scores of more than 20, admitted to general ICU of "Sina" Hospital of TUMS and "Shohada" Hospital of Tabriz University of Medical Sciences were enrolled in this study. Exclusion criteria for all patients were ages below 18 and more than 65 years, pregnancy, breast feeding, over 24 hours of sepsis diagnosis and death probability within 28 days due to nonspecific reasons (such as renal or liver failure).

Patients were randomized via block randomization to receive one of the following treatments: standard treatment for severe sepsis (control group) and standard treatment plus Septimeb (intervention group) for 14 days and were also followed up for another 14 days. According to latest international guidelines [31], standard treatments for severe sepsis were implemented as following: early resuscitation within the first 6 hours of admission, appropriate diagnosis studies to ascertain causative organisms before starting antibiotics, early administration of broad spectrum antibiotic therapy, hypotension control with avasopressor, fluid administration to target Central Venous Pressure (CVP) of 8–12 mmHg and central venous oxygen saturation (Sa O_2) > 95%, low dose steroid, glycemic control(blood glucose <150 mg/dl), target hemoglobin values of 7–9 g/dl in absence of coronary artery disease or acute hemorrhage, lung protection ventilation and standard prophylactic measures for deep vein thrombosis (DVT) and Stress-related Mucosal Damage (SRMD).

Patients in intervention group received 240mg (4 ml) of Septimeb in 150 ml of DW 5%, infused over 1.5 hours on the first day. All hemodynamic data were monitored during the infusion and in case of any negative hemodynamic deterioration, dermal rash, urticaria or anaphylactic reaction, the infusion discontinued. Then 360mg (6 ml) of the drug was infused in 150 ml of DW5%, everyday for 14 days. The time gap between the beginnings of treatment with intervention and the diagnosis of sepsis was also noted to evaluate possible impact of the onset of intervention on mortality.

Demographic data and clinical information were obtained at the beginning (Table 1). APACHE scores, sequential organ failure assessment (SOFA), and simplified acute physiology score (SAPS) were calculated daily. Higher scores indicate more severe illness and a higher number of therapeutic interventions.

Table 1 Demographic and baseline characteristic of patients

	Control group (N:14)	Septimeb group (N:16)	P value
Age (year)	45.69 ± 20.67	39.56 ± 16.46	0.38
Male, No.	10	15	0.18
APACHE II	24.76 ± 4.14	27.56 ± 7.39	0.23
SOFA	8.92 ± 1.97	9.25 ± 2.32	0.69
SAPS	47.69 ± 11.61	43.68 ± 11.21	0.35

Data are mean ± SD. APACHE: Acute Physiologic And Chronic Health Evaluation. SAPS: Simplified Acute Physiologic Score. SOFA: Sequential Organ Failure Assessment.

Mortality during ICU stay and mortality during 14 days were recorded. The standard treatment of sepsis was continued throughout ICU stay of patients.

Sample collection and handling

All patients had central venous catheters and arterial lines for blood sampling. For all patients there were seven scheduled time points to assess IL-2, TNF-α, total antioxidant power (TAP), Matrix Metalloproteinase2 (MMP2) and Platelet Growth Factor (PGF). The levels were analyzed via commercially available enzyme-linked immunosorbent assay kit (BenderMed system, Vienna, Austria). The first sample was taken on ICU admission and prior to initiation of the therapy. Other samples were obtained on days of 1, 2, 3, 7, 10, and 14 post therapies. Blood samples were collected into vacutainer tubes containing EDTA.

The samples were spun at 3000 × g for 15 minutes in order to remove cells and cellular debris. The cell free supernatant and plasma were stored at −80°C until the time of analysis.

Statistical analysis

All data were expressed as mean ± SD. Univariate comparisons of baseline characteristics were performed by the independent student's t-test for parametric data and Mann-Whitney's t-test for non-parametric data. To assess differences between the time points in each treatment group, repeated-measure analysis of variance was done to analyze changes in levels of the biomarkers. Pearson's chi square and Kaplan-meier (Log rank) tests analyzed the differences of survival rates among the two groups. *P*-values less than 0.05 were considered statistically significant.

Result

Thirty patients with severe sepsis and APACHE scores of over 20 were enrolled in this study (13 patients in control group and 16 in intervention group). Demographic and baseline values for APACHE, SOFA and SAPS scores have been summarized in Table 1. The differences in age and sex were not significant between two groups (P= 0.38 and 0.18, respectively). Differences in baseline values for APACHE, SOFA and SAPS scores were not statistically significant either (Table 1).

Compared to controls, Septimeb was effective in improving APACHE (P= 0.229), SOFA (P=0.335) and SAPS (P= 0.059) scores in 14 days but the trend was not statistically significant (Figures 1, 2 and 3). But the score differences between the 14th and first day by LOCF method (Last Observation Carried Forward), showed that adding Septimeb was significantly more effective than standard treatment (Table 2).

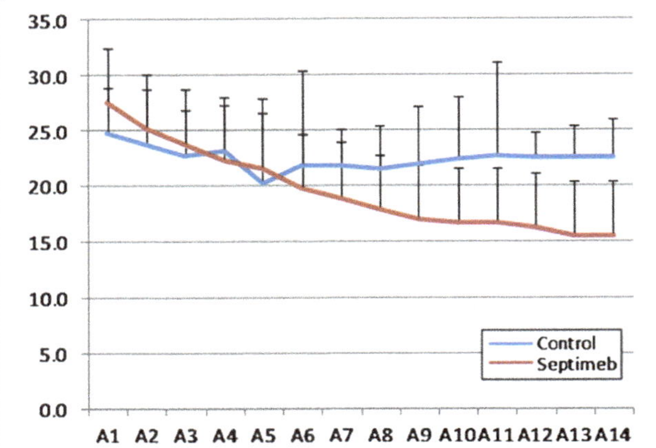

Figure 1 Changes of patients APACHE II score in different days of study. Difference between two groups is not significant (P= 0.266). A: APACHE (Acute Physiologic And Chronic Health Evaluation) 1–14: day 1–14.

The mean survival time was 9.84 (7.32-12.36, CI: 95%) days in control group and 12.93 (11.49-14.3, CI: 95%) days in Septimeb group. The difference in survival time was significant (P=0.019) (Figure 4). In the intervention group, the mortality rate was 18.8% during 28 days while it was 53.8% in control group, the difference was statistically significant (P=0.048).

The changes in the levels of biomarkers including IL-2 (P= 0.35), TNF- α (P= 0.66), TAP (P= 0.92), MMP 2 (P= 0.62) and PGF (P= 0.45) were not different among two groups (Figures 5, 6, 7, 8 and 9). None of the time points (0,1, 2, 3, 7,10 and 14 days) showed significant differences between two groups (p>0.05).

Discussion

The results of this study show that Septimeb, as an adjutant to standard treatment of severe sepsis could reduce mortality rates in patients, but has not significant anti-inflammatory effects.

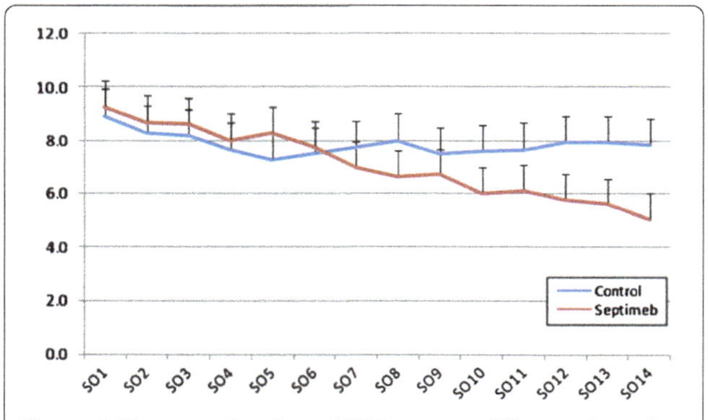

Figure 2 Changes of patients SOFA score in different days of study. Difference between two groups is not significant (P= 0.335). SO: SOFA (Sequential Organ Failure Assessment) 1–14: day 1–14.

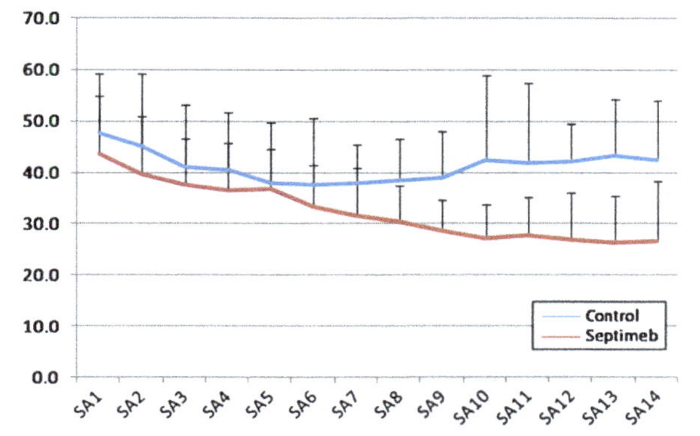

Figure 3 Changes of patients SAPS score in different days of study. Difference between two groups is not significant (P= 0.059). SA: SAPS (Simplified Acute Physiologic Score) 1–14: day 1–14.

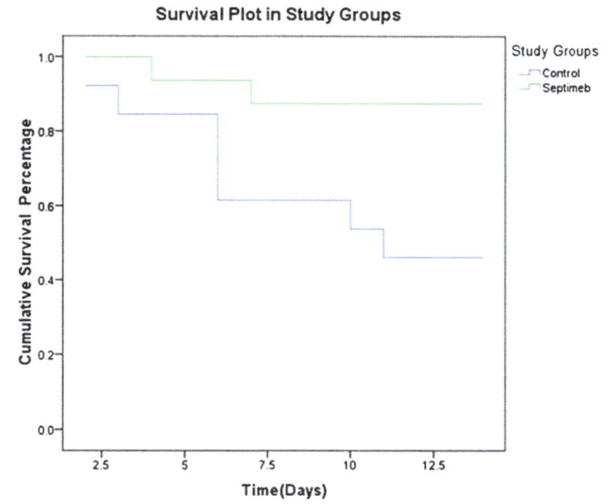

Figure 4 Changes of patient's survival during study period. The differences in survival time was significant (P=0.019).

Despite great advancements in understanding the pathophysiology of sepsis and development of novel therapeutic approaches, mortality of sepsis remains unacceptably high [32]. As mentioned earlier, immune system and inflammatory cytokines have a key role in pathogenesis of sepsis and several studies evaluated the effect of different immunomodulatory treatment on severe sepsis, but fail to improve survival of patients [11-19,21-23,33]. Among immunomodulatory agents, the activated protein C and corticosteroids are the only approved treatment for sepsis. According to the results of PROWESS trial [34,35] and a Meta-analysis [36] about the ineffectiveness of activated protein C on survival of patients with sepsis, Food and Drug Administration (FDA) withdrew this drug from the market and therefore currently there is no specific treatment for severe sepsis.

Previous studies have shown that monovalent therapies could not restore immunostasis in severe sepsis, so the need of drugs with polyvalent activities such as botanical immune-drugs seems inevitable [24,37]. Botanical immunodrugs e.g. Chinese remedy and green tea have been found to have dose-dependent attenuate bacterial endotoxin-induced HMGBI release [38,39]. Septimeb is a new herbal-derived remedy that has been suggested to be able to stimulate lymphocytes in order to produce cytokines in HIV positive patients and also inhibit TNF alpha and increase interferon gamma and Interleukin 2 [40,41]. The phase I and II trial studies with IMOD™ shows this drug is safe and has no mutagenic or allergenic potentials. Based on the results of this study, Septimeb (a more potent form of IMOD) reduced APACHE, SOFA and SAPS scores, as quantitative indices of clinical status [29,30]. Improvements of these scores by Septimeb confirm the potential of this drug in alleviation of the severity of sepsis and consequently reduced mortality rates of patients.

The results of previous study [30] did not show any improvement in survival of septic patients, but in the current study Septimeb decreased mortality rate significantly, this could be because of larger sample size in this study.

Immunotherapy must be applied early during the development of immune-dysfunction following trauma or acute onset of infection, to ensure that all cellular components of immune system will be protected. There is a much earlier temporal relationship between inflammation and the onset of organ dysfunction. Mean biomarker levels during 72 hours were significantly greater in hospital non-survivors [42]. Supporting evidence showed that the initial inflammatory response directly correlates to early, but not late sepsis mortality [8]. A complex interaction of cytokines and cytokine-neutralizing molecules probably determines the clinical presentation and course of sepsis. Intervening in this sequence of events to modify the host inflammatory responses may be a beneficial treatment strategy for sepsis, but currently tested anticytokine therapies have been

Table 2 Change in patient's APACHE, SAPS and SOFA score from 1st day to 14th day study

	Control group (N:14)	Septimeb group (N:16)	P value
APACHE mean difference between 14th and first day±SD	−1.7(±9.8)	−12.7(±7.9)	0.003
SOFA mean difference between 14th and first day	−0.5(±2.3)	−4(±3.3)	0.013
SAPS mean difference between 14th and first day	−3(±12.9)	−18(±16.6)	0.003

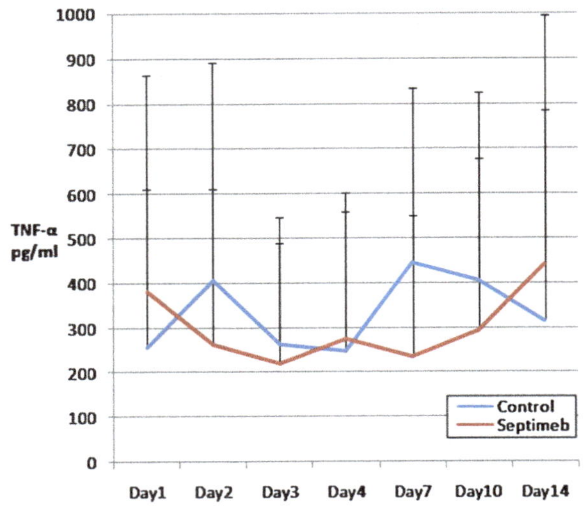

Figure 5 Changes in blood TNF-α level in different days of study. Data are mean ± SE. **Difference between two groups is not significant at P>0.05.

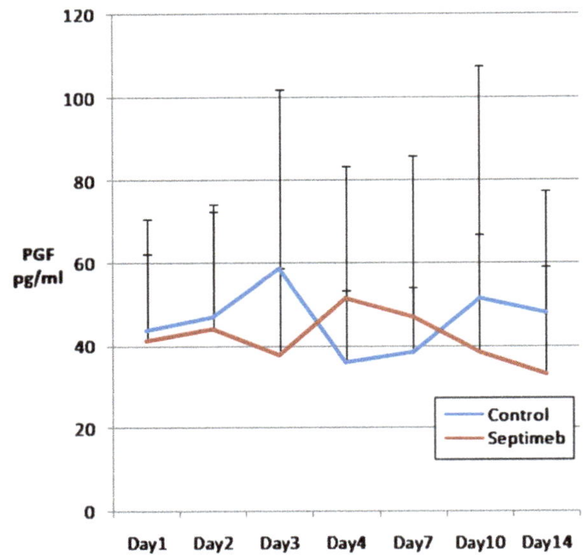

Figure 7 Changes in blood PGF levels in different days of study. Data are mean ± SE. **Difference between two groups is not significant at P>0.05.

largely unsuccessful [20]. Levels of inflammatory biomarkers didn't change significantly by Septimeb and positive effect of Septimeb on mortality rate might be due to other mechanisms. The main problems in severe sepsis are O_2 extraction and O_2 consumption. The critical importance of tissue oxygenation was addressed by a study in which patients in the earliest stages of sepsis were treated by aggressive management with fluids, blood transfusion and inotropic agents to optimize hemodynamic function [43]. After macrocirculatory resuscitation, many patients still demonstrate multisystem organ dysfunction and shock. The recent landscape of sepsis research is focusing on two separate mechanisms that may explain the persistence of the shock state. The first is the role of the microcirculation in the body, and the mixed response of various circulatory beds to the sepsis. The second is that the cells and mitochondria receiving adequate perfusion and oxygenation may still have a decreased ability to properly utilize energy to form ATP, referred to as cytopathic hypoxia [44], that can lead to profound metabolic alterations and the inability to supply energy to the tissues. These two represent attractive

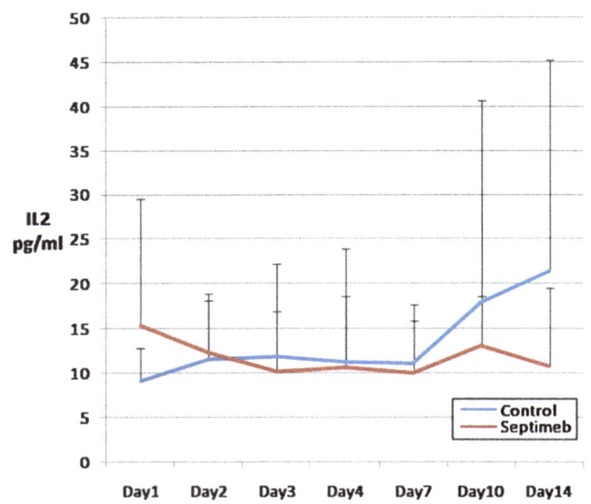

Figure 6 Changes in blood IL-2 level in different days of study. Data are mean ± SE. **Difference between two groups is not significant at P>0.05.

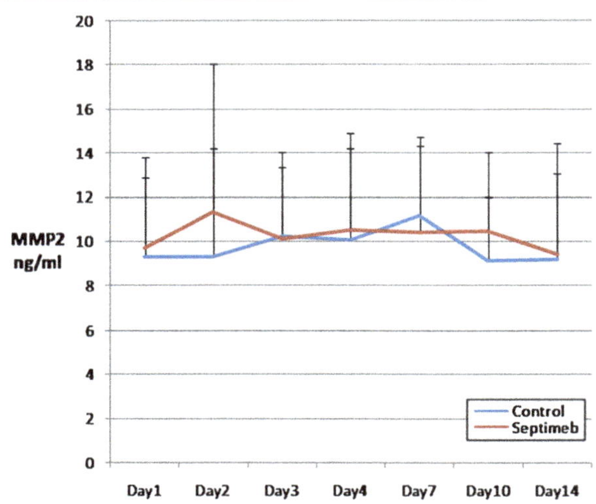

Figure 8 Changes in blood MMP-2 level in different days of study. Data are mean ± SE. **Difference between two groups is not significant at P>0.05.

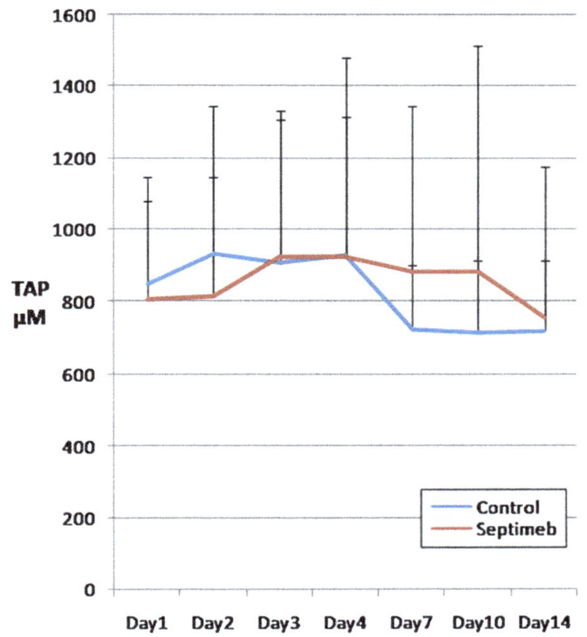

Figure 9 Changes in blood TAP level in different days of study. Data are mean ± SE. **Difference between two groups is not significant at P>0.05.

targets for novel adjunctive resuscitative agents in the treatment of septic shock. Therefore improving tissue oxygenation could be a possible mechanism of Septimeb in reduction of sepsis mortality.

Fortunately, Septimeb showed no adverse effects on coagulation factors like platelet count, prothrombin time, partial thromboplastin time, fibrinogen, and D-dimer. Hemodynamic instability and anaphylactic reactions were not observed during infusion. It could be a safe adjutant to other standard treatments of sepsis [45].

Conclusion

Despite several limitations of this study, especially the small sample size, Septimeb shows positive effects on survival of patients with severe sepsis, considering the withdrawal of activated protein C from markets. Additional studies with adequate sample size is recommended to be performed with Septimeb, but regarding the results and also limited side effects of Septimeb, it could be considered as an adjutant along with other standard measures for treatment of severe sepsis.

Competing interests

The authors have no financial interest to declare. There is no conflict of interest to declare.

Authors' contribution

EK: study design, patient selection, Sample collection and handling, sample analyzing via commercially available enzyme-linked immunosorbent assay kit, draft the manuscript. MA: study design, patient selection, Sample collection and handling, draft the manuscript and revising it. AH: study design, patient selection, Sample collection and handling, revising manuscript. MA: study design, sample analyzing via commercially available enzyme-linked immunosorbent assay kit, draft the manuscript and revising it. KK: study design, patient selection, Statistical analysis, draft the manuscript and revising it. SM: study design, patient selection, Sample collection and handling, draft the manuscript and revising it. AN: study design, patient selection, Sample collection and handling, draft the manuscript and revising it. MB: sample analyzing via commercially available enzyme-linked immunosorbent assay kit, draft the manuscript and revising it. HH: patient selection, Sample collection and handling, analysis and interpretation of data, draft the manuscript and revising it. LK: patient selection, Sample collection and handling, analysis and interpretation of data, draft the manuscript and revising it. MRJ: analysis and interpretation of data , draft the manuscript and revising it. MM: study design, patient selection, Sample collection and handling, sample analyzing via commercially available enzyme-linked immunosorbent assay kit, Statistical analysis, analysis and interpretation of data, draft the manuscript and revising it. All authors read and approved the final manuscript.

Acknowledgement

We gratefully thankful from nurses and ICU staff of Sina and Shohada hospital. We also thanks Iranian ministry of health which financially supported the study.

Author details

[1]Faculty of Pharmacy and Pharmaceutical Sciences Research Centre, Tehran University of Medical Sciences, Tehran, Iran. [2]Faculty of Pharmacy, Ahvaz Jondishapour University of Medical Sciences, Ahvaz, Iran. [3]Department of Anesthesiology and Critical Care Medicine, Faculty of Medicine, Tabriz University of Medical Sciences, Tabriz, Iran. [4]Department of Anesthesiology and Critical Care Medicine, Sina Hospital, Faculty of Medicine, Tehran University of Medical Sciences, Tehran, Iran. [5]Department of Public Health, School of Public Health, Zanjan University of Medical Sciences, Zanjan, Iran. [6]Clinical Pharmacy Department, Faculty of Pharmacy and Research Center for Rational Use of Drugs, Tehran University of Medical Sciences, Tehran, Iran. [7]Clinical Pharmacy Department, Faculty of Pharmacy, Tabriz University of Medical Sciences, Tabriz, Iran.

References

1. Moreno RP, Metnitz B, Adler L, Hoechtl A, Bauer P, Metnitz PGH: **Sepsis mortality prediction based on predisposition, infection and response.** *Intensive Care Med* 2008, **34**:496–504.
2. Vesteinsdottir E, Karason S, Sigurdsson SE, Gottfredsson M, Sigurdsson GH: **Severe sepsis and septic shock: a prospective population-based study in Icelandic intensive care units.** *Acta Anaesthesiol Scand* 2011, **55**:722–731.
3. Caille V, Bossi P, Grimaldi D, Vieillard-Baro A: **[Physiopathology of severe sepsis].** *Presse Med* 2004, **33**:256–261. discussion 269.
4. Bozza FA, Salluh JI, Japiassu AM, Soares M, Assis EF, Gomes RN, Bozza MT, Castro-Faria-Neto HC, Bozza PT: **Cytokine profiles as markers of disease severity in sepsis: a multiplex analysis.** *Critical Care* 2007, **11**:R49.
5. Mousavi S, Mojtahedzadeh M, Abdollahi M: **Place of iron chelators like desferrioxamine and deferasirox in management of hyperoxia-induced lung injury: A systematic review.** *Int J Pharmacol* 2010, **6**:326–337.
6. Shiehmorteza M, Ahmadi A, Abdollahi M, Nayebpour M, Mohammadi M, Hamishehkar H, Najafi A, Pazoki M, Mojtahedzadeh M: **Recombinant human erythropoietin reduces plasminogen activator inhibitor and ameliorates pro-inflammatory responses following trauma.** *DARU J Pharmaceut Sci* 2011, **19**:159–165.
7. Soltan-Sharifi MS, Mojtahedzadeh M, Najafi A, Khajavi MR, Rouini MR, Moradi M, Mohammadirad A, Abdollahi M: **Improvement by N-acetylcysteine of acute respiratory distress syndrome through increasing intracellular glutathione, and extracellular thiol molecules and anti-oxidant power: evidence for underlying toxicological mechanisms.** *Hum Exp Toxicol* 2007, **26**:697–703.
8. Gogos CA, Drosou E, Bassaris HP, Skoutelis A: **Pro-versus anti-inflammatory cytokine profile in patients with severe sepsis: a marker for prognosis and future therapeutic options.** *J Infect Dis* 2000, **181**:176–180.

9. Dimopoulou I, Orfanos S, Kotanidou A, Livaditi O, Giamarellos-Bourboulis E, Athanasiou C, Korovesi I, Sotiropoulou C, Kopterides P, Ilias I: **Plasma pro-and anti-inflammatory cytokine levels and outcome prediction in unselected critically ill patients.** *Cytokine* 2008, **41**:263–267.
10. Hamishehkar HB MT, Abdollahi M, Ahmadi A, Ahmadi A, Mahmoodpour, Mirjalili MR, Abrishami R, Khoshayand MR, Eslami K, Kanani M, Baeeri M, Mojtahedzadeh M: **Identification of enhanced cytokine generation following sepsis. Dream of magic bullet for mortality prediction and therapeutic evaluation.** *DARU* 2010, **18**:155–162.
11. Keh D, Goodman S, Sprung CL: **Corticosteroid therapy in patients with severe sepsis and septic shock.** *Semin Respir Crit Care Med* 2004, **25**:713–719.
12. Minneci PC, Deans KJ, Natanson C: **Corticosteroid therapy for severe sepsis and septic shock.** *JAMA* 2009, **302**:1643. author reply 1644–1645.
13. Panacek EA, Marshall JC, Albertson TE, Johnson DH, Johnson S, MacArthur RD, Miller M, Barchuk WT, Fischkoff S, Kaul M, *et al*: **Efficacy and safety of the monoclonal anti-tumor necrosis factor antibody F(ab')2 fragment afelimomab in patients with severe sepsis and elevated interleukin-6 levels.** *Crit Care Med* 2004, **32**:2173–2182.
14. Reinhart K, Menges T, Gardlund B, Harm Zwaveling J, Smithes M, Vincent JL, Tellado JM, Salgado-Remigio A, Zimlichman R, Withington S, *et al*: **Randomized, placebo-controlled trial of the anti-tumor necrosis factor antibody fragment afelimomab in hyperinflammatory response during severe sepsis: The RAMSES Study.** *Crit Care Med* 2001, **29**:765–769.
15. Knaus WA, Harrell FE Jr, LaBrecque JF, Wagner DP, Pribble JP, Draper EA, Fisher CJ Jr, Soll L: **Use of predicted risk of mortality to evaluate the efficacy of anticytokine therapy in sepsis. The rhIL-1ra Phase III Sepsis Syndrome Study Group.** *Crit Care Med* 1996, **24**:46–56.
16. Suputtamongkol Y, Intaranongpai S, Smith MD, Angus B, Chaowagul W, Permpikul C, Simpson JA, Leelarasamee A, Curtis L, White NJ: **A double-blind placebo-controlled study of an infusion of lexipafant (Platelet-activating factor receptor antagonist) in patients with severe sepsis.** *Antimicrob Agents Chemother* 2000, **44**:693–696.
17. Vincent JL, Spapen H, Bakker J, Webster NR, Curtis L: **Phase II multicenter clinical study of the platelet-activating factor receptor antagonist BB-882 in the treatment of sepsis.** *Crit Care Med* 2000, **28**:638–642.
18. Angstwurm MW, Engelmann L, Zimmermann T, Lehmann C, Spes CH, Abel P, Strauss R, Meier-Hellmann A, Insel R, Radke J, *et al*: **Selenium in Intensive Care (SIC): results of a prospective randomized, placebo-controlled, multiple-center study in patients with severe systemic inflammatory response syndrome, sepsis, and septic shock.** *Crit Care Med* 2007, **35**:118–126.
19. Valenta J, Brodska H, Drabek T, Hendl J, Kazda A: **High-dose selenium substitution in sepsis: a prospective randomized clinical trial.** *Intensive Care Med* 2011, **37**:808–815.
20. Abrishami RA A, Abdollahi M, Moosivand A, Khalili H, Najafi A, Gholami K, Hamishehkar H, Yazdi AP, Mojtahedzadeh M: **Comparison the inflammatory effects of early supplemental parenteral nutrition plus enteral nutrition versus enteral nutrition alone in critically ill patients.** *daru* 2010, **18**:103–106.
21. Bernard GR: **Drotrecogin alfa (activated) (recombinant human activated protein C) for the treatment of severe sepsis.** *Crit Care Med* 2003, **31**:S85–93.
22. Hack CE, Ogilvie AC, Eisele B, Jansen PM, Wagstaff J, Thijs LG: **Initial studies on the administration of C1-esterase inhibitor to patients with septic shock or with a vascular leak syndrome induced by interleukin-2 therapy.** *Prog Clin Biol Res* 1994, **388**:335–357.
23. Peng Z, Pai P, Han-Min W, Jun Z, Hong-Bao L, Rong L, Chen H: **Evaluation of the effects of pulse high-volume hemofiltration in patients with severe sepsis: a preliminary study.** *Int J Artif Organs* 2010, **33**:505–511.
24. Patwardhan B, Gautam M: **Botanical immunodrugs: scope and opportunities.** *Drug Discov Today* 2005, **10**:495–502.
25. Paydary K, Emamzadeh-Fard S, Khorshid H, Kamali K, Seyed AS, Mohraz M: **Safety and Efficacy of Setarud (IMOD (TM)) Among People Living with HIV/AIDS. A Review.** *Recent patents on anti-infective drug discovery* 2012, **7**:66–72.
26. Mohammadirad AK-KH, Gharibdoost F, Abdollahi M: **etarud (IMODTM) as a multiherbal drug with promising benefits in animal and human studies: A comprehensive review of biochemical and cellular evidences.** *Asian J Anim Vet Adv* 2011, **6**:1185–1192.
27. Mohraz M, S B, F M, K K, c R: **Evaluation of safety and efficacy of IMOD inb patients with HIV/AIDS.** *Iranian J Allergy Asthma Immunol* 2007, **6**:10.
28. Mohraz M, Khairandish P, Kazerooni PA, Davarpanah MA, Shahhosseiny MH, Mahdavian B, Vaziry S, Shahriary S, Kamali K, Khorshid KHR, *et al*: **A clinical trial on the efficacy of IMOD in AIDS patients.** *Daru-J Pharmaceut Sci* 2009, **17**:277–284.
29. Keirandish PMM, khorram Khorshid H, Heshmat R, Gharibdust F: **Aphase I clinical trial to determine the maximum tolerated dose and toxicity of IMOD in HIV infected asymptomatic patiets in Iran.** *Iranian J Allergy, Asthma Immunol* 2007, **6**:5.
30. Mahmoodpoor A, Eslami K, Mojtahedzadeh M, Najafi A, Ahmadi A, Dehnadi-Moghadam A, Mohammadirad A, Baeeri M, Abdollahi M: **Examination of Setarud (IMOD (TM)) in the management of patients with severe sepsis.** *Daru-Journal of Faculty of Pharmacy* 2010, **18**:23–28.
31. Hicks P, Cooper DJ: **The Surviving Sepsis Campaign: International guidelines for management of severe sepsis and septic shock: 2008.** *Crit Care Resusc* 2008, **10**:8.
32. Dombrovskiy VY, Martin AA, Sunderram J, Paz HL: **Rapid increase in hospitalization and mortality rates for severe sepsis in the United States: a trend analysis from 1993 to 2003.** *Crit Care Med* 2007, **35**:1244–1250.
33. Busund R, Koukline V, Utrobin U, Nedashkovsky E: **Plasmapheresis in severe sepsis and septic shock: a prospective, randomised, controlled trial.** *Intensive care medicine* 2002, **28**:1434–1439.
34. Dhainaut JF, Laterre PF, LaRosa SP, Levy H, Garber GE, Heiselman D, Kinasewitz GT, Light RB, Morris P, Schein R: **The clinical evaluation committee in a large multicenter phase 3 trial of drotrecogin alfa (activated) in patients with severe sepsis (PROWESS): Role, methodology, and results.** *Critical care medicine* 2003, **31**:2291–2301.
35. Laterre PF, Levy H, Clermont G, Ball DE, Garg R, Nelson DR, Dhainaut JF, Angus DC: **Hospital mortality and resource use in subgroups of the Recombinant Human Activated Protein C Worldwide Evaluation in Severe Sepsis (PROWESS) trial*.** *Critical care medicine* 2004, **32**:2207.
36. Wiedermann C, Kaneider N: **A meta-analysis of controlled trials of recombinant human activated protein C therapy in patients with sepsis.** *BMC emergency medicine* 2005, **5**:7.
37. Reshetnikov EA, Baranov GA, Chuvanov MV, Skalozub O, Reshetnikov EA, Baranov GA, Chuvanov MV, Skalozub OI: **[Immunotherapy in complex treatment of surgical sepsis].** *Khirurgiia (Mosk)* 2008, **7**:11–14.
38. Li W, Ashok M, Li J, Yang H, Sama AE, Wang H: **A major ingredient of green tea rescues mice from lethal sepsis partly by inhibiting HMGB1.** *PLoS One* 2007, **2**:e1153.
39. Wheeler DS, Lahni PM, Hake PW, Denenberg AG, Wong HR, Snead C, Catravas JD, Zingarelli B: **The green tea polyphenol epigallocatechin-3-gallate improves systemic hemodynamics and survival in rodent models of polymicrobial sepsis.** *Shock* 2007, **28**:353–359.
40. Abedi-valugerdi MAN, Khorram Khorsid H, Tavasoti Kheiry M, Garibdust F: **In vivo and ex vivo immune response on herbal drug IMOD in animal experiments.** *Iranian J Allergy Asthma Immunol* 2007, **6**:9.
41. Rezvanfar MA, Ahmadi A, Baeeri M, Abdollahi M: **Inhibition of tumor necrosis factor-alpha and nitrosative/oxidative stresses by Setarud (IMOD®); a molecular mechanism of protection against letrozole-induced polycystic ovary.** *Toxicology Letters* 2011, **205**:S246.
42. Bauer M: **[The physiopathology of sepsis. Current concepts].** *Anaesthesist* 1996, **45**:312–322.
43. Cavazzoni SLZ, Dellinger RP: **Hemodynamic optimization of sepsis-induced tissue hypoperfusion.** *Critical Care* 2006, **10**:S2.
44. Levy R: **Mitochondrial dysfunction, bioenergenic impairment, and metabolic down-regulation in sepsis.** *shock* 2007, **28**:24–28.
45. Khairandish P, Mohraz M, Farzamfar B, Abdollahi M, Shahhosseiny MH, Madani H, Sadeghi B, Heshmat R, Gharibdoust F, Khorram-Khorshid HR: **Preclinical and phase 1 clinical safety of Setarud (IMOD (TM)), a novel immunomodulator.** *Daru-J Pharmaceut Sci* 2009, **17**:148–156.

4

Synthesis and antibacterial activity of novel levofloxacin derivatives containing a substituted thienylethyl moiety

Negar Mohammadhosseini[1,2], Zahra Alipanahi[1], Eskandar Alipour[1], Saeed Emami[3], Mohammad Ali Faramarzi[4], Nasrin Samadi[4], Nika Khoshnevis[4], Abbass Shafiee[2] and Alireza Foroumadi[2*]

Abstract

Background and the purpose of the study: Piperazinyl quinolones such as ciprofloxacin, ofloxacin and levofloxacin are an important group of quinolone antimicrobials which are widely used in the treatment of various infectious diseases. In the present study, we synthesized a new series of levofloxacin derivatives and evaluated their antibacterial activities.

Methods: The *N*-substituted analogs of levofloxacin **6a–j** were prepared by nucleophilic reaction of *N*-desmethyl levofloxacin **11** with thienylethyl bromide derivatives **8** or **9**. All target compounds were tested using conventional agar dilution method in comparison to levofloxacin and *N*-desmethyl levofloxacin and their MIC values were determined against a panel of Gram-positive and Gram-negative bacteria.

Results: All compounds showed significant antibacterial activities against Gram-positive bacteria (MIC = 0.04-6.25 μg/mL); however, the activity against Gram-negative bacteria was lower (MIC = 1.56–100 μg/mL). As is evident from the data, oxime derivatives **6e**, **6h** and **6i** are superior in inhibiting the growth of Gram-positive bacteria (MIC = 0.04–0.19 μg/mL), and their activities were found to be 5–25 times better than *N*-desmethyl levofloxacin **11** and equal or better than levofloxacin **4**.

Conclusion: We have designed and synthesized novel quinolone derivatives bearing functionalized thienylethyl moiety on the piperazine ring of levofloxacin. The results of antibacterial screening against Gram-positive and Gram-negative bacteria revealed that the introduction of functionalized thienylethyl moiety on the piperazine ring of levofloxacin can improve the activity against Gram-positive bacteria. Gram-positive bacteria are responsible for a wide range of infectious diseases, and rising resistance in this group is causing increasing concern. Thus, this study introduces structural features of levofloxacin scaffold for development of new candidates in the field of anti-Gram positive chemotherapy

Keywords: Antibacterial activity, Quinolones, Levofloxacin, Thiophene derivatives, Oximes

Introduction

Fluoroquinolones which are synthetic antibacterial agents are useful for the treatment of urinary tract infections, soft tissue infections, respiratory infections, typhoid fever, sexually transmitted diseases, bone-joint infections, community-acquired pneumonia, acute bronchitis, and sinusitis [1].

Fluoroquinolones consist of a bicyclic ring structure in which there is a substitution at position *N*-1; most of the current agents have a carboxyl group at position 3, a keto group at position 4, a fluorine atom at position 6 and a nitrogen heterocyclic moiety at the C-7 position [2]. Piperazine substitution at C-7 position has resulted in a wide range of clinically useful fluoroquinolone antibacterial agents namely norfloxacin (**1**), ciprofloxacin (**2**), ofloxacin (**3**) and levofloxacin (**4**) [3,4]. Fluoroquinolones with 7-piperazinyl moiety have been reported to possess potent antibacterial activity [5,6]. Levofloxacin, a chiral

* Correspondence: aforoumadi@yahoo.com
[2]Department of Medicinal Chemistry, Faculty of Pharmacy and Pharmaceutical Sciences Research Center, Tehran University of Medical Sciences, Tehran, Iran
Full list of author information is available at the end of the article

version of the earlier drug ofloxacin, is a successful fluoroquinolone antibacterial that departs from the typical quinolones substructure by having a fused ring connecting the N_1 to C_8 position [7]. This ring is connected with an ether moiety at C_8 [8]. Levofloxacin has been reported to be active in vitro against both Gram-positive and Gram-negative bacteria. Two major targets have been identified for levofloxacin activity, topoisomerase II (DNA-gyrase) in Gram-negative bacteria and topoisomerase IV in Gram-positive bacteria [9]. According to the inhibition mechanisms of the quinolones, the site near the C-7 substituent is regarded as drug-enzyme interaction domain and controls the spectrum and selectivity of quinolone molecule [10]. Over the past few years, we were particularly interested in the synthesis and evaluation of *N*-substituted 7-piperazinyl quinolones [5] for their antibacterial activities [11-16]. Although the nature of the C-7 substituent was known to influence quinolone activity in bacteria, we identified that addition of a certain bulky group as a particular chemical modification is permitted at the C-7 position of the piperazine ring and allows manipulation of selectivity and potency. Previously, we described the synthesis and antibacterial activity of certain piperazinyl quinolones (Figure 1), with 2-(thiophen-3-yl)-2-oxoethyl or 2-(thiophen-3-yl)-2-oxyiminoethyl moieties attached to the piperazine ring at the C-7 position [12]. In the present study, we have aimed to achieve new quinolone antibacterial, by preparing the levofloxacin derivatives **6a–j** carrying a 2-thienyl-2-oxoethyl or a 2-thienyl-2-oxyiminoethyl moiety attached to the piperazine ring at C-10 position (Figure 1).

Material and methods

Chemistry

Chemicals and all solvents used in this study were purchased from Merck AG and Aldrich Chemical. Melting points were determined on a Kofler hot stage apparatus and are uncorrected. The IR spectra were obtained on a Shimadzu 470 spectrophotometer (potassium bromide disks). ^{1}H-NMR spectra were measured using a Bruker 400 spectrometer, and chemical shifts are expressed as δ (ppm) with tetramethylsilane as internal standard. Merck silica gel 60 F254 plates were used for analytical TLC. Yields are of purified product and were not optimized. The intermediate compounds **9** were prepared according to the literature [12,14]. *N*-Desmethyl levofloxacin was prepared as previously described method [17]. The synthetic route for achieving the target compounds **6a–j** was depicted in Figure 2.

General procedure for the synthesis of compounds 6a–j

A mixture of thienylethyl bromide derivatives **8** or **9** (0.55 mmol), *N*-desmethyl levofloxacin **11** (174 mg, 0.5 mmol) and $NaHCO_3$ (42 mg, 0.5 mmol) in DMF (5 mL) was stirred at room temperature for 6–10 h. After consumption of *N*-desmethyl levofloxacin **11** (monitored by TLC), water (20 mL) was added and the precipitate was filtered, washed with water and crystallized from methanol-chloroform (9:1) to give compound **6a–j**.

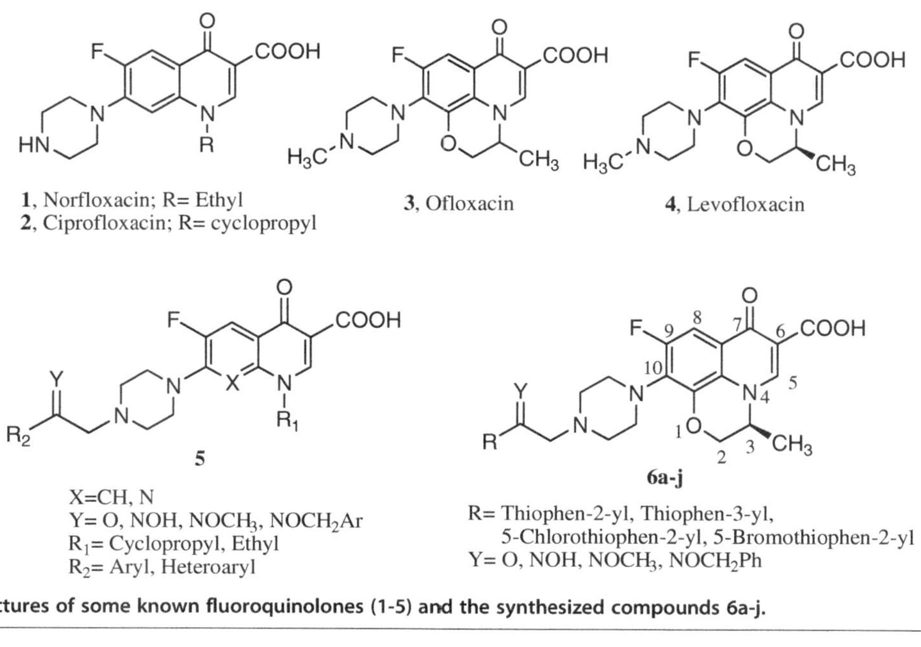

Figure 1 The structures of some known fluoroquinolones (1-5) and the synthesized compounds 6a-j.

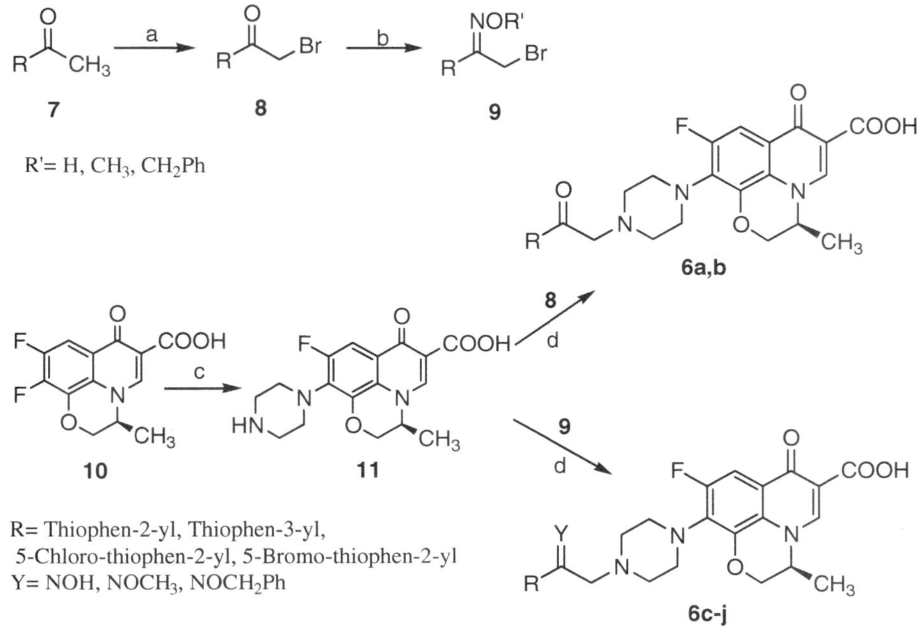

Figure 2 Synthesis of levofloxacin derivatives 6a–j. *Reagents and conditions* :(**a**) $CuBr_2$, $CHCl_3$–EtOAc, reflux;(**b**) $HONH_2{\cdot}HCl$ or$MeONH_2{\cdot}HCl$ or $BnONH_2{\cdot}HCl$, MeOH, r.t.; (**c**) piperazine; (**d**) DMF, $NaHCO_3$, r.t.

10-(4-(2-(5-bromothiophen-2-yl)-2-oxoethyl)piperazin-1-yl)-9-fluoro-3-methyl-7-oxo-3,7-dihydro-2H-[1,4]oxazino[2,3,4-Ij]quinoline-6-Carboxylic acid (6a)

Yield: 31%; mp 165–166°C; IR (KBr) cm^{-1}: 1622, 1721 (C = O). ^{1}H-NMR (DMSO-d_6): 1.45 (d, 3H, CH_3, $J = 6.0$ Hz), 3.26–3.33 (m, 4H, piperazine), 3.38–3.42 (m, 4H, piperazine), 3.49 (s, 2H, CH_2), 3.75 (s, 1H, CH_2), 4.39 (d, 1H, CH_2, $J = 10.9$ Hz), 4.60 (d, 1H, CH_2, $J = 10.9$ Hz), 4.87 (m, 1H, CH-Me), 7.53 (d, 1H, thiophene, $J = 5.0$ Hz), 7.58–7.65 (m, 1H, thiophene), 7.81 (d, 1H, H_8, $J = 11.9$ Hz), 8.99 (s, 1H, H_5), 15.17 (s, 1H, COOH).

10-(4-(2-(5-chlorothiophen-2-yl)-2-oxoethyl)piperazin-1-yl)-9-fluoro-3-methyl-7-oxo-3,7-dihydro-2H-[1,4]oxazino[2,3,4-Ij] quinoline-6-Carboxylic acid (6b)

Yield: 26%; mp 156–157°C; IR (KBr) cm^{-1}: 1620, 1719 (C = O). ^{1}H-NMR (DMSO-d_6): 1.43 (d, 3H, CH_3, $J = 6.2$ Hz), 3.27–3.34 (m, 4H, piperazine), 3.36–3.41 (m, 4H, piperazine), 3.47 (s, 2H, CH_2), 3.77 (s, 1H, CH_2), 4.40 (d, 1H, CH_2, $J = 11.0$ Hz), 4.59 (d, 1H, CH_2, $J = 11.0$ Hz), 4.85 (m, 1H, CH-Me), 7.52 (d, 1H, thiophene, $J = 5.0$ Hz), 7.56–7.64 (m, 1H, thiophene), 7.79 (d, 1H, H_8, $J = 12.1$ Hz), 8.98 (s, 1H, H_5), 15.21 (s, 1H, COOH).

10-(4-(2-(5-chlorothiophen-2-yl)-2-(methoxyimino)ethyl) piperazin-1-yl)-9-fluoro-3-methyl-7-oxo-3,7-dihydro-2H-[1,4] oxazino[2,3,4-Ij]quinoline-6-Carboxylic acid (6c)

Yield: 24%; mp 180–181°C; IR (KBr) cm^{-1}: 1626, 1717 (C = O). ^{1}H-NMR (DMSO-d_6): 1.62 (d, 3H, CH_3, $J = 5.3$ Hz), 2.47–2.70 (m, 4H, piperazine), 3.34–3.42 (m, 4H, piperazine), 3.51 and 3.96 (two s, 2H, CH_2, *E*- and *Z*-isomers), 4.04 and 4.07 (two s, 3H, OMe, *E*- and *Z*-isomers), 4.31–4.37 (m, 1H, CH_2), 4.42–4.52 (m, 1H, CH_2), 4.47–4.51 (m, 1H, CH-Me), 7.04 and 7.08 (two d, 1H, thiophene, *E*- and *Z*-isomers, $J = 4.0$ Hz), 7.63 and 7.69 (two d, 1H, thiophene, *E*- and *Z*-isomers, $J = 4.0$ Hz), 7.73 (d, 1H, H_8, $J = 12.3$ Hz), 8.61 (s, 1H, H_5), 15.01 (s, 1H, COOH).

10-(4-(2-(benzyloxyimino)-2-(5-chlorothiophen-2-yl) ethyl) piperazin-1-yl)-9-fluoro-3-methyl-7-oxo-3, 7-dihydro-2H-[1, 4]oxazino [2, 3, 4-ij]quinoline-6-carboxylic acid (6d)

Yield: 15%; mp 143–144°C; IR (KBr) cm^{-1}: ^{1}H-NMR (DMSO-d_6): 1.62 (d, 3H, CH_3, $J = 6.6$ Hz), 2.47–2.72 (m, 4H, piperazine), 3.28–3.43 (m, 4H, piperazine), 3.50 and 3.65 (two s, 2H, CH_2, *E*- and *Z*-isomers), 4.34 (d, 1H, CH_2, $J = 6.6$ Hz), 4.47 (d, 1H, CH_2, $J = 6.6$ Hz), 5.19 and 5.26 (two s, 2H, OCH_2, *E*- and *Z*-isomers), 5.32 (s, 1H, CH-Me), 6.82 and 6.84 (two d, 1H, thiophene, *E*- and *Z*-isomers, $J = 4.0$ Hz), 6.91 and 6.94 (two d, 1H, thiophene, *E*- and *Z*-isomers, $J = 4.0$ Hz), 7.36–7.40 (m, 5H, phenyl), 7.74 (d, 1H, H_8, $J = 10.0$ Hz), 8.61(s, 1H, H_5), 15.00 (s, 1H, COOH).

9-fluoro-10-(4-(2-(hydroxyimino)-2-(thiophen-2-yl)ethyl) piperazin-1-yl)-3-methyl-7-oxo-3,7-dihydro-2H-[1,4]oxazino [2,3,4-Ij]quinoline-6-Carboxylic acid (6e)

Yield: 16%; mp 314–315°C; IR (KBr) cm^{-1}: 1623 (C = O). ^{1}H-NMR (DMSO-d_6): 1.40–1.58 (m, 3H, CH_3), 2.45-78 (m, 4H, piperazine), 2.85–3.00 (m, 4H, piperazine), 3.51 (s, 2H, CH_2), 4.35 (d, 1H, CH_2, J = 10.4 Hz), 4.57 (d, 1H, CH_2, J = 10.4 Hz), 4.58–4.49 (m, 1H, CH-Me), 7.20–7.40 (m, 1H, thiophene), 7.56 (d, 1H, H_8, J = 11.6 Hz), 7.66–7.76 (m, 1H, thiophene), 7.82–7.90 (m, 1H, thiophene), 8.96 (s, 1H, H_5), 11.95 (s, 1H, NOH), 15.20 (s, 1H, COOH).

9-fluoro-10-(4-(2-(methoxyimino)-2-(thiophen-2-yl)ethyl) piperazin-1-yl)-3-methyl-7-oxo-3,7-dihydro-2H-[1,4]oxazino [2,3,4-Ij]quinoline-6-Carboxylic acid (6f)

Yield: 19%; mp 224–225°C; IR (KBr) cm^{-1}: 1719 (C = O). ^{1}H-NMR (DMSO-d_6): 1.43 (d, 3H, CH_3, J = 4.3 Hz), 2.53–2.63 (m, 4H, piperazine), 3.23–3.31(m, 4H, piperazine), 3.50 and 3.66 (two s, 2H, CH_2, *E*- and *Z*-isomers), 3.89 (s, 3H, OCH_3), 4.36 (d, 1H, CH_2, J = 8.8 Hz), 4.57 (d, 1H, CH_2, J = 8.8 Hz), 4.90–4.94 (m, 1H, CH-Me), 7.08–7.23 (m, 1H, thiophene), 7.54 and 7.76 (two d, 1H, thiophene, *E*- and *Z*-isomers, J = 4.2 Hz), 7.79 and 7.83 (two d, 1H, thiophene, *E*- and *Z*-isomers, J = 4.2 Hz), 7.91 (d, 1H, H_8, J = 10.0 Hz), 8.96 (s, 1H, H_5), 15.00 (s, 1H, COOH).

10-(4-(2-(benzyloxyimino)-2-(thiophen-2-yl)ethyl)piperazin-1-yl)-9-fluoro-3-methyl-7-oxo-3,7-dihydro-2H-[1,4]oxazino [2,3,4-Ij]quinoline-6-Carboxylic acid (6g)

Yield: 17%; mp 157–158°C; IR (KBr) cm^{-1}: 1720 (C = O). ^{1}H-NMR (DMSO-d_6): 1.44(d, 3H, CH_3, J = 7.5 Hz), 2.53–2.61 (m, 4H, piperazine), 3.23–3.38 (m, 4H, piperazine), 3.50 and 3.69 (two s, 2H, CH_2, *E*- and *Z*-isomers), 4.65–4.80 (m, 1H, CH_2), 4.90–4.97 (m, 1H, CH-Me), 5.17 and 5.28 (two s, 2H, OCH_2, *E*- and *Z*-isomers), 7.06–7.22(m, 1H, thiophene), 7.30–7.42 (m, 5H, phenyl), 7.52 and 7.59 (d, 1H, thiophene, J = 4.4 Hz, *Z*-isomer), 7.77 and 7.89 (two d, 1H, thiophene, *E*- and *Z*-isomers, J = 4.4 Hz), 7.94 (d, 1H, H_8, J = 10.0 Hz), 8.96 (s, 1H, H_5), 15.01 (s, 1H, COOH).

9-fluoro-10-(4-(2-(hydroxyimino)-2-(thiophen-3-yl) ethyl) piperazin-1-yl)-3-methyl-7-oxo-3,7-dihydro-2H-[1,4]oxazino [2,3,4-ij]Quinoline-6-carboxylic Acid (6h)

Yield: 22%; mp 354–356°C; IR (KBr) cm^{-1}: 1631, 1719 (C = O). ^{1}H-NMR (DMSO-d_6): 1.40–1.48 (m, 3H, CH_3), 2.53–2.60 (m, 4H, piperazine), 3.37–3.43 (m, 4H, piperazine), 4.31–4.38 (m, 1H, CH_2), 4.52–4.60 (m, 1H, CH_2), 4.84–4.92 (m, 1H, CH-Me), 7.50–7.60 (m, 2H, thiophene), 7.72 (d, 1H, thiophene, J = 4.5 Hz), 8.38–8.43 (m, 1H, H_8), 8.94 (s, 1H, H_5), 11.37 (s, 1H, NOH), 15.19 (s, 1H, COOH).

9-fluoro-10-(4-(2-(methoxyimino)-2-(thiophen-3-yl)ethyl) piperazin-1-yl)-3-methyl-7-oxo-3,7-dihydro-2H-[1,4]oxazino [2,3,4-Ij]quinoline-6-Carboxylic acid (6i)

Yield: 18%; mp 156–157°C; IR (KBr) cm^{-1}: 1630, 1721 (C = O). ^{1}H-NMR (DMSO-d_6): 1.42 (d, 3H, CH_3, J = 4.8 Hz), 2.51–2.65 (m, 4H, piperazine), 3.24–3.32 (m, 4H, piperazine), 3.52 (s, 2H, CH_2), 3.91 (s, 3H, OCH_3), 4.37 (d, 1H, CH_2, J = 8.7 Hz), 4.59 (d, 1H, CH_2, J = 8.7 Hz), 4.91–4.95 (m, 1H, CH-Me), 7.07–7.13 (m, 1H, thiophene), 7.54 (d, 1H, thiophene, J = 4.0 Hz), 7.85 (d, 1H, thiophene, J = 4.0 Hz), 7.90 (d, 1H, H_8, J = 10.3 Hz), 8.98 (s, 1H, H_5), 15.20 (s, 1H, COOH).

10-(4-(2-(benzyloxyimino)-2-(thiophen-3-yl) ethyl) piperazin-1-yl)-9-fluoro-3-methyl-7-oxo-3, 7-dihydro-2H-[1,4]oxazino [2,3,4-ij]quinoline-6-carboxylic acid (6j)

Yield: 17%; mp 162–163°C; IR (KBr) cm^{-1}: 1621, 1716 (C = O). ^{1}H-NMR (DMSO-d_6): 1.43 (d, 3H, CH_3, J = 6.8 Hz), 2.40–2.67 (m, 4H, piperazine), 3.17–3.44 (m, 4H, piperazine), 3.54 and 3.65 (two s, 2H, CH_2, *E*- and *Z*-isomers), 4.54–4.58 (m, 1H, CH_2), 4.90–4.93 (m, 1H, CH-Me), 5.14 and 5.28 (two s, 2H, OCH_2, *E*- and *Z*-isomers), 7.06–7.20 (m, 1H, thiophene), 7.39 (d, 1H, thiophene, J = 4.0 Hz, *Z*-isomer), 7.44 (d, 1H, thiophene, J = 4.0 Hz, *Z*-isomer), 7.48–7.68 (m, 5H, phenyl), 7.68 (d, 1H, thiophene, J = 4.0 Hz, *E*-isomer), 8.31 (d, 1H, thiophene, J = 4.0 Hz, *Z*-isomer), 8.38 (d, 1H, thiophene, J = 4.4 Hz, *E*-isomer), 8.01 (s, 1H, H_8), 8.96 (s, 1H, H_5), 15.01 (s, 1H, COOH).

Antimicrobial activity

Compounds **6a–j** were screened for their antibacterial activity against Gram-positive (*Staphylococcus aureus* ATCC 6538, *Staphylococcus epidermidis* ATCC 12228, *Bacillus subtilis* ATCC 6633) and Gram-negative (*E. coli* ATCC 8739, *Pseudomonas aeruginosa* ATCC 9027, *Klebsiella pneumoniae* ATCC 10031) bacteria by the conventional agar dilution method [18]. Two-fold serial dilutions of the compounds and reference drugs (levofloxacin and *N*-desmethyl levofloxacin) were prepared in Mueller-Hinton agar. Drugs (10.0 mg) were dissolved in DMSO (1 mL) and the solution was diluted with water (9 mL). Further progressive double dilution with melted Mueller-Hinton agar was performed to obtain the required concentrations of 100, 50, 25, 12.5, 6.25, 3.12, 1.56, 0.78, 0.39, 0.19, 0.09, 0.04, 0.02 and 0.01 μg/mL. Petri-dishes were inoculated with $1–5 \times 10^4$ colony-forming units (cfu) and incubated at 37°C for 18 h. The minimum inhibitory concentration (MIC) was defined as the lowest concentration of the test compound, which resulted in no visible growth on the plate. To insure that the solvent had no effect on bacterial growth, a control test was performed with test medium supplemented with DMSO at the same dilutions as used in the experiment.

Results and discussion

As summarized in Figure 2, the *N*-substituted analogs of levofloxacin **6a–j** were prepared by nucleophilic reaction of *N*-desmethyl levofloxacin **11** with thienylethyl bromide derivatives **8** or **9** employing reaction sequences previously described by us for the preparation of other *N*-substituted

Table 1 In vitro antibacterial activities (MICs in μg/mL) of compounds 6a–j

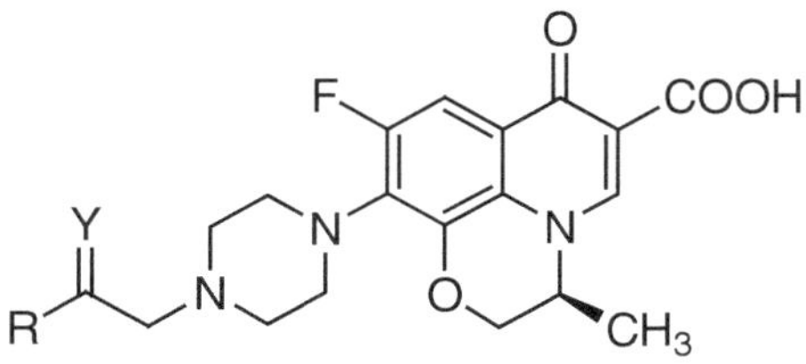

Compound	R	Y	*S. aureus*	*S. epidermidis*	*B. subtilis*	*E. coli*	*P. aeruginosa*	*K. pneumoniae*
6a	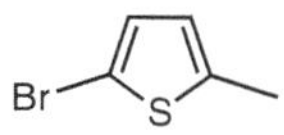	O	0.19	0.19	0.19	12.5	100	100
6b	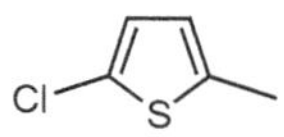	O	0.39	0.19	0.09	1.56	6.25	1.56
6c	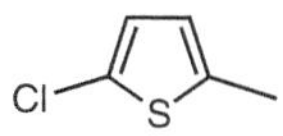	$NOCH_3$	0.78	0.39	0.19	50	50	12.5
6d	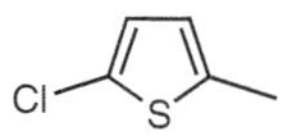	NOBn	3.125	1.56	0.78	50	100	100
6e	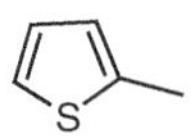	NOH	0.19	0.19	0.19	3.125	25	3.125
6f	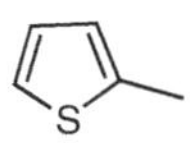	$NOCH_3$	0.39	0.19	0.09	50	100	25
6g	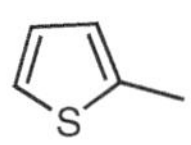	NOBn	6.25	3.125	0.78	100	100	50
6h	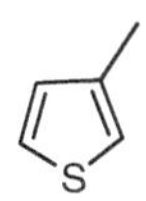	NOH	0.19	0.09	0.04	3.125	12.5	3.125
6i	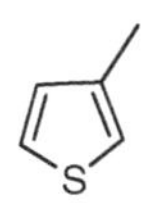	$NOCH_3$	0.19	0.19	0.09	100	100	50
6j	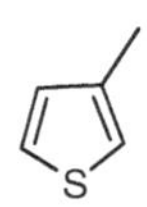	NOBn	6.25	3.125	0.39	50	100	25
Levofloxacin			0.25	0.25	0.5	0.03	4	0.25
***N*-Desmethyl levofloxacin**			4	1	1	0.012	>4	0.25

piperazinyl quinolones. Thus, the oxime derivatives **9** were synthesized by the reaction of ketone **8** with hydroxylamine hydrochloride or *O*-methylhydroxylamine hydrochloride or *O*-benzylhydroxylamine hydrochloride [12,14]. On the other hand, the piperazinyl quinolone (**11**, *N*-desmethyl levofloxacin) was prepared according to the known method

[17], by the reaction of piperazine with 9,10-difluoro-2,3-dihydro-3-methyl-7-oxo-7H-pyrido[1,2,3-de][1,4]benzoxazine-6-carboxylic acid **10**. Reaction of *N*-desmethyl levofloxacin **11** with thienyl ethyl bromide derivatives **8** or **9** in DMF, in the presence of $NaHCO_3$ at room temperature afforded corresponding ketones **6a,b** and oxime derivatives **6c–j**, respectively.

The minimum inhibitory concentrations (MICs, μg/mL) obtained for compounds **6a–j** are presented in Table 1. In general, Table 1 reveals that higher susceptibilities were observed with Gram-positive and poorer susceptibilities with Gram-negative bacteria. The MIC values of ketones **6a,b** and oximes **6c–j** against Gram-positive strains indicate that most compounds possessed a comparable or better activity (MIC = 0.04–3.12 μg/mL) with respect to *N*-desmethyl levofloxacin **11** and levofloxacin **4** (MIC = 0.25–4 μg/mL). As is evident from the data, oximes **6e**, **6h** and **6i** followed by ketone **6a** are superior in inhibiting the growth of Gram-positives (MIC = 0.04–0.19 μg/mL), and their activities were found to be 5–25 times better than *N*-desmethyl levofloxacin **11** and equal or better than levofloxacin **4**. In general, most compounds showed weak to good activity (MIC = 1.56–100 μg/mL) against Gram-negative bacteria. Compound **6b** was the most potent against *E. coli, Pseudomonas aeruginosa* and *Klebsiella pneumonia* (MIC = 1.56–6.25 μg/mL). Comparison between MIC values of 2-thienyl drivatives **6e–g** and 3-thienyl compounds **6h–j** revealed that the corresponding regioisomers have a same antibacterial activity and this modification cannot improve the activity. Also, etherification of oximes by methyl or benzyl groups dramatically diminished the activity against Gram-negatives. However, by *O*-methylation, the activity against Gram-positive bacteria was maintained. In addition, by comparison of 5-chlorothiophene derivatives **6c,d** and corresponding unsubstituted analogs **6f,g** it could be concluded that halogen substituent is not important for activity.

Competing interests
The author(s) declare that they have no competing interests.

Authors' contribution
NM: Synthesis of some target compounds (15%). ZA: Synthesis of the intermediates and some target compounds (10%). EA: Collaboration in identifying of the structures of target compounds (10%). SE: Collaboration in design and identifying of the structures of target compounds, manuscript preparation (10%). MAF: Evaluation of the antibacterial activities (10%). NS: Evaluation of the antibacterial activities (10%). NK: Evaluation of the antibacterial activities (5%). AS: Collaboration in identifying of the structures of target compounds (10%). AF: Design of target compounds and management of the synthetic and pharmacological parts (20%). All authors read and approved the final manuscript.

Acknowledgements
This work was supported by grants from Research Council of Tehran University of Medical Sciences and Iran National Science Foundation (INSF).

Author details
[1]Department of Chemistry, North Tehran Branch, Islamic Azad University, Tehran, Iran. [2]Department of Medicinal Chemistry, Faculty of Pharmacy and Pharmaceutical Sciences Research Center, Tehran University of Medical Sciences, Tehran, Iran. [3]Department of Medicinal Chemistry and Pharmaceutical Sciences Research Center, Faculty of Pharmacy, Mazandaran University of Medical Sciences, Sari, Iran. [4]Department of Pharmaceutical Biotechnology, Faculty of Pharmacy, Tehran University of Medical Sciences, Tehran, Iran.

References
1. Efthimiadou EK, Katsaros N, Karaliota A, Psomas G: **Synthesis, characterization, antibacterial activity, and interaction with DNA of the vanadyl-enrofloxacin complex.** *Bioorg Med Chem Lett* 2007, **17**:1238–1242.
2. Emami S, Shafiee A, Foroumadi A: **Structural features of new quinolones and relationship to antibacterial activity against Gram-positive bacteria.** *Mini Rev Med Chem* 2006, **6**:375–386.
3. Sarro AD, Sarro GD: **Adverse reactions to fluoroquinolones. An overview on mechanistic aspects.** *Curr Med Chem* 2001, **8**:371–384.
4. Anderson VE, Osheroff N: **Type II topoisomerases as targets for quinolone antibacterials.** *Curr Pharm Des* 2001, **7**:339–355.
5. Fang KC, Chen YL, Sheu JY, Wang TC, Tzeng CC: **Synthesis, antibacterial, and cytotoxic evaluation of certain 7-substituted norfloxacin derivatives.** *J Med Chem* 2000, **43**:3809–3812.
6. Pandeya SN, Sriram DV, Nath G, DeClercq E: **Synthesis, antibacterial, antifungal and anti-HIV activities of norfloxacin Mannich bases.** *Eur J Med Chem* 2000, **35**:249–255.
7. Domagala MJ: **Structure-activity and structure-side-effect relationships for the quinolone antibacterials.** *Antimicrob Chemother* 1994, **33**:685–706.
8. Jeffrey LJ, Almstead JK, Gallagher CP, Hu XE, Kim NK, Taylor CJ, Twinem TL, Cynthia D: **Synthesis and biological testing of non-fluorinated analogues of levofloxacin.** *Bioorg Med Chem Lett* 2003, **13**:2373–2375.
9. Segatore B, Setacci D, Perilli M, Franceschini N, Marchetti F, Amicosante G: **Bactericidal activity of levofloxacin and ciprofloxacin on clinical isolates of different phenotypes of Pseudomonas aeruginosa.** *Int J Antimicrob Agents* 2000, **13**:223–226.
10. Foroumadi A, Mohammadhosseini N, Emami S, Letafat B, Faramarzi MA, Samadi N, Shafiee A: **Synthesis and antibacterial activity of new 7-piperazinylquinolones containing a functionalized 2-(furan-3-yl)ethyl moiety.** *Arch Pharm* 2007, **340**:47–52.
11. Foroumadi A, Ghodsi S, Emami S, Najjari S, Samadi N, Faramarzi MA, Beikmohammadi L, Shirazi FH, Shafiee A: **Synthesis and antibacterial activity of new fluoroquinolones containing a substituted *N*-(phenethyl) piperazine moiety.** *Bioorg Med Chem Lett* 2006, **16**:3499–3503.
12. Letafat B, Emami S, Mohammadhoseini N, Faramarzi MA, Samadi N, Shafiee A, Foroumadi A: **Synthesis and antibacterial activity of new N-[2-(thiophen-3-yl)ethyl]piperazinyl quinolones.** *Chem Pharm Bull* 2007, **55**:894–898.
13. Emami S, Foroumadi A, Faramarzi MA, Samadi N: **Synthesis and antibacterial activity of quinolone-based compounds containing a coumarin moiety.** *Arch Pharm* 2008, **341**:42–48.
14. Shafiee A, Haddad Zahmatkesh M, Mohammadhosseini N, Khalafy J, Emami S, Moshafi MH, Sorkhi M, Foroumadi A: **Synthesis and *in-vitro* antibacterial activity of *N*-piperazinyl quinolone derivatives with 5-chloro-2-thienyl group.** *Daru* 2008, **16**:189–195.
15. Foroumadi A, Emami S, Mansouri S, Javidnia A, Saeid-Adeli N, Shirazi FH, Shafiee A: **Synthesis and antibacterial activity of levofloxacin derivatives with certain bulky residues on piperazine ring.** *Eur J Med Chem* 2007, **42**:985–992.
16. Foroumadi A, Emami S, Davood A, Moshafi MH, Sharifian A, Tabatabaiee M, Tarhimi Farimani H, Sepehri G, Shafiee A: **Synthesis and in-vitro antibacterial activities of N-substituted piperazinyl quinolones.** *Arch Pharm* 1997, **3**:559–563.
17. Atarashi S, Yokohama S, Yamazaki KI, Sakano KI, Imamura M: **Synthesis and antibacterial activities of optically active ofloxacin and its fluoromethyl derivative.** *Chem Pharm Bull* 1987, **35**:1896–1902.
18. Baron EJ, Finegold SM: *Bailey Scott's Diagnostic Microbiology.* 11th edition. St. Louis: The C. V. Mosby Company; 2002:235–236.

5

Synthesis and biological evaluation of propargyl acetate derivatives as anti-mycobacterial agents

Parisa Azerang[1], Ali Hossein Rezayan[2], Soroush Sardari[1*], Farzad Kobarfard[3,4], Mitra Bayat[4] and Kimia Tabib[3]

Abstract

Background: The emergence of multidrug-resistant strains of *Mycobacterium tuberculosis* (Mtb) has intensified efforts to discover novel drugs for tuberculosis (TB) treatment. Targeting the persistent state of Mtb, a condition in which Mtb is resistant to conventional drug therapies, is of particular interest.

Methods: This study is focused on propargyl acetate derivatives. Eight molecules were designed based on propargyl alcohols and different acid anhydrides.

Results: All the synthesized compounds and commercially available ones were evaluated for anti-tuberculosis activity.

Conclusions: Inhibitors against Mtb have been identified and characterized for further development into potential novel anti-tubercular drugs.

Keywords: *Mycobacterium tuberculosis*, BCG, Propargyl alcohol, Acetylenic compounds (propargyl acetate derivatives)

Background

Tuberculosis (TB) is a deadly infectious disease and is the leading cause of death worldwide, killing around 2 million people annually, primarily in developing countries. The World Health Organization (WHO) estimates that over one third of the world's population is infected with TB with approximately 8 million new cases of infection diagnosed every year [1-3]. After human immunodeficiency virus (HIV)/AIDS, TB is the second most common cause of death due to an infectious disease, and current trends suggest that TB will still be among the 10 leading causes of global disease burden in the year 2020 [4]. TB incidence is also on the rise because of the correspondingly high HIV infection rates. These two diseases progress at faster rates in co-infected individuals. The immune systems have been compromised by HIV/AIDS, so individuals fall victims to TB which takes opportunity of their weakened immune systems. There is a great interest in the scientific field to come up with a new drug(s) to combat TB. Tuberculosis is an airborne infectious disease caused by mycobacteria, mainly Mycobacterium tuberculosis (Mtb) [5]. The success of mycobacteria in producing disease relies entirely on its ability to utilize macrophages for its replication and more importantly, the maintenance of viability of host macrophages that sustain mycobacteria.

In the present scenario, due to the emergence of multi-drug resistant tuberculosis (MDR-TB) and association between HIV and TB, Directly Observed Treatment Short course (DOTS) is becoming rapidly ineffective in controlling tuberculosis. Recent reports indicate that, areas where there is a high incidence of MDR-TB, DOTS is failing to control the disease [6]. In such circumstances, the second line drugs are prescribed in combination with DOTS. However, this combination of drugs is very expensive, are less effective and thus has to be administered for a longer duration (e.g. p-amino salicylic acid), has significant side effects (e.g., cycloserine) and some are unavailable in many developing countries (e.g. fluoroquinolones).

Hence, it is clear that there is an urgent need to develop novel anti-TB drugs with improved properties such as enhanced activity against multidrug-resistance, reduced toxicity, shortened duration of therapy, rapid mycobactericidial mechanism of action, ability to

* Correspondence: ssardari@hotmail.com
[1]Drug Design and Bioinformatics Unit, Medical Biotechnology Department, Biotechnology Research Center, Pasteur Institute, Tehran, Iran13164
Full list of author information is available at the end of the article

penetrate host cells and exert anti-mycobacterial effect in the intracellular environment.

Alkynes or acetylenic compounds play an important role as building blocks in many synthetic transformations, and in new materials. In addition acetylenic group is common structural motifs found in various natural products and also great interest in medicinal chemistry and the pharmaceutical industry [7]. It moreover functions as a key pharmacophoric unit in acetylenic antibiotics [8] and its presence in anticancer [9] and anti-tubercular [10] agents is noteworthy.

Due to above-mentioned reasons and as a part of our ongoing research program on the synthetic methods in organic compounds [11,12], and also our drug discovery program [13,14], here a series of new acetylenic compounds (propargyl acetate derivatives) were synthesized and evaluated for anti-tubercular activity.

Methods

General

Infrared spectra were determined with a Perkin-Elmer 843 spectrometer (USA). Proton nuclear magnetic resonance (^1H NMR) spectra and carbon nuclear magnetic resonance (^{13}C NMR) spectra were determined on a Bruker Avance DRX 500 MHz spectrometer (Germany) and chemical shifts are reported as δ (ppm) in $CDCl_3$ solution (0.05% v/v TMS). GC/MS spectra were obtained using Agilent 7000 Triple Quad (USA). (EI at 70 eV). The chemicals used in this work were purchased from Merck (Germany), Fluka (Germany) and Sigma-Aldrich (USA) Chemical Companies.

In vitro evaluation of anti-mycobacterial activity

In vitro anti-mycobacterial activity evaluations of the compounds were done by the broth microtiter dilution method) against BCG (1173P2) and ethambutol were used as standard controls.

The test compounds were initially dissolved in DMSO to give a concentration of 1 or 2 mg/L. All wells of micro plates received 100 μL of freshly prepared Middle broke 7H9 medium (Himedia, India), except first column. 200 μL of distilled water was added to the first column of 96 well plates to minimize evaporation of the medium in the test wells during incubation. Then 100 μL of test compounds with desired concentrations (1000 or 2000 μL) were added to the wells of the first row (each concentration was assayed in duplicate) and serial dilution was made from the first row to the last. Microbial suspension of BCG (1173P2) (100 μL), which had been prepared with standard concentration of 0.5 Mcfarland and diluted with 1:10 proportion by the distilled water, was added to all test wells. Plates were then sealed and incubated for 4 days at 37°C. After that 12 μl Tween 80 10% and 20 μl Alamar blue 0.01% (Himedia, India) were added to each test well. The results were assessed after 24 and 48 hours. A blue color was interpreted as no bacterial growth, and color change to pink was scored as bacterial growth. Wells with a well-defined pink color were scored as positive for growth. The MIC (minimum inhibitory concentration) was defined as the lowest drug concentration, which prevented a color change from blue to pink. Ethambutol (Irandaru, Tehran) were used as positive control and DMSO as negative control [15].

General procedure for the preparation of propargyl acetate derivatives 3a-h

To a magnetically stirred solution of anhydride (1.2 mmol) was added 3 drops of concentrated sulfuric acid and mix thoroughly holding the large test tube containing the acetic anhydride in cold water. Then, the alcohol (1 mmol) was added to it in several increments and the reaction mixture stirred at room temperature. After, the reaction mixture was placed in hot water at about 70°C to complete the reaction; the progress of the reaction was monitored by TLC (ethyl acetate/*n*-hexane, 2:1). The purification of product was done according to the literature [16].

Prop-2-ynyl acetate (3a): Yellow liquid (yield 65%). ^1H NMR (500 MHz, $CDCl_3$): δ_H (ppm) 2.07 (3H, s, CH_3), 2.46 (1H, t, $^4J_{HH}$ = 2.5 Hz, ≡CH), 4.64 (1H,d, $^4J_{HH}$ = 2.5 Hz, OCH_2). ^{13}C NMR (125 MHz, $CDCl_3$): δ_C (ppm) 30.7 (CH_3), 51.9 (OCH_2), 74.8 and 77.6 (two acetylenic carbons), 170.1 (C = O). IR (KBr) (ν_{max},cm^{-1}): 3468, 3296, 2948, 2125, 1733. GC EI-MS, m/z: 99 ($M^{+\cdot} + H^+$, 3%).

But-3-yn-2-yl acetate (3b): Yellow liquid (yield 70%). ^1H NMR (500 MHz, $CDCl_3$): δ_H (ppm) 1.49 (3H, d, CH_3), 2.06 (3H, s, CH_3), 2.44 (1H, s, ≡CH), 5.39-5.43 (1H, m, OCH). ^{13}C NMR (125 MHz, $CDCl_3$): δ_C (ppm) 21.00 (CH_3), 21.2 (CH_3), 60.0 and 82.1 (two acetylenic carbons), 72.8 (OCH), 169.8 (C = O). IR (KBr) (ν_{max},cm^{-1}): 3480, 3308, 2999, 2131, 1739. GC EI-MS, m/z: 113 ($M^{+\cdot} + H^+$, 10%).

3-Methylpent-1-yn-3-yl acetate (3c): Yellow liquid (yield 63%). ^1H NMR (500 MHz, $CDCl_3$): δH (ppm) 1.02 (3H, t, $^3J_{HH}$ = 7.4 Hz, CH_3), 1.06 (3H, s, CH_3), 1.84 (2H, q, $^3J_{HH}$ = 7.4 Hz, CH_2), 2.03 (3H, s, CH_3), 2.54 (1H, s, ≡CH). IR (KBr) (ν_{max},cm^{-1}): 3306, 2967, 2867, 2135, 1716. GC EI-MS, m/z: 140 ($M^{+\cdot}$, 10%).

Oct-1-yn-3-yl acetate (3d): Yellow liquid (yield 60%). ^1H NMR (500 MHz, $CDCl_3$): δH (ppm) 0.88 (3H, t, $^3J_{HH}$ = 7.0 Hz, CH_3), 1.30 (2H, m, CH_2), 1.43 (2H, m, CH_2), 1.75 (2H, m, CH_2), 2.07 (3H, s, CH_3), 2.44 (1H, d, $^4J_{HH}$ = 2.5 Hz, ≡CH), 5.32 (H, t of d, $^3J_{HH}$ = 5.0 Hz, $^4J_{HH}$ = 2.5 Hz, OCH). ^{13}C NMR (125 MHz, $CDCl_3$): δ_C (ppm) 13.9 (CH_3), 20.9 (CH_3), 22.2 (CH_2), 24.4 (CH_2), 31.0 (CH_2), 34.4 (CH_2), 63.7 and 77.2 (two acetylenic carbons), 82.0 (OCH_2), 169.9 (C = O). IR (KBr) (ν_{max},cm^{-1}): 3300, 2964, 2874, 2132, 1740. GC EI-MS, m/z: 168 ($M^{+\cdot}$, 10%).

But-3-ynyl acetate (3e): Yellow liquid (yield 80%). ^1H NMR (500 MHz, $CDCl_3$): δ_H (ppm) 2.01 (1H, t, $^4J_{HH}$ = 3.0 Hz, ≡CH), 2.10 (3H, s, CH_3), 2.54 (2H, t of d, $^3J_{HH}$ = 6.5 Hz, $^4J_{HH}$ = 3.0 Hz, CH_2), 4.19 (2H, t, $^3J_{HH}$ = 7.0 Hz, OCH_2).^{13}C NMR (125 MHz, $CDCl_3$): δ_C (ppm) 18.8 (CH_3), 20.7 (CH_2), 61.7 and 70.1 (two acetylenic carbons), 80.0 (OCH_2), 170.8 (C = O). IR (KBr) (ν_{max},cm^{-1}): 3315, 3028, 2900, 2290, 1738. GC EI-MS, m/z: 113 ($M^{+\cdot}$ + H^+, 10%).

Prop-2-ynyl heptanoate (3f): Yellow liquid (yield 78%). ^1H NMR (500 MHz, $CDCl_3$): δ_H (ppm) 1.31 (3H, t, $^3J_{HH}$ = 7.5 Hz, CH_3), 1.63 (8H, m, 4CH_2), 2.33 (2H, t, $^3J_{HH}$ = 8.0 Hz, CH_2), 4.45 (1H, t, $^4J_{HH}$ = 2.0 Hz, ≡CH), 4.65 (2H, d, $^4J_{HH}$ = 2.0 Hz, OCH_2). ^{13}C NMR (125 MHz, $CDCl_3$): δ_C (ppm) 13.8 (CH_3), 22.2, 24.4, 31.1, 33.8, (4CH_2), 51.6 and 74.6, (two acetylenic carbons), 77.7 (OCH_2), 172.9 (C = O). IR (KBr) (ν_{max},cm^{-1}): 3291, 2932, 2865, 2128, 1738. GC EI-MS, m/z: 168 ($M^{+\cdot}$, 10%).

Oct-1-yn-3-yl heptanoate (3g): liquid (yield 55%). ^1H NMR (500 MHz, $CDCl_3$): δ_H (ppm) 0.89 (6H, m, 2CH_3), 1.31 (4H, m), 1.43 (4H, m), 1.63 (4H, m), 1.75 (4H, m), 2.37 (2H, m), 2.42 (1H, d, $^4J_{HH}$ = 2.5 Hz, ≡CH), 5.34 (1H, t of d, $^3J_{HH}$ = 6.5 Hz, $^4J_{HH}$ = 2.0 Hz, OCH). IR (KBr) (ν_{max},cm^{-1}): 3310, 2963, 2872, 2127, 1736. GC EI-MS, m/z: 239 ($M^{+\cdot}$, 10%).

But-3-ynyl heptanoate (3h): Yellow liquid (yield 70%). ^1H NMR (500 MHz, $CDCl_3$): δ_H (ppm) 0.87 (3H, t, $^3J_{HH}$ = 7.0 Hz, CH_3), 1.30 (4H, m, CH_2), 1.61 (2H, m, CH_2), 1.98 (1H, t, $^4J_{HH}$ = 2.5 Hz, ≡CH), 2.32 (2H, m, CH_2), 2.50 (2H, t of d, $^3J_{HH}$ = 7.0 Hz, $^4J_{HH}$ = 3.0 Hz, CH_2), 4.16 (2H, t, $^3J_{HH}$ = 7.0 Hz, OCH_2). ^{13}C NMR (125 MHz, $CDCl_3$): δ_C (ppm) 13.9 (CH_3), 19.0, 22.3, 24.4, 31.2, 34.14 (5CH_2), 61.9 and 69.9 (two acetylenic carbons), 80.1(OCH_2), 173.6 (C = O). IR (KBr) (ν_{max},cm^{-1}): 3304, 2961, 2868, 2126, 1735. GC EI-MS, m/z: 182 ($M^{+\cdot}$, 5%).

Results and discussion

Esterification of alcohols using acid anhydrides in the presence of acid or base catalyst has been known and extensively used by organic chemists for nearly 100 years [17]. Hydroxyl compounds are often converted to acetate derivatives for protection or characterization of the structure. For this purpose, acetic anhydride is commonly employed with an acid or base catalyst, such as zinc chloride, concentrated sulphuric acid, anhydrous sodium [18] acetate or, most often, pyridine [19].

In the present work, propargyl acetate derivatives 3a-h were prepared by acylation of propargyl alcohols 1 with acid anhydrides 2 in H_2SO_4 (Scheme 1) [20].

The reactions are straightforward and as indicated in Scheme 1, treatment of various propagyl alcohols 1 with acid anhydrides 2 in H_2SO_4 led to products 3a-h. To explore the scope and variety of biological activity for products of this reaction, we have examined various

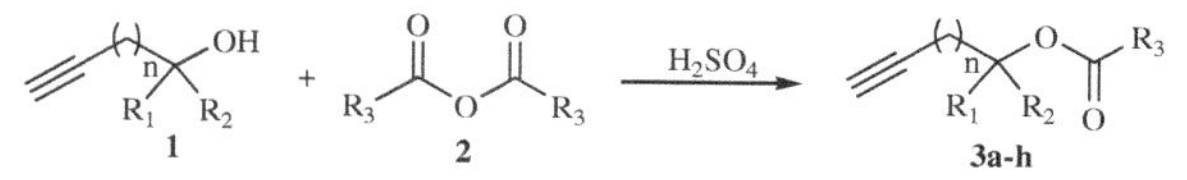

n = 1 or 2
R_1 = H, Me, Et, pentyl
R_2 = H, Me
R_3 = Me, isopropyl, hexyl

Scheme 1 Synthesis of propargyl acetate derivatives.

primary, secondary and tertiary propagyl alcohols in the presence of aliphatic and aromatic acid anhydrides in H_2SO_4 at room temperature. As indicated Figure 1, the reaction proceeds efficiently and led to highly functionalized propargyl acetate derivatives 3a–h in good yields.

The structures of compounds 3a–h were deduced from their ^1H NMR and ^{13}C NMR spectroscopic data. For example, the ^1H NMR spectrum of 3a exhibited a singlet at 2.07 (CH_3), a triplet at 2.46 ($^4J_{HH}$ = 2.5Hz) for acetylenic hydrogen (≡CH) and a doublet at 4.64 ($^4J_{HH}$ = 2.5 Hz, OCH_2). The ^1H decoupled ^{13}C NMR spectrum of 3a showed 5 distinct resonances, and partial assignment of these resonances is given in experimental section.

All the synthesized compounds were evaluated for anti-tubercular activity and the results are summarized in Figure 1.

Compounds 3a-h have almost the same activity except 3 g that is slightly stronger; it shows that the changing of R_1, R_2 and R_3 is not important in these compounds. Therefore, we did not synthesis more derivatives from these compounds. In continuation of the work, we investigated different groups of organic compounds that all of these compounds containing acetylenic group in difference situation, such as alcohols (4–10), acetylenic compounds (11–16), esters (17–20), acids (21), and anhydrides (22–25) (without acetylenic group). In these compounds (4–25), the nature and location of mentioned functional group can affect the anti-bacterial activity of acetylenic compounds. As can be seen from Figure 2, among these acetylenic compounds (11,12,15, 16) and esters (17–20), have almost similar effect and more bioactivity than others. It seems that replacement of alkyne hydrogen with an alkyl or aryl group in case of compounds 12 and 16 and a balanced hydrophobicity playing with special features, in case of compounds 11 and 15 have beneficial effect on the bioactivity. However, it is necessary to examine the possible mechanism of action in detail to clear the reason for the variations of activity.

It is interesting to note that comparison of compounds 3a-h in Figure 1 and 17–20 in Figure 2 which are ester shows that 17–20 more active than 3a-h (3.87 vs 125). This can be because of difference in structure of two classes of esters. The main structural difference between 3a-h and 17–20 is that in 17–20 the ester group is

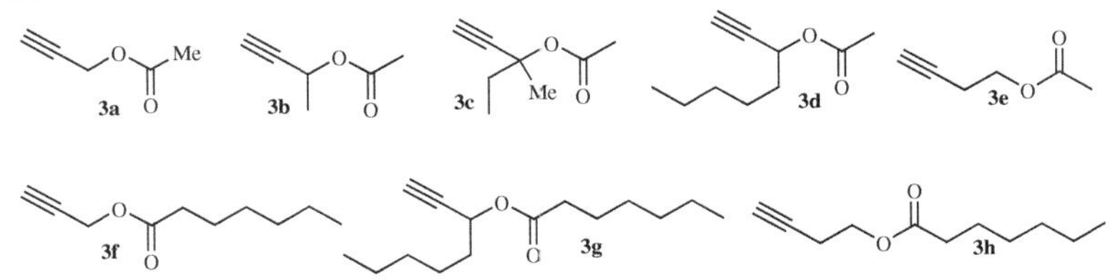

Entry	R1	R2	R3	MIC (μg/ml) 24/48 (hours)
3a	H	H	Methyl	125/125
3b	H	Methyl	Methyl	125/125
3c	Methyl	Ethyl	Methyl	125/125
3d	H	Pentyl	Methyl	125/125
3e	H	H	Methyl	125/125
3f	H	H	Hexyl	125/125
3g	H	Pentyl	Hexyl	62.50/62.50
3h	H	H	Hexyl	125/125
Ethambutol				0.75/0.75
DMSO				6.5/6.5% (v/v)

Figure 1 Synthesized propargyl acetate derivatives and their MIC.

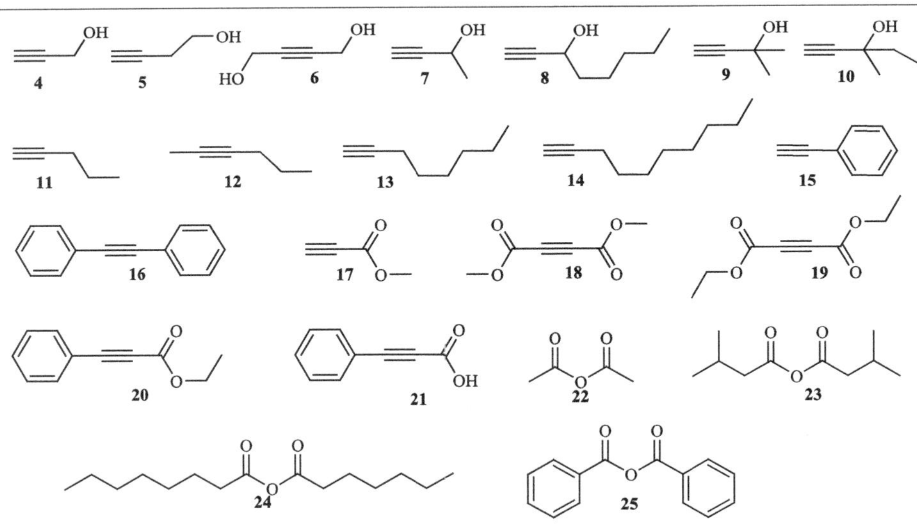

Compounds	4	5	6	7	8	9	10	11	12	13	14
MIC (μg/ml) 24/48 (hours)	125/ 125	125/ 125	125/ 125	125/ 125	125/ 125	125/ 125	125/ 125	3.87/ 15.5	3.87/ 31.25	125/ 125	62.50/ 125

Compounds	15	16	17	18	19	20	21	22	23	24	25
MIC (μg/ml) 24/48 (hours)	3.87/ 31.25	31.25/ 31.25	3.87/ 7.75	3.87/ 7.75	7.75/ 7.75	7.75/ 7.75	62.5/ 125	250/ 500	125/ 250	125/ 500	125/ 500

Ethambutol=0.75/0.75,
DMSO=6.5/6.5% (v/v)

Figure 2 Commercially available substrates and their MIC (minimal inhibition concentration).

terminal whilst in 3a-h is internal. The conjugation of double bond with the triple bond and the resulting dipole moment is a feature that can explain this difference. The same effect can play a role for the better activity of compounds 15 and 16.

Conclusions

In conclusion, the synthesized new class of propargyl acetate derivatives and commercially available compounds were evaluated for anti-tuberculosis activity. Among them, 11, 12, 15, 17 and 18 exhibited promising activity against of *M. bovis*.

Competing interests

The authors declare that they have no competing interests.

Authors' contribution

First person: synthesis of the molecules, bioassay and writing some parts of the draft, second person: preparation of the draft, third person: design of the molecules and PI, fourth person: interpretation of MS and IR spectra, fifth person: obtaining MS spectra, sixth person: obtaining IR spectra. All authors read and approved the final manuscript.

Acknowledgements

We gratefully acknowledge the Pasteur Institute of Iran and Ministry of Health and Medical Education in Iran for partial funding of this project as part of grant number 456.

Author details

[1]Drug Design and Bioinformatics Unit, Medical Biotechnology Department, Biotechnology Research Center, Pasteur Institute, Tehran, Iran13164. [2]Department of Life Science Engineering, Faculty of New Science and Technology, University of Tehran, Tehran, Iran. [3]Department of Medicinal Chemistry, School of Pharmacy, Shahid Beheshti University of Medical Sciences, Tehran, Iran. [4]Phytochemistry Research Centre, Shahid Beheshti University of Medical Sciences, Tehran, Iran.

References

1. Dye C, Scheele S, Dolin P, Pathania V, Raviglione MC: **Consensus statement. Global burden of tuberculosis: estimated incidence, prevalence, and mortality by country. WHO global surveillance and monitoring project.** *JAMA* 1999, **282:**677–686.
2. Muthukrishnan M, Mujahid M, Yogeeswari P, Sriram D: **Syntheses and biological evaluation of new triazole-spirochromone conjugates as inhibitors of Mycobacterium tuberculosis.** *Tetrahedron Lett* 2011, **52:**2387–2389.
3. Agrawal YK, Bhatt HG, Raval HG, Oza PM, Vaidya HB, Manna K, Gogoi P: **Emerging trends in tuberculosis therapy.** *J Sci Indus Res* 2007, **66:**191–208.
4. Murray CJ, Salomon JA: **Modeling the impact of global tuberculosis control strategies.** *Proc Natl Acad Sci USA* 1998, **95:**13881–13886.
5. Kuma V, Abbas AK, Fausto N, Mitchell R: *Robbins Basic Patholog. 8th Edition.* London: Elsevier Health Sciences; 2007.
6. Kimerling ME, Kluge H, Vezhnina N, Iacovazzi T, Demeulenaere T, Portaels F: **Inadequacy of the current WHO re-treatment regimen in a central Siberian prison: treatment failure and MDR-TB.** *Int J Tuberc Lung Dis* 1999, **3:**451–453.
7. Hans RH, Guantai EM, Lategan C, Smith PJ, Wanc B, Franzblau SG, Gut J, Rosenthal PJ, Chibale K: **Synthesis, antimalarial and antitubercular activity of acetylenic chalcones.** *Bioorg Med Chem Lett* 2010, **20:**942–944.
8. Maretina IA, Trofimov BA: **Enediyne antibiotics and their models: new potential of acetylene chemistry.** *Russ Chem Rev* 2006, **75:**825–845.
9. Siddiq A, Dembitsky V: **Acetylenic anticancer agents.** *Anticancer Agents Med Chem* 2008, **8:**132–170.
10. Deng S, Wang Y, Inui T, Chen SN, Farnsworth NR, Cho S, Franzblau SG, Pauli GF: **Anti-TB polyynes from the roots of Angelica sinensis.** *Phytother Res* 2008, **22:**878–882.
11. Shaabani A, Rezayan AH, Kishipour S, Sarvary A, Heidary M, Ng SW: **Synthesis of highly stable unusual charge-separated pyridinium-, isoquinolinium-, quinolinium-, and N-methylimidazoliumtetronic acid zwitterions.** *Tetrahedron* 2009, **65:**6063–6068.
12. Shaabani A, Sarvary A, Ghasemi S, Rezayan AH, Ghadari R, Ng SW: **An environmentally benign approach for the synthesis of bifunctional sulfonamide-amide compounds via isocyanide-based multicomponent reactions.** *Green Chem* 2011, **13:**582–585.
13. Soltani S, Dianat S, Sardari S: **Forward modeling of the coumarin antifungals; SPR/SAR based perspective.** *Avicenna J Med Biotech* 2009, **1:**95–103.
14. Mehravar M, Sardari S: **Screening of antimicrobial membrane-active metabolites of soil microfungi by using chromatic phospholipid/polydiacetylene vesicles.** *J Mycol Med* 2011, **21:**188–197.
15. Camacho-Corona MR, Ramirez-Cabrera MA, Santiago OG, Garza-Gonzalez E, Palacios Idel P, Luna-Herrera J: **Activity against drug resistant-tuberculosis strains of plants used in Mexican traditional medicine to treat tuberculosis and other respiratory diseases.** *Phytother Res* 2008, **22:**82–85.
16. Pearson AL, Roush WJ: *Handbook of Reagents for Organic Synthesis: Acetylating Agents and Protecting Groups.* Chichester: John Wiley; 1999.
17. Verley A, Bolsing F: **Esterbildung und Bestimmung von Alkoholen resp.** *Phenolen Ber Dtsch Chem Ges* 1901, **34:**3354.
18. Secen H, Kalpar AH: **An efficient acetylation of primary and secondary aliphatic alcohols with acetic anhydride in the presence of graphite.** *Turk J Chem* 1999, **23:**27–30.
19. March J: *Advanced Organic chemistry: Reactions, mechanisms, and structure. 4th Edition.* New York: the University of Michigan, Wiley; 1992.
20. Krause P, Hilterhaus L, Fieg G, Liese A, Bornscheuer U: **Chemically and enzymatically catalyzed synthesis of C6–C10 alkyl benzoates.** *Eur J Lipid Sci Technol* 2009, **111:**194–201.

Umbelliprenin is cytotoxic against QU-DB large cell lung cancer cell line but anti-proliferative against A549 adenocarcinoma cells

Narges Khaghanzadeh[1,2], Zahra Mojtahedi[1*], Mohammac Ramezani[3], Nasrollah Erfani[1] and Abbas Ghaderi[1,2]

Abstract

Background: Umbelliprenin is a natural compound, belonging to the class of sesquiterpene coumarins. Recently, umbelliprenin has attracted the researchers' attention for its antitumor activities against skin tumors. Its effect on lung cancer is largely unknown. The aim of our study was to investigate the effects of this natural compound, which is expected to have low adverse effects, on lung cancer.

Methods: The QU-DB large cell and A549 adenocarcinoma lung cancer cell lines were treated with umbelliprenin. IC_{50} values were estimated using methyl thiazolely diphenyl-tetrazolium bromide (MTT) assay, in which a decrease in MTT reduction can occur as a result of cell death or cell proliferation inhibition. To quantify the rate of cell death at IC_{50} values, flow cytometry using Annexin V-FITC (for apoptotic cells), and propidium iodide (for necrotic cells) dyes were employed.

Results: Data from three independent MTT experiments in triplicate revealed that IC_{50} values for QU-DB and A549 were 47 ± 5.3 μM and 52 ± 1.97 μM, respectively. Annexin V/PI staining demonstrated that umbelliprenin treatment at IC_{50} induced 50% cell death in QU-DB cells, but produced no significant death in A549 cells until increasing the umbelliprenin concentration to IC_{80}. The pattern of cell death was predominantly apoptosis in both cell lines. When peripheral blood mononuclear cells were treated with 50 μM and less concentrations of umbelliprenin, no suppressive effect was observed.

Conclusions: We found cytotoxic/anti-proliferative effects of umbelliprenin against two different types of lung cancer cell lines.

Keywords: Annexin, IC_{50}, Lung cancer, MTT assay, Propidium Iodide, Umbelliprenin

Background

Lung cancer is one of the most common causes of cancer related deaths in most countries [1]. In Iran, lung cancer is the third most frequent cancer in both men and women [2]. The current 5 year survival of lung cancer is about 10–15% mostly being attributed to late diagnosis and inefficient therapy [3,4]. The limited success and significant side effects of lung cancer treatment with classic chemotherapeutic agents has led researchers to find more efficient drugs with fewer side effects [5,6].

* Correspondence: mojtahediz@sums.ac.ir
[1]Shiraz Institute for Cancer Research, Shiraz University of Medical Sciences, School of Medicine, Shiraz, Iran
Full list of author information is available at the end of the article

Umbelliprenin is synthesized by various *Ferula* plant species such as *Citrus Limon* [7]. It is a prenylated compound that belongs to the class of sesquiterpene coumarins, and possesses a similar structure to auraptene, a compound whose antitumor activities have largely been investigated [8]. Recently, umbelliprenin has attracted the researchers' attention for its antitumor activities. It has been shown that the cell susceptibility to umbelliprenin decreased in the order M4Beu (metastatic pigmented malignant melanoma) > A549 (non-small cell lung carcinoma) ≈ PC3 (androgen resistant prostate carcinoma) > PA1 (ovary teratocarcinoma) > human primary fibroblasts [9]. The anti-tumor effect of umbelliprenin has also been demonstrated in vivo in a mouse skin tumor model in which oral administration of umbelliprenin significantly delayed the formation of papilloma [10]. Umbelliprenin also showed an inhibitory effect on the matrix metalloproteinases activity [11]. Matrix metalloproteinases are critical enzymes in cancer metastatic cascade, such as migration, angiogenesis, and invasiveness [12,13]. Despite inhibitory effects of umbelliprenin on tumor cells, treatment of peripheral blood mononuclear cells (PBMNCs) with this compound protected them against DNA and chromosome damage induced by H_2O_2 [12-14].

Methyl thiazolely diphenyl-tetrazolium bromide (MTT) assay is frequently employed to determine the in vitro index of cytotoxicity (IC). In metabolically active cells, the reduction of water soluble MTT into an insoluble purple formazan results in accumulation of purple formazan crystals in cells. After solubilization of these crystals, the comparison of the optical density (OD) between treated and untreated cells gives a relative estimation of IC at different doses [15]. For determination of whether decreased MTT reduction is either due to the cell death or decrease in cell proliferation, other complementary tests such as staining with fluorescent dyes annexin V-FITC for apoptotic cells and propidium iodide (PI) for necrotic cells are frequently performed. The sum of apoptotic and necrotic cells represents the total rate of cell death [16].

The effect of umbelliprenin on lung cancer is poorly understood. Here, we employed MTT assay and annexin V/PI staining to investigate the effects of umbelliprenin on lung cancer cells. The A549, a human pulmonary adenocarcinoma cell line, and QU-DB, a human large cell carcinoma line, as well as PBMNCs were treated with umbelliprenin. IC_{50} was defined as the umbelliprenin concentration that resulted in a 50% decrease in the OD of the test compound compared to that of untreated cells. Then, annexin V/PI staining determined whether (i) the decrease in MTT reduction is due to the cell death or suppression of cell proliferation, and (ii) apoptosis or necrosis is the main cause of cell death.

Materials and methods

Cell culture

The study was approved by the Ethic Committee of Shiraz University of Medical Sciences. Two human lung cancer cell lines including A549 (adenocarcinoma) and QU-DB (large cell) were obtained from the National Cell Bank of Iran (NCBI), Pasteur Institute of Iran, Tehran, Iran. PBMCs were obtained from healthy volunteers by Ficoll-Hypaque density sedimentation. All the cells were cultured in RPMI-1640 medium supplemented with 10% heat inactivated fetal bovine serum (FBS) (Gibco/BRL, Germany), penicillin 100 U/ml. and streptomycin 100 µg/ml (Biosera, UK). They were maintained at 37°C in a 5% CO_2 incubator and the media were changed every two day.

Isolation of human peripheral blood mononuclear cells

Participants were informed that blood samples will be used for a research project as healthy individuals, and their written consent was obtained. Fifteen ml heparinized blood samples were collected from healthy volunteers (n=3, aged 30–35). Whole blood samples were diluted 1:1 with PBS, layered onto Ficoll-Paque (1.077 g/ml) at a volume ratio of 2:1 and centrifuged at 400 g for 30 min at 20°C. The PBMCs layer was collected and washed twice at 1500 rpm for 10 min with RPMI-1640 medium. The supernatant was removed and the cells were resuspended in RPMI-1640 medium containing 10% FBS, 1% penicillin and 100 µg/ml streptomycin. Cell viability was tested (>98% viable cells) using the trypan-blue dye exclusion method.

Umbelliprenin preparation

Umbelliprenin ($C_{24}H_{30}O_3$, MW: 366) was synthesized as previously described [17]. Umbelliprenin was first dissolved in DMSO, and then this stock was dilluted in CM10 media at 37°C immediately before use to obtain a maximum DMSO concentration of 0.5% (v/v).

MTT assay

Exponentially growing cells (T75 flasks) of A549 (5000 cells/well), and QU-DB (7000 cells/well) as well as PBMNCs (1 x 10^5 cells/well) were cultured onto 96-well plates in RPMI-1640 containing 10% FBS. Cells were allowed to attach for 24 h before treatment. Then, lung cancer cell lines were treated with fresh medium containing umbelliprenin at different concentrations (10, 20, 50, 100, 200 µM). For PBMNCs, media containing umbelliprenin were added at the time of cell seeding in culture plates. ConA (2.5 µg/ml) treated PBMNCs were used as a positive control for umbelliprenin. 0.5% DMSO and untreated cells were used as the control of solvent and negative control, respectively, in all experiments. Wells containing medium with different concentrations of umbelliprenin without cells were used as the control of compound. The plates were incubated for 24, 48 and 72 h. Then, 5 mg/ml MTT (sigma) was added into each well, and the plates were incubated for 4 h (37°C, 5% CO_2). Media containing MTT were removed and DMSO was added in each well to dissolve the formazan crystals. Absorbance of the wells was read at 570 nm (A_{570}) after 30 min of incubation at room temperature (RT). At least three independent experiments were done in triplicate for each experiment.

Annexin V/PI assay on lung cancer cell lines

To determine the extent of apoptosis and necrosis as well as total cell death (apoptosis + necrosis) induced by umbelliprenin on human lung cancer cell lines, annexin V/PI staining (FITC Annexin V Apoptosis Detection Kit

I, BD Pharmingen, USA) was used. Briefly, the cells in the exponential phase were treated with IC_{50} concentration of umbelliprenin for each cell lines. After 48 h, the cells were trypsinized [18-20] (0.25% trypsin with a longer incubation time was used for gentle dissociation of the attached cells), and washed twice with PBS. The pellets were resuspended in 1X binding buffer. After the addition of annexin V-FITC, the cells were incubated for 15 min at RT in the dark. PI dye was added at the last 5 min of total incubation time. Flowcytometry was done within one hour using FACSCalibur flow cytometer (BD Biosciences, USA).

Statistical analysis

Dose–response curves and IC_{50} values were determined using Curve Expert software, ver.1.3 and expressed as mean ± standard deviation (SD) from at least three independent experiments. Statistical tests including One-way ANOVA, Tukey multiple comparison or unpaired Student's *t* tests were performed using GraphPad Prism, ver.5 software. A *p* value of less than 0.05 was considered as significant.

Results

MTT assay on lung cancer cell lines

Using MTT assay, we demonstrated that umbelliprenin has antitumor activity on both A549 and QU-DB cell lines, and that activity was dose and time-dependent. The umbelliprenin concentration resulting in 50% of cell cytotoxicity/proliferation inhibition was considered as IC_{50}. These values for A549 and QU-DB were found to be 52 ± 1.97 and 47 ± 5.3 µM, respectively. The data represent the mean ± SD of at least three independent experiments done in triplicate. One way ANOVA analysis revealed a significant difference between umbelliprenin treated cells and 0.5% DMSO treated cells in all experiments ($p < 0.05$). Figure 1 displays the summary of these experiments on both A549 and QU-DB cells.

MTT assay on PBMNCs

PBMNCs were used to determine the effects of umbelliprenin on a normal, immune cell. In contrast to suppressory effects of umbelliprenin at 10, 20, and 50 µM on lung cancer cell lines, these concentrations caused no inhibition on PBMNCs with even a higher proliferative index compared to DMSO treated cell. However, at higher doses (100 and 200 µM), umbelliprenin showed some inhibitory activity on PBMNCs. Figure 2 indicates the summary of these experiments on PBMNCs.

Annexin V/PI cell death (apoptosis + necrosis) and trypan blue staining on lung cancer cell lines

For flow cytometry assays, cells were initially studied at their IC_{50} values estimated using MTT. Annexin V/PI staining at IC_{50} of umbelliprenin as compared to DMSO treated controls after 48 h did not show any statistically significant apoptosis or necrosis for A549 cell line. A statistically significant cell death compared to controls was observed after increasing umbelliprenin concentration to IC_{80} (88 µM). The predominant cell death was apoptosis. QU-DB cells were more susceptible to death induced by umbelliprenin than A549 cells, as they showed 50% cell death after 48 h treatment at IC_{50} (50 µM). The dominant cell death was also apoptosis. Figure 3 shows the result of annexin V/PI experiments on both A549 and QU-DB cell lines. Annexin V positive cells detected on FL1, indicated the apoptotic cells. PI positive cells were detected on FL2 and showed death by the necrosis. As it is indicated in Figure 3, the total death rate, either apoptosis or necrosis, at IC_{50} after 48 h for QU-DB was 46.98% ± 8.7% (An^+ = 41.7%, An^+/PI^+ = 4.5%, and PI^+ = 0.7%), and for A549 at IC_{80} after 48 h was 17.22% ± 6.29 (An^+ = 15.9%, An^+/PI^+ = 0.39%, and PI^+ = 1.74%). These values are the subtraction of the death rate in the control group from treated group in each quadrant. The percentages of PI positive cells were less than 5% for both cell lines, and the dominant cell death type was apoptosis.

Our flowcytometry results were in accordance with trypan blue viability test. At IC_{50} value, approximately half of QU-DB cells were dead, however, even at IC_{80}, more than 50% of A549 cells were still viable in comparison to controls.

Discussion

Lung cancers are divided into small cell lung carcinoma and non-small cell lung cancer (NSCLC). The majority of lung cancer cases (about 80%) are NSCLC [1]. There are three major subtypes for NSCLC: adenocarcinoma, squamous cell and large call carcinoma (LCC). The latter has the poorest prognosis of NSCLC, followed by adenocarcinoma [21].

Umbelliprenin has been recently recognized as a compound with antitumor activities [9,10]. The data regarding its effects on lung cancer are limited to a few studies [9]. Here we evaluated the effects of this compound on lung cancer cell lines QU-DB and A549 as well as PBMNCs from healthy individuals using MTT assay. Treatment of A549 and QU-DB cells with umbelliprenin at different doses and intervals showed that umbelliprenin significantly suppressed lung cancer cell lines, and this suppression was in a time-dose dependent manner. These lung cancer cell lines showed approximately similar IC_{50} values (≈50µM) using MTT assay. However, we observed the proliferative effects of umbelliprenin on PBMNCs at 10, 20, and 50 µM doses.

To realize whether the decreased MTT reduction of cancer cell lines caused by umbelliprenin is due to cell

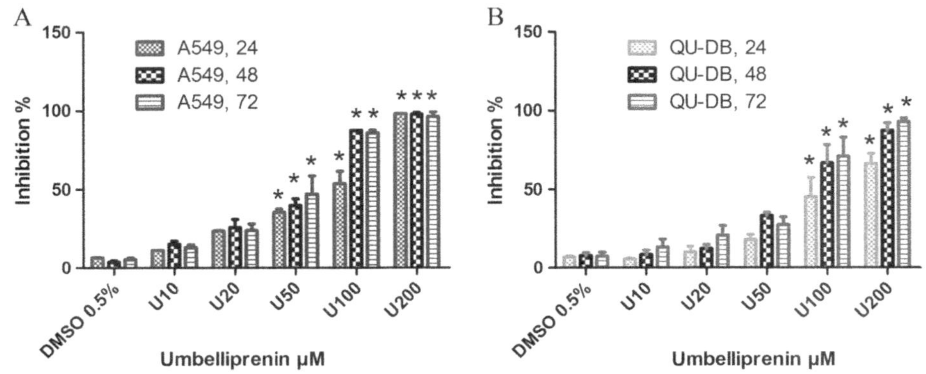

Figure 1 (A) A549 cells and (B) QU-DB cells after 24, 48, and 72 h incubation with umbelliprenin. One way ANOVA and Tukey's Multiple Comparison Tests revealed a significant difference between umbelliprenin treated and 0.5% DMSO treated cells. (*) Represents statistical significance ($p< 0.05$).

death or proliferation inhibition, we analyzed cell death using annexin V/PI staining that simultaneously quantifies apoptosis (Annexin V+) and necrosis (PI+). Apoptosis was added up to necrosis to quantify the total death rate. In this study, the percentage of necrosis was less than 5% in all experiments. Consistent with our MTT assay, QU-DB cells showed approximately 50% cell death at IC_{50} concentration after 48 h of umbelliprenin treatment compared to DMSO control cells ($p=0.002$). The total death rate induced by umbelliprenin was 46.98% ± 8.7%, of which 41.7% (An^+), 4.5% (An^+/PI^+), and 0.7% (PI^+) were related to early apoptosis, late apoptosis and necrosis, respectively. The pattern of cell death was in favor of apoptosis than necrosis. For A549 cell line, we did not observe a significant difference in death rate between treated and untreated cells until we increased the concentration of umbelliprenin to IC_{80}

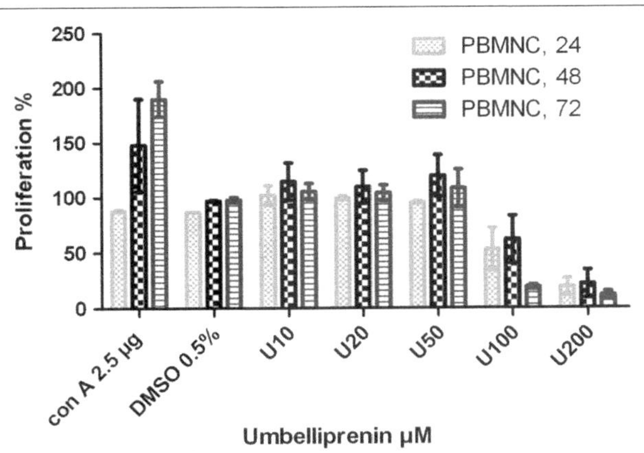

Figure 2 PBMNCs after 24, 48, and 72 h incubation with different concentrations of umbelliprenin. At 10, 20, and 50 μM, umbelliprenin showed no cytotoxicity or a mild proliferation effects on PBMNCs, but at higher doses it showed cytotoxic/anti-proliferative effects. 0.5% DMSO was used as the solvent control and Con A 2.5 μg/ml as a positive control for proliferation.

($p=0.022$). The dominant cell death pattern in this experiment was also apoptosis. The total death rate induced by umbelliprenin was 17.22 ± 6.29, of which early apoptosis, late apoptosis and necrosis patterns constituted 15.9%, 0.39%, and 1.74% death cell types, respectively. These flowcytometry results were partly in agreement with trypan blue viability test in which the number of dead cells was higher in QU-DB than A549 at IC_{50} value calculated using MTT colorimetric assay. Our results indicate that umbelliprenin probably suppresses these cell lines with different pathways. Umbelliprenin is more cytotoxic against QU-DB, a large cell lung cancer cell line compared to A549 adenocarcinoma cell line.

Anti-cancer compounds have been divided into two broad categories according to their ability to damage DNA (cytotoxic), and/or inhibiting either nucleotide biosynthesis or mitosis (anti-proliferative) [22]. Umbelliprenin is structurally related to coumarin family [8]. Coumarin family has been shown both anti-proliferative and cytotoxic effects in different cell lines and situations. Coumarins can exert anti-proliferative effects through inhibition of tubulin polymerization, and induction of cell cycle arrest at G2/M transition of mitotic cell cycle [23]. Coumarins can also induce apoptosis and cell death by mitochondrial dependent and independent mechanisms. They may increase the reactive oxygen species level and release of cytochrome *c* to the cytosol. Several transcription factors, pro-apoptotic and apoptotic molecules are involved in these pathways. For example, it has been shown that apoptotic effects of a coumarin on A549 cells is mediated through pro-apoptotic function of NF-kB by induction of Bax and p53 expression, and reduction of several signaling molecules such as Erk1/Erk2, p38 and JNK [24].

Data regarding the molecular mechanisms of umbelliprenin, itself, are limited. The presence of the aliphatic

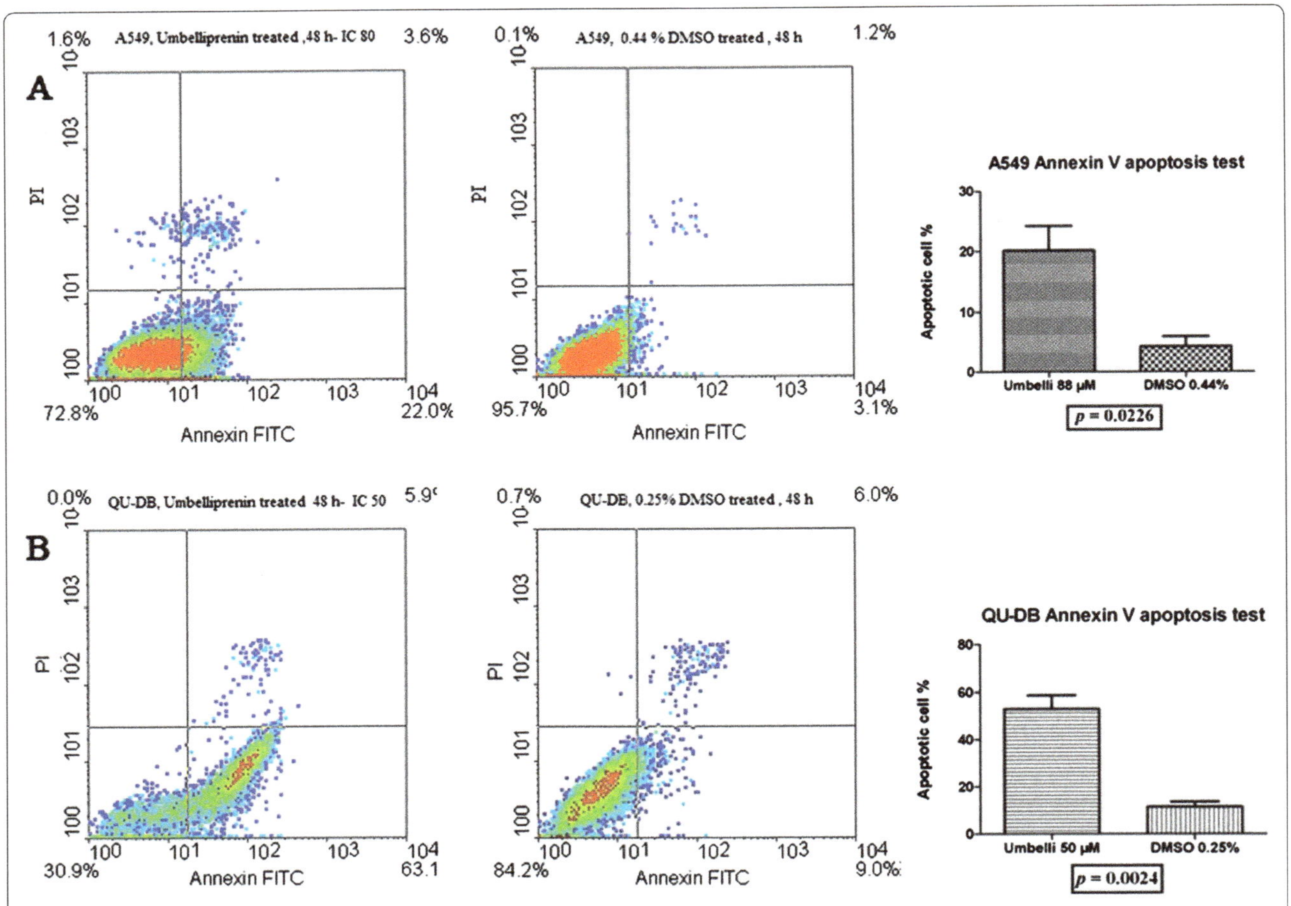

Figure 3 Annexin V/PI staining. (A) A549 cell treated by umbelliprenin or DMSO after 48 h. The apoptosis rate was significantly different between umbelliprenin treated A549 cells compared to DMSO treated cells at IC_{80} of umbelliprenin (p=0.022). **(B)** QU-DB cell was treated by umbelliprenin or DMSO after 48 h. Umbelliprenin induced apoptosis in QU-DB cells at IC_{50} (50 μM) value after 48 h (p=0.002). Numbers adjacent to outlined squares indicate the percentage of cells in each cuadrant. LL: Viable cells (Annexin V −/ PI −), LR: early apoptotic cells (Annexin V +/ PI −), UL: late necrotic cells (Annexin V −/ PI +) and UR: late apoptotic/necrotic cells (Annexin V +/ PI +).

sesquiterpenoid group linked at C7-OH is related to umbelliprenin cytotoxic effects, but the main mechanism in this regard is unknown [9]. Along with umbelliprenins' cytotoxicity effects on various cancer cell lines, its anti-proliferative effects on M4Beu cells via cell cycle arrest in G1 phase has been shown before [9]. Other cancer chemopreventive activity of umbelliprenin can be related to its anti-oxidant activity [14] and its anti-inflammatory effects. Umbelliprenin can inhibit the function of 5-lipoxygenase and reduce the production of lipoxygenase carcinogenic products [25]. All of known functions of this compound can lead us to further understanding of its anti-cancer effects.

The apoptotic and anti-proliferative effects of umbelliprenin on two lung cancer cell lines were demonstrated in the present study using MTT and annexin V/PI assays; some limitations still exist. Pairing of MTT and annexin V/PI methods with other tests such as cell cycle analysis by DNA content using PI staining and RNase A [9], or laser scanning confocal microscopy which monitors several mitochondrial events during apoptosis such as permeability transition and Ca2+ fluxes might be further informative regarding anti-proliferative or cytotoxic effects of umbelliprenin [26]. It will be also interesting to uncover the signalling pathways which promote umbelliprenin-induced apoptosis in lung cancer in future studies.

Conclusions

Using MTT assay and annexin V/PI staining, we demonstrated that umbelliprenin can induce apoptosis in both QU-DB large cell lung cancer and A549 adenocarcinoma cell line but at different doses. The ability of umbelliprenin to induce lymphocyte proliferation along with the induction of apoptosis or inhibition of proliferation in cancer cells makes this compound an attractive compound with fewer side effects for future anti-cancer studies.

Abbreviations

MTT: Methyl thiazolely diphenyl-tetrazolium bromide; PBMNCs: Peripheral blood mononuclear cells; IC: Index of cytotoxicity; OD: Optical density; PI: Propidium iodide; FBS: Fetal bovine serum; An: Annexin V.

Competing interests

The authors declare that they have no competing interests.

Authors' contributions

The role of each author: NK (nkhaghan@sums.ac.ir): Design, data acquisition and analysis, and drafting the manuscript ZM and AG (ghaderia@gmail.com): Design, data analysis, revising the manuscript, and final approval of the manuscript. MR (RamezaniM@mums.ac.ir): Design, revising the manuscript, final approval of the manuscript. NE (erfanin@sums.ac.ir): Data acquisition. All authors read and approved the final manuscript.

Acknowledgments

This work was based on Khaghanzadeh N PhD thesis submitted to the Shiraz University of Medical Sciences, and was funded by grants from Shiraz University of Medical Sciences (89-5291) and Shiraz Cancer Research Center (ICR-87-503). This study was partly supported by Mashhad University of Medical Sciences. No conflict of interest is declared by all authors.

Author details

[1]Shiraz Institute for Cancer Research, Shiraz University of Medical Sciences, School of Medicine, Shiraz, Iran. [2]Department of Immunology, Shiraz University of Medical Sciences, School of Medicine, Shiraz, Iran. [3]Pharmaceutical Research Center, School of Pharmacy, Mashhad University of Medical Sciences, Mashhad, Iran.

References

1. Pirker R, Minar W: **Chemotherapy of advanced non-small cell lung cancer.** *Front Radiat Ther Oncol* 2010, **42**:157–163.
2. Masoompour SM, Yarmohammadi H, Rezaianzadeh A, Lankarani KB: **Cancer incidence in southern Iran, 1998–2002: Results of population-based cancer registry.** *Cancer Epidemiol* 2011, **35**:e42–e47.
3. Reade CA, Ganti AK: **EGFR targeted therapy in non-small cell lung cancer: potential role of cetuximab.** *Biologics* 2009, **3**:215–224.
4. Gabrielson E: **Worldwide trends in lung cancer pathology.** *Respirology* 2006, **11**:533–538.
5. Avery EJ, Kessinger A, Ganti AK: **Therapeutic options for elderly patients with advanced non-small cell lung cancer.** *Cancer Treat Rev* 2009, **35**:340–344.
6. Francis H, Solomon B: **The current status of targeted therapy for Non-small cell lung cancer.** *Intern Med J* 201C, **40**:611–618.
7. Iranshahi M, Kalategi F, Sahebkar A, Sardashti A, Schneider B: **New sesquiterpene coumarins from the roots of Ferula flabelliloba.** *Pharm Biol* 2003, **41**:431–433.
8. Genovese S, Epifano F: **Auraptene: a natural biologically active compound with multiple targets.** *Curr Drug Targets* 2011, **12**:381–386.
9. Barthomeuf C, Lim S, Iranshahi M, Chollet P: **Umbelliprenin from Ferula szowitsiana inhibits the growth of human M4Beu metastatic pigmented malignant melanoma cells through cell-cycle arrest in G1 and induction of caspase-dependent apoptosis.** *Phytomedicine* 2008, **15**:103–111.
10. Iranshahi M, Sahebkar A, Takasaki M, Konoshima T, Tokuda H: **Cancer chemopreventive activity of the prenylated coumarin, umbelliprenin, in vivo.** *Eur J Cancer Prev* 2009, **18**:412–415.
11. Shahverdi AR, Saadat F, Khorramizadeh MR, Iranshahi M, Khoshayand MR: **Two matrix metalloproteinases inhibitors from Ferula persica var. persica.** *Phytomedicine* 2006, **13**:712–717.
12. Stetler-Stevenson WG, Hewitt R, Corcoran M: **Matrix metalloproteinases and tumor invasion: from correlation and causality to the clinic.** *Semin Cancer Biol* 1996, **7**:147–154.
13. John A, Tuszynski G: **The role of matrix metalloproteinases in tumor angiogenesis and tumor metastasis.** *Pathol Oncol Res* 2001, **7**:14–23.
14. Soltani F, Mosaffa F, Iranshahi M, Karimi G, Malekaneh M, Haghighi F, Behravan J: **Evaluation of antigenotoxicity effects of umbelliprenin on human peripheral lymphocytes exposed to oxidative stress.** *Cell Biol Toxicol* 2009, **25**:291–296.
15. Mosmann T: **Rapid colorimetric assay for cellular growth and survival: application to proliferation and cytotoxicity assays.** *J Immunol Methods* 1983, **65**:55–63.
16. Chen GG, Sin FL, Leung BC, Ng HK, Poon WS: **Differential role of hydrogen peroxide and staurosporine in induction of cell death in glioblastoma cells lacking DNA-dependent protein kinase.** *Apoptosis* 2005, **10**:185–192.
17. Askari M, Sahebkar A, Iranshahi M: **Synthesis and Purification of 7-Prenyloxycoumarins and Herniarin as Bioactive Natural Coumarins.** *Iranian Journal of Basic Medical Sciences* 2009, **12**:63–69.
18. Chen Z, Jin K, Gao L, Lou G, Jin Y, Yu Y, Lou Y: **Anti-tumor effects of bakuchiol, an analogue of resveratrol, on human lung adenocarcinoma A549 cell line.** *Eur J Pharmacol* 2010, **643**:170–179.
19. Clarke R, Lund E, Johnson II, Pinder A: **Apoptosis can be detected in attached colonic adenocarcinoma HT29 cells using annexin V binding, but not by TUNEL assay or sub-G0 DNA content.** *Cytometry* 2000, **40**:252.
20. Kim JM, Stapleton F, Willcox MD: **Induction of apoptosis in human corneal epithelial cells in vitro.** *Aust N Z J Ophthalmol* 1999, **27**:214–217.
21. Cole SP, Campling BG, Dexter DF, Holden JJ, Roder JC: **Establishment of a human large cell lung tumor line (QU-DB) with metastatic properties in athymic mice.** *Cancer* 1986, **58**:917–923.
22. Keskin O, Bahar I, Jernigan RL, Beutler JA, Shoemaker RH, Sausville EA, Covell DG: **Characterization of anticancer agents by their growth inhibitory activity and relationships to mechanism of action and structure.** *Anticancer Drug Des* 2000, **15**:79–98.
23. Kim SN, Kim NH, Park YS, Kim H, Lee S, Wang Q, Kim YK: **7-Diethylamino-3 (2'-benzoxazolyl)-coumarin is a novel microtubule inhibitor with antimitotic activity in multidrug resistant cancer cells.** *Biochem Pharmacol* 2009, **77**:1773–1779.
24. Goel A, Prasad AK, Parmar VS, Ghosh B, Saini N: **Apoptogenic effect of 7,8-diacetoxy-4-methylcoumarin and 7,8-diacetoxy-4-methylthiocoumarin in human lung adenocarcinoma cell line: role of NF-kappaB, Akt, ROS and MAP kinase pathway.** *Chem Biol Interact* 2009, **179**:363–374.
25. Iranshahi M, Askari M, Sahebkar A, Hadjipavlou-Litina D: **Evaluation of antioxidant, anti-inflammatory and lipoxygenase inhibitory activities of the prenylated coumarin umbelliprenin.** *DARU* 2009, **17**:99–103.
26. Elmore S: **Apoptosis: a review of programmed cell death.** *Toxicol Pathol* 2007, **35**:495–516.

Synthesis, *in vitro* antifungal evaluation and *in silico* study of 3-azolyl-4-chromanone phenylhydrazones

Adile Ayati[1], Mehraban Falahati[2], Hamid Irannejad[1] and Saeed Emami[1*]

Abstract

Background: The currently available antifungal drugs suffer from toxicity, greatest potential drug interactions with other drugs, insufficient pharmacokinetics properties, and development of resistance. Thus, development of new antifungal agents with optimum pharmacokinetics and less toxicity is urgent task. In the search for new azole antifungals, we have been previously described azolylchromanone oxime ethers as rigid analogs of oxiconazole. In continuation of our work, we incorporated phenylhydrazone moiety instead of oxime ether fragment in azolylchromanone derivatives.

Methods: The 3-azolyl-4-chromanone phenylhydrazones were synthesized via ring closure of 2-azolyl-2'-hydroxyacetophenones and subsequent reaction with phenylhydrazine. The biological activity of title compounds was evaluated against different pathogenic fungi including *Candida albicans*, *Saccharomyces cerevisiae*, *Aspergillus niger*, and *Microsporum gypseum*. Docking stucy, *in silico* toxicity risks and drug-likeness predictions were used to better define of title compounds as antifungal agents.

Results: The *in vitro* antifungal activity of compounds based on MIC values revealed that all compounds showed good antifungal activity against *C. albicans*, *S. cerevisiae* and *M. gypseum* at concentrations less than 16 μg/mL. Among the test compounds, 2-methyl-3-imidazolyl derivative **3b** showed the highest values of drug-likeness and drug-score.

Conclusion: The 3-azolyl-4-chromanone phenylhydrazones considered as analogs of 3-azolyl-4-chromanone oxime ethers basically designed as antifungal agents. The antifungal activity of title compounds was comparable to that of standard drug fluconazole. The drug-likeness data of synthesized compounds make them promising leads for future development of antifungal agents.

Keywords: Azole antifungals, Antifungal activity, 1*H*-imidazole, 1,2,4-triazole, Chroman-4-one, Hydrazone

Introduction

Recently, the incidence of life-threatening fungal diseases has dramatically increased due to the rising number of immunocompromised patients, increased use of anti-cancer drugs, and immunosuppressive therapy for organ transplantation [1]. On the other hand, the currently available antifungal drugs suffer from toxicity, greatest potential drug interactions with other drugs, insufficient pharmacokinetics properties, and development of resistance [2]. Consequently, it is urgent to develop new broad-spectrum antifungal agents with optimum pharmacokinetics and less toxicity.

Several antifungal drugs, including azoles, polyenes, echinocandins and allylamines have been developed to overcome the fungal infections [3]. However, in comparison to the large number of antibacterial drugs the number of clinically available antifungal agents is rather low. Azole antifungals such as ketoconazole, fluconazole, voriconazole, and posaconazole, which inhibit fungal cytochrome P-450 dependent 14α-demethylase, are among the most investigated compounds with respect to their clinical impact and individual mechanism of action

* Correspondence: sd_emami@yahoo.com
[1]Department of Medicinal Chemistry and Pharmaceutical Sciences Research Center, Faculty of Pharmacy, Mazandaran University of Medical Sciences, Sari, Iran
Full list of author information is available at the end of the article

[4]. These antifungal drugs contain imidazole or triazole heterocycles and act through a mechanism in which the heterocyclic nitrogen atom (N-3 of imidazole or N-4 of triazole) binds to the heme iron atom in cytochrome P-450 enzymes. Particularly, the triazole derivatives have a greater affinity for fungal cytochrome P-450 enzymes than for mammalian ones contributing to a favorable safety profile [5].

In the search for new azole antifungals, we have been described azolylchromanone oxime ethers (Figure 1) as rigid analogs of oxiconazole [6-8]. The chroman scaffold also found in some natural flavonoids possessing antifungal activity [9-11]. In continuation of our work, we incorporated phenylhydrazone moiety instead of oxime ether fragment in azolylchromanone derivatives (Figure 1). This modification was made on the basis of zinoconazole, a well-known azole antifungal possessing phenylhydrazone substructure (Figure 2). Thus we describe here, the synthesis and antifungal activity of 3-azolyl-4-chromanone phenylhydrazones. Furthermore, docking study and *in silico* toxicity risks and drug-likeness predictions were used to better define of title compounds as antifungal agents.

Material and methods

Chemistry

All chemical reagents and solvents were purchased from Merck AG Chemical (Germany) and used without further purification. The progress of reactions and the purity of compounds were checked by TLC analysis on silica gel 60 F254 plates (Merck) and visualization was done with UV light (254 nm). Melting points were determined in open glass capillaries using Bibby Stuart Scientific SMP3 apparatus (Stuart Scientific, UK) and are uncorrected. The IR spectra were recorded on FT-IR (PerkinElmer, USA) spectrophotometer using KBr disks. ^{1}H-NMR spectra were recorded using a Bruker 400 (Rheinstatten, Germany) spectrometer, and chemical shifts are expressed as δ (ppm) with tetramethylsilane as internal standard. The MS spectra were obtained with a Finnigan MAT TSQ-70 spectrometer (Finnigan MAT, Germany).

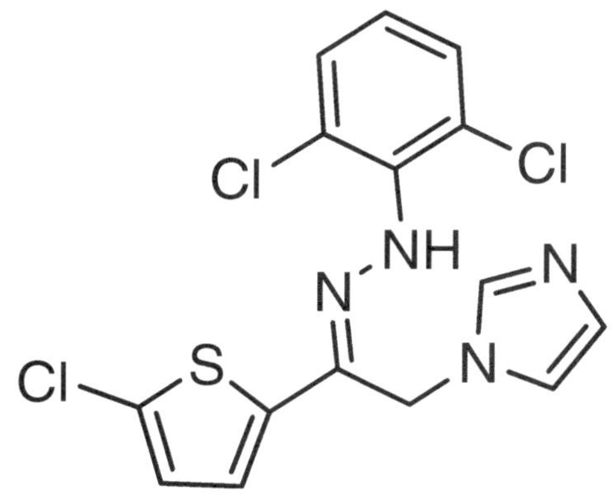

Figure 2 Zinoconazole, a well-known azole antifungal bearing phenylhydrazone substructure.

General procedure for the synthesis of 3-azolyl-4-chromanone derivatives 2a-c

Compounds **2a-c** was synthesized from 2-azolyl-2'-hydroxyacetophenones **1a-c** according to the literature methods [6-8].

General procedure for the synthesis of phenyhydrazone derivatives 3a-c

Phenylhydrazine hydrochloride was added to a solution of compound **2** (0.5 mmol) in methanol (4 mL) and the solution was stirred at room temperature. The completion of the reaction was checked by TLC. After consumption of compound **2** (3–7 days), water was added and the mixture was left in refrigerator overnight. The precipitated solid was separated by filtration and washed with water. The product was re-crystallized from methanol.

2,3-Dihydro-3-(1H-1,2,4-triazol-1-yl)-4H-1-benzopyran-4-one phenylhydrazone (**3a**)

Yield 55 %; IR (KBr, cm^{-1}) 3418, 3238, 3128, 1703, 1603, 1561, 1497, 1478, 1459, 1278, 1261, 1216, 1138,

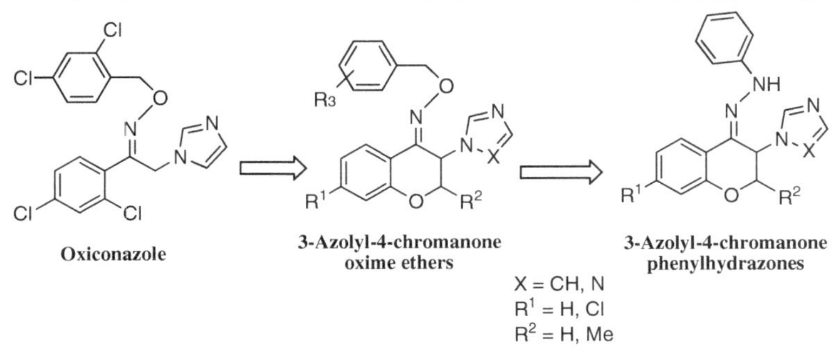

Figure 1 Structures of azolylchromanone oxime ethers as rigid analogs of oxiconazole and designed compounds 3-azolyl-4-chromanone phenylhydrazones.

1055, 831, 763, 691, 678. ^{1}H NMR (400 MHz, DMSO-d_6) δ 4.44 (m, 1 H), 4.82-4.87 (m, 1 H), 5.99 (dd, 1 H, $J = 10.8$ and 6.6 Hz), 6.79-6.90 (m, 2 H), 7.04 (t, 2 H, $J = 7.2$ Hz), 7.12-7.26 (m, 3 H), 7.66 (dt, 1 H, $J = 7.4$ and 2.0 Hz), 7.83 (dd, 1 H, $J = 7.6$ and 2.0 Hz), 8.43 (s, 1 H), 8.64 (s, 1 H), 10.05 (s, 1H). Anal. Calcd for $C_{17}H_{15}N_5O$: C, 66.87; H, 4.95; N, 22.94. Found: C, 66.98; H, 5.14; N, 22.71.

trans-2,3-Dihydro-3-(1H-imidazol-1-yl)-2-methyl-4H-1-benzopyran-4-one phenylhydrazone (**3b**)

Yield 62%; m.p. 228–230°C; IR (KBr, cm^{-1}) 3444, 3246, 1603, 1567, 1498, 1457, 1295, 1255, 1220, 1124, 834, 750, 696. ^{1}H NMR (400 MHz, DMSO-d_6) δ 1.16 (d, 3 H, $J = 6.4$ Hz), 5.19 (dq, 1 H, $J = 12.4$ and 6.4 Hz), 5.88 (d, 1 H, $J = 12.8$ Hz), 6.75 (d, 2 H, $J = 7.2$ Hz), 6.83 (t, 1 H, $J = 8.0$ Hz), 6.92 (t, 2 H, $J = 8.0$ Hz), 7.01 (d, 1 H, $J = 8.0$ Hz), 7.11 (t, 1 H, $J = 7.6$ Hz), 7.14-7.36 (m, 3 H), 7.68 (t, 1 H, $J = 8.4$ Hz), 8.07 (d, 1 H, $J = 7.6$ Hz), 10.34 (s, 1 H). Anal. Calcd for $C_{19}H_{18}N_4O$: C, 71.68; H, 5.70; N, 17.60. Found: C, 71.50; H, 5.79; N, 17.86.

7-Chloro-2,3-dihydro-3-(1H-imidazol-1-yl)-4H-1-benzopyran-4-one phenylhydrazone (**3c**)

Yield 58%; m.p. 192–194°C; IR (KBr, cm^{-1}) 3444, 1602, 1560, 1497, 1418, 1252, 1163, 1082, 814, 754, 696. MS (*m/z*, %) 338 (M^+, 25), 270 (100), 207 (10), 154 (15), 105 (28), 77 (78), 67 (37). Anal. Calcd for $C_{18}H_{15}ClN_4O$: C, 63.81; H, 4.46; N, 16.54. Found: C, 63.66; H, 4.28; N, 16.57.

Antifungal activity

The antifungal activities of title compounds **3a-c** and **2b** were tested against several representative pathogenic fungi including *Candida albicans* PTCC 5027 and *Saccharomyces cerevisiae* PTCC 5177 (as yeast), *Microsporum gypseum* PTCC 5070 (as a dermatophyte) and *Aspergillus niger* PTCC 5012 (as a mould) using agar dilution method [12]. Stock solutions of tested compounds were prepared in DMSO and serially diluted. Sabouraud Dextrose Agar was used for fungal growth. Inocula containing approximately 10^5 CFUs/mL of fungi were prepared from broth cultures in log phase growth. Fungal plates were made in triplicate and incubated at 30°C about 24–48 h for yeast, about 72 h for moulds and about 168 h for dermatophytes. The MIC value was defined as lowest concentration of the antifungal agent at which the test strain does not demonstrate visible growth. The reported MICs are representative of at least two independent experiments.

Docking study

Crystal structure of cytochrome P450 14α-sterol demethylase (Cyp51) from *Mycobacterium tuberculosis* in complex with fluconazole (ID 1EA1) was provided from the Protein Data Bank and prepared for docking calculations using AutoDock Tools 1.5.4 with default settings. Docking was performed using AutoDock vina, and standard parameters were used. Water molecules were not included. The binding site was defined to any residues with 10 Å distant from the co-crystallized fluconazole in the complex crystal structure of the enzyme [13].

In silico drug-likeness and toxicity predictions

OSIRIS Property Explorer [14] was used to estimate the risks of side effects, such as mutagenic, tumorigenic, irritant and reproductive effects, as well as drug-relevant properties including cLog*P*, Log*S* (solubility), MW, drug-likeness and overall drug-score.

Results and discussion

Chemistry

The synthetic route to phenylhydrazone derivatives **3a-c** was illustrated in Scheme 1. The starting 2-azolyl-2'-hydroxyacetophenones **1a-c** was prepared from corresponding 2-bromo-2'-hydroxyacetophenones according to the literature method [15]. Cyclization of compounds **1a-c** with paraformaldehyde or acetaldehyde in refluxing acetic acid gave 3-azolyl-4-chromanones **2a-c** [6-8]. The synthesis of hydrazone derivative **3a** was first attempted by reaction of 3-triazolyl-4-chromanone **2a** with phenylhydrazine hydrochloride in refluxing methanol in the presence of Na_2CO_3 as a base, which resulted in poor yield with mixture of unknown degraded products. Since the condensation reactions of amines and hydrazines with ketones are commonly catalyzed by acids or bases, thus the alternative condition was using hydrochloride salt of phenylhydrazine in the absence of a base. Accordingly, the reaction of compound **2a-c** with phenylhydrazine hydrochloride in methanol at room temperature

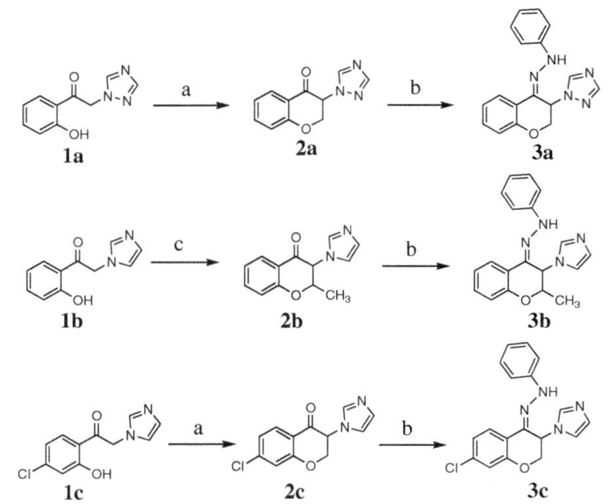

Scheme 1 Synthetic routes to phenylhydrazone derivatives 3a-c. (**a**) paraformaldehyde, AcOH, reflux; (**b**) phenylhyrazine hydrochloride, MeOH, r.t.; (**c**) acetaldehyde, AcOH, 90°C.

afforded final compounds **3a-c** in a mild condition. It seems that the acid released by hydrochloride salt of phenylhydrazine is adequate for catalyzing the condensation reaction.

Theoretically, the reactivity of chromanone derivatives toward N-nucleophiles like substituted hydrazine related to two sites; carbonyl group and C-2 position (Scheme 2). The attack of hydrazine to the C-2 position of chroman ring could result in ring opening and subsequent pyrazoline formation.

Previously, the reaction of chromanone and flavanone derivatives with substituted hydrazines has been investigated in different conditions [16,17]. Kállay et al. have been reported that the flavanone hydrazones are predominantly obtained under acidic conditions while alkaline conditions give the pyrazolines and the 2-hydroxychalcone derivatives due to the ring cleavage of the hetero ring of chromanone [16]. Similarly, in our experiment with 3-azolyl-4-chromanones, the hydrazone derivatives were predominantly obtained under mild acidic conditions, but in the presence of weak base Na_2CO_3, possibly produced a mixture of corresponding hydrazone, acyclic *N*-substituted hydrazine and pyrazoline derivatives which was difficult to separate and characterize (Scheme 2).

The structures of compounds **3a-c** were properly characterized by IR, ^{1}H NMR or Mass spectroscopy as well as elemental analyses. For example, elemental analysis proved the molecular formula of compound **3b** as $C_{19}H_{18}N_4O$. The IR spectra of compound **3b** did not show any absorption due to the presence of C = O group and a broad band was found in 3444 cm^{-1} due to the presence of a N – H bond. The ^{1}H NMR spectrum of **3b** showed a singlet at 10.34 for NH, a double at 8.07 (J = 7.6 Hz) and a triplet at 7.68 (J = 8.4 Hz) for H-5 and H-7 of chroman ring, respectively. The resonance for imidazole protons was observed as a multiplet at the range of 7.14-7.39 ppm. The H-6 and H-8 of chroman ring resonated as a triplet at 7.11 and a doublet at 7.01 ppm. Five protons related to the phenyl group appeared at 6.92, 6.83 and 6.75 ppm. The aliphatic protons of chroman (H-3 and H-2) resonated as a doublet at 5.88 and a doublet of quartet at 5.19 ppm. A doublet appeared at 1.16 ppm, assigned to the methyl protons.

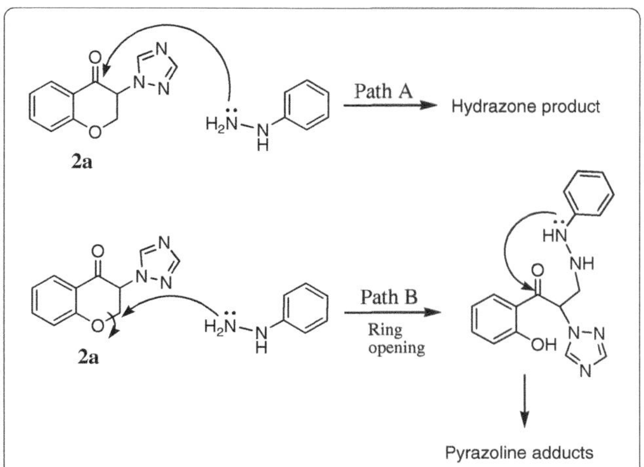

Scheme 2 Possible reactivity of 3-triazolylchroman-4-one derivative 2a toward phenylhydrazine.

Antifungal activity

The antifungal activities of title compounds **3a-c** were tested against several representative pathogenic fungi. The resulting MICs (minimum inhibitory concentrations) of hydrazone compounds were compared with those of fluconazole as a reference antifungal agent and intermediate compound **2b** (Table 1). The results revealed that 2-methyl-3-imidazolylchroman-4-one (**2b**) showed no activity against *Saccharomyces cerevisiae, Aspergillus niger* and *Microsporum gypseum* (MIC >64 μg/mL). Its activity against *Candida albicans* was weak. Compounds **3a,b** exhibited good growth inhibitory activity against different fungal strains with MIC values of 8–16 μg/mL. The 7-chloro-3-imidazolyl derivative **3c** also showed good antifungal activity against *Candida albicans, Saccharomyces cerevisiae* and *Microsporum gypseum* (MIC = 16 μg/mL), but its activity against *A. niger* was moderate. The MIC values of fluconazole against test strains were 8–32 μg/mL. Thus, the antifungal activity of title compounds was comparable to that of standard drug fluconazole. By comparing the MIC values of hydrazone derivative **3b** and its ketone counterpart **2b**, it is revealed that the introduction of phenylhydrazone on chroman ring improves the antifungal activity against all strains.

Previously, we have described azolylchromanone oxime ethers as conformationally restricted analogs of oxiconazole (Figure 1). Many of these derivatives exhibit high activity against different fungal strains [6-8]. In this work, we replaced *O*-benzyloxime ether fragment in azolylchromanone derivatives by phenylhydrazone moiety. The comparison of MIC values of triazole derivative **3a** with its *O*-benzyloxime ether counterpart demonstrates that replacement of *O*-benzyloximino moiety with

Table 1 *In vitro* antifungal activity of compounds 3a-c in comparison with 2b and fluconazole

Compound	Tested fungi (MICs in μg /mL)			
	C. albicans	*S. cerevisiae*	*A. niger*	*M. gypseum*
2b	64	>64	>64	>64
3a	16	16	16	8
3b	8	16	16	16
3c	16	16	64	16
Fluconazole	8	32	32	32

hyrazone can increase antifungal potency. However, in the cases of **3b** and **3c**, their *O*-benzyloximino analogs have a better profile of antifungal activity.

Docking study

Azole antifungals such as fluconazole inhibit fungal cytochrome P-450 dependent 14α-demethylase [4]. With the aim of rationalizing the antifungal activity data obtained, docking study was performed for the selected derivatives **2b** and **3a** in order to investigate the possible interactions with cytochrome P450 14α-sterol demethylase from *Mycobacterium tuberculosis* (Mycobacterium P450 DM). Because no experimental data are available for the target enzyme Candida P450 DM in the Protein Data Bank, the crystallographic structure of the complex between Cytochrome P450 14α-sterol demethylase from *Mycobacterium tuberculosis* (Mycobacterium P450 DM) and fluconazole (ID 1EA1) was used for the docking study [18].

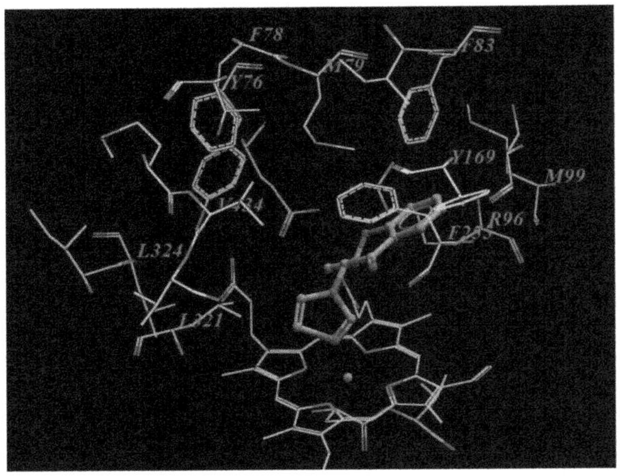

Figure 4 Compound 2b (ball and stick) in the active site of Mycobacterium P450 DM. For clarity, only the amino acids with 10 Å distant from the compound **2b** are shown.

Figure 3 shows the docked reference compound fluconazole in the active site of the same enzyme for validation of our docking protocol and confirmation of the biological data. Figures 4 and 5 show complex between the enzyme's active site and compounds **2b** and **3a**, respectively. The aromatic part of chroman ring of the both compounds is situated in a lipophilic region and interacts with Phe255, Met99, Phe83 and Met79. Oxygen atom (sp^3 hybridized) of the chroman ring is oriented towards the polar region of the enzyme constituted by Arg96 and Arg95. The phenyl attached to the hydrazone moiety is inserted into a hydrophobic pocket above the heme ring formed by ceiling residues Met79, Phe78, Phe255, Val434, Leu321 and Tyr76. The azole ring of both compounds **2b** and **3a** are positioned above the porphyrine plan, with a ring nitrogen atom coordinated to the heme iron. The distance between nitrogen atom of compounds **2b** and **3a** and the heme iron is 2.6 Å and 2.8 Å, respectively.

It has been previously reported that hydrophobic interactions with Val434 is responsible for the potent inhibitory activity of antifungals against *Aspergillus niger* whereas hydrophobic interactions with Leu321, Ile323, Leu324 may be responsible for an enhanced inhibitory activity against *Candida albicans* and other Candida spp. [18]. As shown in Figures 4 and 5, these interactions only can be seen with compound **3a** prototype bearing lipophilic phenylhydrazone side chain and not with compound **2b**; explaining the major potency differences observed in obtained results between **2b** and compounds **3a-c**.

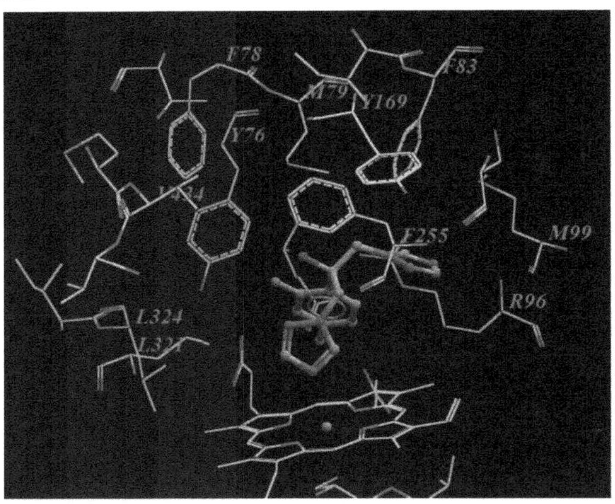

Figure 3 Computed binding geometry of the reference compound fluconazole (ball and stick) in the active site of Mycobacterium P450DM.

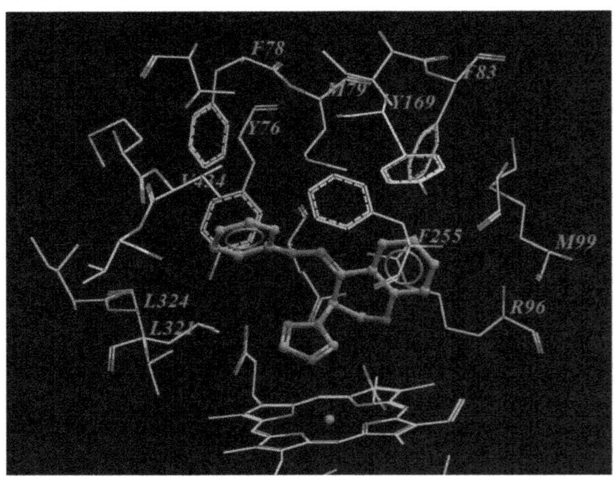

Figure 5 Compound 3a (ball and stick) in the active site of Mycobacterium P450 DM. For clarity, only the amino acids with 10 Å distant from the compound **3a** are shown.

Table 2 Toxicity risks and physicochemical properties of compounds 3a-c in comparison with fluconazole, predicted by OSIRIS Property Explorer

Compound	Toxicity risks				Physicochemical properties				
	Mutagenic	Tumorigenic	Irritant	Reproductive effect	CLogP	Slobility	MW	Drug likeness	Drug-score
3a	(±)	(+)	(−)	(±)	4.18	−3.07	305	1.33	0.26
3b	(±)	(+)	(−)	(−)	4.46	−2.78	318	2.81	0.34
3c	(±)	(+)	(−)	(±)	4.79	−3.14	338	0.17	0.2
Flu	(−)	(−)	(−)	(±)	−0.21	−2.17	306	−1.13	0.46

In silico drug-likeness and toxicity predictions

Currently, several approaches have been developed to assess drug-likeness of bioactive compounds based on topological descriptors, fingerprints of molecular structure or other properties such as molecular weight, water solubility and cLog*P* [19]. In this work, open-source program OSIRIS Property Explorer [14] was used to predict the fragment-based drug-likeness of title compounds and comparing them with fluconazole. OSIRIS program involves the database of traded drugs and commercially available compounds (Fluka) assumable as non drug-like dataset to assess the occurrence frequency of each fragment in the individual structure. The program estimated the risks of side effects, such as mutagenic, tumorigenic, irritant and reproductive effects, as well as drug-relevant properties including cLog*P*, Log*S* (solubility), MW and drug-likeness. Moreover, the overall drug-score was estimated by combining outcome of cLog*P*, Log*S*, MW, toxicity risks and drug-likeness. Drug-score is a measure of compound's potential to meet the criteria of a possible drug candidate [14].

The *in silico* drug-relevant properties obtained by OSIRIS Property Explorer are given in Table 2. Interestingly, the potential drug-likeness values of compounds **3a-c** were significantly higher than that of fluconazole, which showed a negative value of −1.13. As shown in Table 2, compounds **3a-c** had high *in silico* tumorigenic and medium mutagenic toxicity risks due to the phenylhydrazone moiety. However, the *in silico* prediction by OSIRIS Property Explorer showed that the introduction of chlorine on phenylhydrazone can reduce the risk of tumorigenic and mutagenic toxicities. Generally, the drug-score values of compounds **3a-c** (0.2-0.34) were less than that of fluconazole (0.46). Among the final compounds, 2-methyl-3-imidazolyl derivative **3b** showed the highest values of drug-likeness and drug-score.

Conclusion

In conclusion, a series of 3-azolyl-4-chromanone phenylhydrazones were synthesized via ring closure of 2-azolyl-2'-hydroxyacetophenones and subsequent reaction with phenylhydrazine. These compounds considered as analogs of 3-azolyl-4-chromanone oxime ethers basically designed as antifungal agents. The *in vitro* antifungal activity of compounds based on MIC values revealed that all compounds showed good antifungal activity against *Candida albicans*, *Saccharomyces cerevisiae* and *Microsporum gypseum* at concentrations less than 16 μg/mL. The antifungal activity of title compounds was comparable to that of standard drug fluconazole. The biological data and docking study demonstrated that the introduction of phenylhydrazone moiety on chroman ring improves the antifungal activity. The 2-methyl-3-imidazolyl derivative **3b** which showed the highest drug-likeness and drug-score values serves as a lead for future development of antifungal agents.

Competing interests

The authors declare that they have no competing interests.

Authors' contribution

AA participated in the synthesis of compounds. MF performed antifungal activity evaluation. HI participated in the molecular modeling study and performed the docking analysis. SE participated in the design of compounds, supervision of synthetic and computational parts, identifying of the structures of target compounds, accomplishing drug-likeness predictions and manuscript preparation. All authors read and approved the final manuscript.

Acknowledgements

This work was supported by grants from Research Council of Mazandaran University of Medical Sciences and Iran National Science Foundation (INSF).

Author details

[1]Department of Medicinal Chemistry and Pharmaceutical Sciences Research Center, Faculty of Pharmacy, Mazandaran University of Medical Sciences, Sari, Iran. [2]Department of Parasitology, Faculty of Medicine, Tehran University of Medical Sciences, Tehran, Iran.

References

1. Pappas PG: **The role of azoles in the treatment of invasive mycoses: review of the Infectious Diseases Society of America guidelines.** *Curr Opin Infect Dis* 2011, **24**:S1–S13.
2. Nosanchuk JD: **Current status and future of antifungal therapy for systemic mycoses.** *Recent Patents on Anti-Infective Drug Discovery* 2006, **1**:75–84.
3. Odds FC: **Antifungal agents: their diversity and increasing sophistication.** *Mycologist* 2003, **17**(Part 2):51–55.
4. Kathiravan MK, Salake AB, Chothe AS, Dudhe PB, Watode RP, Mukta MS, Gadhwe S: **The biology and chemistry of antifungal agents: a review.** *Bioorg Med Chem* 2012, http://dx.doi.org/10.1016/j.bmc.2012.04.045.
5. Shalini K, Kumar N, Drabu S, Sharma PK: **Advances in synthetic approach to and antifungal activity of triazoles.** *Beilstein J Org Chem* 2011, **7**:668–677.
6. Emami S, Falahati M, Banifatemi A, Moshiri K, Shafiee A: **Stereoselective synthesis and *in vitro* antifungal evaluation of (*E*)- and**

(*Z*)-imidazolylchromanone oxime ethers. *Arch Pharm Pharm Med Chem* 2002, **335**:318–324.

7. Emami S, Falahati M, Banifatemi A, Amanlou M, Shafiee A: **(*E*)- and (*Z*)-1,2,4-triazolylchromanone oxime ethers as conformationally constrained antifungals.** *Bioorg Med Chem* 2004, **12**:3971–3976.
8. Emami S, Falahati M, Banifatemi A, Shafiee A: **Stereoselective synthesis and antifungal activity of (*Z*)-trans-3-azolyl-2-methylchromanone oxime ethers.** *Bioorg Med Chem* 2004, **12**:5881–5889.
9. Weidenbörner M, Jha HC: **Antifungal spectrum of flavone and flavanone tested against 34 different fungi.** *Mycol Res* 1997, **101**:733–736.
10. Pretorius JC: **Flavonoids: a review of its commercial application potential as anti-infective agents.** *Curr Med Chem Anti-Infective Agents* 2003, **2**:335–353.
11. Wei DG, Yang GF, Wan J, Zhan CG: **Binding model construction of antifungal 2-Aryl-4-chromanones.** *J Agric Food Chem* 2005, **53**:1604–1611.
12. Massa S, Di Santo R, Retico A, Simonetti N, Fabrizi G, Lamba D: **Antifungal agents. 1. Synthesis and antifungal activities of estrogen-like imidazole and triazole derivatives.** *Eur J Med Chem* 1992, **27**:495–502.
13. Banfi E, Scialino G, Zampieri D, Mamolo MG, Vio L, Ferrone M, Fermeglia M, Paneni MS, Pric S: **Antifungal and antimycobacterial activity of new imidazole and triazole derivatives. A combined experimental and computational approach.** *J Antimicrob Chemother* 2006, **58**:76–84.
14. *Organic Chemistry Portal.*; 2012. Available at http://www.organic-chemistry.org/prog/peo/. Accessed May 22.
15. Emami S, Foroumadi A, Falahati M, Lotfali E, Rajabalian S, Ebrahimi SA, Farahyar S, Shafiee A: **2-Hydroxyphenacyl azoles and related azolium derivatives as antifungal agents.** *Bioorg Med Chem Lett* 2008, **18**:141–146.
16. Kállay F, Janzsó G, Koczor I: **The reactions of flavanone with substituted hydrazines.** *Tetrahedron* 1967, **23**:4317–4321.
17. Léavai A: **Synthesis of 2-pyrazolines by the reactions of α, β-unsaturated aldehydes, ketones, and esters with diazoalkanes, nitrile imines, and hydrazines.** *J Heterocyclic Chem* 2002, **39**:1–13.
18. Patel PD, Patel MR, Kocsis B, Kocsis E, Graham SM, Warren AR, Nicholson SM, Billack B, Fronczek FR, Talele TT: **Design, synthesis and determination of antifungal activity of 5(6)-substituted benzotriazoles.** *Eur J Med Chem* 2010, **45**:2214–2222.
19. Tetko IV: **Computing chemistry on the web.** *Drug Discov Today* 2005, **10**:1497–1500.

8

In vitro and *in vivo* activities of ticarcillin-loaded nanoliposomes with different surface charges against *Pseudomonas aeruginosa* (ATCC 29248)

Amir Gharib[1*†], Zohreh Faezizadeh[1†] and Masoud Godarzee[2†]

Abstract

Background: *Pseudomonas aeruginosa* exhibits multiple antibiotic resistance mechanisms. Different studies have shown that entrapment of antibiotics into liposomes could increase their anti-*Pseudomonas* activity. The objectives of this study were to prepare ticarcillin loaded-nanoliposomes with variable surface charges and evaluate their *in vitro* and *in vivo* efficacies against *Pseudomonas aeruginosa* (ATCC 29248).

Methods: Ticarcillin-loaded nanoliposomes with positive, negative and neutral surface charges were prepared by extrusion method. Ticarcillin encapsulation efficacies for different formulations were measured by HPLC method. Minimum inhibitory concentration (MIC) of ticarcillin nanoliposomal forms against strain ATCC 29248 were determined by broth dilution method. The killing rate of *Pseudomonas aeruginosa* was exposed to various concentrations of ticarcillin in free and nanoliposomal forms were analyzed. Ultimately, *in vivo* therapeutic efficacy of nanoliposomes in burned mice skin infected with strain ATCC 29248 was investigated.

Results: The encapsulation efficacies for ticarcillin-loaded cationic nanoliposomes were significantly higher (76% ± 0.17) than those of neutral (55% ± 0.14) and anionic (43% ± 0.14) nanoliposomes. The MIC of free, cationic, neutral and anionic nanoliposomal forms of ticarcillin against ATCC 29248 were to 24, 3, 6 and 48 mg/L, respectively. The killing rates of ticarcillin-loaded cationic nanoliposomes were higher than those of free and other drug formulations. Treatment by ticarcillin-loaded nanoliposomes with positive, neutral and negative surface charges resulted in almost 100, 60 and 20% survival rates, respectively.

Conclusion: Our data suggested that cationic ticarcillin-loaded nanoliposomes because of high effectiveness would be a good choice to treatment of *Pseudomonas aeruginosa* infections.

Keywords: Ticarcillin, Nanoliposome, Pseudomonas aeruginosa, Killing rate, Surface charge

Background

Pseudomonas aeruginosa is an opportunistic pathogen causing severe, acute and chronic nosocomial infections in hospitals, especially burn units [1]. Since *P. aeruginosa* can rapidly disseminate from the burn wound sites into the blood stream the clinical outcome in these patients can lead to sepsis, which is often fatal [2]. The major problem associated with *Pseudomonas* infection is resistance to conventional antibiotics. Therefore, there is the compelling need to develop novel drug delivery to overcome this resistance [3]. Ticarcillin is an antibiotic belonging to the carboxypenicillin subgroup of third-generation penicillins and covers gram-negative bacteria such as *P. aeruginosa*, but nowadays, this drug is susceptible to degradation by *P. aeruginosa* beta-lactamases [4,5]. Like other antibiotics, increasing time and usage have led to resistance to ticarcillin and so, a delivery system that reducing the ticarcillin-resistant while increasing its therapeutic index is of great interest, and nanoliposomes can provide these benefits [6,7]. Liposomes are spherical and colloidal vesicles that may range from a tens nanometer to several micrometers in size [8,9]. The alterations of liposomal lipids can lead to production of

* Correspondence: amirgharib@gmail.com
†Equal contributors
1Department of Laboratory Sciences, Borujerd Branch, Islamic Azad University, Borujerd, Iran
Full list of author information is available at the end of the article

liposomes with variable surface charges [10,11]. Positively or negatively charged liposomes were obtained using both phosphatidylcholine and cholesterol, in combination with stearylamine or dicetylphosphate, respectively [12,13]. Later studies demonstrated that encapsulation of antibiotics into liposomal formulations with different surface charges markedly alters their pharmacokinetics, increasing half-lives and effectiveness [14,15]. Variable results were reported on the *in vitro* and *in vivo* antibacterial activity of liposomal antibiotics against bacteria [7,9]. While some antibiotics such as amikacin are only slowly released from the liposomal carrier, other drugs including ciprofloxacin leak out rapidly [15]. According to the literature, manipulation of physicochemical characteristics of liposomes, like particle size, surface charge, sensitivity to pH changes and bilayer rigidity can have marked effects on the *in vitro* and *in vivo* behavior of antibiotics loaded liposomes and therefore have a major impact on therapeutic success [1,7,14]. The effectiveness of ticarcillin-loaded in nanoliposomes with deferent surface charges yet was not studied. The primary objective of this study was to prepare the ticarcillin-loaded nanoliposomes with three different (neutral, negative and positive) surface charges and evaluate *in vitro* antibacterial activity of their against *P. aeruginosa* (ATCC 29248). A secondary objective was to investigate the therapeutic efficacy of prepared nanoliposomes using a mouse burn model.

Methods

Materials

Ticarcillin, stearylamine, dicetylphosphate, cholesterol and egg lecithin was purchased from Sigma Chemical Company (St. Louis, USA) and chloroform, methanol, ammonium acetate and Muller-Hinton broth was purchased from Merck (Darmstadt, Germany).

Microorganism

P. aeruginosa (ATCC 29248) was purchased from American Type Culture Collection (Rockville, MD, USA). For experimentation, this strain was inoculated onto blood agar plates and incubated for 24 h at 37°C.

Preparation of nanoliposomes

Nanoliposomes were prepared by extrusion method as previously described [16]. Briefly, egg lecithin and cholesterol in the molar ratio of 4:1 were dissolved in chloroform and dried to a lipid film with a rotary evaporator (Brinkman, Toronto, Canada) under N_2 flow and vacuum at 30°C. The dried lipids were dispersed by agitation in 6 ml of an aqueous solution of ticarcillin (10 mg/ml in PBS, pH 7.4) and sonicated at 4°C in ultrasonic bath (Braun-sonic 2000, Burlingame, USA). At finally, ticarcillin-loaded neutral nanoliposomes were obtained by extruding of respective suspension through a polycarbonate membrane with 100 nm-sized pores for 12 times and separating excess free drug and larger lipid aggregation by centrifugation (100000 g for 30 min). Cationic and anionic ticarcillin-loaded nanoliposomes were prepared and optimized by added stearylamine and dicetylphosphate in nanoliposomal membrane formulations in molar ratios of 0.5, 1, 2 and 3, respectively. Control nanoliposomes were prepared similarly, but PBS (pH 7.4) was used instead of the ticarcillin solution.

Determination of encapsulation efficacy

The content of ticarcillin in prepared nanoliposomes was determined by HPLC as described previously [17]. Then, the percentage of drug loading was calculated as:

$$\begin{aligned}&\text{Amount of ticarcillin in nanoliposomes}\\ &\quad\times\ \text{Total volume tested}\\ &\quad\times\ 100/\text{Total sample volume}\\ &\quad\times\ \text{Initial amount of ticarcillin}\end{aligned}$$

Particle size, zeta-potential and polydispersity index determination

Mean particle size, zeta-potential and polydispersity index of nanoliposomes was evaluated by the reported method using Malvern zetasizer (Malvern instrument, Worcestershire, UK) apparatus [11].

Antimicrobial susceptibility testing

The MICs of free and variable ticarcillin-loaded nanoliposomes for *P. aeruginosa* (ATCC 29248) were determined by the broth dilution technique as recommended by CLSI (formerly NCCLS) [18]. Bacterial cell suspensions of ~ 5×10^5 cells/ml were diluted in Muller-Hinton broth and dispensed (100 μl) into a microtiter tray containing serial two-fold dilutions of ticarcillin. The tray was then incubated for 24 h at 37°C. The MIC was recorded to be the lowest concentrations of ticarcillin in free and nanoliposomal forms that prevented visible bacterial growth and expressed in μg/ml.

Time-kill studies

Time kill studies were preformed in triplicate in 10 ml tubes containing 2 ml of Mueller-Hinton broth as described previously [19]. In brief, 100 μl of *P. aeruginosa* suspension were resuspended in 10 ml of Mueller-Hinton broth and incubated overnight at 37°C, and adjusted to a McFarland standard of 0.5. Then, 100 μl of this standardized inoculum were added to separate culture tubes containing 1 ml of Mueller-Hinton broth with 1 ml ticarcillin solutions in free and different nanoliposomal forms at 1, 2 and 4 times the MIC and incubated at 37°C. At finally, colony counts were performed onto Trypticase soy agar (TSA) plates at 0, 2, 4, 6 and 24 h and the results were expressed as log colony forming unit (CFU)/ml.

In vivo study

In vivo therapeutic efficacies of ticarcillin-loaded nanoliposomes were tested by a described method [20], with some modification. In brief, sixty male BALB/c mice (20–22 g) obtained from the National Institute of Pasture, Iran. Animals were handled according to the national guidelines of the laboratory animal and housed in separate and pathogen- free cages and received food and water *ad libitum* [21]. All groups were anesthetized with ketamine-xylazine mixture (50 mg/kg each, given intramuscularly), and their backs were shaved. To induce burn in the backs of mice, a brass bar (10 by 10 by 100 mm) was heated in boiling water for 15 min and applied on the shaved back of the animals for 45 s. Then, 50 μl of the bacterial inoculum (containing 10^9 CFU of total bacteria) was applied subcutaneously into the sites of the burn on the animal's back. The mice were divided into 5 groups. All groups were treated topically as follows: Group 1 received cationic ticarcillin-loaded nanoliposomes (75 mg/kg/12h); group 2 received neutral ticarcillin-loaded nanoliposomes (75 mg/kg/12h); group 3 received anionic ticarcillin-loaded nanoliposomes (75 mg/kg/12h); group 4 received anionic ticarcillin-loaded nanoliposomes (75 mg/kg/12h); group 5 received empty nanoliposomes (75 mg/kg/12h), and group 6 received physiological saline (1 ml/kg/12h); for 7 days starting from the 3rd day post infection. Two days after the last dose the surviving animals were anesthetized and sacrificed by cervical dislocation and the liver, kidney, spleen and skin of mice were removed under sterile conditions and homogenized for 5–10 min in PBS (2 ml/g). The homogenates were serially diluted and plated for growth in TSA. The inoculated plates were then incubated at 37°C for 24 h and the colony forming unit (CFU) was counted.

Data analysis

The results were expressed as means ± standard errors of means. The data of killing rate study were statistically evaluated by paired Student's *t*-test, and *P value* of less than 0.05 was considered significant. The survival rates of control and treated mice were determined by using chi-squared with Yates correction and by Fisher's exact test. Therefore, these data were used to prepare of cationic and anionic ticarcillin-loaded nanoliposomes.

Results

Encapsulation efficacy

The results showed that encapsulation efficacies of ticarcillin in cationic, neutral and anionic nanoliposomal forms were 76% ± 0.17, 55% ± 0.21 and 43% ± 0.14, respectively. Tables 1 and 2 shows the highest encapsulation efficacies of ticarcillin into cationic and anionic nanoliposomes were obtained by the addition of 1 molar of stearylamine and dicetylphosphate to formulations, respectively.

Table 1 Influence of stearylamine molarity in encapsulation efficacy*

	Molarity of stearylamine			
	0.5	1	2	3
Encapsulation efficacy	70 ± 0.14	76% ± 0.17**	67 ± 0.32	63 ± 0.18

* The Data are expressed as Mean ± S.E.M.
** Significant difference ($p < 0.05$).

Particle size, zeta-potential and polydispersity index analysis

Table 3 shows the mean particle size, zeta-potential and polydispersity index of empty and ticarcillin loaded-nanoliposomes with variable surface charges. Size homogeneity of empty and loaded-nanoliposomes suggested that ticarcillin was entrapped into lipid bilayer, according to the previous studies [14,21]. Zeta-potential of nanoliposomes revealed that prepared nanoparticles have appropriate stability in aqueous dispersion [22].

Bacterial susceptibilities

The MICs values ticarcillin in either free or nanoliposomal forms for *P.aeruginosa* (ATCC 29248) was shown in Table 4. The MICs of free, cationic and neutral nanoliposomal forms of ticarcillin were higher than anionic formulation, respectively.

Time-killing study

The killing curves of ticarcillin in free and encapsulated forms at 1, 2 and 4 times the MICs was shown in Figure 1. In all conditions free ticarcillin was more effective on reduced bacterial counts as compared with ticarcillin encapsulated in anionic nanoliposomes (Figure 1). At one times of MIC only ticarcillin encapsulated in cationic nanoliposomes could eliminate of *P. aeruginosa* after 24 h (Figure 1-A). At two times of MIC both ticarcillin encapsulated in cationic and neutral nanoliposomes eradicated the bacteria after 6 and 24 h, respectively (Figure 1-B). At four times of MIC, both ticarcillin in free and encapsulated in cationic and neutral nanoliposomes could

Table 2 Influence of dicetylphosphate molarity in encapsulation efficacy*

	Molarity of dicetylphosphate			
	0.5	1	2	3
Encapsulation efficacy	38 ± 0.34	43% ± 0.14**	34 ± 0.11	27 ± 0.30

* The Data are expressed as Mean ±S.E.M.
** Significant difference ($p < 0.05$).

Table 3 Particle size, zeta-potential and polydispersity index of empty and ticarcillin-loaded nanoliposomes

Formulations	Mean particle size (nm)	Zeta-potential (mV)	Polydispersity index
Empty			
Neutral liposomes	94.9 ± 0.15	−1.1 ± 0.27	0.22 ± 0.01
Anionic liposomes	93.2 ± 0.36	−15.7 ± 0.95	0.23 ± 0.04
Cationic liposomes	95.3 ± 0.49	+20.1 ± 0.52	0.25 ± 0.02
Loaded			
Neutral liposomes	95.2 ± 0.31	−1.1 ± 0.27	0.23 ± 0.02
Anionic liposomes	92.6 ± 0.44	−15.2 ± 0.86	0.26 ± 0.01
Cationic liposomes	96.1 ± 0.14	+21.8 ± 0.13	0.25 ± 0.03

eliminate the *P.aeruginosa* (ATCC 29248) after 4, 8 and 24 h, respectively (Figure 1-C).

Therapeutic efficacy test

The treatment of the *P. aeruginosa*-infected burned mice with ticarcillin-loaded cationic nanoliposomes compared to control animals showed significant reduction in CFU values in evaluated organs, especially in skin, spleen and liver (Table 5). It was found that mortality of mice as control (without AmB administrated) was 100% after 7 days, whereas mice treated with ticarcillin in free and encapsulated in cationic, neutral and anionic nanoliposomes showed the increase in survival rate of 30, 100, 60 and 20%, respectively.

Discussion

The use of liposomes as antibiotic carrier systems has been widely investigated [11,20]. However, the main problems associated with application of liposomes as carriers for antibiotics is insufficient quantities in the target site [1,18]. In addition, the preparation of antibiotic-loaded liposomes with high encapsulation efficacy may not be easy because the variable interactions between antibiotics and bilayer lipids can occur [2,11]. For the elimination of this problem, investigators were changed lipids in liposomal membrane formulation. In this report, we evaluated the potential of incorporation of ticarcillin into cationic, neutral and anionic nanoliposomes. The results showed that ticarcillin can be encapsulated into three kinds of nanoliposomes with variable entrapment efficacy. It has been shown that the highest encapsulation efficiencies occur when lipids and loaded drugs have opposite charges [13,15]. In this case, we previously reported that superoxide dismutase (SOD) with negative surface charge has high encapsulation efficacy in cationic liposomes [12]. Whereas the electric charge of ticarcillin in the pH 7.4 is negative [20], it probably makes the encapsulation efficacy of ticarcillin in cationic nanoliposomes were higher than neutral and anionic nanoliposomes, respectively. Our results suggest that entrapped of ticarcillin in neutral and cationic nanoliposomal forms enhanced the antipseudomonal activity of its compared to free ticarcillin. Our data fits well with some other studies. We previously studied that amikacin-loaded neutral liposomes displayed stronger bactericidal activity than the free drug [9]. Furthermore, it has been reported that encapsulated of cephalexin in liposomes with neutral and negative surface charges could protect the drug from hydrolysis by *staphylococcal* β-lactamase as well [22]. Several hypotheses, including increased electrostatic impulsion and protection of the antibiotics from bacterial enzymes may explain the mechanism of enhanced antimicrobial activities of liposomal formulations [7,14,23]. Additionally, the molecular configuration of antibiotics within liposomes could play an important role in these cases [18]. The time-kill assays confirmed that higher potency of cationic and neutral nanoliposomal forms of ticarcillin than free antibiotics. These results are in accordance with previous findings, which reported that a significantly higher killing rate of *P. aeruginosa* with meropenem and gentamicin-loaded cationic liposomes were occurred [24]. So, we hypothesized that electrostatic interaction between the outer membrane lipopolysaccharides of *P. aeruginosa* and cationic nanoliposome loaded-ticarcillin could enhance the mechanism of drug entry into this microorganism cell. Burns, wounds, and other exposed tissues are particularly susceptible to microbial contamination and infections [25,26]. It is proven that potential mortality from burn wound infections, even with aggressive antibiotic therapy, may approach or exceed 50% [27]. Treatment of

Table 4 *In vitro* antimicrobial activities of free and nanoliposomal forms of ticarcillin for *P. aeruginosa* (ATCC 29248)

	Minimum inhibitory concentration (mg/L)			
Drugs	**Free ticarcillin**	**Tticarcillin-loaded nanoliposomes**		
		Cationic	**Neutral**	**Anionic**
Microorganism				
***P. aeruginosa* (ATCC 29248)**	24	3	6	48

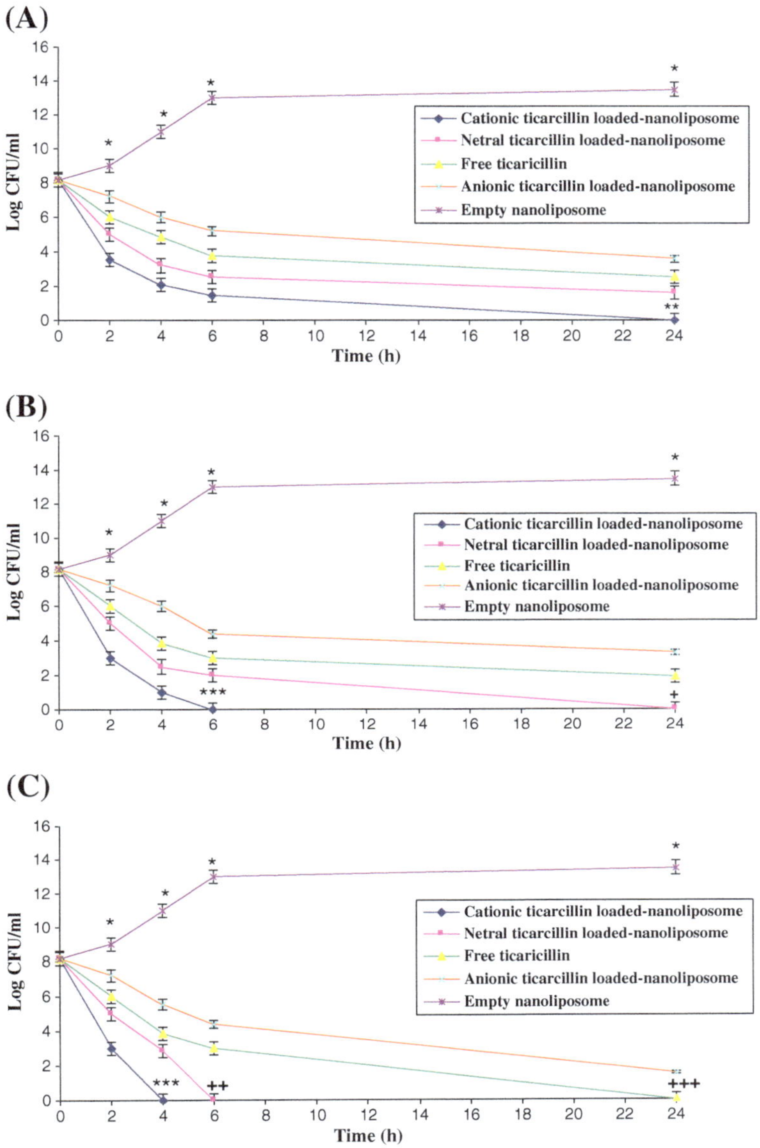

Figure 1 Killing curves for *P. aeruginosa* (ATCC 29248) was exposed to various concentrations (A=1×MIC, B=2×MIC and C=4×MIC) of ticarcillin in free and neutral, negative and positive nanoliposomal forms. *Significant difference between killing rate of empty nanoliposomes versus free and another loaded nanoliposomes (p<0.01), **Significant difference between killing rate of cationic nanoliposomes versus free and another loaded nanoliposomes (p<0.05), ***Significant difference between killing rate of cationic nanoliposomes versus free and another loaded nanoliposomes (p<0.01), $^{+}$Significant difference between killing rate of neutral nanoliposomes versus free and anionic nanoliposomes (p<0.05), $^{++}$Significant difference between killing rate of free drug versus anionic nanoliposomes (p<0.05). $^{+++}$Significant difference between killing rate of cationic nanoliposomes versus free and another loaded nanoliposomes (p<0.01).

mice with ticarcillin-loaded in cationic nanoliposomes resulted in 100% survival rate and in almost complete eradication of the bacteria from the spleens, livers, and skins of infected animals. These results may be due to the optimal antibiotic delivery that reported by several investigators [20,28]. When cationic liposomes containing antibiotics are applied topically; they may interact with the cell membranes of exposed tissues and therefore, protects the burn wound tissues from further bacterial contamination [29].

Conclusion

In vitro and *in vivo* testing of nanoliposomes indicated that ticarcillin-loaded in cationic nanoliposomes have a stronger protective effect against *P. aeruginosa* infection compared to free, neutral and anionic ticarcillin

Table 5 The survival rate of infected burned mice and colony-forming units (CFUs) of *P. aeruginosa* (ATCC 29248) in different organs

Treatment	Tissue/Organ	Log CFU/ Gram tissue (n=3)	Percentage of survival mice (n=10)
Control without drug administration (received physiological saline, Topically)	Liver	3.211 ± 0.5	None survived
	Kidney	3.750 ± 0.3	
	Spleen	3.829 ± 0.6	
	Skin	3.690 ± 0.2	
Empty nanoliposomes (1 mg Kg^{-1}, Topically)	Liver	3.355 ± 0.4	None survived
	Kidney	3.960 ± 0.8	
	Spleen	3.764 ± 1.5	
	Skin	3.590 ± 1.3	
Free ticarcillin (1 mg Kg^{-1}, Topically)	Liver	2.315 ± 0.04	30
	Kidney	2.198 ± 0.07	
	Spleen	2.312 ± 1.3	
	Skin	2.420 ± 0.04	
Anionic ticarcillin-loaded nanoliposome (1 mg Kg^{-1}, Topically)	Liver	2.715 ± 0.8	20
	Kidney	2.910 ± 0.2	
	Spleen	2.650 ± 1.4	
	Skin	2.680 ± 1.1	
Neutral ticarcillin-loaded nanoliposome (1 mg Kg^{-1}, Topically)	Liver	1.712 ± 0.6	60
	Kidney	2.045 ± 0.1	
	Spleen	1.024 ± 1.1	
	Skin	1.362 ± 0.04	
Cationic ticarcillin-loaded nanoliposome (1 mg Kg^{-1}, Topically)	Liver	Nil*	100
	Kidney	1.013 ± 0.07**	
	Spleen	Nil*	
	Skin	Nil*	

The Data are expressed as Mean±Standard error of mean from three separate experiments. Analysis of variance of one-way classification between the treatment means was heterogeneous and the *t*-test values (two-tailed) were significant, * $p < 0.001$ and ** $p < 0.05$.

formulations. Therefore, we suggest that effective formulations would be a good choice for treatment of patients with *P. aeruginosa* infections, especially in burn units of hospitals.

Competing interests
The author(s) declare that they have no competing interests.

Authors' contributions
All authors have read and approved the final manuscript.

Acknowledgments
This study was supported by Islamic Azad University, Borujerd Branch, Iran. The authors would like to acknowledge staffs of the university. The author would like to thank also the University of Tarbiat Modares and its staff members, especially for some technical help and advice.

Author details
[1]Department of Laboratory Sciences, Borujerd Branch, Islamic Azad University, Borujerd, Iran. [2]Department of Biology, Borujerd Branch, Islamic Azad University, Borujerd, Iran.

References
1. Alipour M, Suntres ZE, Lafrenie RM, Omri A: **Attenuation of *Pseudomonas aeruginosa* virulence factors and biofilms by co-encapsulation of bismuth-ethanedithiol with tobramycin in liposomes.** *J Antimicrob Chemother* 2010, **65**:684–693.
2. Moore NM, Flaws ML: **Antimicrobial resistance mechanisms in *Pseudomonas aeruginosa*.** *Clin Lab Sci* 2011, **24**:47–51.
3. Moore NM, Flaws ML: **Epidemiology and pathogenesis of *Pseudomonas aeruginosa* infections.** *Clin Lab Sci* 2011, **24**:43–46.
4. Manuel J, Zhanel GG, de Kievit T: **Cadaverine suppresses persistence to carboxypenicillins in *Pseudomonas aeruginosa* PAO1.** *Antimicrob Agent Chemother* 2010, **54**:5173–5179.
5. Karr JC, Lauretta J, Keriazes G: ***In vitro* antimicrobial activity of calcium sulfate and hydroxyapatite (Cerament Bone Void Filler) discs using heat-sensitive and non-heat-sensitive antibiotics against methicillin-resistant *Staphylococcus aureus* and *Pseudomonas aeruginosa*.** *J Am Podiatr Med Assoc* 2011, **101**:146–152.
6. Slain D, Sarwari AR, Petros KO, McKnight RL, Sager RB, Mullett CJ: **Impact of a multimodal antimicrobial stewardship srogram on *Pseudomonas aeruginosa* susceptibility and antimicrobial use in the intensive care unit setting.** *Crit Care Res Pract* 2011, **2011**:416–426.
7. Pumerantz A, Muppidi K, Agnihotri S, Guerra C, Venketaraman V, Wang J: **Preparation of liposomal vancomycin and intracellular killing of meticillin-resistant *Staphylococcus aureus* (MRSA).** *Int J Antimicrob Agents* 2011, **37**:140–144.

8. Gaffari MA, Dabbagh MA, Gharib A: **Human erythrocyte superoxide dismutase encapsulated in positively charged liposomes.** *Iranian J Pharm Sci* 2005, **1**:153–160.
9. Mirzaee M, Owlia P, Mehrabi MR, Gharib A: ***In Vitro* bactericidal activity of encapsulated amikacin in liposome.** *Iranian J Pathol* 2009, **4**:151–156.
10. Sarbolouki MN, Maghdooni Bagheri P, Saneei V: **The influence of lipid composition and beta-carotene on lipid peroxidation in liposomes.** *DARU J Pharm Sci* 2005, **13**:184–154.
11. Tamaddon AM, Hosseini-Shirazi F, Moghimi HR: **Preparation of oligodeoxynucleotide encapsulatedcationic liposomes and release study with models of cellular membranes.** *DARU J Pham Sci* 2007, **15**:61–70.
12. Zhong Z, Wan Y, Han J, Shi S, Zhang Z, Sun X: **Improvement of adenoviral vector-mediated gene transfer to airway epithelia by folate-modified anionic liposomes.** *Int J Nanomedicine* 2011, **6**:1083–1093.
13. Roychoudhury J, Sinha R, Ali N: **Therapy with sodium stibogluconate in stearylamine-bearing liposomes confers cure against SSG-resistant *Leishmania donovani* in BALB/c mice.** *PLoS One* 2011, **6**:e17376.
14. Huang CM, Chen CH, Pornpattananangkul D, Zhang L, Chan M, Hsieh MF: **Eradication of drug resistant *Staphylococcus aureus* by liposomal oleic acids.** *Biomaterials* 2011, **32**:214–221.
15. Gubernator J: **Active methods of drug loading into liposomes: recent strategies for stable drug entrapment and increased *in vivo* activity.** *Expert Opin Drug Deliv* 2011, **8**:565–580.
16. Maestrelli F, Capasso G, Gonzalez-Rodriguez ML, Rabasco AM, Ghelardini C, Mura P: **Effect of preparation technique on the properties and *in vivo* efficacy of benzocaine-loaded ethosomes.** *J Liposome Res* 2009, **4**:1–8.
17. McWhinney BC, Wallis SC, Hillister T, Roberts JA, Lipman J, Ungerer JP: **Analysis of 12 beta-lactam antibiotics in human plasma by HPLC with ultraviolet detection.** *J Chromatogr B Analyt Technol Biomed Life Sci* 2010, **878**:2039–2043.
18. National Committee for Clinical Laboratory Standards: *Methods for dilution antimicrobial susceptibility tests for bacteria that grow aerobically: approved standard-6th ed.* Wayne, PA: National Committee for Clinical Laboratory Standards; 2003. NCCLS document M7-A6.
19. Shrivastava SM, Saurabh S, Rai D, Dwivedi VK, Chaudhary M: ***In vitro* microbial efficacy of sulbactomax: a novel fixed dose combination of ceftriaxone sulbactam and ceftriaxone alone.** *Cur Drug Ther* 2009, **4**:73–77.
20. Dale RK, Schnell G, Wong JP: **Therapeutic Efficacy of "Nubiotics" against Burn Wound Infection by *Pseudomonas aeruginosa*.** *Antimicrob Agents Chemother* 2004, **48**:2918–2923.
21. Committe on the Care and Use of Laboratory Animals of the Institute of Laboratory Animal Resources: *Commission on Life Sciences National Research Council. Guide for the care and use of laboratory animals.* Washington, D.C: National Academy Press; 1996.
22. Shaffa MW, Dayem SA, Elshemy WM: ***In vitro* antibacterial activity of liposomal cephalexin against *Staphylococcus aureus*.** *Romanian J Biophys* 2008, **18**:293–300.
23. Gharib A, Faezizadeh Z, Mohammad Asghari H: **Preparation and antifungal activity of spray-dried amphotericin B-loaded nanospheres.** *DARU J Pharm Sci* 2011, **19**:351–355.
24. Drulis-Kawa Z, Dorotkiewicz-Jach A, Gubernator J, Gula G, Bocer T, Doroszkiewicz W: **The interaction between *Pseudomonas aeruginosa* cells and cationic PC:Chol:DOTAP liposomal vesicles versus outer-membrane structure and envelope properties of bacterial cell.** *Int J Pharm* 2009, **367**:211–219.
25. Klein DG, Fritsh DE, Amin SG: **Wound infection following trauma and burn injuries.** *Crit Care Nursing N Am* 1995, **7**:627–642.
26. Pruitt BA, McManus AT, Kim SH, Goodwin CW: **Burn wound infections: current status.** *World J Surg* 1998, **22**:135–145.
27. Wurtz RE, Karajovic E, Dacumos, Hanumandass M: **Nosocomial infections in a burn intensive care unit.** *Burns* 1995, **21**:180–184.
28. McVay CS, Velásquez M, Fralick JA: **Phage Therapy of *Pseudomonas aeruginosa* Infection in a Mouse Burn Wound Model.** *Antimicrob Agents Chemother* 2007, **51**:1934–1938.
29. Price CI, Horton JW, Baxter CR: **Liposome delivery of aminoglycosides in burn wounds.** *Surg Gynecol Obstet* 1992, **174**:414–418.

Enhanced antibacterial activity of roxithromycin loaded pegylated poly lactide-co-glycolide nanoparticles

Mona Noori Koopaei[1], Mohamad Shahab Maghazei[1], Seyed Hossein Mostafavi[2], Hossein Jamalifar[3], Nasrin Samadi[3], Mohsen Amini[4], Soheyl Jafari Malek[1], Behrad Darvishi[1], Fatemeh Atyabi[1,2] and Rassoul Dinarvand[1,2*]

Abstract

Background and the purpose of the study: The purpose of this study was to prepare pegylated poly lactide-co-glycolide (PEG-PLGA) nanoparticles (NPs) loaded with roxithromycin (RXN) with appropriate physicochemical properties and antibacterial activity. Roxithromycin, a semi-synthetic derivative of erythromycin, is more stable than erythromycin under acidic conditions and exhibits improved clinical effects.

Methods: RXN was loaded in pegylated PLGA NPs in different drug;polymer ratios by solvent evaporation technique and characterized for their size and size distribution, surface charge, surface morphology, drug loading, in vitro drug release profile, and in vitro antibacterial effects on *S. aureus, B. subtilis, and S. epidermidis*.

Results and conclusion: NPs were spherical with a relatively mono-dispersed size distribution. The particle size of nanoparticles ranged from 150 to 200 nm. NPs with entrapment efficiency of up to 80.0±6.5% and drug loading of up to 13.0±1.0% were prepared. In vitro release study showed an early burst release of about 50.03±0.99% at 6.5 h and then a slow and steady release of RXN was observed after the burst release. In vitro antibacterial effects determined that the minimal inhibitory concentration (MIC) of RXN loaded PEG-PLGA NPs were 9 times lower on *S. aureus*, 4.5 times lower on *B. subtilis*, and 4.5 times lower on *S. epidermidis* compared to RXN solution. In conclusion it was shown that polymeric NPs enhanced the antibacterial efficacy of RXN substantially.

Keywords: Roxithromycin, PLGA, Pegylation, Nanoparticles, Antibacterial

Introduction

Infectious diseases were the important reason of death worldwide at the beginning of the 20th century [1]. An introduction of antibacterial agents leads to the decreases in mortality and morbidity from infectious diseases over the last century. These days, though, resistance to antibiotics has been reaching a critical level, invalidating major antibacterial drugs that are currently used in the clinic [2,3]. Exploring antibacterial NPs is one of the new efforts in addressing this challenge, to which microbial pathogens may not be able to develop resistance. For instance, in recent studies it has been suggested that some metal nanostructures are recognized to have antibacterial activities, which is utilized in controlling infectious diseases [4].

The advantages of NP-based antibacterial drug delivery include improved solubility of poorly water-soluble drugs, sustained and stimuli-responsive drug release, which eventually lowers administration frequency and dose, and prolonged drug half-life and systemic circulation time. Moreover, minimized systemic side effects via targeted delivery of antibacterial drugs as well as combined, synergistic, and resistance-overcoming effects via co delivery of multiple antibacterial drugs can be achieved using NP carriers [5,6].

Among different nanoparticulate systems, polymeric NPs have several unique characteristics for antibacterial drug delivery. Firstly, particle properties such as size, zeta potentials, and drug release profiles can be precisely tuned by selecting different polymer lengths, surfactants,

* Correspondence: dinarvand@tums.ac.ir
[1]Novel Drug Delivery Lab, Faculty of Pharmacy, Tehran University of Medical Sciences, Tehran 1417614411, Iran
[2]Nanotechnology Research Centre, Faculty of Pharmacy, Tehran University of Medical Sciences, Tehran, Iran
Full list of author information is available at the end of the article

and organic solvents during the preparation process. Secondly, polymeric NPs are structurally stable and can be prepared with a narrow size distribution. Thirdly, the surface of polymeric NPs can be functionalized by groups that can be chemically customized with either drug moieties or targeting ligands [5].

Among the different polymers developed to formulate polymeric NPs, PLGA has attracted considerable attention due to its attractive properties: (i) biodegradability and biocompatibility, (ii) FDA and European Medicine Agency approval in drug delivery systems for parenteral administration, (iii) well described formulations and methods of production adapted to various types of drugs e.g. hydrophilic or hydrophobic small molecules or macromolecules, (iv) protection of drug from degradation, (v) possibility of sustained release, (vi) possibility to modify surface properties to provide stealth properties and/or better interaction with biological materials and (vii) possibility to target NPs to specific organs or cells [7].

Poly ethylene glycol (PEG) has been frequently used for the surface treatment of polymeric NPs to create a stealth layer that prolongs the circulation lifetime of NPs in the blood stream. Specifically, the PEG coating forms a hydration layer that retards the reticuloendothelial system (RES) recognitions of NPs through sterically inhibiting hydrophobic and electrostatic interactions with plasma proteins [8]. This minimizes the interface with phagocytic cells and increasing the blood circulation time. Another attractive characteristic of PEG, with admiration to its use for mucosal drug administration, is associated to its mucoadhesion promoting result, a mechanism of chain penetration across the polymer mucosa interface may be the reason for this phenomenon.[9].

Roxithromycin (RXN), a semi-synthetic 14-memberedring macrolide antibiotic derived from erythromycin, has a molecular weight of 837.06. It possesses improved pharmacokinetic properties such as high serum concentrations and a long half-life of about 13 h. Furthermore, this it is more resistant to gastric acid hydrolysis. Because of these properties, together with its spectrum of activity, RXN appears to offer advantages for the treatment of respiratory tract infections [10] . RXN has bitter taste and is very slightly soluble in aqueous medium. The oral bioavailability of RXN is 50% and the low bioavailability of the drug is mainly due to poor aqueous solubility and dissolution behavior [11]. Ciprofloxacin loaded PLGA NPs showed increased antibacterial effect [12]. In another study, it was reported that rifampicin loaded PLGA NPs are remarkably more effective against gram-positive bacteria [13].

In previous study, RXN microspheres with polymers were prepared successfully by the emulsion solvent diffusion method to cover its bitter taste [14]. Preparation and characterization of complexes of RXN with â-cyclodextrin (BCD), hydroxypropyl â-cyclodextrin (HPBCD) to increase the solubility, improve the dissolution properties and improve the antibacterial activity has been also reported so as to increase the efficacy of this narrow spectrum antibiotic [11].

In this study RXN loaded PEG-PLGA NPs were prepared to improve its antibacterial effect. Their physicochemical characters, drug release and in vitro antibacterial effects against *S. aureus*, *B. subtilis*, and *S. epidermidis* were determined.

Methods

Materials

RXN powder (USP) was kindly donated by Shifa PharMed Co, Iran. PLGA (lactide:glycolide, 50:50; Resomer RG 504H, molecular weight 48,000) was purchased from Boehringer Ingelheim (Ingelheim, Germany). Polyvinyl alcohol (molecular weight 22,000) and bifunctional NH2-PEG-OH (average molecular weight 10000) were purchased from Sigma-Aldrich (St Louis, MO). 1-Ethyl-3-(3-dimethylaminopropyl)carbodiimide (EDC), N-hydroxysuccinimide (NHS), Poly vinyl alcohol (PVA), with molecular weight of 95,000 from Acros Organics (Geel, Belgium) and acetone from Merck (Darmstadt, Germany) were used. Mueller-Hinton broth and Mueller-Hinton agar (both from Merck) media were used for microbiological tests. *S.aureus* (ATCC : 6538) , *B. subtilis* (ATCC : 6633), and *S. epidermidis* (ATCC : 12228) were obtained from the stock culture of Department of Drug and Food Control, Faculty of Pharmacy, Tehran University of Medical Sciences, Iran. In all experiments reverse osmosis (RO) purified water was freshly prepared prior to use. All other materials used were of analytical or HPLC grade.

Synthesis of PEG-PLGA

Hydroxylate functionalized PEG-PLGA was synthesized by conjugation of OH-PEG-NH2 to carboxylic group of PLGA [15]. NHS (135 mg, 1.1 mmol) in the presence of EDC (230 mg, 1.2 mmol) was added to a stirred solution of PLGA-COOH (5 g, 0.14 mmol) in methylene chloride (10 mL). The mixture was stirred for 3 hours at 25°C. PLGA-NHS was precipitated with ethyl ether (5 mL) and repeatedly washed in an ice-cold mixture of ethyl ether and methanol to remove the residual NHS. After drying under vacuum, PLGA-NHS (1 g, 0.059 mmol) was dissolved in chloroform (4 mL) followed by addition of NH2-PEG-OH (250 mg, 0.074 mmol) and N, N-diisopropylethylamine (28 mg, 0.22 mmol). The copolymer was precipitated with cold methanol after 12 hours and washed with the same solvent (35 mL) to remove unreacted PEG [15]. The resulting PEG-PLGA block copolymer was dried under vacuum and used for NP preparation without further treatment. The following are the main nuclear magnetic resonance (NMR) peaks of the sample:

1H-NMR (CDCl3 at 300 Hz) d 5.2 (m, (OCH(CH3)C (O)OCH2C(O)n-(CH2CH2O)m), 4.8 (m, (OCH(CH3)C (O)OCH2C(O)n-(CH2CH2O)m), 3.7 (s, (OCH(CH3)C (O)OCH2C(O)n-(CH2CH2O)m), 1.6 (d, (OCH(CH3)C (O)OCH2C(O))n-(CH2CH2O)m.

Preparation of roxithromycin-loaded pegylated PLGA nanoparticles

PEG-PLGA NPs loaded with RXN with different ratios of the drug were prepared by a solvent evaporation method [16,17]. Briefly, known amounts of polymer and RXN were added into a mixture of 1 ml DCM:acetone (3:10), which was suitably stirred to ensure that all material was dissolved. This organic phase was emulsified with 6.7 ml of aqueous solution of PVP (0.5% w/v) by sonication using a probe sonicator (Misonix S4000-010, USA) at amplitude 10 for 5 min. NPs were formed immediately, and gently stirred at room temperature for 5 h to evaporate the organic solvent. The resulting NP suspension was then ultracentrifuged (15,000 rpm for 20 min at room temperature) using a Sigma 3K30 centrifuge. After centrifugation, the NP precipitate was washed using the same volume of distilled water as the supernatant, and again centrifuged at 15,000 rpm for 15 minutes. The washing process was repeated three times in order to remove the adsorbed drugs. To Control of NP during post-formulation treatment, the size and drug loading of NP were studied through the storage in solid-state three months after freeze-drying.

Particle size and zeta potential measurement

The particle size distribution and poly dispersity index (PDI) of NPs were determined by Photon Correlation Spectroscopy (PCS) using a Zetasizer nanoZS (Malvern Instruments, Worcestershire, UK) at 25°C. Zeta potential of NPs was also measured by the same instrument. Before the measurement, all samples were diluted ten times with deionized water to prevent inter particle aggregation. All the measurements were triplicate and Mean±SD is reported.

Drug loading and entrapment efficiency

Lyophilized NPs (2.5 mg) were dissolved in 1 mL of acetonitrile and shaken lightly followed by sonication for 6 minutes. Thereafter, 2 mL of methanol was added to precipitate the polymer. The sample was filtered and the drug quantity in the filtrate was determined by high-pressure liquid chromatography. Drug loading was determined as the ratio of drug content of NPs to the total weight of the NPs. The entrapment efficacy was obtained as the ratio of the amount of RXN incorporated in NPs to the amount used for the preparation of NPs [18]. The experiments were carried out in triplicate.

In vitro drug release

The RXN release profile at pH 7.4 in phosphate-buffered saline and at pH 5.2 in acetate buffer was studied. Five mg of freeze-dried RXN loaded NPs was poured into screw-capped tubes and suspended in 10 mL of phosphate-buffered saline pH 7.4 or acetate buffer pH 5.2. The tubes were placed in a water bath maintained at 37 ± 0.5°C and shaken at 90 cycles/min. At fixed time intervals, the tubes were taken from the water bath and centrifuged at 21,000 g for 15 min. The NPs were resuspended in 10 mL of fresh buffer and placed back into the water bath to continue the release measurements. An aliquot of 9 mL was taken from the supernatant. A volume of 1 mL of methanol was added to precipitate any remaining PLGA, centrifuged for 15 min at 13255 rpm, and analyzed by high-pressure liquid chromatography. The experiments were carried out in triplicate [13].

HPLC analysis was performed at 37°C, using a Knauer apparatus (model K-1001, WellChrom, Berlin, Germany) equipped with a reversed-phase C18 column (25 cm × 0.46 cm internal diameter, pore size 5 μm; Teknokroma, Barcelona, Spain) and eluted isocratically with Mix 307 volumes of acetonitrile and 693 volumes of a 49.1 g/l solution of ammonium dihydrogen phosphate adjusted to PH 5.3 with dilute sodium hydroxide solution. The flow rate was fixed at 1.5 ml/min and detection was obtained by UV detection at 205 nm. The linear regression coefficient determined in the range 0.05–10 μg/ml was 0.9994 (n = 6). The method sensitivity was 0.05 μg/ml (signal to noise ratio, 3:1) [19].

Differential scanning calorimetry (DSC)

DSC was performed to investigate the physical status of RXN in the NPs. DSC scans of RXN, PEG-PLGA, physical mixture of PEG-PLGA and RXN and RXN-loaded NPs were performed on a Mettler DSC 823e equipped with Mettler STARe system software for the data acquisition. The samples were scanned at a speed of 5°C/min in a 30–250°C temperature range.

Surface morphology

Scanning electron microscopy (SEM, Philips XL 30, Philips, The Netherlands) was used to determine the shape and surface morphology of the NPs produced. NPs were coated with gold under vacuum before scanning electron microscopy.

Antibacterial efficacy test

Broth microdilution technique was utilized to determine the MIC of RXN loaded NPs. RXN solution with the same concentration of NPs and drug free NPs, prepared exactly similar to RXN NPs except no drug was added against *S. aureus*, *B. subtilis*, and *S.epidermidis* were used as positive and negative control groups. Drug free NPs were used to ensure the carrier and the ingredients do not have any antibacterial activity. The bacterium obtained in lyophilized form which was cultured in Luria Bertuni agar medium (Scharlau, Spain) after suspending in sterile distilled water. The plate incubated for 24 h at 37°C. Single colony from the plate was transferred into 4 ml fluid of LB medium and incubated over night at 37°C and 200 rpm in shaking incubator. The cells were harvested by centrifugation at 3000 rpm (Behdad, Iran) for 15 min at 4°C. Subsequently, they were washed twice and resuspended in Ringer solution to provide the concentration range of 105–106 CFU/ml for broth dilution method (National Committee for Clinical Laboratory Standards, 1996). A quantity of 12 tubes for each sample and each microbial strain were employed respectively. In each tube 1ml of medium was placed and was autoclaved at 121°C for 15 min. After sterilization, 1 ml of sample was added to the first tube and mixed [13].

Statistical analysis

One-way analyses of variance (ANOVA) were performed for comparison of the results. A value of $P < 0.05$ was considered to be significant.

Results and discussion

Synthesis of PEG-PLGA

In this study PEG-PLGA was synthesized and characterized. The basic chemical structure of PEG-PLGA copolymer was confirmed by 1H-NMR (Figure 1). This figure is very similar to the previously reported spectrum and confirms the synthesis of the PLGA-PEG copolymer. One of the prominent features is a peak at 3.7 ppm, matching the methylene groups of PEG. Overlapping doublets at 1.6 ppm are attributed to the methyl groups of the D- and L-lactic acid repeat units. The multiples at

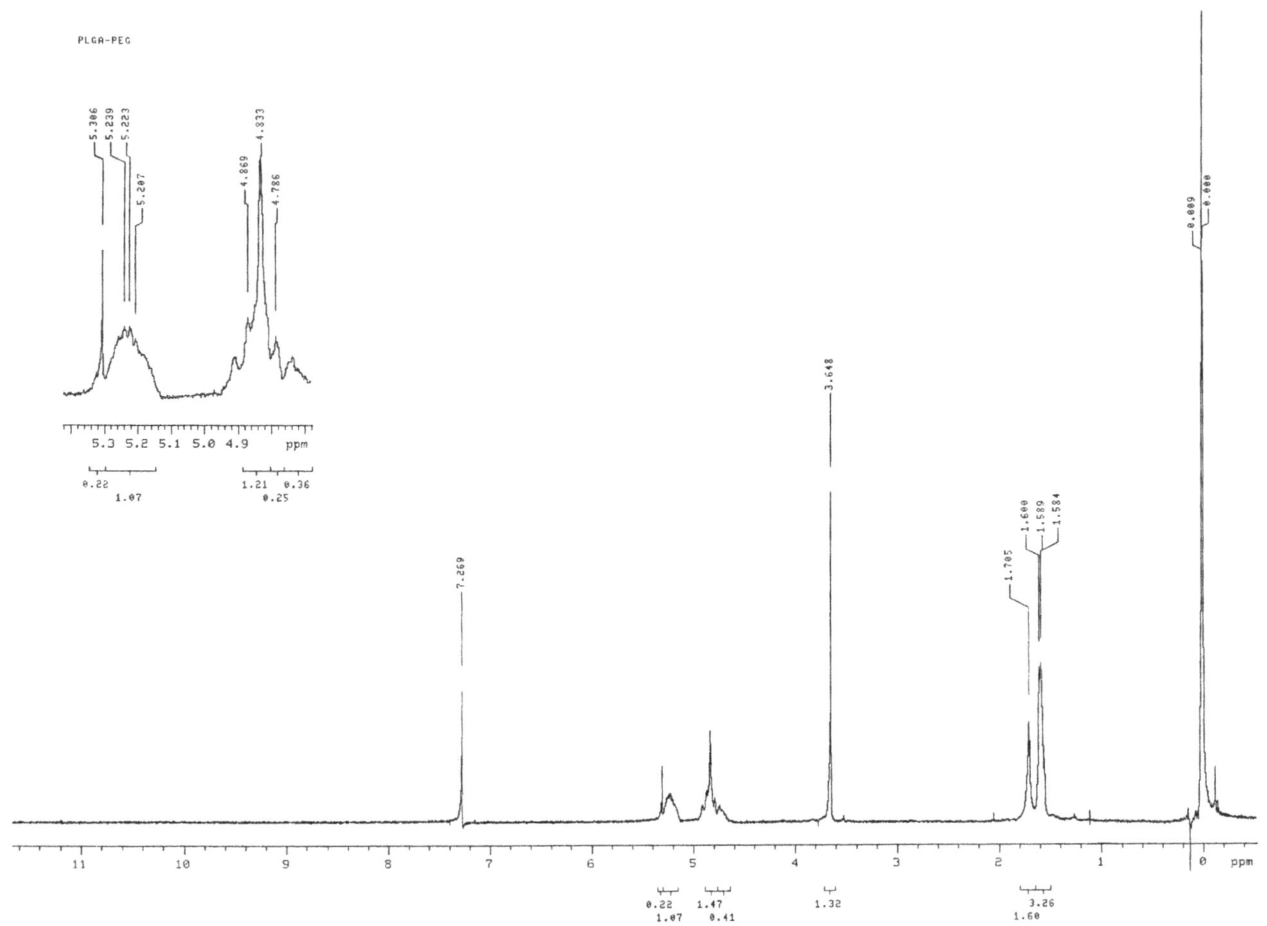

Figure 1 ^{1}H NMR spectrum of PEG–PLGA copolymer.

Table 1 Physicochemical characteristics of the roxithromycin nanoparticles

Sample	RXN-PLGA (mg)	Mean diameter ± SD (nm)	PDI ± SD	Zeta potential ± SD (mV)	Drug loading (%)	Entrapment efficiency (%)
S1	4 -25	152±8.4	0.09±0.10	−1.88±0.72	8.8±1.3	64.0±4.2
S2	5 -25	178±6.3	0.13±0.03	−2.63±0.53	10.5±1.1	73.0±3.8
S3	8.2- 25	196±10.5	0.11±0.05	−6.23±2.10	13.0±1.0	80.0±6.5
S4	10 -20	177±6.7	0.09±0.05	−2.48±0.36	11.0±2.1	34.0±5.5
S5	10- 10	181±11.6	0.93±0.12	−4.02±1.64	12.5±1.8	41.0±4.3

5.2 ppm and 4.8 ppm correspond to the lactic acid -CH and the glycolic acid -CH, respectively, with the high complexity of the peaks resulting from different D-lactic, L-lactic glycolic acid sequences in the polymer backbone [15].

Preparation and characterization of roxithromycin-loaded nanoparticles

Nanoparticles were prepared by sonication-solvent evaporation method. Entrapment efficiencies, drug loading, size, morphology and zeta potential of RXN pegylated NPs are reported in the Table 1. As shown in Table 1, the size of NPs was in the range of 150–200 nm. . Increasing the amount of internal phase, containing drug and polymer, increased the size of nanoparticles. This may be the result of enhanced viscous forces resisting droplet break down by sonication. The viscous forces is in opposition to the shear stresses in the organic phase and the final finishing size and size distribution of particles depends on the net shear stress available presented for droplet breakdown. Narrow range of size distribution was observed for NPs and the prepared NPs exhibited a relative monodisperse distribution. As seen in Figure 2, SEM micrograph of the RXN loaded NPs confirms that NPs are in spherical shape with smooth surfaces (Figure 2). All formulations appeared to be homogenous irrespective of their compositions. The particle size is an important parameter, as the biopharmaceutical properties of nanoparticles can be influenced by its physicochemical properties. The pegylation of nanoparticles increases the blood circulation of nanoparticles which suitable for IV administration [19,20]. The negative zeta potential of the PLGA nanoparticles tends to limit their capability to interact with negatively charged plasmids and intracellular uptake. Pegylation of PLGA helps to adjust the surface charge of the nanoparticles to become less negative. In this study, PLGA-PEG NPs showed less negative zeta potential (−1.9±0.11) than PLGA NPs (−25.4±0.24). It has been proved that the amount of phagocytosis is the lowest when zeta potential is closer to zero [21].

The table also shows an increase in the amount of PLGA resulted in an increase in the drug entrapment. This may be attributed to the higher viscosity of the internal organic phase for higher PLGA ratios, which in turn would decrease the diffusion coefficient of the drug.

DSC was carried out to investigate the effect of the process on thermal behavior of formulations [20]. The DSC scans of samples and the melting point data are presented in Figure 3. At the mentioned scanning rate (5°C/min) pure RXN powder had an endothermic peak at 125°C. However, no melting peak could be detected for the NP formulations. This shows that DTX in the NPs is in an amorphous or disordered crystalline phase, miscible in polymeric NPs. The reduction in enthalpy of

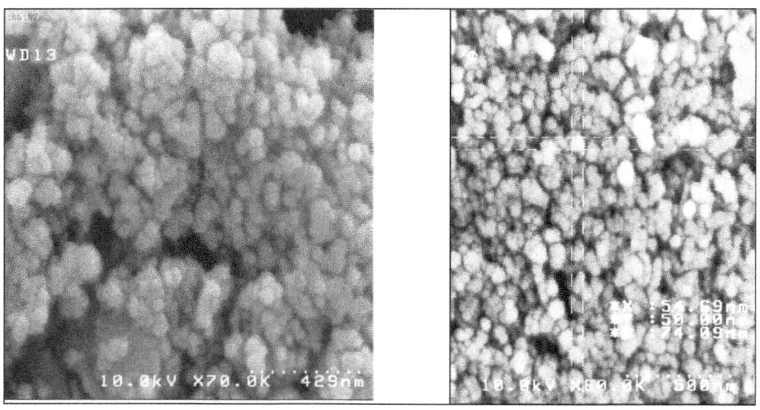

Figure 2 SEM micrographs of nanoparticles showing the shape and the surface characteristics of NPs.

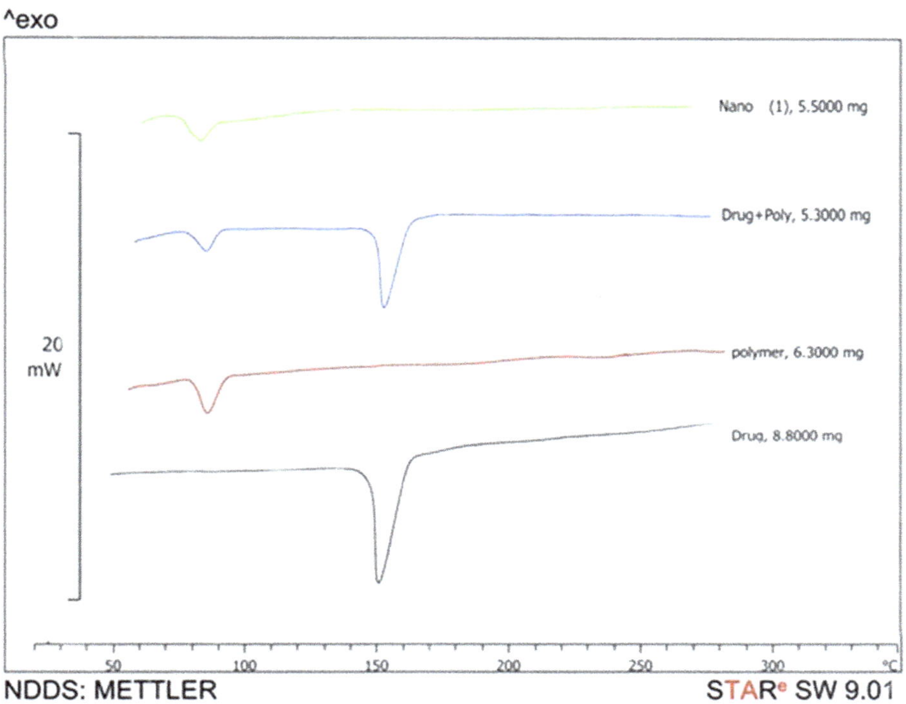

Figure 3 **DSC thermograms of roxithromycin, PEG-PLGA, physical mixture of roxithromycin and polymer, and roxithromycin loaded PEG-PLGA nanoparticles.**

the physical mixture of drug–polymer is due to the presence of smaller amount of drug in the mixture in comparison with pure drug.

NPs when freeze dried with sucrose (10% w/w), as cryoprotectant, were physically stable. No significant changes in size, zeta potential or drug content was detected after freeze dried NPs kept at 4°C for three months.

In vitro roxithromycin release

The profile of in vitro release of RXN from NPs in the acetate buffer (pH 5.2) and phosphate-buffered

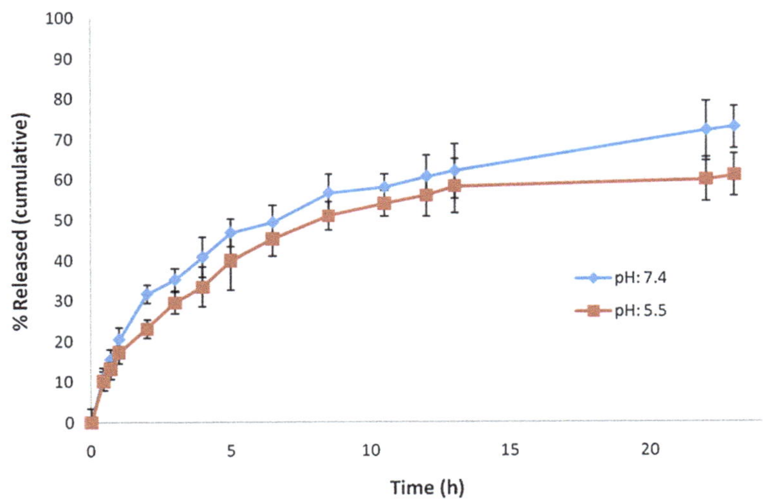

Figure 4 **In vitro roxithromycin release profiles from nanoparticles in acetate buffer (pH 5.5, 37°C) and phosphate-buffered solution (pH = 7.4, 37°C).** Data are represented as mean ± standard deviation (n = 3).

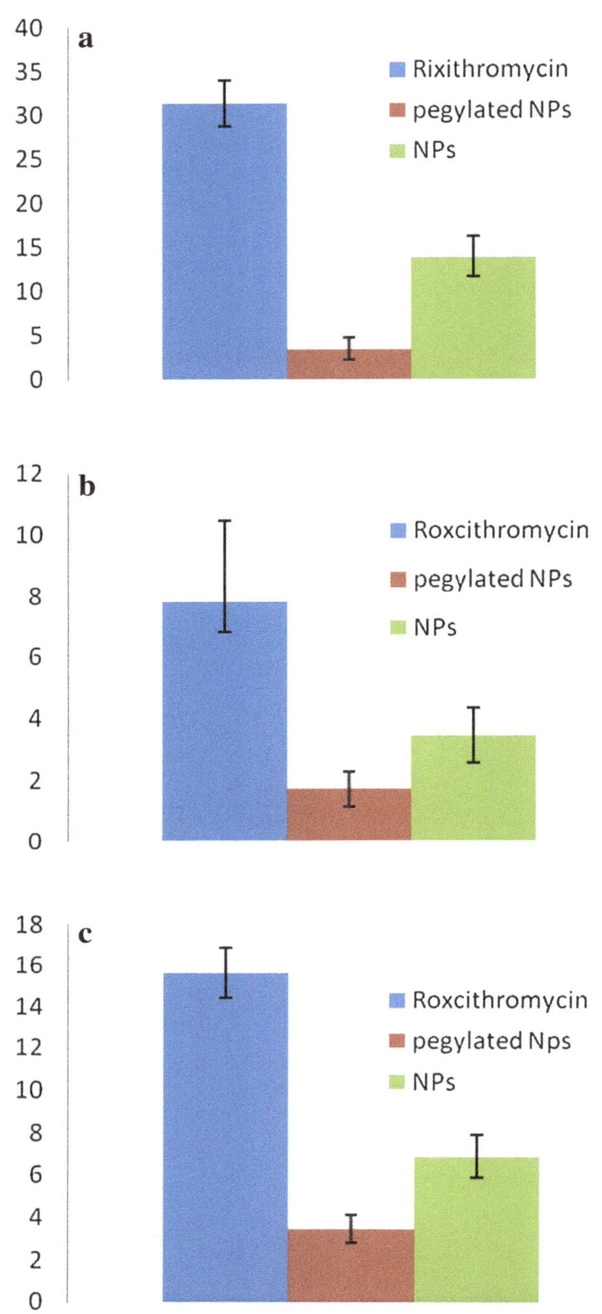

Figure 5 Minimum inhibitory concentrations (MICs) (±SD) of the intact roxithromycin, roxithromycin loaded nanoparticle and pegylated NPs suspensions against *S. aureus* (a), *S. epodermidis* (b) and B. subtilis (c) (n = 3).

saline (pH 7.4) within first day is depicted in Figure 4. During the first hours of release, an early burst release greater than 50% was detected. A slow and steady release of RXN was observed after the burst release. The burst release may be due to the release of RXN loaded on the surface or just beneath the surface of the NPs. Then the sustained release is mainly due to the diffusion of drug molecules through the polymeric matrix of the NPs.

Antibacterial activity of the nanoparticle suspensions

The MIC of PEG-PLGA formulations and RXN powder on *S. aureus, B. subtilis, and S. epidermidis* are reported in Figure 5. Drug free polymeric nanoparticles showed no antibacterial activity which indicates that none of the ingredients have any antibacterial effect. The MIC of RXN loaded PLGA NPs were 2.3 times lower on *S. aureus*, 2.2 times lower on *B. subtilis,* and 2.4 times lower on *S. epidermidis* compared to RXN solution. Consequently, in vitro anti-microbial activity of RXN PLGA NPs is better than the commercialized drug formulations. Additionally, The MIC of RXN loaded PEG-PLGA NPs were 9 times lower on *S. aureus*, 4.5 times lower on both *B. subtilis*, and *S. epidermidis* compared to RXN solution. The higher antibacterial effect of RXN PLGA NPs and PEG-PLGA NPs may have been resulted from higher bacterial adhesion of the NPs. In other studies enhanced antimicrobial activity from PLGA NPs containing antimicrobial agents has been reported [21,22]. The improved the therapeutic effect of the nanoparticulate antibacterial delivery systems may the result of increased drug concentration nearby its target. Moreover, improved penetration of NPs from biological membranes is also generally accepted. For RXN to be effective it should pass the bacterial membrane to reach its intra cellular site of action, subunit 50S of the bacterial ribosome to inhibits the transaction of peptides.

Conclusion

In this study, RXN a semi-synthetic macrolide antibiotic was successfully loaded into PEG-PLGA NPs. MIC tests indicated that antibacterial activity of RXN NPs increased several times compared to RXN aqueous solution against *S. aureus*, *B. subtilis*, and *S. epidermidis*. This allows more efficient therapy compared with the antibiotic in its original form. However, more studies are necessary to be approved in animals to verify the pharmacological activities.

Competing interest

The authors declare that they have no competing interests.

Authors' contributions

MNK conceived the study, synthesized the copolymer and drafted the manuscript. MSM carried out the experiments and assisted MNK in drafting the manuscript. SHM assisted in preparation of nanoparticles. NS Supervised the antibacterial studies. HJ participated in the antimicrobial studies. MA supervised the synthesis and characterization of copolymers. SJM and BD assisted in preparation and characterization of nanoparticles. FA supervised the preparation and characterization of nanoparticles. RD supervised the project and participated in its design and coordination and is the corresponding author of the manuscript. All authors read and approved the final manuscript.

Acknowledgments
The authors would like to thank Nanotechnology Research Centre and the Research Deputy of Tehran university of Medical Sciences for their financial support.

Author details
[1]Novel Drug Delivery Lab, Faculty of Pharmacy, Tehran University of Medical Sciences, Tehran 1417614411, Iran. [2]Nanotechnology Research Centre, Faculty of Pharmacy, Tehran University of Medical Sciences, Tehran, Iran. [3]Department of Drug and Food Control, Faculty of Pharmacy, Tehran University of Medical Sciences, Tehran, Iran. [4]Department of Medicinal Chemistry, Faculty of Pharmacy, Tehran University of Medical Sciences, Tehran, Iran.

References

1. Cohen ML: **Changing patterns of infectious disease.** *Nature* 2000, **406:**762–767.
2. Gold HS, Moellering RC: **Antimicrobial-drug resistance.** *N Engl J Med* 1996, **335:**1445–1453.
3. Walsh C: **Molecular mechanisms that confer antibacterial drug resistance.** *Nature* 2000, **406:**775–781.
4. Huh AJ, Kwon YJ: **Nanoantibiotics: a new paradigm for treating infectious diseases using nanomaterials in the antibiotics resistant era.** *J Control Rel.* 2011, **156**(2):128–145.
5. Zhang L, Pornpattananangkul D, Hu CM, Huang CM: **Development of nanoparticles for antimicrobial drug delivery.** *Curr Med Chem* 2010, **17:**585–594.
6. Zhang L, Gu FX, Chan JM, Wang AZ, Langer RS: **Nanoparticles in medicine: therapeutic applications and developments.** *Clin Pharmacol Ther* 2008, **83**(5):761–769.
7. Danhier F, Ansorena E, Silva JM, Coco R, Le A, Préat V: **PLGA-based nanoparticles :An overview of biomedical applications.** *J Control Rel.* 2012, **161**(2):505–522.
8. Gref R, Domp A, Quellec P, Blunk T, Muller RH, Verbavatz JM, Langer R: **The controlled intravenous delivery of drugs using PEG coated sterically stabilized nanospheres.** *Adv Drug Del Rev.* 1995, **16:**215–233.
9. Tobío M, Sánchez A, Vila A, Soriano I, Evora C, Vila-Jato J, *et al:* **The role of PEG on the stability in digestive fluids and in vivo fate of PEG-PLA nanoparticles following oral administration. Colloids and surfaces.** *B, Biointerfaces* 2000, **18:**315–323.
10. Spencer RC, Wheat PF: **In vitro activity of roxithromycin against Moraxella catarrhalis.** *Diagn Microbiol Infect Dis* 1992, **15**(4 Suppl):63S–65S.
11. Patil R, Thakkar S, Doke S, Boldhane S, Kakade S, Kuchekar B: *Studies on Characterization, Solubility, Dissolution Rate and Antimicrobial Activity of Roxithromycin - Cyclodextrin System.* www.aapsj.org/abstracts/AM_2005/AAPS2005-002259.pdf.
12. Gandomi N, Aboutaleb E, Noori M, Atyabi F, Fazeli MR, Farbod E, *et al:* **Solid lipid nanoparticles of ciprofloxacin hydrochloride with enhanced antibacterial activity.** *J Nanosci Lett.* 2012, **2:**21.
13. Esmaeili F, Hosseini-Nasr M, Rad-Malekshahi M, Samadi N, Atyabi F, Dinarvand R: **Preparation and antibacterial activity evaluation of rifampicin-loaded poly lactide-co-glycolide nanoparticles.** *Nanomedicine: NBM.* 2007, **3**(2):161–167.
14. Gao Y, Cui F, Guan Y, Yang L, Wang Y, Zhang L: **Preparation of roxithromycin-polymeric microspheres by the emulsion solvent diffusion method for taste masking.** *Int J Pharm* 2006, **318**(1–2):62–69.
15. Koopaei MN, Dinarvand R, Amini M, Rabbani H, Emami S, Ostad SN, *et al:* **Docetaxel immunonanocarriers as targeted delivery systems for her2-positive tumor cells: preparation, characterization, and cytotoxicity studies.** *Int J* 2011, **6:**1903–1912.
16. Esmaeili F, Atyabi F, Dinarvand R: **Preparation and characterization of estradiol-loaded PLGA nanoparticles using homogenization-solvent diffusion method.** *DARU* 2008, **16:**196–202.
17. Ebrahimnejad P, Dinarvand R, Sajadi A, Jaafari MR, Nomani AR, Azizi E, *et al:* **Preparation and in vitro evaluation of actively targetable nanoparticles for SN-38 delivery against HT-29 cell lines.** *Nanomedicine: NBM.* 2010, **6**(3):478–485.
18. Kashi TSJ, Eskandarion S, Esfandyari-Manesh M, Marashi SMA, Samadi N, Fatemi SM F, Eshraghi S, Dinarvand R: **Improved drug loading and antibacterial activity of minocycline-loaded PLGA nanoparticles prepared by solid/oil/water ion pairing method.** *Int J Nanomed* 2012, **7:**221–234.
19. Commission CP: *Pharmacopoeia of the People's Republic of China 2010 (Set of 3, English edition)*; 2011.
20. Yadav KS, Sawant KK: **Modified nanoprecipitation method for preparation of cytarabine-loaded PLGA nanoparticles.** *AAPS PharmSciTech* 2010, **11:**1456–465.
21. Peng HS, Liu XJ, Lv GX, Sun B, Kong QF, Zhai DX, Wang Q, Zhao W, Wang GY, Wang DD, Li HL, Jin LHKN: **Voriconazole into PLGA nanoparticles: Improving agglomeration and antifungal efficacy.** *Int J Pharm* 2008, **352:**29–35.
22. Grislain L, Couvreur P, Lenaerts V, Roland M, Deprez Decampaneere D, Speiser P: **Pharmacokinetics and distribution of a biodegradable drug-carrier.** *Int J Pharm* 1983, **15:**335–345.

The effect of semelil (angipars®) on bone resorption and bone formation markers in type 2 diabetic patients

Shirin Hasani-Ranjbar*, Zahra Jouyandeh, Mostafa Qorbani, Mahbubeh Hemmatabadi and Bagher Larijani

Abstract

Background and purpose of the study: Diabetes mellitus has been recognized as a major risk factor for osteoporosis in which bone turnover is affected by different mechanisms. As the morbidity, mortality and financial cost related to osteoporosis are expected to rise in Iran in coming years, and considering the efficacy of Angipars® for improvement of different ulcers which made it a new herbal drug in diabetic foot ulcer, there is a need to evaluate the effect of this new drug on different organs including bone resorption and bone formation markers.

Methods: In this randomized, double- blind clinical trial, 61 diabetic patients were included. The subjects were randomly divided into intervention and control groups. Subjects of intervention group received 100 mg of Angipars® twice a day. Laboratory tests including bone resorption and bone formation markers were performed at baseline and after 3 months.

Result: 31 patients in study group and 30 patients in control group finished the study. The mean age of the study population and the mean disease duration was respectively 51.8 ± 6.2 and 7.5 ± 4.7 years with no significant differences between intervention and control patients. No statistically significant differences between patients and controls were observed in pyridinoline, osteocalcin, urine calcium, bone alkaline phosphatase and tumor necrosis factor (TNF-α). Only urine creatinine level significantly changed between two groups after 3 month of treatment (p-value: 0.029)

Conclusion: In conclusion, the findings of this study indicate that Semelil (Angipars®) had no beneficial or harmful effects on bone. It might be other effects of this new component on bone turnover process which need more studies and more time to be discovered.

Keywords: Diabetes mellitus type 2, Bone turnover markers, Angipars®, Semelil

Introduction

Diabetes mellitus affects skeletal system and bone metabolism through multiple pathways and it has been recognized as a major risk factor for osteoporosis [1]. Besides, osteoporosis is the most prevalent metabolic bone disease, which dramatically decreases the quality of life and increase financial burden on diabetic patients [2,3].

The relationship between diabetes and osteoporosis has been the main subject of many researches. Several mechanisms have been proposed for diabetes-related osteoporosis. Clinical trials uniformly support the fact that new bone formation and bone quality, are altered in both types of diabetes. Bone quality changes may be affected by micro vascular events common in diabetes [4,5]. Poor glycemic control can induce hypercalciuria which has been considered a potential risk factor for osteoporosis in patients with type 2 diabetes [6,7]. Besides, vitamin D deficiency is common in patients with type 2 diabetes. In the study by Dobnig et al., mean serum parathyroid hormone (PTH) and osteocalcin levels were significantly lower in treated type 2 diabetic patients; therefore, bone formation appears to be decreased in diabetes [8]. It is shown that bone metabolism and glucose metabolism are associated with each other through the action of osteocalcin [9]. Also, an

* Correspondence: sh_hasani@sina.tums.ac.ir
Endocrinology and Metabolism Research Institute, Tehran University of Medical Sciences, Tehran, Iran

increase in inflammation and associated cytokines accelerate bone turnover and bone loss in diabetic patients [4].

On the other hand, diabetes mellitus is associated with oxidative reactions. Many studies showed that increase in free oxygen radicals could induce tissue damage and abnormalities in anti-oxidant defenses in diabetes. Oxidative stress can impair the balance between proteolytic enzymes and their inhibitors that may cause or worsen osteoporosis in diabetic patients [10]. In vitro studies have shown that oxidative stress inhibits osteoblastic differentiation and induces osteoblast insults and apoptosis. Thus, oxidative stress may be related to the pathogenesis of diabetic bone disorders [11-13].

Melilotus officinalis (yellow sweet clover) is a species of a plant in the family of *Feabaceae*, native to Eurasia and introduced in North America, Africa and Australia. *Melilotus officinalis* contains coumarin, flavonoides (kampeferol, quercetin glycosides), triterpene saponins and volatile oil. *Melilotus officinalis* has antiphlogistic and antiedematous effects, which explain its use for inflammatory and congestive edema. It increases venous reflux and improves lymphatic kinetics [14]. Recent studies have reported a potential usefulness of administration of *Melilotus officinalis* extract for microcirculation improvement and anti-inflammation effects. Current studies showed that *Melilotus officinalis* (Angipars®) can improve diabetic foot ulcers [15,16]. *This product* also decreased nitric oxide (NO) synthesis [17] which has important effects on bone cell function and plays an important role in cytokine and inflammation induced bone loss [18]. Also it has been shown that coumarin and vitamin-K supplementations increase the serum markers for bone formation (including osteocalcin and bone alkaline phosphatase) and may reduce urinary calcium and hydroxyproline excretion (well-known markers for bone resorption). These supplements are two main components of *M. Officinalis* extracts [19]. As the morbidity, mortality and financial cost related to osteoporosis are expected to rise in Iran in coming years, and considering the efficacy of Angipars® for improvement of different ulcers which made it a new herbal drug in diabetic foot ulcer, there is a need to evaluate the effect of this new drug on different organs including bone. Since there is a need for alternative and complementary pharmacotherapy which has better results and less complications comparing to previous methods and considering the mechanisms involved in diabetes-induced osteoporosis [2,20,21], we decided to conduct a randomized clinical trial to examine the effect of *Melilotus officinalis* extract on bone formation and resorption markers in diabetic patients with osteoporosis.

Materials and methods

A double blind randomized clinical trial was conducted on diabetic patients referred to the Shariati hospital diabetes clinic of the Tehran University of Medical Sciences (TUMS). These patients had previously confirmed diabetes type 2, according to the ADA (American Diabetes Association) criteria. The Participants were enrolled to the study based on the following inclusion and exclusion criteria.

Sixty one diabetic patients, between 40–60 years old, under treatment with life style modification and/or oral hypoglycemic agents and no recent inflammatory and infectious process (at least for the past 4–6 weeks and during the study) were included. Patients with chronic disease such as chronic renal failure (serum creatinine > 270 μmol/L), chronic liver failure and decompensate heart failure were excluded. Other exclusion criteria include: coronary artery bypass graft (CABG), respiratory infectious disease, proliferative retinopathy, pregnant or lactating females, childbearing- aged women without safe contraception methods, diabetic foot ulceration or gangrene, smoking, alcohol abuse, hemoglobin a1c (HgA1C) > 9%, any type of known drug hypersensitivity, malignancy in breast, liver and genital system, vascular disease, fracture history during the past 3 years and use of multivitamin supplements and other traditional drugs in the previous 4–6 weeks, the use of medications that affect bone metabolism, such as corticosteroids, gonadotropin releasing hormone (GnRH) analogous drugs, anticonvulsant, heparin, aluminum-containing antacids, thyroid hormone, thiazides and supplements containing calcium and other minerals. All patients participating in this study were under a same lifestyle and were matched for the drug they used; and also all the patients received just oral agents (metformin/glybenclamide).

Patients' inclusion was completely informative and voluntary. After inclusion of each patient, complete explanation was given about the goal of study, probable side effects of the drug and patients' rights during the research process. Then, written informed consent according to institutional guidelines was obtained before treatment. The study protocol was approved by the Medical Ethics Committee of Medical Sciences/TUMS (code number: 0011).

In this study, sample randomization was based on "Permuted Balanced Block" method by an epidemiologist. Patients were randomly assigned into 2 groups: intervention (n = 31) and control (n = 30). Semelil (Angipars®) was prepared by Pars Roos drug company (Tehran, Iran). In the intervention group, patients received 100 mg of Angipars® capsules twice a day. In the control group, participants received placebo (a non absorbable polymer) with the same dose. All participants were given a similar lifestyle program. The patients were followed for a period of three months.

For the primary assessment, a complete set of evaluations was performed which included:

1. A complete past medical history of the trial patients and an extensive physical examination were done by a trained physician, a dietary questionnaire completed at the beginning and the end of the study.

Table 1 Baseline characteristics of subjects in mean ± SD

Variable	Group A	Group B	P-value
Age (yr)	51.87 ± 6.21	51.43 ± 5.37	0.654
BMI (kg/m2)	28.22 ± 3.97	29.98 ± 5.32	0.269
Lumbar T-score	−0.36 ± 1.04	−0.25 ± 1.39	0.731
Femoral T-score	0.27 ± 0.97	0.21 ± 1.09	0.833
Fasting blood sugar	166.51 ± 51.97	180.80 ± 74.99	0.148
Duration of diabetes	6 (8)	8.5 (6.5)	0.154
Sex (female)	25 (80.6%)	23 (76.7%)	0.762

Group A: Diabetic patients on drug.
Group B: Control group.
BMI: Body Mass Index.
Duration of diabetes is presented as median (IQR).
IQR: 75th – 25th.
Sex is presented as a number (percent).

2. Measurement of bone mineral density and reporting T-score and Z-score at the baseline, to be sure if there is a major difference between patients in groups.
3. Approximately 20 ml blood (after fasting for over 12 hours) was taken from every participant. Blood samples were centrifuged within 3 hours of sampling for 20 minute to obtain serum. Samples were frozen at −80°C and they were immediately sent to the hormone laboratory of Endocrinology and Metabolism Research Institute (EMRI)/ Shariati hospital/ TUMS. Baseline laboratory tests were including a complete blood count, fasting blood sugar, HbA1C, bone alkaline phosphatase, osteocalcin, serum TNF-α, urine calcium and creatinine, urine pyridinoline.
4. Monthly documentation of patient's compliance to therapy and acceptance of side effects.
5. Recording any probable side effects and necessary managements.

The distribution of qualitative variables was assessed by Kolmogorov-Smirnov test. Descriptive statistics, including mean, median frequencies, and percentages, were used to describe the population of study. Mean-Whitney U or *T* test and Chi-square test was performed for comparing quantitative and qualitative variables between groups respectively. The Analysis of covariance (ANCOVA) test was used for comparison outcomes between case and control group. Data were analyzed with SPSS software version 16 (SPSS Inc, Chicago, Illinois). P-values < 0.05 (2-sided test) were considered statistically significant.

Results

Approximately eighty percent (78.7%) of participants were women. The mean age of participants in intervention and placebo group was respectively 51.87 ± 6.21 and 51.43 ± 5.37 years. The baseline characteristics of the participants are shown in Table 1. There was no significant difference in baseline characteristics and bone markers' level between group A and B. After 3 months of treatment, no statistically significant differences between patients and controls were observed in pyridinoline, osteocalcin, urine calcium, bone alkaline phosphatase and TNF- α. Only urine creatinine level significantly changed between two groups after 3 months of treatment (p-value: 0.029). Table 2 shows mean levels of bone markers before, after 3 months and difference values between and within groups in intervention and placebo groups.

Discussion

There are different hypothesis about the mechanisms of diabetic bone disorders including oxidative stress [11]. Increasing number of osteoporotic patients in recent years especially as a complication of diabetes mellitus causes a need for an alternative new pharmacotherapy which has better results and less complications comparing to previous methods [2]. Angipars® (Semelil) a new herbal drug which is derived from a plant named *Melilotus Officinalis* has been investigated as a useful new drug in treatment of diabetic ulcers in a clinical trial study in Iran [22].

Melilotus Officinalis has been proved to be helpful in reducing inflammation, regulation of the immune system

Table 2 Mean levels of bone markers before and after 3 month of treatment in drug (A) and placebo (B) groups

Variables	Group A			Group B			Difference		**P-value
	Baseline	3rd month	*P-value	Baseline	3rd month	*P-value	Group A	Group B	
Pyridinoline	51.17 ± 87.90	13.06 ± 5.81	0.766	41.01 ± 38.94	15.67 ± 11.05	0.268	−40.8 ± 96.5	−28.2 ± 42.6	0.656
Osteocalcin	2.20 ± 0.47	2.5 ± 0.58	0.564	2.22 ± 0.60	2.24 ± 0.82	0.230	0.37 ± 0.80	0.23 ± 0.96	0.390
Urine Calcium	9.09 ± 9.08	8.10 ± 6.98	0.045	6.95 ± 5.03	5.77 ± 6.31	0.044	−1 ± 9.1	0.21 ± 5.9	0.683
Urine Creatinine	120.55 ± 58.59	108.23 ± 48.99	0.273	111.68 ± 72.39	130.39 ± 68.47	0.003	−11.2 ± 64	34.6 ± 49.2	0.029
Bone Alkaline phosphatase	24.9 ± 7	20.8 ± 19.7	0.014	23.8 ± 10.4	20.6 ± 7.5	0.048	−4.5 ± 7	−3 ± 10.8	0.364
TNF-α	91.68 ± 52.92	88.84 ± 55.75	0.006	90.85 ± 27.21	80.94 ± 28.73	0.026	−4.2 ± 26.1	−12.4 ± 28.2	0.267

Group A: Diabetic patients on drug.
Group B: Control group.
*P-value according to paired *T*-test.
** P-value according to ANCOVA test.

and improvement of vascular blood flow which is thought to be due to the inhibitory effect of natural coumarin on oxidative DNA damage and formation [23,24]. No previously human or animal study has been published on the effects of Angipars® on bone markers in diabetic patients. Although Leilei Bao et al. found that some components in *M. Officinalis* were potent inhibitors of osteoclastogenesis which leads to decrease in the resorption capacity of osteoclasts [25], in this study no significant changes were seen in bone markers due to treatment with Angipars®.

Angipars® is a new herbal drug proved being useful in healing diabetic foot ulcers however the exact mechanism of its action is unknown yet. Our study showed that this drug had no adverse effect or beneficial effect on bone formation and bone resorption in diabetic patients.

Actually this study has some limitations including small sample size and short length of the study. It seems to us that a new study should be designed for another 6 months and a higher dose of Angipars® to find out whether it gives better results.

Conclusion

In conclusion, the findings of this study indicate that Angipars® had no beneficial or harmful effects on bone. It might be other effects of this new component on bone turnover process and markers which need more studies and more time to be discovered.

Competing interests

The authors declare that they have no competing interests.

Authors' contributions

Dr SR: Suggesting the main idea of the clinical trial study, preparing the proposal and editing the article (20%). Dr ZJ: Writing the article and abstract (20%). Dr MG: Epidemiologic review and data analysis (20%). Dr MH: Running the study as data collection and other performing process during the study (20%). Dr BL: Main supporter of the study (20%). All authors read and approve the final manuscript.

Acknowledgement

The authors would like to thank all the staff of the Endocrinology and Metabolic Research Center and Pharmaceutical Sciences Research Center and all the individuals who took part in this study. Authors also thank Pars Roos Company that provided Angipars® and placebo. This study was an in house study with no financial support. Authors declare no conflict of interest.

References

1. Leidig-Bruckner G, Zeigler R: **Diabetes mellitus a risk factor for osteoporosis?** *Exp Clin Endocrinol Diabetes* 2001, **109**(suppl2):s493–s514.
2. Reginster JY, Burlet N: **Osteoporosis: a still increasing prevalence.** *Bone* 2006, **38:**S4–S9.
3. Altindag O, Erel O, Soran N, Celik H, Selek S: **Total oxidative/anti-oxidative status and relation to bone mineral density in osteoporosis.** *Rheumatol Int* 2008, **28:**317–321.
4. Schwartz AV: **Diabetes mellitus: does it affect bone?** *Calcif Tissue Int* 2003, **73:**515–519.
5. Vogt MT, Cauley JA, Kuller LH, Nevitt MC: **Bone mineral density and blood flow to the lower extremities: the study of osteoporotic fractures.** *J Bone Miner Res* 1997, **12**(2):283–289.
6. Raskin P, Stevenson MR, Barilla DE, Pak CY: **The hypercalciuria of diabetes mellitus: its amelioration with insulin.** *Clin Endocrinol (Oxf)* 1978, **9:**329–335.
7. Brandi ML: **Bone health and diabetes.** *Medicographia* 2010, **32:**364–369.
8. Dobnig H, Piswanger-Sölkner JC, Roth M, Obermayer-Pietsch B, Tiran A, Strele A, Maier E, Maritschnegg P, Sieberer C, Fahrleitner-Pammer A: **Type 2 diabetes mellitus in nursing home patients: effects on bone turnover, bone mass, and fracture risk.** *J Clin Endocrinol Metab* 2006, **91:**3355–3363.
9. Kanazawa I, Yamaguchi T, Masahiro Y, Yamauchi M, Kurioka S, Yano S, Sugimoto T: **Serum osteocalcin level is associated with glucose metabolism and atherosclerosis parameters in Type 2 diabetes mellitus.** *J Clin Endocrinol Metab* 2009, **94**(1):45–49.
10. Banfi G, Lorio E, Corsi M: **Oxidative stress, free radicals and bone remodeling.** *Clin Chem Lab Med* 2008, **46**(11):1550–1555.
11. Hamada Y, Fujii H, Fukagawa M: **Role of oxidative stress in diabetic bone disorder.** *Bone* 2009, **45:**35–38.
12. Bai XC, Lu D, Bai J, Zheng H, Ke ZY, Li XM, Luo SQ: **Oxidative stress inhibits osteoblastic differentiation of bone cells by ERK and NF-kappaB.** *Biochem Bioph Res Co* 2004, **314:**197–207.
13. Pasco JA, Nicholson GC, Ng F, Henry MJ, Williams LJ, *et al:* **Oxidative stress may be a common mechanism linking major depression and osteoporosis.** *Acta Neuropsychiatr* 2008, **20:**112–116.
14. Abdollahi M, Farzamfar B, Salari P, Khorram Khorshid HR, Larijani B, Farhadi M, Madani SH: **Evaluation of acute and sub-chronic toxicity of semelil (ANGIPARS™), a new phytotherapeutic drug for wound healing in rodents.** *DARU* 2008, **16**(1):7–14.
15. Larijani B, Heshmat R, Bahrami A, Delshad H, Ranjbar Omrani G, Mohammad K, Heidarpour R, Mohajeri Tehrani MR, Kamali K, Farhadi M, Gharibdoust F, Madani SH: **Effects of intravenous semelil (ANGIPARSTM) on diabetic foot ulcers healing: a multicenter clinical trial.** *DARU* 2008, **6**(1):35–40.
16. Larijani B, Hasani Ranjbar S: **Overview of diabetic foot; novel treatments in diabetic foot ulcer.** *DARU* 2008, **16**(supplement 1):1–6.
17. Luminita P-M, Alina Elena P, Pârvu M, Taamas M, Buia R, Puia M: **Effects of melilotus officinalis on acute inflammation.** *Phytother Res* 2002, **16:**316–319.
18. Sheweita SA, Khoshhal KI: **Calcium metabolism and oxidative stress in bone fractures: role of antioxidants.** *Curr Drug Metab* 2007, **8**(5):519–525.
19. Verneer C, Gisbers B, Craciun A, Greonen-Van Dooren M, Knapen M: **Effects of vitamin K on bone mass and bone metabolism.** *J Nutr* 1996, **126:**1187s–1191s.
20. Hasani-Ranjbar S, Larijani B, Abdollahi M: **A systematic review of Iranian medicinal plants useful in diabetes mellitus.** *Arch Med Sci* 2008, **4**(3):285–292.
21. Mehri A, Hasani Ranjbar S, Larijani B, Abdollahi M: **A systematic review of efficacy and safety of urtica dioica in the treatment of diabetes.** *Int J Pharmacol* 2011, **7**(2):161–170.
22. Hemmatabadi M, Abdollahi M, Bakhshayeshi S, Heshmat R, Baeeri M, Azimaraghi O, Larijani B: **Benefits of angipars on oxidant-antioxidant balance in diabetic patients; a randomized, double-blind placebo controlled clinical trial.** *DARU* 2010, **17**(1):50–55.
23. Farzamfar B, Minaie B, Mobtaker M, Salari P, Khorasani R, Abdollahi M: **Effect of electromagnetic form of melilotus officinalis extract on dermal wound healing in diabetic mice.** *Pharmacologyonline* 2008, **2:**246–254.
24. Kaneko T, Tahara S, Takabayashi F: **Inhibitory effect of natural coumarin compounds, esculetin and 25. esculin, on oxidative DNA damage and formation of aberrant crypt foci and tumors induced by 1,2-dimethylhydrazine in rat colons.** *Biol Pharm Bull* 2007, **30**(11):2052–2057.
25. Leilei B, Luping Q, Lei L, Yanbin W, Ting H, Liming X, Qiaoyan Z: **Anthraquinone compounds from morinda officinalis inhibits osteoclastic bone resorption in vitro.** *Chem Biol Interact* 2011, **194:**97–105.

Monitoring of adverse drug reactions associated with antihypertensive medicines at a university teaching hospital in New Delhi

Fowad Khurshid[1,2], Mohammed Aqil[1*], Mohammad Shamshir Alam[1], Prem Kapur[3] and Krishna K Pillai[1]

Abstract

Aim: To monitor the adverse drug reactions (ADRs) caused by antihypertensive medicines prescribed in a university teaching hospital.

Methods: The present work was an open, non-comparative, observational study conducted on hypertensive patients attending the Medicine OPD of Majeedia Hospital, Jamia Hamdard, New Delhi, India by conducting patient interviews and recording the data on ADR monitoring form as recommended by Central Drugs Standard Control Organization (CDSCO), Government of India.

Results: A total of 21 adverse drug reactions were observed in 192 hypertensive patients. Incidence of adverse drug reactions was found to be higher in patients more than 40 years in age, and females experienced more ADRs (n = 14, 7.29%) than males, 7 (3.64%). Combination therapy was associated with more number of adverse drug reactions (66.7%) as against monotherapy (33.3%). Calcium channel blockers were found to be the most frequently associated drugs with adverse drug reactions (n = 7), followed by diuretics (n = 5), and β-blockers (n = 4). Among individual drugs, amlodipine was found to be the commonest drug associated with adverse drug reactions (n = 7), followed by torasemide (n = 3). Adverse drug reactions associated with central nervous system were found to be the most frequent (42.8%) followed by musculo-skeletal complaints (23.8%) and gastro-intestinal disorders (14.3%).

Conclusions: The present pharmacovigilance study represents the adverse drug reaction profile of the antihypertensive medicines prescribed in our university teaching hospital. The above findings would be useful for physicians in rational prescribing. Calcium channel blockers were found to be the most frequently associated drugs with adverse drug reactions.

Keywords: Antihypertensive medicines, Adverse drug reaction, Teaching hospital and Pharmacovigilance

Introduction

Adverse drug reactions have been creating headlines over the last forty years since the thalidomide tragedy. International attention to patient safety has been growing significantly since the publication of the US Institute of Medicine report "To err is human: building a safer health system" [1-3]). There is no standard definition of an adverse drug reaction (ADR). Early studies used their own definitions, which were indistinct and could be interpreted to include intentional and unintentional overdose, as well as some administration errors [4,5]. According to World Health Organization (WHO) "An adverse drug reaction (ADR) is any response to a drug which is noxious and unintended and occurs at doses normally used in man for prophylaxis, diagnosis or therapy of disease or the modification of physiological function" [6]. Food and Drug Administration (FDA) defines a serious adverse event as one in which the patient outcome is death, or life threatening, hospitalization, disability, congenital anomaly or required intervention to prevent permanent impairment or damage [7]. ADRs are a major universal problem and are one of the leading

* Correspondence: aqilmalik@yahoo.com
[1]Faculty of Pharmacy, Jamia Hamdard (Hamdard University), New Delhi 110062, India
Full list of author information is available at the end of the article

causes of mortality and morbidity in health care facilities globally. The incidence of ADR varies with studies. A published meta-analysis of the incidence of adverse drug reactions (ADRs) in hospitalized patients concluded that ADRs rank as the fourth to sixth leading cause of death in the United States and the overall incidence of serious ADR accounted for 6.7% of hospitalized patients [8]. According to a study carried out at a private tertiary care hospital in South India, the incidence of ADRs was found to be 1.8%, out of which 12% of suspected ADRs were severe and 49% ADRs were moderate in severity [9]. A study by Arulmani et al. in India carried out in a secondary care hospital reported an overall 9.8% incidence of ADRs, of which 3.4% of ADRs were associated with hospital admissions [10]. Another study carried out in a tertiary care referral center in South India showed that admissions due to ADRs accounted for 0.7% of total admissions and deaths due to ADRs accounted for 1.8% of total ADRs [11]. Monitoring of ADRs is an ongoing, ceaseless, and continuing process. Though ADR monitoring is still in its infancy in India, this is likely to expand in the times to come. As the newer drugs are striking the Indian market, the need for ADR monitoring is growing more than ever before. Therefore, monitoring of the adverse effects particularly those of serious nature is obligatory [12]. It is important to remember that most ADRs would subside once the offending agent is discontinued or dosage reduced; however, many result in permanent damage. Therefore, it is important to motivate healthcare providers to understand their role and responsibility in the detection, management, documentation, and reporting of ADRs, and all essential activities for optimizing patient safety. The objective of this study was to monitor the ADRs caused by antihypertensive medicines prescribed in our university teaching hospitals.

Methods

The present work was an open, non-comparative, observational study to reports incidence of ADRs due to antihypertensive medicines at our university teaching hospital. The study protocol was assessed and approved by Jamia Hamdard Institutional Review Board (Approval letter No. JHIRB 07/07, February 15, 2007). The study was conducted in patients attending the Medicine outpatient department (OPD) of Majeedia Hospital, a 150 bedded teaching hospital of Jamia Hamdard, New Delhi, India by conducting patient interviews after their informed consent was obtained and recording the data on ADR monitoring form as recommended by Central Drugs Standard Control Organization (CDSCO), Government of India (http://cdsco.nic.in/adr3.pdf). The information collected includes patient information (initials, age, sex, height, weight), suspected adverse event (brief description of the reaction, onset date/stop date of occurrence of events, outcomes of events , treatment receive), suspected medication (name, indication, start date/stop date, dose, frequency, route of administration), Medical history (past/present), concomitant medication, relevant test /laboratory data, other relevant history including pre-existing medical conditions. All hypertensive patients irrespective of age and sex and patients treated with at least one antihypertensive agent were included in the study. Patients who were not treated with antihypertensive agents, all the mentally retarded and unconscious patients (patients depending on other people for medication administration) and drug addicts were excluded from the study. All the data were kept confidential. The study was carried out during the period of February 2007 to May 2007 (4 months) by a registered pharmacist attending the medicine OPD on a daily basis. Study was conducted on 192 eligible patients at Majeedia Hospital who were willing to participate. Furthermore, some patients (n = 13) presenting with ADRs were observed for changes in biochemical parameters based on pathological lab reports.

The estimation of the probability that a drug caused an adverse clinical event is usually based on clinical judgment. For this study, the Naranjo's scale which categorizes the causality relationship into *definite, probable, possible* or *unlikely* was used for the assessment of the exact nature of ADR [13].

Results

During the study period, a total of 192 hypertensive patients visited Majeedia Hospital. Among the 192-hypertensive patients 87 (45.4%) were males and 105 (54.6%) were females. A total of 21 ADRs were observed in 13 out of 192 hypertensive patients. Among the 13 patients reported with ADRs 8 (4.1%) patients were female and 5 (2.6%) were male (Table 1).

Females experienced more ADRs (n = 14, 7.29%) than males, (n = 7, 3.64%). The most vulnerable age group

Table 1 Frequency of different age groups in ADR and non ADR hypertensive patients

Age groups (years)	Patient with ADRs		Patients without ADRs		Total
	Male	Female	Male	Female	
21–30	0	0	12	3	15
31–40	1	0	19	28	48
41–50	1	5	10	33	49
51–60	0	2	23	13	38
61–70	1	0	11	13	25
71–80	2	1	5	7	15
81–90	0	0	2	0	2
Total	**5**	**8**	**82**	**97**	**192**

was 41–50 years with respect to ADRs (n = 6) followed by 71–80 years (n = 3), 51–60 years (n = 2), 31–40 years and 61–70 years (n = 1 each). No ADR was observed in the age group of 21–30 years and 81–90 years.

Out of 192 patients, 87 (45.3%) were receiving monotherapy and 105 (54.7%) were receiving multiple drug therapy. A significant difference in number of ADRs was observed in patients receiving monotherapy (33.3%) than those on combination therapy (66.7%). Calcium channel blockers (CCBs) was found to be the commonest therapeutic class associated with ADRs (n = 7), followed by diuretics (n = 5), β-blockers (n = 4), ARBs (n = 3) and ACE inhibitors (n = 2). Among individual drugs amlodipine was found to be the commonest drug associated with ADRs (n = 7) with one third of total number of reported ADRs. The common complaints with the usage of amlodipine were: abdominal pain, ankle oedema, sedation, pedal oedema, and back pain. Torasemide (a diuretic) was the next drug on the list of suspect drugs with 3 (14%) of total number of ADRs with fatigue, visual impairment and dizziness being the adverse effects. Dry cough was the most frequent ADR observed in our study with ramipril (Table 2).

On Naranjo's probability scale more than half (57%) of the reported ADRs were classified as "possible", 38% as "probable" and ~ 5% as "unlikely". ADRs associated with CNS (n = 9, 42.8%) were found to be most frequent (e. g., dizziness, headache, depression etc.) followed by Musculo-skeletal (n = 5, 23.8%) complaints (e.g., back pain, fatigue ankle and pedal edema) and gastrointestinal (n = 3, 14.3%) disorders (e.g., abdominal pain, anorexia), (Table 3). Majority of ADRs observed in our study were mild (n = 14, 66.6%), which were well tolerated by the patients for example, headache, dizziness etc. followed by moderate (n = 7, 33.3%) ADRs, e.g. insomnia, depression (propranolol), ankle oedema (amlodipine) etc. The offending drug was withdrawn (dechallenged) which reversed the symptoms. None of the ADRs was categorized as severe.

The biochemical parameters of the patients who experienced ADRs were mostly unperturbed. Only one patient who presented with ramipril associated dry cough had elevated Serum glutamate pyruvate transaminase (SGPT) and Serum glutamate oxaloacetate transaminase (SGOT) levels. The blood sugar levels were found to be more than the normal values only in patients with concomitant diabetes mellitus (Table 4).

Discussion

The demographic details of our study population showed female gender predominance over males, which was similar to that reported in other studies found in the literature [10,11,14-18]. This might be due to higher emotion quotient in females, which makes them more

Table 2 Adverse Drug Reactions and the suspected antihypertensive medicine

Suspected Drugs (No. of Prescriptions)	ADRs Experienced	No. of ADRs (%*)	Interventions
Calcium Channel Blockers			
Amlodipine (68)	Ankle edema	02 (2.94%)	Dechallenge
	Abdominal pain	02 (2.94%)	Symptomatic treatment
	Sedation	01 (1.47%)	Symptomatic treatment
	Pedal edema	01 (1.47%)	Symptomatic treatment
	Back pain	01 (1.47%)	Symptomatic treatment
Total		07 (10.29%)	
Diuretics			
Torasemide (18)	Fatigue	01 (5.55%)	Symptomatic treatment
	Visual impairment	01 (5.55%)	Dechallenge
	Dizziness	01 (5.55%)	No change in treatment
Total		03 (16.66%)	
Amiloride (09)	Dizziness	01 (11.11%)	No change in treatment
	Loss of appetite	01 (11.11%)	Symptomatic treatment
Total		02 (22.22%)	
Grand Total		05 (18.51%)	
ACE Inhibitors			
Ramipril (33)	Dry cough	02 (6.06%)	Dechallenge
Total		02 (6.06%)	
Angiotensine Receptor Blockers			
Telmisartan (17)	Dizziness	01 (5.88%)	No change in treatment
Losartan (22)	Dizziness	01 (4.54%)	No change in treatment
Olmesartan (06)	Dizziness	01 (16.66%)	No change in treatment
Total		03 (6.66%)	
Beta-blockers			
Atenolol (34)	Bradycardia	01 (2.94%)	No change in treatment
Metoprolol (12)	Headache	01 (8.33%)	No change in treatment
Propranolol (20)	Insomnia	01 (5.00%)	Dechallenge
	Depression	01 (5.00%)	Dechallenge
Total		04 (6.06%)	

*The percentage of ADRs was calculated from no of prescriptions of suspected drug.

Table 3 Organ system affected due to ADRs

Organ System	No. of ADRs	%* of ADRs
Central Nervous System	09	42.8
Musculo-skeletal System	05	23.8
Gastro-intestinal System	03	14.3
Respiratory System	02	9.5
Eye	01	4.8
Cardiovascular System	01	4.8
Total	**21**	**100**

*The percentage of ADRs was calculated from total no. of observed ADRs.

sensitive to the pharmacological actions of medicines, thus enhancing the probability of ADRs. Rational dose titration may lead to minimization of ADRs in females. Incidence of ADRs was found to be higher in older patients i.e., more than 40 years (n = 12) as compared to younger ones i.e., less than 40 years (n = 1). Compromised organ functions, decreased BMR (basal metabolic rate), concomitant disease conditions and multiple drug regimens might be assigned as likely reasons for higher incidence of ADRs in older patients.

As anticipated, multiple therapies (more than one drug) were associated with more number of ADRs (67%) as against monotherapy (33%). Many epidemiological studies on risk factors for ADRs have shown that patients on multiple therapies were more likely to develop ADR as compared to patients on monotherapy [15,19-21]. Multiple therapies need to be discouraged as these enhance the probability of ADRs due to drug–drug interactions. It is recommended that only the absolutely essential medicines be prescribed in the management of hypertension.

CCBs were the most frequently associated drugs with ADRs. This is consistent with the findings of previous studies [16,22,23]. By contrast β-blockers have also been reported more significantly associated with ADRs than other drug categories [15,24] and the physicians considered discontinuing the treatment more frequently in patients receiving β-blockers in comparison to other drugs [15]. Among individual drugs amlodipine was found to be the commonest drug associated with ADRs. The common complaints with the usage of amlodipine were: abdominal pain, ankle oedema, sedation, pedal oedema, and back pain. Oedema has been reported elsewhere as the most common problem with amlodipine [16] and in other study conducted on 57 patients in Belgium [25]. Also, flushing, dizziness and peripheral oedema have been mentioned as common complaints with CCBs in a review [26]. Torasemide (a diuretic) was associated with fatigue, visual impairment and dizziness being the adverse effects. Dizziness and headache have been reported as common side effects associated with diuretics. These side effects could be related to the fluid or electrolytes imbalance caused by these medicines [26]. Dry cough was the most often ADR observed in our study with ramipril. This is in confirmation of previous reports with almost 44% of patients experiencing dry cough on using ACE inhibitors [22,27]. The adverse effects observed with other medicines were consistent with their pharmacological profiles.

The effects of ADRs on different organs/systems of the body were assessed and classified on the basis of

Table 4 Biochemical parameters of the hypertensive patients exposed to ADRs

S. No	Patient's code	Age (Years)	Sex	Biochemical Parameters							
				SGPT 5–40 IU/L	SGOT 5–40 IU/L	B.Sugar 80–150 mg/dl	B.Urea 15–45 mg/dl	S.Creatinine 0.5–1.4 mg/dl	S.Sodium 136–149 meq/L	S.Potassium 3.5–5.4 meq/L	Chloride 98–108 meq/L
1	HTN 01	38	M	15	12	121	21	0.8	144	4.5	105
2	HTN 02	50	F	37	27	189	32	1.3	144	4.2	106
3	HTN 03	46	M	27	33	159	74	1.8	135	5.1	106
4	HTN 04	73	M	27	33	290	16	0.9	138	4.8	98
5	HTN 05	47	F	16	12	343	15	0.8	139	3.9	102
6	HTN 06	58	F	40	42	122	32	1.0	141	4.4	103
7	HTN 07	45	F	37	28	180	32	1.3	144	4.2	104
8	HTN 08	45	F	26	29	250	38	1.2	140	4.3	100
9	HTN 09	75	M	34	42	148	18	0.9	141	4.5	105
10	HTN 10	80	F	27	29	130	25	1.2	140	4.6	102
11	HTN 11	63	M	27	38	189	30	1.3	140	4.8	104
12	HTN 12	60	F	30	28	110	26	0.9	139	4.3	103
13	HTN 13	50	F	68	81	107	17	1.0	146	4.6	108

B. Sugar: Blood Sugar, **B. Urea**: Blood Urea, **S. Creatinine**: Serum Creatinine, **S. Sodium**: Serum Sodium, **S. Potassium**: Serum Potassium, **SGOT**: Serum glutamate oxaloacetate transaminase, **SGPT**: Serum glutamate pyruvate transaminase.

symptoms reported by the patients who experienced adverse drug reactions. The most common systems associated with ADRs in our study were the central nervous system (CNS) followed by musculo-skeletal complaints. This finding is consistent with previous studies which have reported CNS manifestation [10,18,23,28]. The gastrointestinal system has also been reported to be involved in the majority of ADRs [10,18,23,29]. In our study, this formed the third largest report on ADRs.

The biochemical parameters of the patients who experienced ADRs were mostly unperturbed. Only one patient who presented with ramipril associated dry cough had elevated SGPT and SGOT levels. As the enzymatic levels were altered in an odd patient, it is concluded that the elevated SGPT and SGOT levels might be due to concomitant disease condition(s) and could not be attributed to ramipril administration. One patient receiving torasemide presented with fatigue and visual impairment along with elevated blood urea and serum creatinine levels. Again as the above observation was in merely one patient, the elevated blood urea and serum creatinine levels could be assigned to other pathological conditions and might not have been induced by torasemide. The blood sugar levels were found to be more than the normal values only in patients with concomitant diabetes mellitus.

Conclusion

The above study is a part of ongoing pharmacovigilance program conducted at our university teaching hospital. During this pharmacovigilance study, calcium channel blockers were found to be the most frequently associated drugs with ADRs followed by diuretics, β-blockers, ARBs and ACE inhibitors. As the present study is related to ADR profile of antihypertensive agents, it may be helpful in selection of appropriate medicines for hypertensive patients, enhancing patient adherence with the therapy by selecting medicines of lesser ADRs profile, reducing unnecessary economic burden to the patients due to unwanted effects of the therapy.

Competing interests

The author(s) declare that they have no competing interests.

Authors' contributions

FK collected the data in the Medicine OPD of Majeedia Hospital, New Delhi. MA conceptualized and supervised the research work and is the corresponding author. MSA prepared the manuscript. PK was the hospital clinician attached with the present study. KKP critically reviewed the manuscript internally prior to submission. All authors read and approved the final manuscript.

Acknowledgments

The authors are thankful to all the physicians, laboratory members of the Majeedia Hospital and the patients who participated in the present study. The authors also thank Mohammed S. Alsultan, PharmD, PhD, Associate professor of Clinical Pharmacy, King Saud University, Saudi Arabia for reviewing the manuscript.

Author details

[1]Faculty of Pharmacy, Jamia Hamdard (Hamdard University), New Delhi 110062, India. [2]Pharmacoeconomics and Outcomes Research Unit; Department of Clinical Pharmacy, College of Pharmacy, King Saud University, P.O Box: 2457, Riyadh 11451, Saudi Arabia. [3]Majeedia Hospital, Jamia Hamdard (Hamdard University), New Delhi 110062, India.

References

1. Homsted L: **Institute of Medicine report: to err is human: building a safer health care system.** *Fla Nurse* 2000, **48**:6.
2. American College of Clinical Pharmacology response to the Institute of Medicine report, American College of Clinical Pharmacology response to the Institute of Medicine report "To err is human: building a safer health system": **The Public Policy Committee.** *J Clin Pharmacol* 2000, **40**:1075–1078.
3. Stefl ME: **To Err is Human: Building a Safer Health System in 1999.** *Front Health Serv Manage* 2001, **18**:1–2.
4. Cluff LE, Thornton GF, Seidl LG: **Studies on the Epidemiology of Adverse Drug Reactions. I. Methods of Surveillance.** *JAMA* 1964, **188**:976–983.
5. Ogilvie RI, Ruedy J: **Adverse drug reactions during hospitalization.** *Can Med Assoc J* 1967, **97**:1450–1457.
6. International drug monitoring: the role of national centres: **Report of a WHO meeting.** *World Health Organ Tech Rep Ser* 1972, **498**:1–25.
7. Kessler DA: **Introduction: Med Watch using FDA form 3500, a new approach to reporting medication and device adverse effects and products problem.** *JAMA* 1993, **269**:2765–2768.
8. Lazarou J, Pomeranz BH, Corey PN: **Incidence of adverse drug reactions in hospitalized patients: a meta-analysis of prospective studies.** *JAMA* 1998, **279**:1200–1205.
9. Sriram S, Ghasemi A, Ramasamy R, Devi M, Balasubramanian R, Ravi TK, *et al*: **Prevalence of adverse drug reactions at a private tertiary care hospital in south India.** *J Res Med Sci* 2011, **16**:16–25.
10. Arulmani R, Rajendran SD, Suresh B: **Adverse drug reaction monitoring in a secondary care hospital in South India.** *Br J Clin Pharmacol* 2008, **65**:210–216.
11. Ramesh M, Pandit J, Parthasarathi G: **Adverse drug reactions in a south Indian hospital–their severity and cost involved.** *Pharmacoepidemiol Drug Saf* 2003, **12**:687–692.
12. Dhikav V, Singh S, Anand KS: **Adverse drug reaction monitoring in India.** *JIACM* 2004, **5**:27–33.
13. Naranjo CA, Busto U, Sellers EM, Sandor P, Ruiz I, Roberts EA, *et al*: **A method for estimating the probability of adverse drug reactions.** *Clin Pharmacol Ther* 1981, **30**:239–245.
14. Sharma H, Aqil M, Imam F, Alam MS, Kapur P, Pillai KK: **A pharmacovigilance study in the department of medicine of a university teaching hospital.** *Pharm Pract* 2007, **5**:46–49.
15. Olsen H, Klemetsrud T, Stokke HP, Tretli S, Westheim A: **Adverse drug reactions in current antihypertensive therapy: a general practice survey of 2586 patients in Norway.** *Blood Press* 1999, **8**:94–101.
16. Aqil M, Imam F, Hussain A, Alam MS, Kapur P, Pillai KK: **A pharmacovigilance study for monitoring adverse drug reactions with antihypertensive agents at a South Delhi hospital.** *Int J Pharm Pract* 2006, **14**:311–313.
17. Hussain A, Aqil M, Alam MS, Khan MR, Kapur P, Pillai KK: **A pharmacovigilance study of antihypertensive medicines at a South delhi hospital.** *Indian J Pharm Sci* 2009, **71**:338–341.
18. Mohebbi N, Shalviri G, Salarifar M, Salamzadeh J, Gholami K: **Adverse drug reactions induced by cardiovascular drugs in cardiovascular care unit patients.** *Pharmacoepidemiol Drug Saf* 2010, **19**:889–894.
19. Guidelines Committee: **European Society of Hypertension- European Society of Cardiology guidelines for the management of arterial hypertension.** *J Hypertens* 2003, **21**:1011–1053.
20. Kearney PM, Whelton M, Reynolds K, Whelton PK, He J: **Worldwide prevalence of hypertension: a systematic review.** *J Hypertens* 2004, **22**:11–19.
21. Caranasos GJ, Stewart RB, Cluff LE: **Drug-induced illness leading to hospitalization.** *JAMA* 1974, **228**:713–717.

22. Basak SC, Ravi K, Manavalan R, Sahoo RK: **A study of adverse drug reactions to antihypertensive drugs perceived by patients in a rural hospital.** *Ind J Pham Sci* 2004, **66:**814–818.
23. Gholami K, Ziaie S, Shalviri G: **Adverse drug reactions induced by cardiovascular drugs in outpatients.** *Pharm Pract* 2008, **6:**51–55.
24. Malhotra S, Karan RS, Pandhi P, Jain S: **Pattern of use and pharmacoeconomic impact of antihypertensive drugs in a north Indian referral hospital.** *Eur J Clin Pharmacol* 2001, **57:**535–540.
25. Biston P, Melot C, Degaute JP, Clement D, Quoidbach A: **Prolonged antihypertensive effect of amlodipine: a prospective double-blind randomized study.** *Blood Press* 1999, **8:**43–48.
26. Ferrari A: **Headache: one of the most common and troublesome adverse reactions to drugs.** *Curr Drug Saf* 2006, **1:**43–58.
27. Woo KS, Nicholls MG: **High prevalence of persistent cough with angiotensin converting enzyme inhibitors in Chinese.** *Br J Clin Pharmacol* 1995, **40:**141–144.
28. Jha N, Bajracharya O, Namgyal T: **Prevalence of adverse drug reactions with commonly prescribed drugs in different hospitals of Kathmandu valley.** *Kathmandu Univ Med J* 2007, **5:**504–510.
29. Suh DC, Woodall BS, Shin SK: **Hermes-De Santis ER. Clinical and economic impact of adverse drug reactions in hospitalized patients.** *Ann Pharmacother* 2000, **34:**1373–1379.

12

Synthesis and biological evaluation of novel benzyl piperazine derivatives of 5-(5-nitroaryl)-1,3,4-thiadiazoles as Anti-*Helicobacter pylori* agents

Negar Mohammadhosseini[1], Parastoo Saniee[2], Ameneh Ghamaripour[3], Hassan Aryapour[3], Farzaneh Afshar[4], Najmeh Edraki[1], Farideh Siavoshi[2], Alireza Foroumadi[1] and Abbas Shafiee[1*]

Abstract

Background and the purpose of the study: *Helicobacter pylori* is recognized as the main cause of gastritis and gastroduodenal ulcers and classified as class 1 carcinogen pathogen. Different 1,3,4-thiadiazole derivatives bearing 5-nitroaryl moiety have been shown considerable anti- *H. pylori* activity. In attempt to find new and potent derivatives of described scaffold, a new series of 1-(substituted benzyl)-4-(5-(5-nitroaryl-2-yl)-1,3,4-thiadiazol-2-yl) piperazine derivatives were synthesized and evaluated against three metronidazole-resistant isolates of *H. pylori* using paper disk diffusion bioassay test.

Methods: The title compounds were prepared through the reaction of 1-(5-(5-nitroaryl-2-yl)-1,3,4-thiadiazol-2-yl) piperazine **5a-b** and substituted benzyl chloride in DMF. The inhibitory activity of the new derivatives **6a-q** against three metronidazole-resistant isolates of *H. pylori* was evaluated by the disc diffusion method and compared with the commercially available standard drug metronidazole.

Results and discussion: The results of SAR study indicated that the potency and anti-*H. pylori* activity profile of synthesized derivatives is mainly attributed to the substituted nitroaryl moiety at the C-5 position of 1,3,4-thiadiazole ring. Most of 1,3,4-thiadiazole derivatives bearing 5-nitrofuran moiety at C-5 position of central thiadiazole ring, demonstrated more promising anti-*H. pylori* than the 5-nitrothiophen counterpart.

Conclusion: The most potent nitrofuran derivative containing 3-methoxybenzyl piperazine pendant at the C-2 position of 1,3,4-thiadiazole ring (compound **6i**), demonstrated strong anti-*H. pylori* potential at studied concentrations 100-25 μg/disk (IZD > 20 mm) against all studied metronidazole- resistant isolates of *H. pylori*.

Keywords: Anti-*Helicobacter pylori* activity, 1,3,4-Thiadiazole, Nitrofuran, Nitrothiophen

Introduction

Helicobacter pylori, an spiral-shaped Gram-negative bacterium, has been considered as the leading cause of gastritis and gastroduodenal ulcer in developing countries. *H. pylori* is also classified as the class 1 carcinogen pathogen because of its epidemiological relationship to gastric adenocarcinoma and gastric mucosa-associated lymphoid tissue lymphoma [1-3]. Therefore; treatment of *Helicobacter pylori* requires targeted therapeutic strategy.

Different studies show that eradication of *H. pylori* infection resulted to ulcer healing and reduced prevalence of gastric cancer [4]. However, treatment of this infection is complicated and successful eradication of this organism is continuously requiring a combination regime using a minimum of two different antibiotics plus proton pump inhibitor (PPI) agent [3,5,6].

Although several combination therapy regimes using various anti-bacterial agents through different duration of therapy are proposed for eradication of *H. pylori* infection, emergence of resistance strains is a growing global concern. Clinical evaluation of current therapeutic

* Correspondence: ashafiee@ams.ac.ir
[1]Department of Medicinal Chemistry, Faculty of Pharmacy and Pharmaceutical Sciences Research Center, Tehran University of Medical Sciences, Tehran 14176, Iran
Full list of author information is available at the end of the article

agents indicated the incidence of drug-drug interaction, infection relapses and side effects of common drugs [7,8]. These factors have been the rationale for the development of new anti- *Helicobacter pylori* drugs and search for novel therapeutic molecules that offer better protection and decreased relapse towards resistant strains.

Nitrofuran and nitrothiophene heterocyclic derivatives have been extensively studied in therapy against different microbial infections [9-11]. Moreover, the antimicrobial and anti-Helicobacter property of 1,3,4-thiadiazole moiety is well established and attachment of this antimicrobial scaffold with nitro-hetrocyclic moieties would accommodate the bioresponses and antimicrobial activity depending on the type of substituted group and position of attachment [12-14]. In our previous works, we have investigated the anti-Helicobacter potential of different 5-(5-nitroaryl)-1,3,4-thiadiazole scaffold bearing different C-2 attached pendants. Among different nitroheterocycles, 5-nitrofuran, 5-nitrothiophen and 5-nitroimidazole moieties are preferable for substitution at C-5 position of 1,3,4-thiadiazole ring. These nitroheteroaromatic moieties mimic the nitroaromatic part of nitroheterocyclic drugs such as metronidazole and furazolidon (Figure 1) [11,14-17]. In continuation of our research program to find a novel antibacterial agent [18], we have previously demonstrated the considerable antibacterial activity of 5-nitroimidazole-based 1,3,4-thiadiazoles bearing cyclic amine functionality such as pyrrolidine and piperazine derivatives at the C-2 position of thiadiazole ring against resistant strains of *Helicobacter pylori* [15]. In order to find the structural requirement of cyclic amine derivatives of 5-(nitroaryl)-1,3,4-thiadiazole as anti-*H. pylori* agents, herein, we describe the synthesis and anti-*Helicobacter* evaluation of a new series of 5-(nitrothienyl) and 5-(nitrofuryl)-1,3,4-thiadiazoles containing different piperazine side chain at 2-position of 1,3,4-thiadiazole ring system (Figure 1).

Material and methods

Chemistry

A Kofler hot stage apparatus was used for the measurement of reported melting. The IR spectra were recorded on a Nicollet FT-IR Magna 550 spectrometer. The ^1H NMR spectra were recorded on a Varian FT-400 MHz or Bruker FT-500 MHz spectrometer and chemical shifts (δ) are reported in ppm relative to internal tetramethylsilane. The

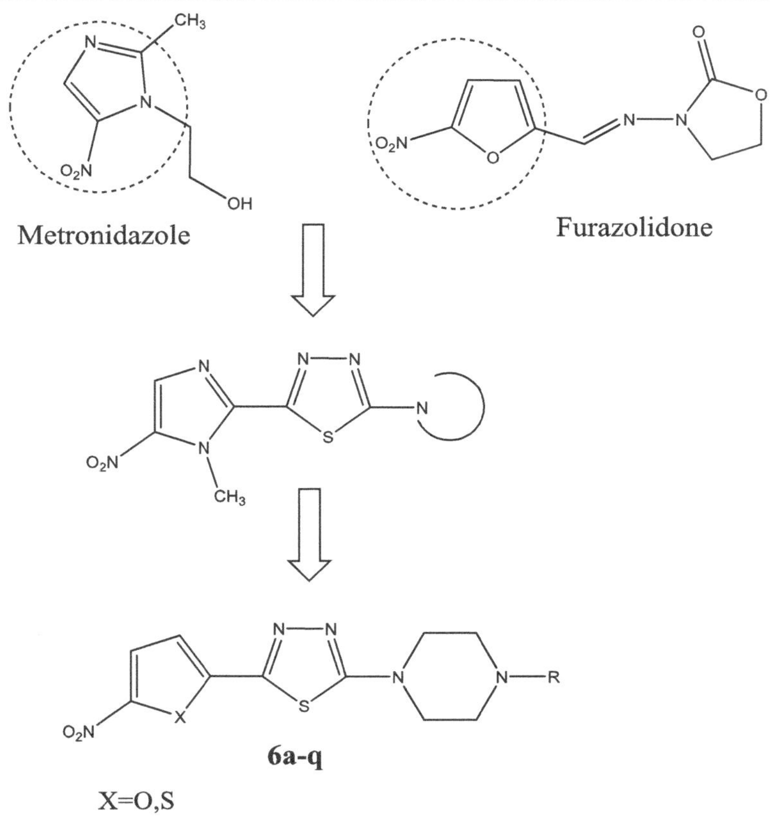

Figure 1 Chemical structure of current nitroheterocyclic drugs (Metronidazole and Furazolidone) used in the treatment of *H.pylori* infection and designed 5-(nitroaryl)-1,3,4-thiadiazoles bearing piperazine derivatives 6a-q.

mass spectra were run on a Agilent 1100/Bruker Daltonic (Ion trap) VL instrument. at 70 eV. Fross- Heraeus CHN-O rapid analyzer was used for elemental analysis of synthesized compounds and the results are within ± 0.4% of the theoretical values. Analytical thin-layar chromatography (TLC) on Merck silicagel 60 F254 plates using various mobile phases of different polarities was performed in order to confirm the purity of final products.

General method for the synthesis of 1-substitutedbenzyl-4-(5-(5-nitroaryl-2-yl)-1,3,4-thiadiazol-2-yl)piperazine 6a-q

To a mixture of 1-(5-(5-nitroaryl-2-yl)-1,3,4-thiadiazol-2-yl)piperazine **5a-b** (1.0 mmol) and different benzyl chloride derivatives (1.0 mmol) in DMF (15 mL), $NaHCO_3$ (0.21 mmol) was added and the resulted mixture was stirred at room temperature overnight. After completion of the reaction, water was added, and the resulted precipitate was filtered off, washed with water, and crystallized from ethanol.

1-(2-nitrobenzyl)-4-(5-(5-nitrothiophen-2-yl)-1,3,4-thiadiazol-2-yl)piperazine (6a)

Yield 40%; m.p. 219-221°C; IR(KBr): 1343, 1527 cm^{-1} (NO_2); ^{1}H-NMR($CDCl_3$) δ: 2.48-2.64 (m, 4H, piperazine), 3.48-3.63 (m, 2H, CH_2), 3.48-3.63 (m, 4H, piperazine), 7.16 (bs, 1H, thiophene), 7.45 (bs, 1H, phenyl), 7.52-7.60 (m, 2H, phenyl), 7.80-7.92 (m, 2H, phenyl-thiophene); MS: m/z (%) 432 (M^+, 1), 415 (21), 241 (15), 191 (81), 172 (15), 136 (100), 120 (33), 91 (34), 69 (93), 42 (25). Anal. Calcd. For $C_{17}H_{16}N_6O_4S_2$: C, 47.21; H, 3.73; N, 19.43; Found: C, 47.03; H, 3.51; N, 19.67.

1-(3-nitrobenzyl)-4-(5-(5-nitrothiophen-2-yl)-1,3,4-thiadiazol-2-yl)piperazine (6b)

Yield 33%; m.p. 205-206°C; IR(KBr): 1344, 1528 cm^{-1} (NO_2); ^{1}H-NMR($CDCl_3$) δ: 2.26-2.69 (m, 4H, piperazine), 3.60-3.72 (m, 4H, piperazine and 2H, CH_2), 7.16 (bs, 1H, thiophene), 7.58 (t, 1H, phenyl, J = 7.5Hz), 7.68 (bs, 1H, phenyl), 7.86 (bs, 1H, thiophene), 8.15 (bs, 1H, phenyl), 8.24 (s, 1H, phenyl); MS: m/z (%) 432 (M^+, 2), 241 (14), 191 (88), 172 (14), 155 (16), 136 (100), 111 (16), 90 (60), 73 (18), 56 (47). Anal. Calcd. For $C_{17}H_{16}N_6O_4S_2$: C, 47.21; H, 3.73; N, 19.43; Found: C, 47.54; H, 3.61; N, 19.83.

1-(4-nitrobenzyl)-4-(5-(5-nitrothiophen-2-yl)-1,3,4-thiadiazol-2-yl)piperazine (6c)

Yield 60%; m.p. 232-234°C; IR(KBr): 1340, 1509 cm^{-1} (NO_2); ^{1}H-NMR($CDCl_3$) δ: 2.35-2.50 (m, 4H, piperazine), 3.40-3.60 (m, 4H, piperazine and 2H, CH_2), 7.02 (s, 1H, thiophene), 7.37 (d, 2H, phenyl, J = 7.6Hz), 7.70 (s, 1H, thiophene), 8.02 (d, 2H, phenyl, J = 7.6 Hz); MS: m/z (%)432 (M^+, 16), 415 (16), 395 (46), 368 (11), 313 (11), 296 (14), 241 (32), 191 (100), 172 (33), 155 (12), 136 (77), 106 (31), 78 (37), 56 (30). Anal. Calcd. For $C_{17}H_{16}N_6O_4S_2$ C, 47.21; H, 3.73; N, 19.43; Found: C, 47.56; H, 3.99; N, 19.07.

1-(2,6-difluorobenzyl)-4-(5-(5-nitrothiophen-2-yl)-1,3,4-thiadiazol-2-yl)piperazine (6d)

Yield 31%; m.p. 198-199°C; IR(KBr): 1343, 1503 cm^{-1} (NO_2); ^{1}H-NMR($CDCl_3$) δ: 2.64-2.76 (m, 4H, piperazine), 3.60-3.71 (m, 4H, piperazine), 3.79 (s, 2H, CH_2), 6.92 (t, 3H, phenyl, J = 7.6Hz), 7.14 (d, 1H, thiophene, J = 3.6Hz), 7.85 (d, 1H, thiophene, J = 3.6Hz); MS: m/z (%) 423 (M^+, 2), 182 (100), 166 (30), 127 (100), 111 (15), 83 (21), 57 (31), 41 (23). Anal. Calcd. For $C_{17}H_{15}F_2N_5O_2S_2$: C, 48.22; H, 3.57; N, 16.54; Found: C, 48.49; H, 3.34; N, 16.16.

1-(2,4,5-trifluorobenzyl)-4-(5-(5-nitrothiophen-2-yl)-1,3,4-thiadiazol-2-yl)piperazine (6e)

Yield 33%; m.p. 213-215°C; IR(KBr): 1342, 1513 cm^{-1} (NO_2); ^{1}H-NMR($CDCl_3$) δ: 2.64 (bs, 4H, piperazine), 3.59 (s, 2H, CH_2), 3.65 (bs, 4H, piperazine), 6.90-7.00 (m, 1H, phenyl), 7.12 (bs, 1H, thiophene), 7.20-7.38 (m, 1H, phenyl), 7.87 (bs, 1H, thiophene); MS: m/z (%) 441 (M^+, 5), 241 (13), 200 (86), 182 (19), 145 (100), 128 (11), 69 (11), 42 (14). Anal. Calcd. For $C_{17}H_{14}F_3N_5O_2S_2$: C, 46.25; H, 3.20; N, 15.86; Found: C, 45.88; H, 3.44; N, 16.03.

1-(2,5-diChlorobenzyl)-4-(5-(5-nitrothiophen-2-yl)-1,3,4-thiadiazol-2-yl)piperazine (6f)

Yield 93%; m.p. 210-211°C; IR(KBr): 1344, 1504 cm^{-1} (NO_2); ^{1}H-NMR($CDCl_3$) δ: 2.65-2.74 (m, 4H, piperazine), 3.60-3.74 (m, 2H, CH_2 and 4H, piperazine), 7.13-7.32 (m, 3H, phenyl-thiophene), 7.50 (s, 1H, phenyl), 7.86 (d, 1H, thiophene, J = 3.6 Hz); MS: m/z (%) 459 (M^++4, 0.4), 457 (M^++2, 3), 455 (M^+, 4), 214 (93), 192 (18), 159 (100), 123 (18). Anal. Calcd. For $C_{17}H_{15}Cl_2N_5O_2S_2$: C, 44.74; H, 3.31; N, 15.35; Found: C, 44.51; H, 3.70; N, 15.67.

1-(3,4-dichlorobenzyl)-4-(5-(5-nitrothiophen-2-yl)-1,3,4-thiadiazol-2-yl)piperazine (6g)

Yield 36%; m.p. 183-185°C; IR(KBr): 1343, 1508 cm^{-1} (NO_2); ^{1}H-NMR($CDCl_3$) δ: 2.51-2.63 (m, 4H, piperazine), 3.52 (s, 2H, CH_2), 3.60-3.68 (m, 4H, piperazine), 7.13-7.24 (m, 2H, phenyl-thiophene), 7.40 (dd, 2H, phenyl), 7.85 (s, 1H, thiophene); MS: m/z (%) 459 (M^++4, 0.5), 457 (M^++2, 3), 455 (M^+, 5), 241 (18), 214 (81), 159 (100), 124 (16), 89 (12), 56 (19). Anal. Calcd. For $C_{17}H_{15}Cl_2N_5O_2S_2$: C, 44.74; H, 3.31; N, 15.35; Found: C, 44.46; H, 3.62; N, 15.14.

1-(4-bromobenzyl)-4-(5-(5-nitrothiophen-2-yl)-1,3,4-thiadiazol-2-yl)piperazine (6h)

Yield 50%; m.p. 207-208°C; IR(KBr): 1343, 1509 cm^{-1} (NO_2); ^{1}H-NMR($CDCl_3$) δ: 2.53-2.68 (m, 4H, piperazine), 3.52 (s, 2H, CH_2), 3.60-3.69 (m, 4H, piperazine),

7.14-7.20 (m, 3H, phenyl-thiophene), 7.44-7.50 (m, 2H, phenyl), 7.85 (s, 1H, thiophene); MS: m/z (%) 467 (M^++2, 13), 465 (M^+, 14), 296 (16), 280 (14), 265 (10), 254 (41), 239 (100). Anal. Calcd. For $C_{17}H_{16}BrN_5O_2S_2$: C, 43.78; H, 3.46; N, 15.02; Found: C, 43.94; H, 3.74; N, 14.78.

1-(3-methoxybenzyl)-4-(5-(5-nitrofuran-2-yl)-1,3,4-thiadiazol-2-yl)piperazine (6i)

Yield 54%; m.p. 126-127°C; IR(KBr): 1355, 1536 cm^{-1} (NO_2); ^{1}H-NMR($CDCl_3$) δ: 2.63 (t, 4H, piperazine, J = 5.1 Hz), 3.57 (s, 2H, CH_2), 3.67 (t, 4H, piperazine, J = 5.1Hz), 3.83 (s, 3H, OCH_3), 6.84-6.87 (m, 1H, phenyl), 6.92-6.95 (m, 2H, phenyl), 7.17 (d, 1H, furan, J = 3.7 Hz), 7.21-7.23 (m, 1H, phenyl), 7.44 (d, 1H, furan, J = 3.7 Hz); MS: m/z (%) 401 (M^+, 7), 176 (86), 147 (13), 121 (100), 91 (24), 57 (18), 40 (14). Anal. Calcd. For $C_{18}H_{19}N_5O_4S$: C, 53.85; H, 4.77; N, 17.45; Found: C, 53.97; H, 4.54; N, 17.79.

1-(2-nitrobenzyl)-4-(5-(5-nitrofuran-2-yl)-1,3,4-thiadiazol-2-yl)piperazine (6j)

Yield 43%; m.p. 197-199°C; IR(KBr): 1353,1529 cm^{-1} (NO_2); ^{1}H-NMR($CDCl_3$) δ: 2.62 (t, 4H, piperazine, J = 5.1 Hz), 3.62 (t, 4H, piperazine, J = 5.1 Hz), 3.89 (s, 2H, CH_2), 7.17 (d, 1H, furan, J = 3.8 Hz), 7.44 (d, 1H, furan, J = 3.8 Hz),7.45-7.48 (m, 1H, phenyl), 7.56-7.59 (m, 2H, phenyl), 7.85 (d, 1H, phenyl, J = 7.8 Hz); MS: m/z (%) 416 (M^+, 2), 399 (46), 381 (13), 225 (18), 191 (86), 166 (14), 136 (100), 105 (12), 78 (44), 56 (19). Anal. Calcd. For $C_{17}H_{16}N_6O_5S$:C, 49.03; H, 3.87; N, 20.18; Found: C, 49.28; H, 3.64; N, 20.42.

1-(3-nitrobenzyl)-4-(5-(5-nitrofuran-2-yl)-1,3,4-thiadiazol-2-yl)piperazine (6k)

Yield 50%; m.p. 144-146°C; IR(KBr): 1353, 1529 cm^{-1} (NO_2); ^{1}H-NMR($CDCl_3$) δ: 2.66 (t, 4H, piperazine, J = 5.0 Hz), 3.69 (t, 4H, piperazine, J = 5.0 Hz), 3.71 (s, 2H, CH_2), 7.18 (d, 1H, furan, J = 3.9 Hz), 7.44 (d, 1H, furan, J = 3.9 Hz), 7.54 (t, 1H, phenyl, J = 7.9 Hz), 7.71 (d, 1H, phenyl, J = 7.9 Hz), 8.17 (d, 1H, phenyl, J = 7.9 Hz), 8.26 (bs, 1H, phenyl); MS: m/z (%) 416 (M^+, 7), 399 (12), 225 (19), 191 (100), 166 (20), 136 (86), 90 (37), 57 (21), 40 (18). Anal. Calcd. For $C_{17}H_{16}N_6O_5S$: C, 49.03; H, 3.87; N, 20.18; Found: C, 48.88; H, 3.56; N, 20.44.

1-(4-nitrobenzyl)-4-(5-(5-nitrofuran-2-yl)-1,3,4-thiadiazol-2-yl)piperazine (6l)

Yield 50%; m.p. 212-213°C; IR(KBr): 1348, 1505 cm^{-1} (NO_2); ^{1}H-NMR($CDCl_3$) δ: 2.65 (t, 4H, piperazine, J = 5.1 Hz), 3.69(s, 2H, CH_2), 3.70 (t, 4H, piperazine, J = 5.1 Hz), 7.18 (d, 1H, furan, J = 3.9 Hz), 7.44 (d, 1H, furan, J = 3.9 Hz), 7.56 (d, 2H, phenyl, J = 8.6 Hz), 8.23 (d, 2H, phenyl, J = 8.6 Hz); MS: m/z (%) 416 (M^+, 9), 399 (13), 225 (21), 191 (100), 166 (12), 136 (87), 106 (36), 78 (49), 60 (11), 42 (40). Anal. Calcd. For $C_{17}H_{16}N_6O_5S$: C, 49.03; H, 3.87; N, 20.18; Found: C, 49.31; H, 3.58; N, 20.36.

1-(2,6-difluorobenzyl)-4-(5-(5-nitrofuran-2-yl)-1,3,4-thiadiazol-2-yl)piperazine (6m)

Yield 50%; m.p. 176-179°C; IR (KBr): 1353, 1540 cm^{-1} (NO_2); ^{1}H-NMR($CDCl_3$) δ: 2.69 (t, 4H, piperazine, J = 4.6 Hz), 3.67 (t, 4H, piperazine, J = 4.6 Hz), 3.79 (s, 2H, CH_2), 6.93 (t, 2H, phenyl, J = 7.4 Hz), 7.16 (d, 1H, furan, J = 3.8 Hz), 7.28-7.38 (m, 1H, phenyl), 7.43 (d, 1H, furan, J = 3.8 Hz); MS: m/z (%) 407 (M^+, 5), 182 (85), 149 (11), 127 (100), 69 (11), 42 (11). Anal. Calcd. For $C_{17}H_{15}F_2N_5O_3S$:C, 50.12; H, 3.71;N, 17.19; Found: C, 50.35; H, 3.45; N, 17.54.

1-(2,4,5-trifluorobenzyl)-4-(5-(5-nitrofuran-2-yl)-1,3,4-thiadiazol-2-yl)piperazine (6n)

Yield 41%; m.p. 174-175°C; IR(KBr): 1355, 1517 cm^{-1} (NO_2); ^{1}H-NMR($CDCl_3$) δ: 2.65 (t, 4H, piperazine, J = 5.2 Hz), 3.60 (s, 2H, CH_2), 3.68 (t, 4H, piperazine, J = 5.2 Hz), 6.84-6.86 (m, 1H, phenyl), 7.18 (d, 1H, furan, J = 3.8 Hz), 7.25-7.26 (m, 1H, phenyl), 7.74 (d, 1H, furan, J = 3.8 Hz); MS: m/z (%) 425 (M^+, 6), 225 (13), 200 (94), 166 (11), 145 (100), 82 (12). Anal. Calcd. For $C_{17}H_{14}F_3N_5O_3S$: C, 48.00; H, 3.32; N, 16.46; Found: C, 48.35; H, 3.44; N, 16.18.

1-(2,5-dichlorobenzyl)-4-(5-(5-nitrofuran-2-yl)-1,3,4-thiadiazol-2-yl)piperazine (6o)

Yield 92%; m.p. 165-167°C; IR(KBr): 1353, 1549 cm^{-1} (NO_2); ^{1}H-NMR($CDCl_3$) δ: 2.71 (t, 4H, piperazine, J = 4.6 Hz), 3.67 (s, 2H, CH_2), 3.68 (t, 4H, piperazine, J = 4.6 Hz), 7.17 (d, 1H, furan, J = 3.6 Hz), 7.22 (dd, 1H, phenyl, J = 8.5 Hz, J = 2.0 Hz), 7.32 (d, 1H, phenyl, J = 8.5 Hz, J = 2.0 Hz), 7.45 (d, 1H, furan, J = 3.6 Hz), 7.51 (d, 1H, phenyl, J = 2.0 Hz); MS: m/z (%) 443 (M^++4, 0.4), 441 (M^++2, 3), 439 (M^+, 6), 313 (12), 236 (16), 214 (95), 192 (16), 159 (100), 123 (16), 99 (13), 82 (16), 57 (20), 40 (16). Anal. Calcd. For $C_{17}H_{15}Cl_2N_5O_3S$: C, 46.37; H, 3.43; N, 15.91; Found: C, 46.65; H, 3.67; N, 15.69.

1-(3,4-dichlorobenzyl)-4-(5-(5-nitrofuran-2-yl)-1,3,4-thiadiazol-2-yl)piperazine (6p)

Yield 62%; m.p. 161-162°C; IR(KBr): 1353, 1503 cm^{-1} (NO_2); ^{1}H-NMR($CDCl_3$) δ: 2.62 (t, 4H, piperazine, J = 5.0 Hz), 3.53 (s, 2H, CH_2), 3.67 (t, 4H, piperazine, J = 5.0 Hz), 7.17 (d, 1H, furan, J = 3.8 Hz), 7.19 (dd, 1H, phenyl, J = 8.3 Hz, J = 2.0 Hz), 7.41-7.45(m, 2H, phenyl), 7.47 (d, 1H, furan, J = 3.8 Hz); MS: m/z (%) 443 (M^++4, 0.5), 441 (M^++2, 3), 439 (M^+, 5), 273 (12), 238 (11), 214 (93), 159 (100), 123 (16), 100 (7), 82 (13), 56 (15). Anal. Calcd. For $C_{17}H_{15}Cl_2N_5O_3S$: C, 46.37; H, 3.43; N, 15.91; Found: C, 46.68; H, 3.16; N, 16.09.

1-(4-bromobenzyl)-4-(5-(5-nitrofuran-2-yl)-1,3,4-thiadiazol-2-yl)piperazine (6q)

Yield 28%; m.p. 192-193°C; IR(KBr): 1353, 1508 cm^{-1} (NO_2); ^{1}H-NMR($CDCl_3$) δ: 2.61 (t, 4H, piperazine, J = 5.0 Hz), 3.54 (s, 2H, CH_2), 3.66 (t, 4H, piperazine, J = 5.0 Hz), 7.17 (d, 1H, furan, J = 3.9 Hz), 7.23 (d, 2H, phenyl, J = 8.3Hz), 7.44 (d, 1H, furan, J = 3.9 Hz), 8.25 (d, 2H, phenyl, J = 8.3 Hz); MS: m/z (%) 451 (M^++2, 1), 449 (M^+, 2), 210 (20), 169 (100), 90 (44), 56 (22), 40 (21). Anal. Calcd. For $C_{17}H_{16}BrN_5O_3S$: C, 45.34; H, 3.58; N, 15.55; Found: C, 45.59; H, 3.92; N, 15.27.

Biological activity

Patients and bacterial strains

Different isolates of *H. pylori* were obtained from 160 dyspeptic patients consisted of 78 men and 82 women whose mean ages were 48 and 43 years, respectively. Based on the endoscopic diagnosis, the patients were classified into three groups: gastritis (124, 77.5%), ulcers (32, 20%) and cancer.

Antral biopsies demonstrating positive urease tests were transported to the microbiology lab in semisolid (0.1% agar) normal saline. The biopsies were cultured using selective medium containing brucella agar (Merck), 7% defibrinated sheep blood, vancomycin (5 mg/L), trimethoprim (5 mg/L), polymyxin B (50 mg/L), and amphotericin B (4 mg/L). Incubation of cultured isolates was performed at 37°C under microaerobic conditions (CO_2 incubator; Heraeus, Germany). After 3–5 days, all cultures were examined for observation of pinpoint (1–2 mm) glistening colonies. Identification of *H. pylori* isolates was carried out according to the spiral microscopic appearance, Gram negative stain and some biochemical examinations such as urease, oxidase and catalase positive test and negative activities of nitrate and H_2S.

The protocol of this research was approved by Pharmaceutical Sciences Research Center ethics committee (number 90-3-29: 1-1).

Consent

Written informed consent was obtained from the patient for the publication of this report.

Antimicrobial susceptibility test

Antimicrobial susceptibility test was performed using disk diffusion method (DDM). Recruited antibiotics included metronidazole, tetracycline. In the first step of the susceptibility evaluation, one hundred and ten strains were recruited. As a result of remarkable resistance of different studied bacterial isolates to recruited antibiotics and in attempt to increase the accuracy of the metronidazole resistant rates, in the second step of our study, an additional fifty strains of *H. Pylori* isolates were recruited for susceptibility testing with metronidazole (32, 16, 8, and 4 µg/mL) and with 2, 1, and 0.5 µg/mL of tetracycline. The susceptibility tests were repeated twice for the resistant strains. Bacterial suspensions were prepared in normal saline with the turbidity of Mac-Farland standard No.2 (equivalent to 6 × 108cell/mL). 100 µl of each bacterial suspension were inoculated in the surface of non- selective blood agar plates and the culture plates were allowed to dry at room temperature (10 min). Sterile blank disks were deposited on the surface of inoculated plates. 10 µL of each antibiotic dilution was poured into a blank disk. Moreover, control plates with growth positive bacterial culture were prepared using the introduction of 10 µl of the antibiotic solvent into the blank disks.

Plates were incubated at described condition and the inhibition zone diameters (IZD) were examined after 3–5 days. Susceptible and resistant isolates of *H.pylori* demonstrated IZDs ≥20 mm and ≤10 mm for metronidazole, respectively. The antibacterial activities of target compounds were evaluated against three metronidazole-resistant isolates of *H. pylori.* All experiments were performed in triplicate and the mean of IZDs produced by test compounds in four concentrations (100, 50, 25 and 12.5 µg/mL) was considered as antibacterial activity.

Anti-Helicobacter pylori activity assay

As mentioned earlier, the growth inhibitory potential of test compounds was evaluated against three metronidazole resistant isolates of *H. pylori* by the filter paper disk diffusion method at 37°C, under microqerophilic condition on selective Brucella agar with 7% defibrinated horse blood. Four concentrations of titled compounds in dimethylsulfoxide (DMSO) were used for evaluation of anti *Helicobacter* activity assay. Blank standard disks (6 mm in diameter) were deposited on the surface of test plates and impregnated with 10 μL of different concentrations of target compounds. Test plates were incubated at 37°C for 3–5 days and the inhibition zone around each disk (average diameter) was measured. The control disks were impregnated with 10 μL of DMSO. All antibacterial activity experiments were performed in triplicate and the antibacterial activity was expressed as the mean of IZDs (mm) produced by the test compounds at each evaluated concentration.

Result and discussion

Chemistry

The synthetic pathway for the target compounds **6a-q** is depicted in the Scheme 1. A mixture of 5-nitroaryl-2-carboxaldehyde diacetate **1a-b** with thiosemicarbazide was refluxed in ethanol to afford thiosemicarbazone **2a-b**. Amino-1,3,4-thiadiazoles **3a-b,** were synthesized through the oxidative cyclization of **2a-b** in presence of ammonium ferric sulfate. In the next step, diazotization of **3a-b** in hydrochloric acid and in the presence of copper powder

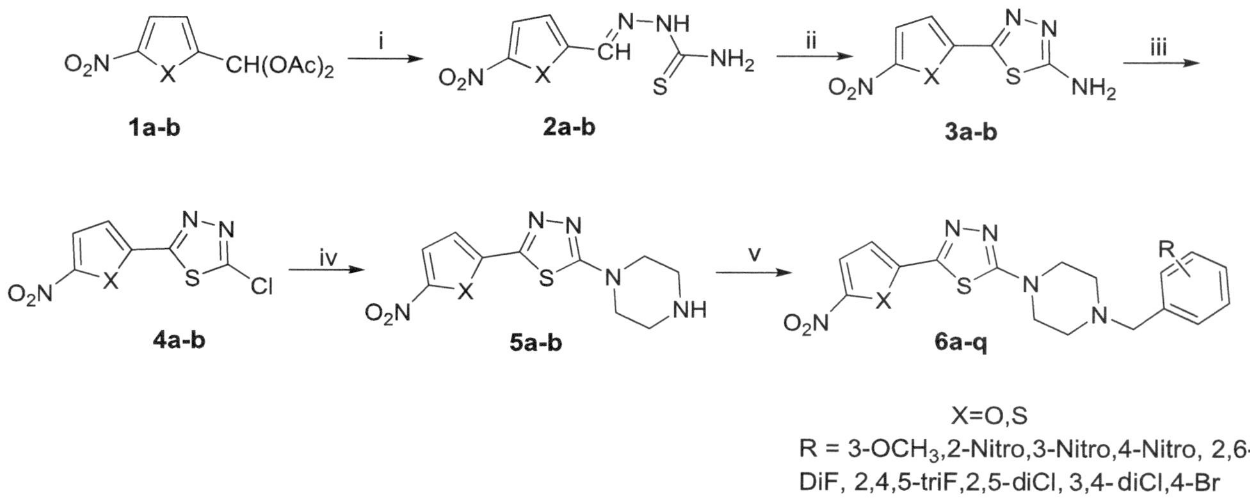

Scheme 1 Reagents and conditions: (i) thiosemicarbazide, EtOH, HCl, reflux, 1.5 h; (ii) $NH_4Fe(SO_4)_2$, $12H_2O$, H_2O reflux, 25 h; (iii) $NaNO_2$, HCl, Cu, °C→ rt, 3 h; (iv) Piperazine hydrate, EtOH, $NaHCO_3$ 1 h; (v) DMF, Substituted benzyl chloride, 4 h.

yielded chloro-1,3,4-thiadiazole **4a-b**. 1-(5-(5-nitroaryl-2-yl)-1,3,4-thiadiazol-2-yl)piperazine **5a-b** were prepared through the reaction of chloro-1,3,4-thiadiazole derivatives **4a-b** with piperazine hydrate in stirred ethanol.

The prepared key intermediates **5a-b** were further reacted with different substituted benzyl chlorides in refluxing DMF to give the corresponding 1-substituted-benzyl-4-(5-(5-nitroaryl-2-yl)-1,3,4-thiadiazol-2-yl)piperazine **6a-q**. The structures of compounds **6a-q** were determined using spectroscopic methods including mass spectrometry, ^{1}H NMR, IR, and elemental analysis. The chemical structure of target compounds are shown in Figure 2.

Anti-*Helicobacter pylori* activity and structure-activity relationship study

The *in vitro* anti-Helicobacter activity of synthesized derivatives was determined by paper disk diffusion bioassay against three metronidazole resistant *H. pylori* isolates. The average of inhibition zone diameters (IZD) of compounds against three isolates at four different concentrations (100, 50, 25 and 12.5 μg/ disk) is summarized in Figure 2. The anti-*H. pylori* activity of target derivatives could be simply categorized as follows: strong response, zones range diameter >20 mm; moderate response, zone diameter 16–20 mm; weak response, zone diameter 11–15 mm; and little or no response, zone diameter <10 mm [15].

Investigation of the IZD of studied compounds revealed that the target derivatives demonstrated a wide spectrum of anti-*H. pylori* activity varied from little (IZD <10 mm) to strong (IZD >20 mm) response at concentration of 100 μg/disk against metronidazole resistant strains. In view of the obtained data, the following structure-activity relationship might be developed:

Assessment of nitroheterocyclic moiety

Based on the substituted nitroaromatic group, the studied 1,3,4-thiadiazole derivatives could be classified into two groups: Nitrothiophen **6a-h** and nitrofuran **6i-q** derivatives. The results of anti-*H. pylori* activity indicated that the inhibitory responses of test compounds is mainly attributed to the substituted nitroaryl moiety at the C-5 position of 1,3,4-thiadiazole ring. While all of nitrothiophene derivatives **6a-h** demonstrated weak (IZD = 11–15 mm) to little (IZD <10 mm) inhibitory response at concentration of 100 μg/disk against three metronidazole resistant isolates, most of nitrofurane derivatives **6i-q** showed strong (IZD > 20 mm) to moderate (IZD = 16–20) growth inhibitory potential at the same concentration.

It could be concluded that nitrofuran **6i-q** derivatives of 1,3,4-thiadiazole scaffold, are more potent than the nitrothiophen **6a-h** counterpart.

Investigation of substituted group into the benzyl piperazine pendant

In order to find the structural requirement of substituted moiety at C-2 position of 1,3,4-thiadiazole scaffold,

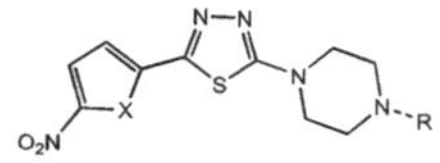

Compound	X	R	Average of Inhibition Zone Diameters (range, mm)[a]			
			100 μg/disk	50 μg/disk	25 μg/disk	12.5 μg/disk
6a	S	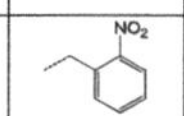	14.7 (11-16)	10 (9-10)	6 --	6 --
6b	S	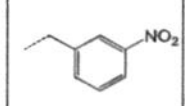	12 (10-14)	6 --	6 --	6 --
6c	S	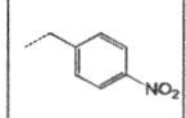	15 (11-18)	11 (9-11)	6 --	6 --
6d	S	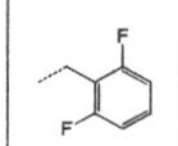	13 (10-15)	6 --	6 --	6 --
6e	S	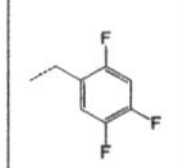	13.5 (10-15)	6 --	6 --	6 --
6f	S	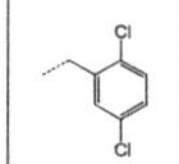	14 (12-16)	6 --	6 --	6 --
6g	S	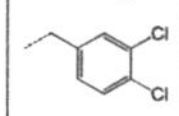	13.5 (15-14)	6 --	6 --	6 --
6h	S	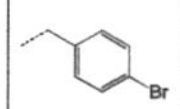	14 (11-16)	6 --	6 --	6 --
6i	O	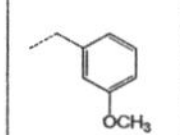	28 (25-30)	24 (21-28)	21.5 (16-24)	20 (15-22)
6j	O	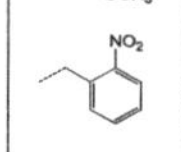	16 (12-20)	8 (6-13)	3.6 (6-11)	6 --
6k	O	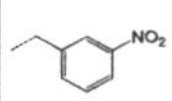	22 (19-25)	19.5 (18-20)	17 (15-20)	16 (14-18)
6l	O	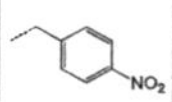	11 (10-11)	6 --	6 --	6 --
6m	O	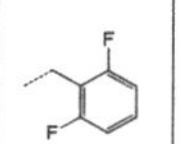	20 (17-22)	19 (17-21)	17 (15-20)	14.5 (12-18)
6n	O	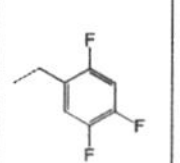	23 (22-24)	21 (20-22)	19 (15-21)	17 (13-20)
6o	O	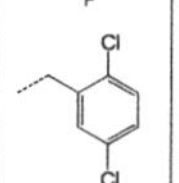	12 (12-17)	5 (6-15)	4 (6-12)	3.6 (6-11)
6p	O	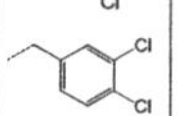	16 (12-19)	11.5 (11-12)	4 (6-11)	3.3 (6-10)
6q	O	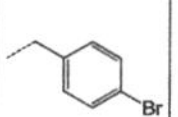	18 (11-25)	13 (6-22)	12 (6-20)	10.5 (6-18)

[a] The anti-Helicobacter pylori activity was determined by the paper disk diffusion bioassay. All tests were performed in triplicate and the antibacterial activity was expressed as the mean of inhibition zone diameters (mm) produced by title compounds.

Figure 2 Average of inhibition zone diameters of compounds 6a-q at four different concentrations against three metronidazole resistant *H. pylori* isolates.

different benzyl piperazine derivatives were substituted at the described position. Among the nitrofuran derivatives **6i-q**, 3-methoxybenzyl piperazine derivative **6i,** demonstrated strong anti-*H. pylori* potential at studied concentrations 100–25 μg/disk (IZD > 20 mm) against studied isolates. Investigation of the growth inhibitory potential of the nitrofuran series **6i-q** revealed that substitution of nitro group at the *meta* position of the benzyl piperazine side chain, resulted in compound with strong (IZD = 20 mm) to moderate (IZD = 16–20 mm) growth inhibitory potential at 100 and 50–12.5 μg/disk, respectively. However, introduction of nitro substitute at *ortho* or *para* position of the benzyl piperazine pendant, resulted in compound with diminished inhibitory potential against resistant strains of *H. pylori* isolates (compounds **6j** (IZD = 16 mm, moderate response) and **6l** (IZD = 11 mm, weak response) respectively). Moreover, substitution of fluorine groups at different positions of benzyl pieperzine side chain influenced the growth inhibitory potential of compounds which is mainly dependent on the position and number of substituted fluorine groups; compound **6n** containing 2,4,5-triflouro benzyl piperazine pendant at C-2 position of 5-nitrofuran-1,3,4-thiadiazole scaffold, produced strong inhibitory response at 100 and 50 μg/disk (IZD =23 and 21 mm, respectively); while the anti-*H. pylori* potential of 2,5-difluoro benzyl piperazine counterpart was diminished to weak (IZD = 12 mm) to no response (IZD = 5 mm) at 100 and 50 μg/disk, respectively.

Conclusion

A novel series of 5-(5-nitroaryl)-1,3,4-thiadiazole derivatives containing various benzyl piperazine moiety at C-2 position of 1,3,4-thiadiazole ring were synthesized and evaluated against three metronidazole-resistant isolates of *H.pylori* using paper disk diffusion bioassay test. Structure-activity relationship study of these derivatives indicated that 1,3,4-thiadiazole derivatives bearing 5-nitrofuran moiety at C-5 position of central thiadiazole ring, demonstrated more promising anti-*H. pylori* than the 5-nitrothiophen counterpart. The most potent nitrofuran derivative had 3-methoxybenzyl piperazine pendant at the C-2 position of 1,3,4-thiadiazole ring. The results indicated that the anti-*H. pylori* potential of the nitrofurane derivatives of 1,3,4-thiadiazole scaffold is mainly attributed to the type and position of the substituted group at the benzyl piperazine pendant. Future studies may be aimed at designing more potent derivatives of these series in order to investigate the structure-activity relationship of cyclic amine derivatives of 5-(nitroaryl)-1,3,4-thiadiazole derivatives as Anti-*H. pylori* agents.

Competing interests

The authors declare that they have no competing interests.

Authors' contributions

NM: Synthesis of some target compounds. PS: Evaluation of the antibacterial activities (10%). AG: Evaluation of the antibacterial activities. HA: Evaluation of the antibacterial activities (10%). FA: Synthesis of the intermediates and some target compounds. NE: Collaboration in identifying of the structures of target compounds. FS: Evaluation of the antibacterial activities. AF: Collaboration in design and identifying of the structures of target compounds, manuscript preparation. AS: Design of target compounds and management of the synthetic and pharmacological parts. All authors read and approved the final manuscript.

Acknowledgements

This work was financially supported by grants from Research Council of Tehran University of Medical Sciences grant No.90/d/425/236 and Iran National Science Foundation (INSF).

Author details

[1]Department of Medicinal Chemistry, Faculty of Pharmacy and Pharmaceutical Sciences Research Center, Tehran University of Medical Sciences, Tehran 14176, Iran. [2]Department of Microbiology, Faculty of Sciences, University of Tehran, P.O. Box: 14155–6455, Tehran, Iran. [3]Department of Biology, Faculty of Science, Golestan University, Gorgan, Iran. [4]Department of Chemistry, Science and Research Branch, Islamic Azad University, Arak, Iran.

References

1. Marshall BJ, Warren JR: **Unidentified curved bacilli in the stomach of patients with gastritis and peptic ulceration.** *Lancet* 1984, **1**(8390):1311–1315.
2. Bardhan PK: **Epidemiological features of *H. pylori* infection in developing countries.** *Clin Infect Dis* 1997, **25**:973–978.
3. Gisbert JP, Pajares JM: **Treatment of *H. pylori* infection: the past and the future.** *Eur J Intern Med* 2010, **21**:357–359.
4. Sepulveda AR, Coelho LG: ***H. pylori* and gastric malignancies.** *Helicobacter* 2002, **7**:37–42.
5. Egan BJ, Katicic M, O'Connor HJ, O'Mora n CA: **Treatment of *H. pylori*.** *Helicobacter* 2007, **12**:31–37.
6. Petersen AM, Krogfelt KA: ***H. pylori*: an invading microorganism? A review.** *FEMS Immunol Med Microbiol* 2003, **36**:117–126.
7. Gisbert JP: **Review: second-line rescue therapy of *H. pylori* infection.** *Therap Adv Gastroenterol* 2009, **2**:331–356.
8. Kivi M, Tindberg Y, Sörberg M, Casswall TH, Befrits R, Hellström PM, Bengtsson C, Engstrand L, Granström M: **Concordance of *H. pylori* strains within families.** *J Clin Microbiol* 2003, **41**:5604–5608.
9. Nair MD, Nagarajan K: **Nitroimidazoles as chemotherapeutic agents.** *Prog Drug Res* 1983, **27**:163–252.
10. Foroumadi A, Pournourmohammadi S, Soltani F, Asgharian-Rezaee M, Dabiri S, Kharazmi A, Shafiee A: **Synthesis and in vitro leishmanicidal activity of 2-(5-nitro-2-furyl) and 2-(5-nitro-2-thienyl)-5-substituted-1,3,4-thiadiazoles.** *Bioorg Med Chem Lett* 2005, **15**:1983–1985.
11. Foroumadi A, Emami S, Pournourmohammadi S, Kharazmi A, Shafiee A: **Synthesis and in vitro leishmanicidal activity of 2-(1-methyl-5-nitro-1H-imidazol-2-yl)-5-substituted-1,3,4-thiadiazole derivatives.** *Eur J Med Chem* 2005, **40**:1346–1350.
12. Tahghighi A, Razmi S, Mahdavi M, Foroumadi P, Ardestani SK, Emami S, Kobarfard F, Dastmalchi S, Shafiee A, Foroumadi A: **Synthesis and anti-leishmanial activity of 5-(5-nitrofuran-2-yl)-1,3,4-thiadiazol-2-amines containing N-[(1-benzyl-1H-1,2,3-triazol-4-yl)methyl] moieties.** *Eur J Med Chem* 2012, **50**:124–128.
13. Poorrajab F, Ardestani SK, Emami S, Behrouzi-Fardmoghadam M, Shafiee A, Foroumadi A: **Nitroimidazolyl-1,3,4-thiadiazole-based anti-leishmanial agents: synthesis and in vitro biological evaluation.** *Eur J Med Chem* 2009, **44**:1758–1762.
14. Foroumadi A, Sorkhi M, Moshafi MH, Safavi M, Rineh A, Siavoshi F, Shafiee A, Emami S: **2-Substituted-5-nitroheterocycles: in vitro anti- *H. pylori* activity and structure-activity relationship study.** *Med Chem* 2009, **5**:529–534.
15. Moshafi MH, Sorkhi M, Emami S, Nakhjiri M, Yahya-Meymandi A, Negahbani AS, Siavoshi F, Omrani M, Alipour E, Vosooghi M, Shafiee A, Foroumadi A: **5-Nitroimidazole-based 1,3,4-thiadiazoles: heterocyclic analogs of metronidazole as anti- *H. pylori* agents.** *Arch Pharm* 2011, **344**:178–183.
16. Mirzaei J, Siavoshi F, Emami S, Safari F, Khoshayand MR, Shafiee A, Foroumadi A: **Synthesis and in vitro anti- *H. pylori* activity of N-[5-(5-nitro-2-heteroaryl)-1,3,4-thiadiazol-2-yl]thiomorpholines and related compounds.** *Eur J Med Chem* 2008, **43**:1575–1580.
17. Foroumadi A, Rineh A, Emami S, Siavoshi F, Massarrat S, Safari F, Rajabalian S, Falahati M, Lotfali E, Shafiee A: **Synthesis and anti- *H. pylori* activity of 5-(nitroaryl)-1,3,4-thiadiazoles with certain sulfur containing alkyl side chain.** *Bioorg Med Chem Lett* 2008, **18**:3315–3320.
18. Mohammadhosseini N, Alipanahi Z, Alipour E, Emami S, Faramarzi M, Samadi N, Khoshnevis N, Shafiee A, Foroumadi A: **Synthesis and antibacterial activity of novel levofloxacin derivatives containing a substituted thienylethyl moiety.** *DARU* 2012, **20**:16.

13

Hepatoprotective effect of silyamarin in individuals chronically exposed to hydrogen sulfide; modulating influence of TNF-α cytokine genetic polymorphism

Ali Mandegary[1*], Arastoo Saeedi[2], Aziz Eftekhari[1], Vahideh Montazeri[1] and Elham Sharif[3]

Abstract

Background and the purpose of the study: Silymarin, a standardized extract of the milk thistle (*Silybum marianum*), is believed to exert some of its hepatoprotective effects though inhibition of free radicals and inflammation. In this study the effect of some pro- and anti-inflammatory cytokines and also antioxidant genes polymorphisms on the hepatoprotective effects of silymarin in the occupationally exposed individuals to hydrogen sulfide (H_2S) in the sour natural gas refinery was investigated.

Methods: We genotyped seven polymorphisms in six genes reported by others as modifiers of oxidative stress (NQO1, mEPXH1, GSTT1 and GSTM1) and inflammation (TNF-α and TGF-β1) for an association in effect of decreasing in liver function tests (LFTs). The LFTs of 77 sour gas refinery workers were measured before and after administration of silymarin (140 mg, three times per day for 1 month).

Results: A significant reduction of blood AST, ALT and ALP was observed after 30 days of consumption ($p < 0.001$). The decreasing effect of silymarin on ALT in the subjects with high producer genotype (A allele carriers) was less than low producers. There were no significant associations between TGF-β1 and the studied genes of oxidative stress pathway and the effectiveness of silymarin.

Conclusion: This is the first report about the effectiveness of silymarin in the subjects exposed chronically to H_2S. Meanwhile, the modulatory effect of TNF-α on the effectiveness of silymarin might be used for individualize therapy.

Keywords: Silymarin, Hepatoprotective, Hydrogen sulfide, Occupational toxicology, Polymorphism

Introduction

The workers of natural gas refineries are exposed to potentially toxic substances like hydrogen sulfide (H_2S) and benzene. Recently we have shown that the oxidative stress biomarkers increased in the workers of sweet and, in higher levels, sour gas refineries [1]. Meanwhile the levels of liver function tests (LFTs) were high in the H_2S exposed subjects [1]. Although pathogenesis of liver toxicity induced by H_2S has not been elucidated so far, there is experimental evidence that induction of oxidative stress plays a key role [2,3]. Several observations suggest that increased reactive oxygen species (ROS) and resulting oxidative stress is a critically important determinant of liver injury [4,5]. Oxidative stress is involved in the release of pro-inflammatory mediators (cytokines and chemokines) and injury to the liver cells [4,5]. Silymarin, a mixture of flavonolignans isolated from *Silybum marianum* (milk thistle), has been used to treat liver diseases for hundreds of years [6,7]. The hepatoprotective effect of silymarin is mainly due to its strong antioxidant activity and scavenging the free radicals [8]. It also effectively inhibits the inflammation [9,10], which can also damage the liver [6,11]. Silybin is an effective antioxidant, conserving GSH in liver cells while stabilizing the liver cell membranes against oxidative attack [4,12].

* Correspondence: alimandegary@kmu.ac.ir
[1]Department of Pharmacology & Toxicology, School of Pharmacy and Pharmaceutics Research Center, Kerman University of Medical Sciences, Kerman, Iran
Full list of author information is available at the end of the article

There are inter-individual variations in detoxifying enzymes and cytokines that could be translated into differences in susceptibility for xenobiotic toxicity and treatment outcomes [13-17]. So in this study, we decided to investigate the association of polymorphisms in the enzymes involved in general oxidative stress defence including NAD(P)H:quinone oxidoreductase-1 (NQO1), Glutathione S-transferases (GST) M1 and T1, and microsomal epoxide hydrolase (EPHX1) enzymes and the two most important cytokines involved in the pathogenesis of liver disease with the basis of inflammation, namely tumor necrosis factor-α (TNF-α) and transforming growth factor-β1 (TGF-β1) cytokines and the treatment outcome of silymarin in the subjects chronically exposed to H_2S.

Materials and methods

Materials

Silymarin containing tablets (Livergol) was purchased from Goldaru, Isfahan, Iran. PCR master mix was obtained from CinnaClone (Iran). Ethylenediamine tetraacetic acid (EDTA), Tris, agarose, Sodium Dodecyl Sulfate (SDS), isopropanol and ethanol were purchased from Merck (Germany). Proteinase K and DNA ladder were obtained from Fermentas (Germany).

Study subjects

In this cross-sectional study, 77 employees of sour gas refinery were recruited. According to local authorities, the atmospheric concentration of H_2S in the place was 10–15 ppm [1]. The eligibility criteria for the cases were as follow: working at least 5 years in the refinery and no history of liver disease. Demographic data, general health conditions, lifestyle, years of employment and smoking habits were registered in a questionnaire. Written informed consent was obtained from the subjects after describing the aim of the study. The study was conducted according to the declaration of Helsinki and subsequent revisions and approved by the Ethical Committee of Kerman University of Medical Sciences (No: 91/91/k, KMU). The liver function tests (LFTs) including aspartate aminotransferase (AST) and alanine aminotransferase (ALT) and alkaline phosphatase (ALP) were determined before and after administration of silymarin at the dosage of 150 mg three times per day (Livergol, Goldaru, Esfahan, Iran).

DNA extraction and GST genotyping

DNA was extracted from 5 ml peripheral blood using Miller method [18]. The subjects were genotyped for the deletion in GSTM1 and GSTT1 by a multiplex polymerase chain reaction (PCR). The PCR conditions and primers were as described previously [19]. TNF-α -308G/A and TGF-β1 codon 10 and codon 25 genotyping methods were based on the PCR-ARMS, and were similar to those previously described [20]. The amplified fragments were 184-bp, 241-bp and 233-bp respectively for TNF-α, TGF-β1 codon 10 and 25. EPXH1 exon 4 (His139Arg), NQO1 (C609T) and TNF-α (G-308A, for confirmation of PCR-ARMS for TNF-α -308G/A) genotyping methods were based on PCR-RFLP and as described before [21-23]. The products of each PCR reaction and digestion were resolved by electrophoresis on 3% agarose gels stained with ethidium bromide. Reliability and validity of the PCR and RFLP methods were assessed through re-conducting the genotype assays using at least a 10% sample of our DNA samples. The polymorphisms of heterozygous, homozygous and wild-type TNF-α which obtained by PCR-ARMS were re-checked with PCR-RFLP method. In addition, for TGF-β1 the method was also assessed through re-conducting the genotype assays using most of DNA samples with mutations (both heterozygous and homozygous). The results for all re-assessments were 100% concordant.

Statistical analysis

For the comparison of continuous variables, we firstly checked the assumption that they were normally distributed. If the distribution was normal, the results were expressed as means and standard error (SE) and a classical t-test or one-way ANOVA was used accordingly. According to the genes polymorphisms, genotypes were collapsed into two categories: homozygous (common genotypes) versus heterozygous + variant homozygous and they were coded as follow: GSTM1*0 (code 0) and GSTM1-positive (code 1), GSTT1*0 (code 0) and GSTT1-positive (code 1), NQO1 CC allele (code 0) and CT/TT alleles (code 1), EPXH exon 4 AA allele (code 0) and AG/GG alleles (code 1), TGF-β1 codon 10 TT allele (code 0, high producer) and TC/CC alleles (code 1, low producer), and TGF-β1 codon 25 GG allele (code 0, high producer) and GC/CC alleles (code 1, low producer). Combination of TGF-β1 codons 10 and 25 was as follow: TT/GG (code 0, high producer) and all other combinations (code 1, low producer). Simple and multiple linear regression was used to screen the independent variables including genetic polymorphism to best predict the value of the LFTs and LFTs difference. Age and BMI variables believed to potentially confound the association with LFTs' level were included in the multivariate model. The significance (P) of genetic polymorphisms factors from multivariate analysis was considered as adjusted p-value. Differences between LFTs before and after administration of silymarin were analyzed using paired-sample t-test. For all the tests, a p-value less than 0.05 was considered to be significant. All analyses were conducted using SPSS statistical software (version 11.5).

Results

Significant decreases in AST ($P < 0.01$), ALT ($P < 0.001$) and ALP ($P < 0.001$) were observed by use of silymarin

(Figure 1). The mean ± SE of AST before and after using were 39.8 ± 0.78 and 29.7 ± 0.07 U L^{-1} (Figure 1A). A significant (P < 0.001) decrease in ALT was observed after administration of silymarin (66.4 ± 1.4 U L^{-1} before versus 30.5 ± 0.9 U L^{-1} after (Figure 1B). After use of silymarin, the ALP level decreased significantly (P < 0.001). The mean ± SE values before and after were 231.2 ± 5.9 and 209.2 ± 4.8 U L^{-1} (Figure 1C).

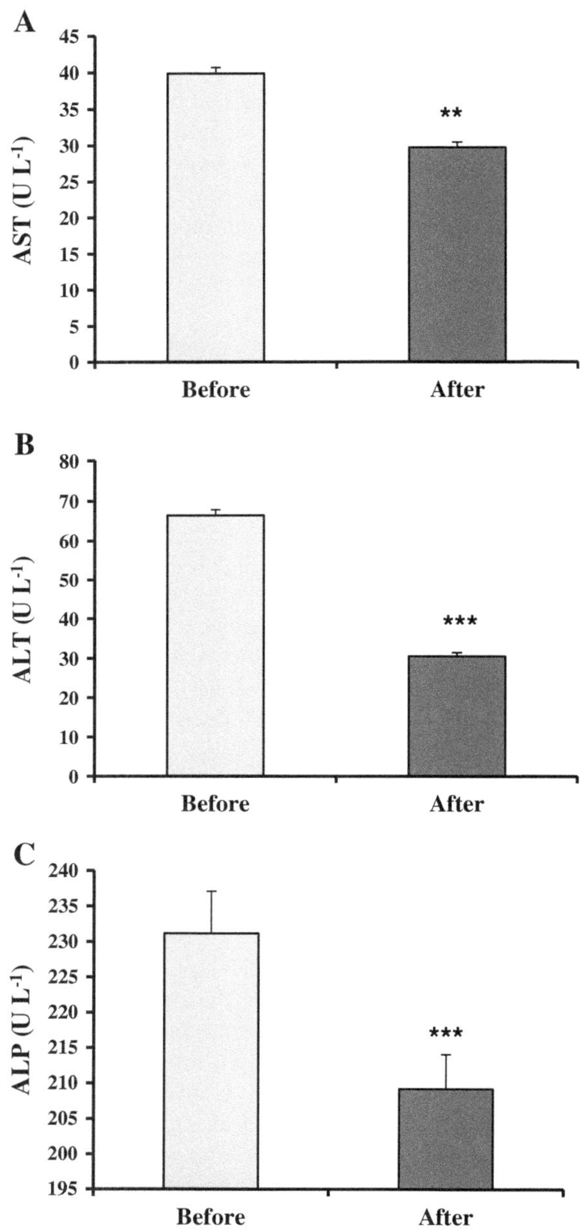

Figure 1 Effect of the consumption of silymarin on serum LFTs. AST (**A**), ALT (**B**) and ALP (**C**) levels in the chronically H_2S exposed subjects (n = 77) were measured before and after administration of silymarin. Results are expressed as mean ± SE. ** *p* < 0.001 and *** *p* < 0.001 compared with before treatment by Pair sample t-test.

Simple and multivariate linear regression were performed to analyze the association of GSTM1, GSTT1, NQO1 and EPXH1 genes polymorphisms with changes in LFTs after administration of silymarin (Table 1). There was no association between the abovementioned genes' polymorphisms and decreasing in LFTs after administration of silymarin.

Simple and multivariate linear regression were performed to analyze the association of TNF-α, TGF-β1 codon 10, TGF-β1 codon 25 and combination of these two codons polymorphisms with changes in LFTs after administration of silymarin (Table 2). TNF-α G-308A polymorphism was significantly associated with deceasing in the AST (p = 0.04) and ALT (p = 0.003). These results show that decreasing in the AST and ALT levels are lower in the subjects with high producer TNF-α genotype. These associations remained significant after adjustment with age and BMI. There was also negative significant association between TGF-β1 codon 10 polymorphisms and decreasing in ALP that this association was abolished when age and BMI added to the model.

Discussion

In light of our recent study demonstrating increase in the LFT levels in the workers exposed chronically to H_2S, we became interested in determining whether a well-known hepatoprotective natural product like silymarin could decrease the LFTs in the subjects and if the genetics of the subjects could determine responding to treatment. Administration of silymarin (140 mg tablets, thrice per day for 1 - month) significantly reduced the LFTs in the subjects. The hepatoprotective mechanisms of silymarin on H_2S-induced elevation of LFTs have not been addressed so far. Recently we have also shown that stress oxidative biomarkers were higher in the workers in exposure to H_2S [1]. Lines of evidence demonstrate that stress oxidative is one of the main mechanisms for the toxic effect of xenobiotics on the liver [4,15,24]. Antioxidant activity and scavenging the free radicals have been reported as the main mechanism for the hepatoprotective effect of silymarin [6].

Our data showed significant association (B = −8.30, CI: -13.73,-2.86) between the polymorphism of TNF-α G-308A and the changes in ALT and AST after administration of silymarin (Table 2). In other words, decrease in ALT and AST in the high TNF-α producers treated with silymarin is significantly lower than low producers. TNF-α is a pro-inflammatory cytokine involved in the pathogenesis of variety of liver injuries [25]. TNF-α, in concert with other cytokines, mediates the recruitment of neutrophils to the liver that induce inflammation and cell death [26]. Production of TNF-α is under genetic control which determined by a number of single nucleotide polymorphisms in this gene. The G-308A polymorphism in the promoter of the gene is the most studied one that has been linked to higher TNF-α production [27,28] as homozygosity for

Table 1 Association of oxidative stress related genes polymorphisms with changes in LFTs' levels by consumption of silymarin

LFT	Gene	Unadjusted		Adjusted	
		B (CI)	p-value	B (CI)	p-value
AST	NQO1	−0.73 (−3.38, 4.84)	0.72	−0.05 (−4.10, 3.92)	0.98
	GSTM1	−0.58 (−4. 02, 3.03)	0.75	−0.64 (−4.25, 2.97)	0.72
	GSTT1	1.27 (−3.10, 5.64)	0.56	1.92 (−2.55, 6.38)	0.40
	EPXH4	1.34 (−3.10, 5.77)	0.54	1.72 (−2.73, 6.17)	0.44
ALT	NQO1	0.87 (−4.20, 5.92)	0.73	0.79 (−4.40, 5.98)	0.76
	GSTM1	−4.24 (−8. 62, 0.13)	0.05	4.21 (−8.67, 0.25)	0.06
	GSTT1	1.30 (−4.23, 6.83)	0.64	1.22 (−4.50, 6.92)	0.65
	EPXH4	1.04 (−3.02, 4.67)	0.54	0.89 (−4.46, 6.24)	0.74
ALP	NQO1	−12.83 (−39.89, 14.22)	0.35	−2.64 (−20.22, 14.95)	0.76
	GSTM1	1.21 (−23.79, 26.21)	0.92	2.27 (−13.67, 18.22)	0.77
	GSTT1	21.28 (−8.93, 51.50)	0.16	10.21 (−9.46, 29.87)	0.30
	EPXH4	−14.20 (−47.62, 19.22)	0.40	1.73 (−17.78, 21.24)	0.86

Multivariate regression: Parameters adjusted for age and BMI;
B: Partial regression coefficient.

TNF1 (TNF1/TNF1) is associated with low production (TNF-α^{Lo}), whereas the TNF1/TNF2 and TNF2/TNF2 genotypes are high producers (TNF-α^{Hi}). The effect of TNF-α on the production of ROS was also shown elsewhere [25]. TNF-induced ROS production activates JNK (c-jun N-terminal kinase) by oxidizing and inactivating several members of the MAP kinase phosphates (MKPs). Taking together, one might relate the less hepatoprotective effect of an antioxidant compound like silymarin in high producer of TNF-α to higher production of ROS in these subjects.

Our data also showed no association between the polymorphisms of TGF-β and some of detoxifying enzymes and the changes in LFTs after administration of silymarin. Univariate regression analysis showed a significant association between TGF-β1 gene polymorphism at codon 10 and ALP levels that this association was abolished after adjusting the regression with confounders like age and BMI. This is in consistent with the previous reports about the role of BMI on the LFTs [29].

Conclusion

Administration of silymarin (140 mg tablets, thrice per day for 1 month) significantly reduced the LFTs in the subjects exposed chronically to H_2S. Meanwhile, increasing the dose of silymarin in the high TNF-α producers to obtain therapeutic effects might be needed.

Table 2 Association of inflammation related cytokines polymorphisms with changes in LFTs' levels by consumption of silymarin

LFT	*Gene*	*Unadjusted*		*Adjusted*	
		B (CI)	p-value	B (CI)	p-value
AST	TNF-α	−4.27 (−8.57, 0.03)	0.05	−4.58 (−8.97, -0.21)	**0.04***
	TGF-β1 codon 10	−0.77 (−5. 17, 3.61)	0.72	−0.07 (−4.56, 4.41)	0.97
	TGF-β1 codon 25	2.78 (−3.36, 8.93)	0.36	2.79 (−3.40, 8.98)	0.37
	TGF-β1 codons 10/25	0.99 (−3.04, 5.03)	0.62	1.37 (−2.73, 5.46)	0.50
ALT	TNF-α	−8.30 (−13.73, -2.86)	**0.003***	−8.93 (−14.62, -3.23)	**0.003***
	TGF-β1 codon 10	−3.62 (−8.92, 1.67)	0.17	−3.43 (−9.00, 2.14)	0.22
	TGF-β1 codon 25	5.87 (−1.29, 13.03)	0.10	5.94 (−1.36, 13.24)	0.10
	TGF-β1 codons 10/25	−0.33 (−5.28, 4.63)	0.89	0.03 (−5.11, 5.24)	0.99
ALP	TNF-α	−6.17 (−41.08, 28.75)	0.72	−0.85 (−21.93, 20.21)	0.93
	TGF-β1 codon 10	−31.45 (−61.31, -1.59)	0.03	−9.05 (−27.43, 8.32)	0.33
	TGF-β1 codon 25	16.67 (−25.38, 58.73)	0.43	−12.00 (−37.17, 13.17)	0.34
	TGF-β1 codons 10/25	−16.16 (−44.41, 12.07)	0.25	−8.65 (−24.63, 7.33)	0.28

Multivariate regression: Parameters adjusted for age and BMI. *Significant effect. B: Partial regression coefficient.

Competing interests

The authors declare that they have no competing interests.

Authors' contributions

AM participated in the design of the study, performed the statistical analysis, participated in the sequence alignment and drafted the manuscript. AS carried out sampling and carried out genotyping of some genes. AE carried out genotyping of some genes and filed the data. VM carried out genotyping of some genes. ESh carried out DNA extraction and helped to draft the manuscript. All authors read and approved the final manuscript.

Acknowledgements

This works is supported by Deputy of Research, Kerman University of Medical Sciences. The authors would like to thank Ms. Maryam Sezavar and Dr. Samaneh Soleymani for their helps. This article also has been derived from the thesis of MSc students (AS and AE) in Kerman University of medical Sciences, Faculty of Pharmacy, Kerman, Iran.

Author details

[1]Department of Pharmacology & Toxicology, School of Pharmacy and Pharmaceutics Research Center, Kerman University of Medical Sciences, Kerman, Iran. [2]Physiology Research Center, Kerman University of Medical Sciences, Kerman, Iran. [3]Herbal and Traditional Medicines Research Center, Kerman University of Medical Sciences, Kerman, Iran.

References

1. Mandegary A, Sezavar M, Saeedi A, Amirheidari B, Naghibi B: **Oxidative stress induced in the workers of natural gas refineries, no role for GSTM1 and GSTT1 polymorphisms.** *Hum Exp Toxicol* 2012, **31**:1271–1279.
2. Eghbal MA, Pennefather PS, O'Brien PJ: **H2S cytotoxicity mechanism involves reactive oxygen species formation and mitochondrial depolarisation.** *Toxicology* 2004, **203**:69–76.
3. Attene-Ramos MS, Wagner ED, Gaskins HR, Plewa MJ: **Hydrogen sulfide induces direct radical-associated DNA damage.** *Mol Cancer Res* 2007, **5**:455–459.
4. Ha HL, Shin HJ, Feitelson MA, Yu DY: **Oxidative stress and antioxidants in hepatic pathogenesis.** *World J Gastroenterol* 2010, **16**:6035–6043.
5. Jaeschke H: **Reactive oxygen and mechanisms of inflammatory liver injury: Present concepts.** *J Gastroenterol Hepatol* 2011, **26**(Suppl 1):173–179.
6. Pradhan SC, Girish C: **Hepatoprotective herbal drug, silymarin from experimental pharmacology to clinical medicine.** *Indian J Med Res* 2006, **124**:491–504.
7. Saller R, Brignoli R, Melzer J, Meier R: **An updated systematic review with meta-analysis for the clinical evidence of silymarin.** *Forsch Komplementmed* 2008, **15**:9–20.
8. Tsai JH, Liu JY, Wu TT, Ho PC, Huang CY, Shyu JC, Hsieh YS, Tsai CC, Liu YC: **Effects of silymarin on the resolution of liver fibrosis induced by carbon tetrachloride in rats.** *J Viral Hepat* 2008, **15**:508–514.
9. De La Puerta R, Martinez E, Bravo L, Ahumada MC: **Effect of silymarin on different acute inflammation models and on leukocyte migration.** *J Pharm Pharmacol* 1996, **48**:968–970.
10. Katiyar SK: **Silymarin and skin cancer prevention: anti-inflammatory, antioxidant and immunomodulatory effects (Review).** *Int J Oncol* 2005, **26**:169–176.
11. Luster MI, Simeonova PP, Gallucci RM, Bruccoleri A, Blazka ME, Yucesoy B: **Role of inflammation in chemical-induced hepatotoxicity.** *Toxicol Lett* 2001, **120**:317–321.
12. Shaker E, Mahmoud H, Mnaa S: **Silymarin, the antioxidant component and Silybum marianum extracts prevent liver damage.** *Food Chem Toxicol* 2010, **48**:803–806.
13. Fabris C, Soardo G, Falleti E, Toniutto P, Vitulli D, Federico E, Del Forno M, Mattiuzzo M, Gonano F, Pirisi M: **Relationship among hepatic inflammatory changes, circulating levels of cytokines, and response to IFN-alpha in chronic hepatitis C.** *J Interferon Cytokine Res* 1998, **18**:705–709.
14. Bidwell J, Keen L, Gallagher G, Kimberly R, Huizinga T, McDermott MF, Oksenberg J, McNicholl J, Pociot F, Hardt C, D'Alfonso S: **Cytokine gene polymorphism in human disease: on-line databases.** *Genes Immun* 1999, **1**:3–19.
15. Czaja MJ: **Cell signaling in oxidative stress-induced liver injury.** *Semin Liver Dis* 2007, **27**:378–389.
16. Abbas Z, Moatter T, Hussainy A, Jafri W: **Effect of cytokine gene polymorphism on histological activity index, viral load and response to treatment in patients with chronic hepatitis C genotype 3.** *World J Gastroenterol* 2005, **11**:6656–6661.
17. Lopez P, Gomez J, Mozo L, Gutierrez C, Suarez A: **Cytokine polymorphisms influence treatment outcomes in SLE patients treated with antimalarial drugs.** *Arthritis Res Ther* 2006, **8**:R42.
18. Miller SA, Dykes DD, Polesky HF: **A simple salting out procedure for extracting DNA from human nucleated cells.** *Nucleic Acids Res* 1988, **16**:1215.
19. Mandegary A, Rostami S, Alimoghaddam K, Ghavamzadeh A, Ghahremani MH: **Gluthatione-s-transferase T1-null Genotype predisposes adults to acute promyelocytic leukemia; a case–control study.** *Asian Pacific J Cancer Prev* 2011, **12**:1279–1282.
20. Perrey C, Turner SJ, Pravica V, Howell WM, Hutchinson IV: **ARMS-PCR methodologies to determine IL-10, TNF-alpha, TNF-beta and TGF-beta 1 gene polymorphisms.** *Transpl Immunol* 1999, **7**:127–128.
21. Cheng SL, Yu CJ, Chen CJ, Yang PC: **Genetic polymorphism of epoxide hydrolase and glutathione S-transferase in COPD.** *Eur Respir J* 2004, **23**:818–824.
22. Naoe T, Takeyama K, Yokozawa T, Kiyoi H, Seto M, Uike N, Ino T, Utsunomiya A, Maruta A, Jin-nai I, Kamada N, Kubota Y, Nakamura H, Shimazaki C, Horiike S, Kodera Y, Saito H, Ueda R, Wiemels J, Ohno R: **Analysis of genetic polymorphism in NQO1, GST-M1, GST-T1, and CYP3A4 in 469 Japanese patients with therapy-related leukemia/ myelodysplastic syndrome and de novo acute myeloid leukemia.** *Clin Cancer Res* 2000, **6**:4091–4095.
23. Wilson AG, Symons JA, McDowell TL, McDevitt HO, Duff GW: **Effects of a polymorphism in the human tumor necrosis factor alpha promoter on transcriptional activation.** *Proc Natl Acad Sci USA* 1997, **94**:3195–3199.
24. Videla LA: **Oxidative stress signaling underlying liver disease and hepatoprotective mechanisms.** *World J Hepatol* 2009, **1**:72–78.
25. Schwabe RF, Brenner DA: **Mechanisms of Liver Injury. I. TNF-alpha -induced liver injury: role of IKK, JNK, and ROS pathways.** *Am J Physiol Gastrointest Liver Physiol* 2006, **290**:G583–589.
26. Marcos M, Gomez-Munuera M, Pastor I, Gonzalez-Sarmiento R, Laso FJ: **Tumor necrosis factor polymorphisms and alcoholic liver disease: a HuGE review and meta-analysis.** *Am J Epidemiol* 2009, **170**:948–956.
27. Wilson AG, di Giovine FS, Blakemore AI, Duff GW: **Single base polymorphism in the human tumour necrosis factor alpha (TNF alpha) gene detectable by NcoI restriction of PCR product.** *Hum Mol Genet* 1992, **1**:353.
28. Kroeger KM, Carville KS, Abraham LJ: **The −308 tumor necrosis factor-alpha promoter polymorphism effects transcription.** *Mol Immunol* 1997, **34**:391–399.
29. Choi JW: **Association between elevated serum hepatic enzyme activity and total body fat in obese humans.** *Ann Clin Lab Sci* 2003, **33**:257–264.

4-Aryl-4*H*-naphthopyrans derivatives: one-pot synthesis, evaluation of Src kinase inhibitory and anti-proliferative activities

Ali Rafinejad[1], Asal Fallah-Tafti[1], Rakesh Tiwari[2], Amir Nasrolahi Shirazi[2], Deendayal Mandal[2], Abbas Shafiee[1], Keykavous Parang[2], Alireza Foroumadi[1] and Tahmineh Akbarzadeh[1*]

Abstract

Background: A series of 2-amino-4-aryl-4*H*-benzo[h or f]chromene-3-carbonitrile derivatives were synthesized and evaluated for inhibition of Src kinase and cell proliferation in breast carcinoma (BT-20) cell lines.

Methods: The one-pot, three-component reaction of α or β-naphthol, malonitrile and an aromatic aldehyde in the presence of diammonium hydrogen phosphate was afforded the corresponding 2-amino-4-aryl-4*H*-benzo[h or f] chromene-3-carbonitrile derivatives, All target compounds were evaluated for inhibition of Src kinase and cell proliferation in breast carcinoma (BT-20) cell lines.

Results: Among all tested compounds, unsubstituted 4-phenyl analog **4a** showed Src kinas inhibitory effect with IC_{50} value of 28.1 μM and was the most potent compound in this series. In general, the compounds were moderately active against BT-20. 3-Nitro-phenyl **4e** and 3-pyridinyl **4h** derivatives inhibited the cell proliferation of BT-20 cells by 33% and 31.5%, respectively, and found to be more potent compared to doxorubicin (25% inhibition of cell growth).

Conclusion: The data indicate that 4-aryl-4*H*-naphthopyrans scaffold has the potential to be optimized further for designing more potent Src kinase inhibitors and/or anticancer lead compounds.

Keywords: Anticancer activity, Carbonitrile, Naphthopyrans, Protein kinase, Src kinase

Introduction

c-Src kinase is one of the most widely studied member of the Src (acronym of sarcoma) family of non-receptor protein tyrosine kinases (PTKs). c-Src acts as a critical component in a number of signaling pathways that control cell growth, proliferation, invasion, and apoptosis [1-3]. Previous studies have shown that c-Src kinase is highly regulated and is active only at low levels in most normal cells while it is upregulated in many human cancers [4,5]. Most recently emerging data reveals that the predominant consequences of increased c-Src activity in tumor cells results in reduction of cell adhesion, facilitation of motility, and thereby promotion of an invasive phenotype [6]. Interest in designing c-Src kinase inhibitors as a treatment for cancer and in particular, as an antiinvasion strategy has been increased in the last decade. The current popularity of Src kinases as drug targets is due to several factors including the positive correlation between the development of cancer and the upregulation of Src activity and reduction of cancer progression by inhibition of Src kinase in several types of cancer [7-10].

Several c-Src kinase inhibitors have been identified over the years [11]. Src kinase inhibitor scaffolds span a variety of structural classes, including staurosporine as a standard nonselective protein kinase inhibitor, pyrazolopyrimidine (e.g., PP1, PP2) [12,13], anilinoquinazoline [14,15], and quinolinecarbonitrile [16-18] derivatives. The Saracatinib (AZD0530) [15,19] and Bosutinib (SKI-606) [20,21] with anilinoquinazoline and 3-quinolinecarbonitrile cores, respectively (Figure 1), are among potent Src kinase

* Correspondence: akbarzad@tums.ac.ir
[1]Department of Medicinal Chemistry, Faculty of Pharmacy and Drug Design & Development Research Center, Tehran University of Medical Sciences, Tehran, Iran
Full list of author information is available at the end of the article

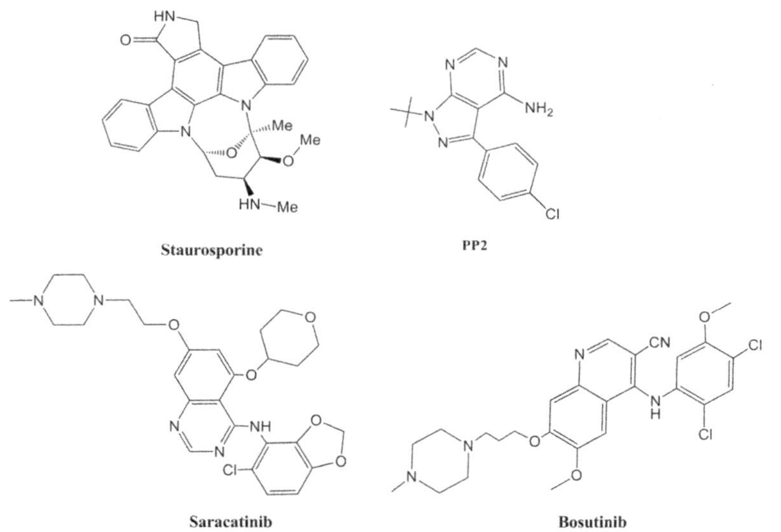

Figure 1 Chemical structures of some of the Src kinase inhibitors.

inhibitors, which are currently in clinical development for the treatment of a wide range of tumor types. Since ATP binding region is strongly conserved among protein kinases, designing selective Src kinase inhibitors is still a great challenge. Therefore, research is needed to explore new scaffolds which selectively inhibit Src kinase domain.

Recently emerging data support the hypothesis that the presence of a nitrile group in different scaffolds, such as quinolinecarbonitrile (e.g., Bosutinib), and benzylidene-malononitriles (tyrophostins (acronym of tyrosine phosphorylation inhibitors)), is crucial for protein kinase inhibitory activity [22]. Compound **A** (Figure 2) [23] with

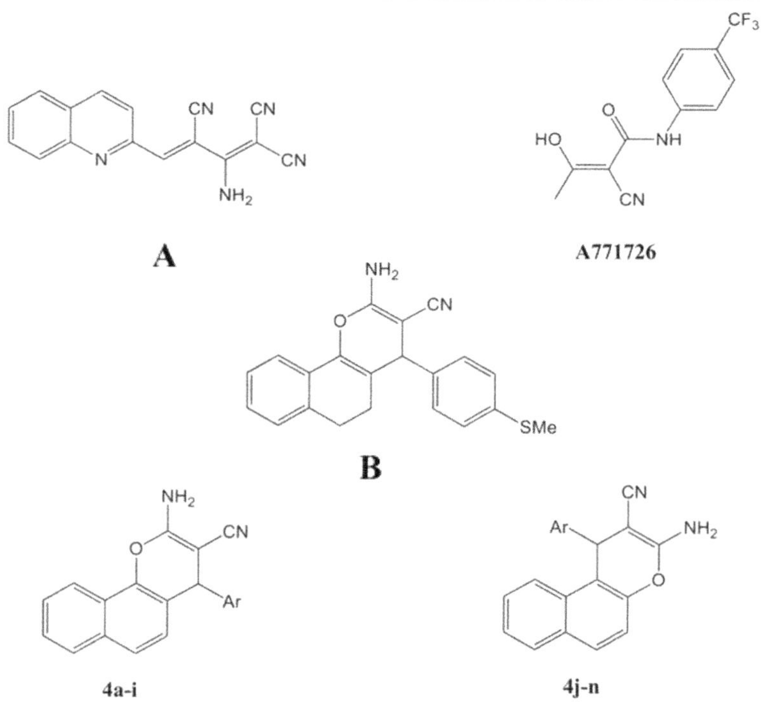

Figure 2 Benzylidene-malononitrile(tyrophstin) derivative as protein kinase inhibitor (A), Chemical structures of A771726, active metabolite of Leflunomide, antiproliferative 4-aryl-*4H*-5,6-dihydronaphtho[1,2-b]pyran (compound B), and synthesized 4-Aryl-*4H*-Naphthopyrans (4a-n).

2-quinoline tyrophostin structure exhibit IC_{50} in the low molecular range (IC_{50}= 1.7 μM) against EFGR. Furthermore, A771726 (Figure 2) with cyano hydroxyl β-butenamide, which is the predominant active metabolite of Leflunamide, has been identified as a tyrosine kinase inhibitor and antiproliferative agent [24,25]. This compound was used as a starting lead for designing new antiproliferative compounds that finally led to the identification of 4-aryl-4*H*-5,6-dihydronaphtho[1,2-b]pyran **B** (Figure 2) as a new lead compound with moderate activity on the mesenchymal stem cell proliferation assay (IC_{50} = 13 μM) [25]. Different derivatives of naphthopyranes have been synthesized since then and showed multiple pharmacological effects, such as anti-rheumatoid, anti-diabetic, anti-proliferative, and protease inhibition effects [25,26].

We previously reported synthesis and evaluation of 4-aryl-4*H*-chromene-3-carbonitrile derivatives as Src kinase inhibitors [27]. As part of our efforts to identify new scaffolds as Src kinase inhibitors [28-35], herein we report the synthesis and evaluation of selected 2 or 3-amino-4-aryl-4*H*-benzo[*h* or *f*]chromene-3-carbonitrile derivatives **4a-n** (Figure 2) that contains both nitrile and naphthopyrane cores as Src kinase inhibitors or anti-proliferative agents.

Methods

Materials

All starting materials, reagents, and solvents were purchased from Merck AG (Germany). The purity of the synthesized compounds was confirmed by thin layer chromatography (TLC) using various solvents of different polarities. Merck silica gel 60 F254 plates were applied for analytical TLC. Column chromatography was performed on Merck silica gel (70–230 mesh) for purification of the intermediate and final compounds. Melting points were determined on a Kofler hot stage apparatus (Vienna, Austria) and are uncorrected. ^1H NMR spectra were recorded using a Bruker 500 MHz spectrometer (Bruker, Rheinstatten, Germany), and chemical shifts were expressed as δ (ppm) with tetramethylsilane (TMS) as an internal standard. The IR spectra were obtained on a Shimadzu 470 (Shimadzu, Tokyo, Japan) spectrophotometer (potassium bromide disks). The mass spectra were run on a Finnigan TSQ-70 spectrometer (Thermo Finnigan, West Chester, OH, USA) at 70 eV. Elemental analyses were carried out on a CHN-O-rapid elemental analyzer (Heraeus GmbH, Hanau, Germany) for C, H, and N, and the results were within ± 0.4% of the theoretical values.

General procedure for the peparation of 2-amino-4-aryl-4*H*-naphthopyran-3-carbonitrile derivatives 4a-n

In general, diammonium hydrogen phosphate (DAHR, 0.5 mmol) was added to a mixture of α or β-naphtol (5 mmol), substituted aryl-aldehyde (5 mmol), and malonitrile (5 mmol) in ethanol (10 mL) and water (10 mL). The reaction mixture was stirred at room temperature for 4 h. After cooling, the precipitated solid was filtered, washed with cold ethanol, and crystallized from the same solvent. The synthesized compounds were characterized by IR, ^1H NMR, mass spectrpscopy and elemental analysis. Physicochemical and spectral properties of compounds **4a-n** were consistent with the previously reported data [36,37].

c-Src kinase activity assay

The effect of synthesized compounds on the activity of c-Src kinase was determined by HTScan Src Kinase Assay Kit, catalogue number 7776 from Cell Signaling Technology (Danvers, MA, USA); according to manufacturer's protocol. Streptavidin-coated plates were purchased from Pierce (Rockford, IL, USA). In brief, the kinase reaction was started with the incubation of the 12.5 μL of the reaction cocktail (0.5 ng/μL of GST-Src kinase in 1.25 mM DTT) with 12.5 μL of prediluted compounds (dissolved in 1% DMSO) for 5 min at room temperature. ATP/substrate (25 μL, 20 μM/1.5 uM) cocktail was added to the mixture. The biotinylated substrate (catalogue number 1366) contains the residues surrounding tyrosine 160 (Tyr160) of signal transduction protein and has a sequence of EGIYDVP. The reaction mixture was incubated for 30 min at room temperature. The kinase reaction was stopped with the addition of 50 μL of 50 mM EDTA (pH 8.0). The reaction solution (25 μL) was transferred into 96-well streptavidin plates (Pierce, part number 15125), diluted with 75 μL double distilled water, and incubated at room temperature for 60 min. At the end of the incubation, the wells were washed three times with 200 μL of 0.05% Tween-20 in PBS buffer (PBS/T). After that to each well was added 100 μL of phosphotyrosine antibody (P-Tyr-100) (1:1000 dilution in PBS/T with 1% BSA) and the wells were incubated for another 60 min. After washing three times with 0.05% Tween-20 in PBS/T, the wells were incubated with 100 μL secondary anti-mouse IgG antibody, which was HRP-conjugated (1:500 dilution in PBS/T with 1% BSA) for next 30 min at room temperature. The wells were washed five times with 0.05% Tween-20 in PBS and then were incubated with 100 μL of 3,3',5,5'-tetramethylbenzidine dihydrochloride (TMB) substrate for 5 min. The reaction was stopped by adding 100 μL/well of stop solution to each well and mixed well and read the absorbance at 450 nm using a microplate reader (Molecular devices, spectra Max M2). IC_{50} values of the compounds were calculated using ORIGIN 6.0 (origin lab) software. IC_{50} is the concentration of the compound that inhibited enzyme activity by 50%. All the experiments were carried out in triplicate [27].

Cell culture and cell proliferation assay

Cell culture

Breast carcinoma BT-20 (ATCC no. HTB-19) cell lines were obtained from American Type Culture Collection. Cells were grown on 75 cm^2 cell culture with EMEM medium for breast carcinoma and supplemented with 10% fetal bovine serum (FBS), and 1% penicillin-streptomycin solution (10,000 units of penicillin and 10 mg of streptomycin in 0.9% NaCl) in a humidified atmosphere of 5% CO_2, 95% air at 37°C.

Cell proliferation assay

Cell proliferation assay of compounds was evaluated in BT-20 cells, and was compared with that of doxorubicin (DOX)[38]. Cell proliferation assay was carried out using CellTiter 96 aqueous one solution cell proliferation assay kit (Promega, USA). Briefly, upon reaching about 75-80% confluence, 5000 cells/well were plated in 96-well microplate in 100 μL media. After seeding for 72 h, the cells were treated with 50 μM compound in triplicate. DOX (10 μM) was used as the positive control. Incubation was carried out at 37°C in an incubator supplied with 5% CO_2 for 72 h. At the end of the sample exposure period (72 h), 20 μL CellTiter 96 aqueous solution was added. The plate was returned to the incubator for 1 h in a humidified atmosphere at 37°C. The absorbance of the formazan product was measured at 490 nm using microplate reader. The blank control was recorded by measuring the absorbance at 490 nm with wells containing medium mixed with CellTiter 96 aqueous solution but no cells. Results were expressed as the percentage of the control (DMSO without compound set at 100%). The percentage of cell survival was calculated as (OD value of cells treated with test compound - OD value of culture medium) / (OD value of control cells – OD value of culture medium) × 100%.

Results and discussion

Chemistry

Naphthopyran analogs described here (**4a-n**) were synthesized following the synthetic routes outlined in Figure 3. The compounds were synthesized according to the previously reported general procedure by a one-pot reaction [37] through the condensation of a substituted aromatic aldehyde (**1**), malonitrile, and α or β-naphtol (**3, 5**) in ethanol and water in the presence of diammonium hydrogen phosphate (Figure 4).

Src kinase inhibitory activity

The results of Src kinase inhibitory activity of compounds **4a-n** are shown in Table 1. Compounds **4a**, **4d**, **4i**, **4m**, and **4n** exhibited higher Src kinase inhibitory activity (IC_{50} =28.1– 34.7 μM in following order **4a>4i,4m>4n>4d**) when compared with that of other compounds. Unsubstituted phenyl analog **4a** showed an IC_{50} value of 28.1 μM and was the most potent compound in this series. 2-Chlorophenyl substituted analog **4d** was one of the potent compounds in α-naphthol series with an IC_{50} value of 34.7 μM. Similarly compound **4j** with 3-chlorophenyl substitution was a moderately effective compound in β-naphthol series with an IC_{50} value of 41.7 μM. In addition, 2,3-dichlorophenyl substituted compounds **4f** and **4l** were among potent inhibitors in both α and β-naphthol series of compounds. However, substitution of 2,6-dichlorophenyl in compound **4g** led to loss of inhibitory activity, suggesting that chloro substitution at positions 2 and 6 of phenyl ring is detrimental in Src kinase inhibition. Compounds **4m** and **4n** with 3-hydroxyphenyl and 4-methoxyphenyl moieties, respectively, were among potent compounds in β-naphthol series. 3-Nitrophenyl substitution resulted in loss of activity in compounds **4e** and **4k** in both α and β-naphthol series of compounds. Similarly compounds **4b** (4-F-Ph) and **4c** (3-Br-Ph) did not show any

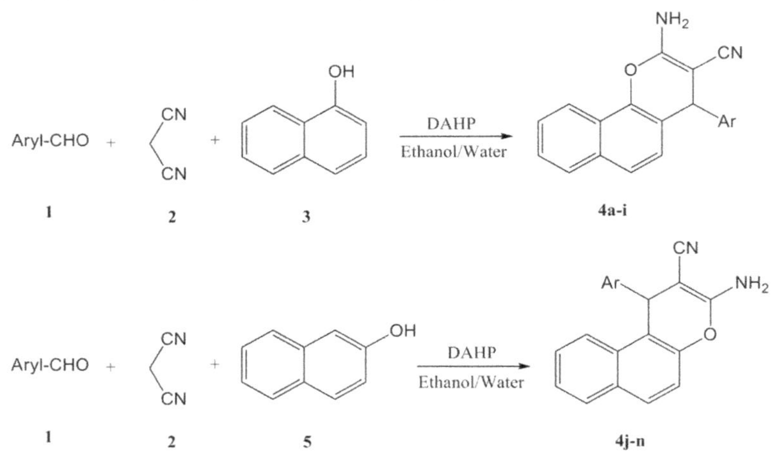

Figure 3 Inhibition of BT-20 cell proliferation by compounds 4a-n (50 μM) after 72 h incubation. The results are shown as the percentage of the control DMSO that has no compound (set at 100%). All the experiments were performed in triplicate.

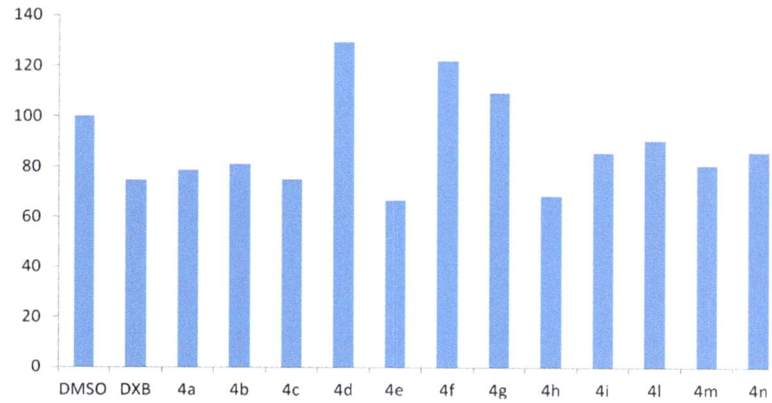

Figure 4 One-pot synthesis of 4-Aryl-4*H*-Naphthopyrans 4a-n.

Table 1 Inhibition of Src Kinase activity by 2-amino-4-aryl-4*H*-naphtopyran-3-carbonitrile derivatives

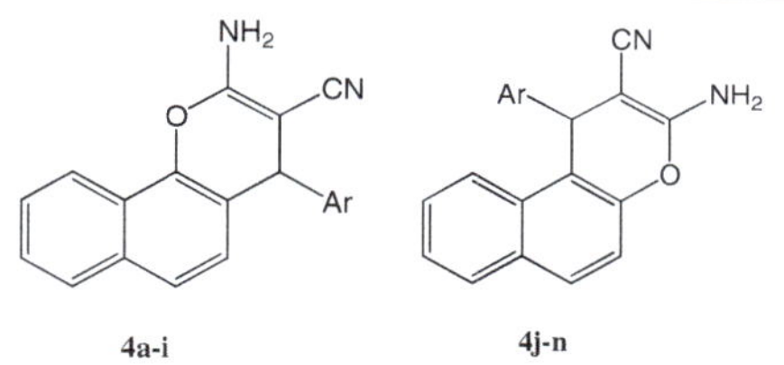

Compounds	Ar	IC_{50} (μM)[a]
4a	Ph	28.1
4b	4-F-Ph	> 150
4c	3-Br-Ph	> 150
4d	2-Cl-Ph	34.7
4e	3-NO_2-Ph	> 150
4f	2,3-di(Cl)-Ph	41.7
4g	2,6-di(Cl)-Ph	> 150
4h	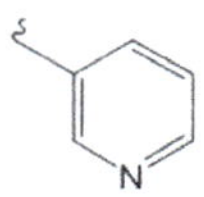	36.5
4i	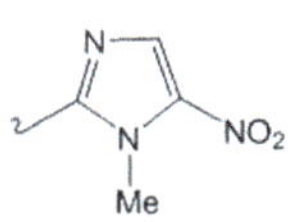	33.8
4j	3-Cl-Ph	41.7
4k	3-NO_2-Ph	> 150
4l	2,3-di(Cl)-Ph	38.9
4m	3-OH-Ph	33.8
4n	4-MeO-Ph	34.5
Staurosporin	-	0.3
PP2	-	2.8

[a]The concentration that inhibited enzyme activity by 50%.

significant inhibitory activity (IC_{50} > 150) against Src kinase. On the other hand, compounds **4h** with pyridine ring substitution and compound **4i** with 1-methylnitroimidazole moiety showed good inhibitory activity against Src kinase compared to other phenyl substituted compounds.

Anti-proliferative activities

The effect of the inhibitors at the concentration of 50 μM on the cell proliferation of breast carcinoma (BT-20) cell line was evaluated (Figure 3). Compounds **4e** and **4h** inhibited the cell proliferation of breast carcinoma cells (BT-20) by 33% and 31.5% (**4h**>**4e**), respectively (Figure 3). Compounds **4e** and **4h** found to be more potent on BT-20 cell proliferation assay compared to doxorubicin, while compound **4c** with 24.8% cell proliferation inhibitory effect against BT-20 cell line was as effective as doxorubicin (25% inhibition of cell growth).

Although compound **4h** was found to be a moderate Src kinase inhibitor and a potent anti-proliferative agent against BT-20 cell line, there were no significant correlation between Src kinase inhibitory potency of the other compounds with their growth inhibition activity against cancer cells. Compounds **4a**, **4d**, **4i**, **4m**, and **4n** with good Src kinase inhibitory activity showed less potency in anti-proliferation assay (0-21%). In contrast, compound **4e** that showed good anti-proliferative effect against breast carcinoma cells was a weak Src kinase inhibitor (IC_{50} > 150 μM). It seems that *in vitro* enzymatic and cell-based assays may not correlate well due to the diversity in solubility and cellular uptake of the compounds. Further studies are required to determine whether these compounds have limited cellular uptakes that lead to their minimal anti-proliferative activities.

Conclusions

A number of 2-amino-4-aryl-4*H*-benzo[h or f]chromene-3-carbonitrile derivatives were prepared and evaluated for Src kinase inhibitory and anticancer activities. In summary, structure-activity relationship studies revealed that the incorporation of less bulkier groups such as unsubstituted phenyl at position of aryl is preferred and well tolerated compared to other groups in generating Src inhibitory activity. The data provide insights for key structural requirements for further optimization of chromene-carbonitrile derivatives as a scaffold and generating more potent and selective Src kinase inhibitors and/or anticancer agents.

Competing interest

The authors declare that there is no conflict of interest related to this publication.

Authors' contributions

AR contributed to the synthesis of some target compounds. AFT contributed to synthesis of the intermediates and some target compounds, and preparation of the manuscript. RK participated in evaluation of the Src Kinase Inhibitory activities. ANS and DM participated in evaluation of the anti-proliferative activities. KP collaborated in management of the pharmacological part, and edition of manuscript. AS contributed in identifying of the structures of target compounds. AF collaborated in design of target compounds. TA participated in designing of target compounds, management of the synthetic and pharmacological parts, and preparation of the manuscript and approval of final article. All authors read and approved the final manuscript.

Acknowledgements

This research was supported financially by Research Council of Tehran University of Medical Sciences grant number: 10826-33-02-89 and American Cancer Society which supported this study through a grant.

Author details

[1]Department of Medicinal Chemistry, Faculty of Pharmacy and Drug Design & Development Research Center, Tehran University of Medical Sciences, Tehran, Iran. [2]Department of Biomedical and Pharmaceutical Sciences, College of Pharmacy, The University of Rhode Island, Kingston, RI, USA.

References

1. Yeatman TJ: **A renaissance for SRC.** *Nat Rev Cancer* 2004, **4**:470–480.
2. Yu CL, Meyer DJ, Campbell GS, Larner AC, Carter-Su C, Schwartz J, Jove R: **Enhanced DNA-binding activity of a Stat3-related protein in cells transformed by the Src oncoprotein.** *Science* 1995, **269**:81–83.
3. Niu G, Wright KL, Huang M, Song L, Haura E, Turkson J, Zhang S, Wang T, Sinibaldi D, Coppola D, Heller R, Ellis LM, Karras J, Bromberg J, Pardoll D, Jove R, Yu H: **Constitutive Stat3 activity up-regulates VEGF expression and tumor angiogenesis.** *Oncogene* 2002, **21**:2000–2008.
4. Russello SV, Shore SK: **SRC in human carcinogenesis.** *Front Biosci* 2004, **9**:139–144.
5. Tsygankov AY, Shore SK: **Src: regulation, role in human carcinogenesis and pharmacological inhibitors.** *Curr Pharm Des* 2004, **10**:1745–1756.
6. Boyer B, Valles AM, Edme N: **Induction and regulation of epithelial-mesenchymal transitions.** *Biochem Pharmacol* 2000, **60**:1091–1099.
7. Johnson FM, Gallick GE: **SRC family nonreceptor tyrosine kinases as molecular targets for cancer therapy.** *Anticancer Agents Med Chem* 2007, **7**:651–659.
8. Nam JS, Ino Y, Sakamoto M, Hirohashi S: **Src family kinase inhibitor PP2 restores the E-cadherin/catenin cell adhesion system in human cancer cells and reduces cancer metastasis.** *Clin Cancer Res* 2002, **8**:2430–2436.
9. Coluccia AM, Benati D, Dekhil H, De Filippo A, Lan C, Gambacorti-Passerini C: **SKI-606 decreases growth and motility of colorectal cancer cells by preventing pp 60(c-Src)-dependent tyrosine phosphorylation of beta-catenin and its nuclear signaling.** *Cancer Res* 2006, **66**:2279–2286.
10. Gonzalez L, Agullo-Ortuno MT, Garcia-Martinez JM, Calcabrini A, Gamallo C, Palacios J, Aranda A, Martin-Perez J: **Role of c-Src in human MCF7 breast cancer cell tumorigenesis.** *J Biol Chem* 2006, **281**:20851–20864.
11. Benati D, Baldari CT: **SRC family kinases as potential therapeutic targets for malignancies and immunological disorders.** *Curr Med Chem* 2008, **15**:1154–1165.
12. Sundaramoorthi R, Shakespeare WC, Keenan TP, Metcalf CA III, Wang Y, Mani U, Taylor M, Liu S, Bohacek RS, Narula SS, Dalgarno DC, van Schravandijk MR, Violette SM, Liou S, Adams S, Ram MK, Keats JA, Weigle M, Sawyer TK, Weigele M: **Bone-targeted Src kinase inhibitors: novel pyrrolo- and pyrazolopyrimidine analogues.** *Bioorg Med Chem Lett* 2003, **13**:3063–3066.
13. Schenone S, Bruno O, Ranise A, Bondavalli F, Brullo C, Fossa P, Mosti L, Menozzi G, Carraro F, Naldini A, Bernini C, Manetti F, Botta M: **New pyrazolo [3,4-d]pyrimidines endowed with A431 antiproliferative activity and inhibitory properties of Src phosphorylation.** *Bioorg Med Chem Lett* 2004, **14**:2511–2517.
14. Ple PA, Green TP, Hennequin LF, Curwen J, Fennell M, Allen J, Lambert-Van Der Brempt C, Costello G: **Discovery of a new class of anilinoquinazoline inhibitors with high affinity and specificity for the tyrosine kinase domain of c-Src.** *J Med Chem* 2004, **47**:871–887.
15. Hennequin LF, Allen J, Breed J, Curwen J, Fennell M, Green TP, Lambert-van Der Brempt C, Morgentin R, Norman RA, Olivier A, Otterbein L, Ple PA, Warin N, Costello G: **N-(5-chloro-1,3-benzodioxol-4-yl)-7-[2-(4-methylpiperazin-1-yl)ethoxy]-5- (tetrahydro-2H-pyran-4-yloxy)quinazolin-4-amine, a novel, highly selective, orally available, dual-specific c-Src/Abl kinase inhibitor.** *J Med Chem* 2006, **49**:6465–6488.
16. Barrios Sosa AC, Boschelli DH, Wu B, Wang Y, Golas JM: **Further studies on ethenyl and ethynyl-4-phenylamino-3-quinolinecarbonitriles: identification of a subnanomolar Src kinase inhibitor.** *Bioorg Med Chem Lett* 2005, **15**:1743–1747.
17. Boschelli DH, Wu B, Ye F, Durutlic H, Golas JM, Lucas J, Boschelli F: **Facile preparation of new 4-phenylamino-3-quinolinecarbonitrile Src kinase inhibitors via 7-fluoro intermediates: identification of potent 7-amino analogs.** *Bioorg Med Chem* 2008, **16**:405–412.
18. Boschelli DH, Wang D, Wang Y, Wu B, Honores EE, Barrios Sosa AC, Chaudhary I, Golas J, Lucas J, Boschelli F: **Optimization of 7-alkene-3-quinolinecarbonitriles as Src kinase inhibitors.** *Bioorg Med Chem Lett* 2010, **20**:2924–2927.
19. Dulsat C, Mealy N, Castaner R: **Saracatinib. Dual Src/ABL kinase inhibitor, Oncolytic.** *Drugs Fut* 2009, **34**:106–114.
20. Boschelli DH, Ye F, Wang YD, Dutia M, Johnson SL, Wu B, Miller K, Powell DW, Yaczko D, Young M, Tischler M, Arndt K, Discafani C, Etienne C, Gibbons J, Grod J, Lucas J, Weber JM, Boschelli F: **Optimization of 4-phenylamino-3-quinolinecarbonitriles as potent inhibitors of Src kinase activity.** *J Med Chem* 2001, **44**:3965–3977.
21. Boschelli DH, Boschelli F: **Bosutinib. Dual Src and Abl kinase inhibitor, treatment of solid tumors, treatment of CML and Ph+ ALL.** *Drugs Fut* 2007, **32**:481–490.
22. Lawrence DS, Niu J: **Protein kinase inhibitors: the tyrosine-specific protein kinases.** *Pharmacol Ther* 1998, **77**:81–114.
23. Brunton VG, Lear MJ, McKeown P, Robins DJ, Workman P: **Synthesis and antiproliferative activity of tyrphostins containing quinoline moieties.** *Anticancer Drug Des* 1996, **11**:463–483.
24. Morin MJ: **From oncogene to drug: development of small molecule tyrosine kinase inhibitors as anti-tumor and anti-angiogenic agents.** *Oncogene* 2000, **19**:6574–6583.
25. Dell CP: **Antiproliferative naphthopyrans: biological activity, mechanistic studies and therapeutic potential.** *Current Med Chem* 1998, **5**:179–194.
26. Wiernicki TR, Bean JS, Dell C, Williams A, Wood D, Kauffman RF, Singh JP: **Inhibition of vascular smooth muscle cell proliferation and arterial intimal thickening by a novel antiproliferative naphthopyran.** *J Pharmacol Exp Ther* 1996, **278**:1452–1459.
27. Fallah-Tafti A, Tiwari R, Shirazi AN, Akbarzadeh T, Mandal D, Shafiee A, Parang K, Foroumadi A: **4-aryl-4H-chromene-3-carbonitrile derivatives: evaluation of Src kinase inhibitory and anticancer activities.** *Med Chem* 2011, **7**:466–472.
28. Fallah-Tafti A, Foroumadi A, Tiwari R, Shirazi AN, Hangauer DG, Bu Y, Akbarzadeh T, Parang K, Shafiee A: **Thiazolyl N-benzyl-substituted acetamide derivatives: synthesis, Src kinase inhibitory and anticancer activities.** *Eur J Med Chem* 2011, **46**:4853–4858.

29. Kumar D, Reddy VB, Kumar A, Mandal D, Tiwari R, Parang K: **Click chemistry inspired one-pot synthesis of 1,4-disubstituted 1,2,3-triazoles and their Src kinase inhibitory activity.** *Bioorg Med Chem Lett* 2011, **21**:449–452.
30. Sharma D, Sharma RK, Bhatia S, Tiwari R, Mandal D, Lehmann J, Parang K, Olsen CE, Parmar VS, Prasad AK: **Synthesis, Src kinase inhibitory and anticancer activities of 1-substituted 3-(N-alkyl-N-phenylamino)propane-2-ols.** *Biochimie* 2010, **92**:1164–1172.
31. Tiwari R, Brown A, Narramaneni S, Sun G, Parang K: **Synthesis and evaluation of conformationally constrained peptide analogues as the Src SH3 domain binding ligands.** *Biochimie* 2010, **92**:1153–1163.
32. Kumar A, Wang Y, Lin X, Sun G, Parang K: **Synthesis and evaluation of 3-phenylpyrazolo[3,4-d]pyrimidine-peptide conjugates as Src kinase inhibitors.** *Chem Med Chem* 2007, **2**:1346–1360.
33. Kumar A, Ye G, Wang Y, Lin X, Sun G, Parang K: **Synthesis and structure-activity relationships of linear and conformationally constrained peptide analogues of CIYKYY as Src tyrosine kinase inhibitors.** *J Med Chem* 2006, **49**:3395–3401.
34. Nam NH, Lee S, Ye G, Sun G, Parang K: **ATP-phosphopeptide conjugates as inhibitors of Src tyrosine kinases.** *Bioorg Med Chem* 2004, **12**:5753–5766.
35. Nam NH, Ye G, Sun G, Parang K: **Conformationally constrained peptide analogues of pTyr-Glu-Glu-Ile as inhibitors of the Src SH2 domain binding.** *J Med Chem* 2004, **47**:3131–3141.
36. Balalaie S, Ramezanpour S, Bararjanian M, Gross JH: **DABCO-catalyzed efficient synthesis of naphthopyran derivatives via One-Pot three-component condensation reaction at room temperature.** *Synthetic Commun* 2008, **38**:1078–1089.
37. Abdolmohammadi S, Balalaie S: **Novel and efficient catalysts for the one-pot synthesis of 3,4-dihydropyrano[c]chromene derivatives in aqueous media.** *Tetrahedron Lett* 2007, **48**:3299–3303.
38. Chhikara BS, St Jean N, Mandal D, Kumar A, Parang K: **Fatty acyl amide derivatives of doxorubicin: synthesis and in vitro anticancer activities.** *Eur J Med Chem* 2011, **46**:2037–2042.

Synthesis, docking and acetylcholinesterase inhibitory assessment of 2-(2-(4-Benzylpiperazin-1-yl)ethyl)isoindoline-1,3-dione derivatives with potential anti-Alzheimer effects

Ahmad Mohammadi-Farani[1], Aram Ahmadi[2,4], Hamid Nadri[3] and Alireza Aliabadi[4*]

Abstract

Background: Alzheimer's disease (AD) as neurodegenerative disorder, is the most common form of dementia accounting for about 50-60% of the overall cases of dementia among persons over 65 years of age. Low acetylcholine (ACh) concentration in hippocampus and cortex areas of the brain is one of the main reasons for this disease. In recent years, acetylcholinesterase (AChE) inhibitors like donepezil with prevention of acetylcholine hydrolysis can enhance the duration of action of acetylcholine in synaptic cleft and improve the dementia associated with Alzheimer's disease.

Results: Design, synthesis and assessment of anticholinesterase activity of 2-(2-(4-Benzylpiperazin-1-yl)ethyl) isoindoline-1,3-dione derivatives showed prepared compounds can function as potential acetylcholinesterase inhibitor. Among 12 synthesized derivatives, compound 4a with *ortho* chlorine moiety as electron withdrawing group exhibited the highest potency in these series ($IC_{50} = 0.91 \pm 0.045$ μM) compared to donepezil ($IC_{50} = 0.14 \pm 0.03$ μM). The results of the enzyme inhibition test (Ellman test) showed that electron withdrawing groups like Cl, F and NO_2 can render the best effect at position *ortho* and *para* of the phenyl ring. But compound 4g with methoxy group at position 3(*meta*) afforded a favorable potency ($IC_{50} = 5.5 \pm 0.7$ μM). Furthermore, docking study confirmed a same binding mode like donepezil for compound 4a.

Conclusions: Synthesized compounds 4a-4l could be proposed as potential anticholinesterase agents.

Keywords: Synthesis, Phthalimide, Acetylcholinesterase (AChE), Anti-Alzheimer, Ellman test, Docking

Background

Alzheimer's disease (AD), is described by Dr. Alois Alzheimer in 1907 as a neurodegenerative disorder. AD as a disease of the central nervous system (CNS) characterized especially by premature senile mental deterioration. AD patients exhibit a significant decrease in cognitive ability and severe behavioral and psychological abnormalities such as irritability, anxiety and depression [1]. AD, one of the most diffuse neurodegenerative pathology among the elderly, causes a progressive impairment in functional performances and continuous reduction in cognitive activities and memory [2-7]. AD is the most common form of dementia accounting for about 50-60% of the overall cases of dementia among persons over 65 years of age, is a neurodegenerative alteration characterized by a low acetylcholine (ACh) in hippocampus and cortex [8]. AD is said to be the leading cause of dementia in elderly patients. Nowadays, with increase of the elderly population, the prevalence of AD is likely to increase. AD persons exert a decrease in mental functions and performances and consequently rendering them incapacitated and unable to perform normal daily activities. Elderly persons are the most common individuals afflicted with this disease. Unfortunately, the true nature or cause of the disease is still unknown and therefore, the development of effective anti-

* Correspondence: aliabadi.alireza@gmail.com
[4]Department of Medicinal Chemistry, Faculty of Pharmacy, Kermanshah University of Medical Sciences, Kermanshah, Iran
Full list of author information is available at the end of the article

alzheimer is one of the encouraging area in current medicinal chemistry researches [1].

Over two decades ago, several autopsy studies inside hippocampus revealed that the levels of the neurotransmitter acetylcholine in patients with Alzheimer's disease are importantly decreased [9]. Currently, the loss of cholinergic function is the only evidentiary finding responsible for cognitive decline. Hence, therapeutical development has focused on this theory. The loss of the basal forebrain cholinergic system is one of the most significant aspects of neurodegeneration in the brains of AD patients, and it is thought to play a central role in producing cognitive impairments [1,2,10,11]. Alzheimer's disease leads to a progressive decline of the cognitive function, executive function losses, memory deficits, and eventually to incapacitating dementia before death. In order to improve cholinergic neurotransmission, different strategies have been investigated including the increase of synthesis or pre-synaptic release of ACh, the stimulation of cholinergic post-synaptic muscarinic and nicotinic receptors, and the reduction of ACh synaptic degradation using AChE inhibitors (e.g., AChEIs or anticholinesterase agents) [12-19].

Acetylcholinesterase inhibitors have beneficial effects on cognitive, functional, and behavioral symptoms of AD. A recent review by the Quality Standard Subcommittee of the American Academy of Neurology investigated important issues in the management of dementia. The reviewers concluded that despite the small average degree of benefit of treatment with acetylcholinesterase inhibitors they should be the first-line treatment in patients with mild to moderate AD [4]. Four cholinesterase inhibitors tacrine, donepezil, rivastigmine, and galantamine are approved by the US Food and Drug Administration (FDA) and are currently in the market (Figure 1) [5].

According to the several reports about the efficacy of phthalimide derivatives in inhibition of AChE, [20-27] (Figure 2) in the current project, we focused on the design and synthesis of new anticholinesterase agents with phthalimide-based structure to reach more active analogs towards inhibition of AChE. Besides, we hope the new analogs to render lower side effects. Improving the pharmacokinetic properties of the designed compounds could be another aim of this study. In fact, phthalimide based compounds have similar pharmacophoric portions like indanone ring of the donepezil and are able to act as peripheral binding site inhibitor of AChE. We also investigated *in silico* binding mode of proposed ligands into the acetylcholinesterase enzyme in comparison with donepezil as reference drug by docking procedure.

Methods

Preliminary design

In the recent years, there are several reports about the potentiality of phthalimide derivatives as potent anticholinesterase agents. In fact, the phthalimide-based compounds can function as inhibitor of the peripheral binding site of AChE enzyme [20-27]. On the other hands, it is well-known in medicinal chemistry that piperazine ring can act as good bioisosteric replacement for piperidine moiety. According to the Figure 3, we designed a new series of donepezil-like analogues with replacement of the indanone and piperidine rings of the donepezil with

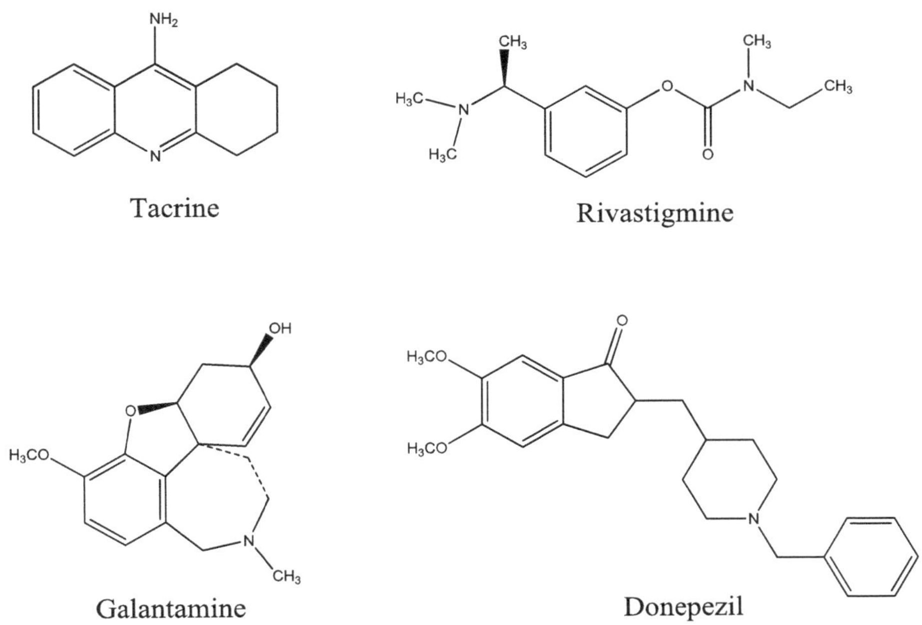

Figure 1 Structures of acetycholinesterase inhibitors in the market.

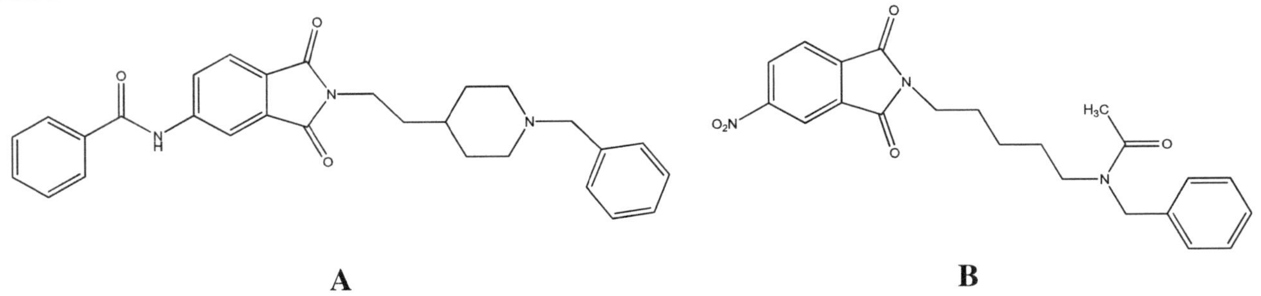

Figure 2 Two structures of phthalimide based anticholinesterase.

phthalimide (or isoindoline-1,3-dione) group and piperazine ring respectively. As illustrated in Figure 3, there are three distinct and critical portions in the structure of donepezil. Part A or peripheral binding site portion is necessary for binding to the AChE enzyme. The phenyl ring of the indanone moiety of donepezil participates in π-π stacking interaction with indole ring of Trp 279 in the active site of AChE. Part B is a linker region as well as an interacting part with Phe 330 in the active site of the AChE. According to the structure activity relationship (SAR) of donepezil-like analogs, the nitrogen atom of the piperidine ring is necessary for binding to the active site of the enzyme and removing of the nitrogen can be detrimental for anticholinesterase activity of the ligand. In fact, the charged nitrogen of the piperidine ring makes a cation-π interaction with Phe 330. Pat C or benzyl moiety unit plays its role through a π-π stacking interaction with indole ring of the Trp 84 [16]. Hence, in the designed compounds (Figure 3), the considering of these three pivotal portions of the donepezil was carried out and subsequently the synthesis of proposed compounds was done.

Chemistry

All chemical substances consisting starter materials, reagents and solvents were purchased from the commercial supplier like Merck and Sigma-Aldrich companies. The purity of the prepared compounds was proved by thin layer chromatography (TLC) using various solvents of different polarities. Merck silica gel 60 F_{254} plates were used for analytical TLC. Column chromatography was applied on Merck silica gel (70–230 mesh) for purification of intermediate and final compounds. ^{1}H-NMR spectra were recorded using a Bruker 400 MHz spectrometer in deutrated solvents, and chemical shifts are expressed as δ (ppm) with tetramethylsilane (TMS) as internal standard. The IR spectra were obtained on a Shimadzu 470 spectrophotometer using potassium bromide (KBr) disks. Melting points were determined

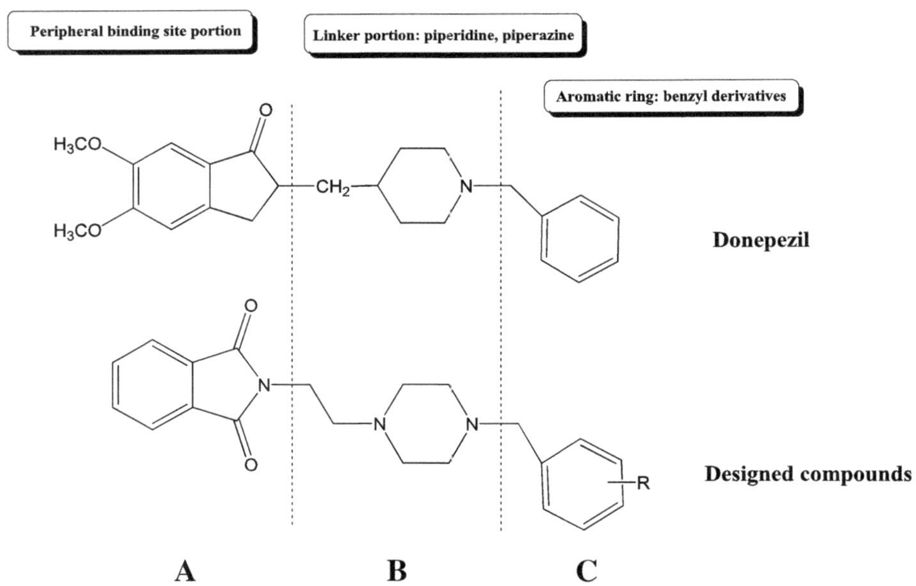

Figure 3 Design of new donepezil-like analogs based on the phthalimide structure.

using Electrothermal 9001 elemental analyzer apparatus and are uncorrected. The mass spectra were run on a Finigan TSQ-70 spectrometer (Finigan, USA) at 70 eV.

Synthesis of 2-(2-(piperazin-1-yl)ethyl)isoindoline-1,3-dione (3)

In a flask 3 g (20 mmol) of Phthalic anhydride, 2.6 ml (20 mmol) *N*-amnioethylpiperazine and 2.9 ml (20 mmol) triethylamine (Et_3N) were mixed in 40 ml of toluene solvent. The reaction mixture was refluxed for 24 hours and the termination of reaction and formation of the desired product was confirmed by thin layer chromatography. The discoloration of the reaction medium and formation of a yellow precipitate was also an indicator of the progress of the reaction. Then, toluene was evaporated under reduced pressure using rotary evaporator apparatus and the obtained yellow viscose and oily residue was washed several times by ethyl acetate (EtOAc) and diethyl ether (Et_2O) [28].

^1H NMR ($CDCl_3$, 400 MHz) δ (ppm): 2.37 (m, 4H, Piperazine), 2.54 (m, 4H, Piperazine), 3.22 (t, 2H, phthalimide-CH_2-CH_2-piperazine), 3.44 (t, 2H, phthalimide-CH_2-CH_2-piperazine), 4.73 (NH, Piperazine), 7.35-7.85 (m, 4H, Phthalimide). IR (KBr, cm^{-1}) ū: 3380, 3330, 3157, 3111, 2924, 1730, 1681, 1521, 1489, 1458, 1328, 1303, 1186, 1143, 1035, 910, 750, 710. MS (*m/z*, %): 259 (M^+, 10), 224 (30), 174 (30), 160 (60), 149 (85), 99 (100), 70 (70), 57 (65), 41 (40).

General procedure for synthesis of compounds 4a-4l:

In a flat-bottom flask equimolar quantities of compound 3 and appropriate derivative of benzyl chloride were added together in dichloromethane (CH_2Cl_2) solvent. The reaction mixture was stirred in room temperature overnight. Then, dichloromethane was evaporated under reduced pressure and the afforded residue was washed by diethyl ether and *n*-hexane. Methanol containing Hydrochloric acid gas was added to the residue to form the related hydrochloride salt of the product [29].

2-(2-(4-(2-Chlorobenzyl)piperazin-1-yl)ethyl)isoindoline-1,3-dione (4a)

^1H NMR (DMSO-d_6, 400 MHz) δ (ppm): 2.36 (m, 8H, Piperazine), 3.33 (t, 2H, CH_2-piperazine), 3.35 (s, 2H, -CH_2-2-Chlorophenyl), 3.61 (t, 2H, -CH_2-Phthalimide), 7.25-7.32 (m, 2H, 2-Chlorophenyl), 7.34-7.44 (m, 2H, 2-Chlorophenyl), 7.46-7.87 (m, 4H, Phthalimide). MS (*m/z*, %): 385 (M^++2, 2), 383 (M^+, 5), 225 (50), 223 (100), 160 (50), 125 (95), 89 (15), 70 (20). IR (KBr, cm^{-1}) ū: 3460, 3051, 2943, 2800, 2762, 1766, 1465, 1438, 1396, 1357, 1300, 1192, 1161, 1107, 1041, 921, 759, 717, 698.

2-(2-(4-(3-Chlorobenzyl)piperazin-1-yl)ethyl)isoindoline-1,3-dione (4b)

^1H NMR (DMSO-d_6, 400 MHz) δ (ppm): 2.34 (m, 4H, Piperazine), 3.35 (t, 2H, -CH_2-piperazine), 3.51 (s, 2H, -CH_2-phenyl), 3.7 (t, 2H, -CH_2-phthalimide), 7.27-7.32 (m, H_2, H_5, 3-Chlorophenyl), 7.41 (d, 1H, J = 8 Hz, H_6-3-Chlorophenyl), 7.45 (d, J = 8 Hz, H_4-3-Chlorophenyl), 7.85 (m, 2H, H_5,H_6-phthalimide), 7.88 (m, 2H, H_4,H_7-phthalimide). IR (KBr, cm^{-1}) ū: 3160, 3113, 2924, 1710, 1681, 1533, 1521, 1489, 1458, 1327, 1303, 1186, 1143, 1037, 715.

2-(2-(4-(4-Chlorobenzyl)piperazin-1-yl)ethyl)isoindoline-1,3-dione (4c)

^1H NMR ($CDCl_3$, 400 MHz) δ (ppm): 2.2 (t, 2H, -N-CH_2-CH_2-NH-, piperazine), 2.5 (t, 2H, -N-CH_2-CH_2-NH-, Piperazine), 2.63 (t, 2H, phthalimide-CH_2-CH_2-piperazine), 3.42 (s, 2H, -CH_2-phenyl), 3.8 (t, 2H, phthalimide-CH_2-CH_2-piperazine), 7.23 (d, 2H, J = 8 Hz, $H_{2,6}$-4-chlorophenyl), 7.30 (d, 2H, J = 8 Hz, $H_{3,5}$-4-chlorophenyl phenyl), 7.76 (m, 4H, Phthalimide). IR (KBr, cm^{-1}) ū: 3400, 3380, 3135, 3111, 2927, 2812, 1703, 1681, 1533, 1521, 1489, 1456, 1328, 1305, 1186, 1143, 1035, 721, 707. MS (*m/z*, %): 384 (M^+ +1, 20), 383 (M^+, 18), 280 (20), 223 (100), 167 (30), 149 (90), 125 (90).

2-(2-(4-(2-Fluorobenzyl)piperazin-1-yl)ethyl)isoindoline-1,3-dione (4d)

^1H NMR (DMSO-d_6, 400 MHz) δ (ppm): 2.4 (m, 4H, piperazine), 3.1 (m, 4H, aliphatic), 3.8 (s, 2H, -CH_2-phenyl), 7.35 (m, 4H, 2-Fluorophenyl), 7.88 (m, 4H, Phthalimide). IR (KBr, cm^{-1}) ū: 3429, 2993, 2924, 2854, 1774, 1716, 1396, 1068, 1010, 721. MS (*m/z*, %): 368 (M^++1, 25), 313 (40), 285 (35), 257 (40), 236 (100), 152 (40), 111 (60), 97 (95), 83 (90), 69 (90), 57 (85), 43 (50).

2-(2-(4-(3-Fluorobenzyl)piperazin-1-yl)ethyl)isoindoline-1,3-dione (4e)

^1H NMR (DMSO-d_6, 400 MHz) δ (ppm): 3.37-3.87 (m, aliphatic), 3.99 (s, 2H, -CH_2-phenyl), 7.29 (d, 1H, J = 8 Hz, H_2-3-Fluorophenyl), 7.49 (m, 1H, H_6-3-Fluorophenyl), 7.66 (d, 1H, J = 8 Hz, H_5-3-Fluorophenyl), 7.68 (d, 1H, J = 8 Hz, H_3-3-Fluorophenyl), 7.86-7.88 (m, 4H, phthalimide). IR (KBr, cm^{-1}) ū: 3371, 2993, 2958, 2924, 2854, 1774, 1712, 1546, 1462, 1404, 1056, 972, 721.

2-(2-(4-(4-Fluorobenzyl)piperazin-1-yl)ethyl)isoindoline-1,3-dione (4f)

^1H NMR (DMSO-d_6, 400 MHz) δ (ppm): 3.99 (m, 12H, aliphatic), 3.96 (s, -CH_2-phenyl), 3.99 (t, 2H, -CH_2-phthalimide), 7.3 (t, 2H, J = 8 Hz, 4-Fluorophenyl), 7.58-7.73 (m, 4-Fluorophenyl), 7.83-7.88 (m, 4H, Phthalimide). IR (KBr, cm^{-1}) ū: 3367, 2997, 2854, 1774, 1716, 1604, 1512, 1462, 1400, 1056, 975, 721.

2-(2-(4-(3-Methoxybenzyl)piperazin-1-yl)ethyl)isoindoline-1,3-dione (4g)

^{1}H NMR (DMSO-d_6, 400 MHz) δ (ppm): 3.2-3.66 (m, aliphatic), 3.79 (s, 3H, -OCH_3), 3.97 (s, 2H, -CH_2-phenyl), 7.1-7.36 (m, 4H, 4-Methoxyphenyl), 7.58-7.66 (m, 4H, Phthalimide). IR (KBr, cm^{-1}) ῡ: 3371, 2993, 1774, 1716, 1612, 1462, 1435, 1400, 1381, 1269, 1056, 972, 906, 798, 721. MS (*m/z*, %): 379 (M^+, 15), 219 (100), 160 (30), 121 (80), 91 (20).

2-(2-(4-(4-Methoxybenzyl)piperazin-1-yl)ethyl)isoindoline-1,3-dione (4h)

^{1}H NMR (DMSO-d_6, 400 MHz) δ (ppm): 3.1-3.78 (m, aliphatic), 3.78 (s, 3H, -OCH_3), 4.4 (s, 2H, -CH_2-phenyl), 7.1 (dd, 4H, $J = 8$ Hz, 4-Methoxyphenyl), 7.43-7.58 (m, 4H, Phthalimide). IR (KBr, cm^{-1}) ῡ: 3429, 2978, 2935, 1778, 1716, 1612, 1516, 1462, 1435, 1400, 1235, 1184, 1072, 1029, 802, 725.

2-(2-(4-(2-Nitrobenzyl)piperazin-1-yl)ethyl)isoindoline-1,3-dione (4i)

^{1}H NMR (DMSO-d_6, 400 MHz) δ (ppm): 2.25-2.35 (m, 8H, Piperazine), 3.35 (t, 2H, -CH_2-piperazine), 3.66 (s, 2H, CH_2-phenyl), 3.68 (t, 2H, -CH_2-phthalimide), 7.4-7.66 (m, 4H, 2-Nitrophenyl), 7.83-7.89 (m, 4H, Phthalimide). IR (KBr, cm^{-1}) ῡ: 3155, 3111, 2956, 2922, 1681, 1521, 1489, 1458, 1327, 1303, 1188, 1141, 1035, 740, 717, 705. MS (*m/z*, %): 394 (M^+, 3), 377 (15), 259 (30), 235 (40), 234 (100), 200 (50), 160 (70), 130 (30), 99 (55), 78 (30) 56 (15).

2-(2-(4-(3-Nitrobenzyl)piperazin-1-yl)ethyl)isoindoline-1,3-dione (4j)

^{1}H NMR (DMSO-d_6, 400 MHz) δ (ppm): 2.51 (m, 4H, Piperazine), 3.53 (t, 2H, -CH_2-piperazine), 3.79 (s, -CH_2-phenyl), 3.85 (t, 2H, -CH_2-phthalimide), 7.6-7.66 (m, 2H, $H_{4,6}$-3-Nitrophenyl), 7.65 (s, 1H, H_2-3-Nitrophenyl), 7.75 (t, $J = 8$ Hz, 1H, H_5-3-Nitrophenyl), 7.85 (m, 2H, $H_{5,6}$-phthalimide), 7.88 (m, 2H, $H_{4,7}$-phthalimide). IR (KBr, cm^{-1}) ῡ: 3425, 2924, 2854, 1774, 1716, 1531, 1435, 1400, 1350, 1060, 806, 721.

2-(2-(4-(4-Nitrobenzyl)piperazin-1-yl)ethyl)isoindoline-1,3-dione (4k)

^{1}H NMR (DMSO-d_6, 400 MHz) δ (ppm): 2.3 (m, 8H, Piperazine), 3.33 (t, 2H, phthalimide-CH_2-$\underline{CH_2}$-piperazine), 3.56 (s, 2H, -CH_2-phenyl), 3.69 (t, 2H, phthalimide-$\underline{CH_2}$-CH_2-piperazine), 7.57 (d, 2H, $J = 8$ Hz, $H_{2,6}$-4-Nitrophenyl), 7.83-7.88 (m, 4H, Phthalimide), 8.19 (d, 2H, $J = 8$ Hz, $H_{3,5}$-4-Nitrophenyl). IR (KBr, cm^{-1}) ῡ: 3157, 3111, 2924, 1775, 1681, 1519, 1489, 1458, 1330, 1303, 1186, 1143, 1037, 750, 710. MS (*m/z*, %): 395 (M^++1, 10), 394 (M^+, 35), 235 (85), 234 (100), 191 (60), 174 (30), 160 (85), 90 (25), 70 (40).

2-(2-(4-Benzylpiperazin-1-yl)ethyl)isoindoline-1,3-dione (4l)

^{1}H NMR (DMSO-d_6, 400 MHz) δ (ppm): 2.51 (m, 4H, Piperazine), 3.55 (m, 8H, aliphatic), 3.99 (s, 2H, -CH_2-phenyl), 7.45-7.68 (m, 4H, phenyl), 7.85 (m, 4H, Phthalimide). IR (KBr, cm^{-1}) ῡ: 3414, 2997, 2924, 1774, 1712, 1635, 1431, 1396, 1064, 721. MS (*m/z*, %): 349 (10), 234 (20), 189 (100), 160 (35), 91 (90).

Anticholinesterase activity assay (Ellman test)

Lyophilized powder of acetylcholinesterase from electric eel source (AChE, E.C. 3.1.1.7, Type V-S, 1000 unit) was purchased from Sigma-Aldrich (Steinheim, Germany). 5,5'-Dithiobis-(2-nitrobenzoic acid), potassium dihydrogen phosphate, dipotassium hydrogen phosphate, potassium hydroxide, sodium hydrogen carbonate, and acetylthiocholine iodide were purchased from Fluka (Buchs, Switzerland). Compounds 4a-4l were dissolved in a mixture of 20 ml distilled water and 5 ml methanol and then diluted in 0.1 M KH_2PO_4/K_2HPO_4 buffer (pH 8.0) to afford a final concentration range. The Ellman test was carried out for assessment of the anticholinesterase activity of intended compounds *in vitro*. Prior to use, all solutions were adjusted to 25°C. To achieve 20-80% inhibition of AChE activity five different concentrations of each compound were tested. The assay solution consisted of a 0.1 M potassium phosphate buffer pH 8.0, with the addition of 0.01 M 5,50-dithio-bis(2-nitrobenzoic acid), 2.5 unit/mL of enzyme solution (AChE, E.C. 3.1.1.7, Type V-S, lyophilized powder, from electric eel) (Sigma Chemical). Compounds 4a-4l were added to the assay solution and preincubated at 25°C with the enzyme for 15 min followed by adding 0.075 M substrate (acetylthiocholine iodide). After rapid and immediate mixing the change of absorption was measured at 412 nm. In order to justify non enzymatic reaction assays were carried out with a blank containing all components except AChE.

The blank reading contained 3 ml buffer, 200 μl water, 100 μl DTNB and 20 μl substrate. The reaction rates were calculated, and the percent inhibition of test compounds was determined. Each concentration was analyzed in triplicate, and IC_{50} values were determined graphically from inhibition curves (log inhibitor concentration vs percent of inhibition). Spectrophotometric measurements were performed on a Cecil BioAquarius CE 7250 Double Beam Spectrophotometer [30].

Docking

ArgusLab 4.0 software was applied to perform molecular docking studies [31,32]. All intended ligands were constructed in arguslab workspace and all ligands 4a-4l were energy minimized by AM1 as semiemperical method. The pdb file of acetylcholinesterase enzyme in complex with donepezil (pdb code: 1EVE) was downloaded from brookhaven protein databank [33]. The geometry

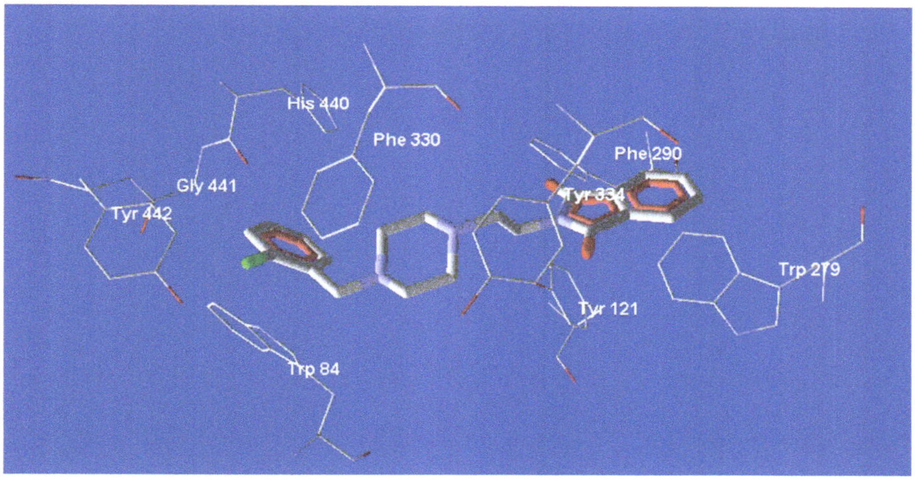

Figure 4 Docked molecule of compound 4a in the active site of AChE (PDB code: 1EVE). The principal amino acids (Trp 279, Phe 330, Trp 84) are evident in the nearby of the docked molecule.

optimization of structure of acetylcholinesterase enzyme was performed using universal force field (UFF) as a molecular mechanic method. The docking process was done for all ligands in the workspace of ArgusLab 4 software after defining the related groups for each ligand and also for related protein. The binding location of donepezil was defined as binding site for finding the best pose and conformation for all ligands. Binding mode and related interactions of all ligands were explored in Molegro molecular viewer software (Figure 4, Figure 5) [34].

Results and discussion

Chemistry

As summarized in the Scheme 1, all intermediate and final compounds 3 and 4a-4l were synthesized with an acceptable to high yield (ranging 61–96%) as listed in Table 1. Compound 3 was obtained through a Gabriel synthetic reaction. Reaction of phthalic anhydride with *N*-aminoethylpiperazine afforded the compound 3 with 61% yield. The reaction was carried out under reflux conditions in toluene solvent. Washing of yellowish oily product was done by ethyl acetate and *n*-hexane. A yellow powder was obtained after trituration. Obtained product was used for synthesis of 4a-4l derivatives. Room temperature stirring of equimolar quantities of compound **3** with appropriate benzyl chloride derivatives afforded 4a-4l derivatives. Dichloromethane was used as solvent and overnight stirring is necessary for achieving an acceptable yield. After evaporation, an oily residue was obtained. Methanolic hydrochloric acid was applied

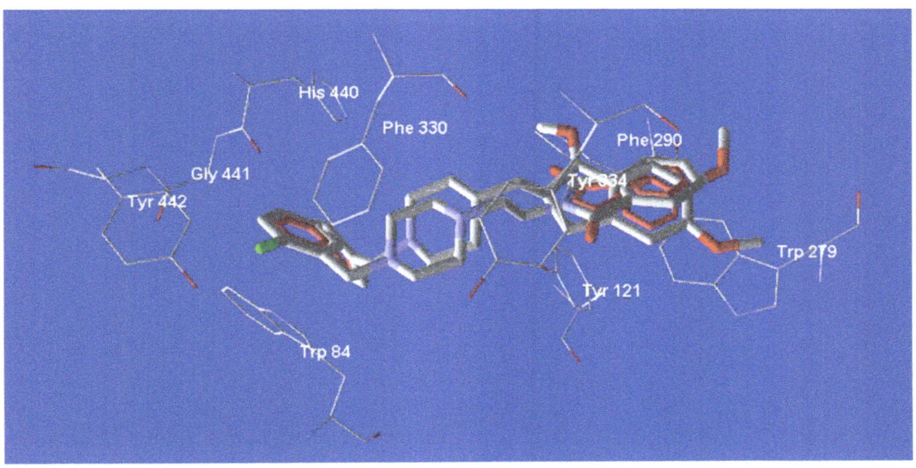

Figure 5 Superimposed structure of compound 4a with donepezil in the active site of AChE. A similar binding mode and interaction like donepezil are observed for compound 4a.

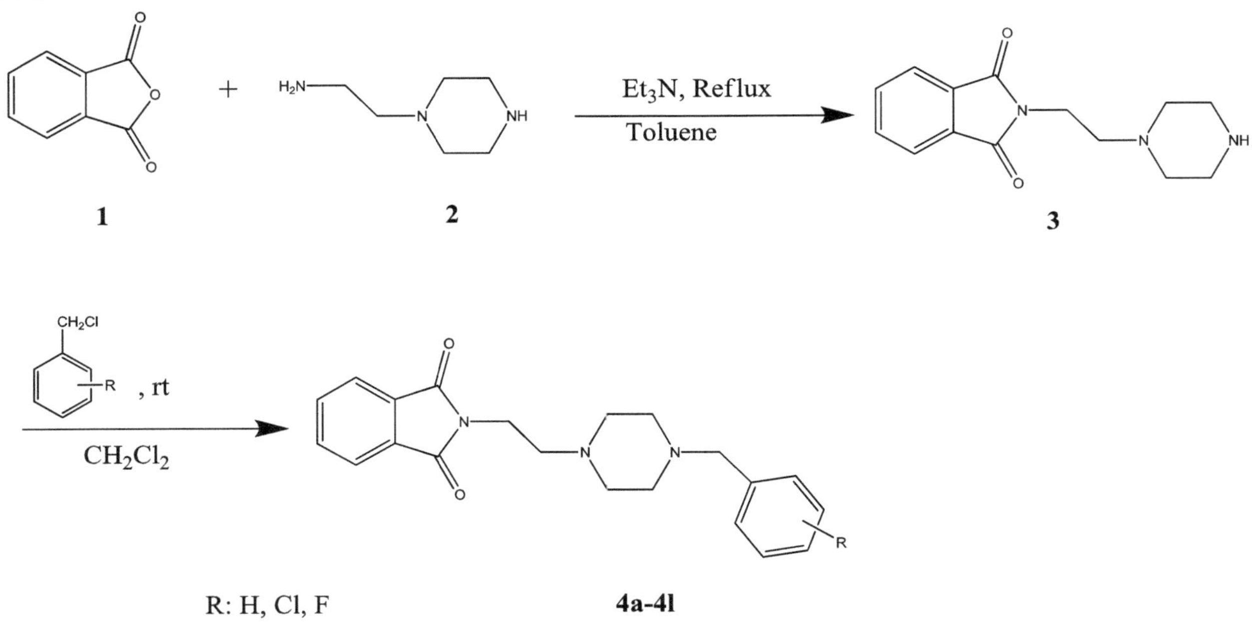

Scheme 1 Synthetic pathway of compounds 4a-4l.

to form the corresponding hydrochloride salt of each derivative. For each compound 2 ml of methanolic solvent was added to the obtained residue and stirred at room temperature for 5–10 minutes. The formed precipitate was filtered, dried and collected.

Different types of substituent consisted of three electron withdrawing substituents (Cl, F, NO_2) and also an electron donating substituent ($-OCH_3$) were synthesized to investigate the electronic effects of various moieties. Furthermore, compound 4l was also synthesized without any group on the phenyl ring to explore the effect of the presence of the substitution on this ring.

Melting points of intermediate and final compounds were obtained using capillary tubes by electrothermal melting point analyzer. A range in melting point was recorded for compounds 3, 4a, 4b, 4f and 4i. In other cases a sharp point was detected and presented in Table 1. ^{1}H NMR, IR and MS spectroscopic methods were applied for characterization and identification of all compounds. Deutrated dimethyl sulfoxide (DMSO-d_6) was used for ^{1}H NMR acquisition and TMS (tetramethyl silane) was applied as internal standard. Infrared spectroscopy was performed for all compounds using KBr disk and outstanding peaks was reported. Molecular ion

Table 1 Properties of synthesized compounds

Compounds	R	Closed formula	MW (g/mol)	mp (°C)	Yield (%)	Appearance
3	-	$C_{14}H_{17}N_3O_2$	259	105-109	61	Yellow
4a	2-Cl	$C_{21}H_{22}$ Cl N_3O_2	383	105-107	81	Creamy
4b	3-Cl	$C_{21}H_{22}$ Cl N_3O_2	383	100-103	74	Creamy
4c	4-Cl	$C_{21}H_{22}$ Cl N_3O_2	383	122	78	Creamy
4d	2-F	$C_{21}H_{22}FN_3O_2$	367	226	96	Yellow
4e	3-F	$C_{21}H_{22}FN_3O_2$	367	225	77	Creamy
4f	4-F	$C_{21}H_{22}FN_3O_2$	367	293-296	77	Yellow
4g	3-OCH_3	$C_{22}H_{25}N_3O_3$	379	259	82	Yellow
4h	4-OCH_3	$C_{22}H_{25}N_3O_3$	379	265	65	Yellow
4i	2-NO_2	$C_{21}H_{22}N_4O_4$	394	118-120	78	Orange
4j	3-NO_2	$C_{21}H_{22}N_4O_4$	394	286	92	Orange
4k	4-NO_2	$C_{21}H_{22}N_4O_4$	394	162	80	Creamy
4l	H	$C_{21}H_{23}N_3O$	349	231	92	Orange

Table 2 Results (IC_{50}, μM) of *in vitro* acetylcholinesterase assay of compounds 4a-4l

Compound	4a	4b	4c	4d	4e	4f	4g	4h	4i	4j	4k	4l	Donepezil
R	2-Cl	3-Cl	4-Cl	2-F	3-F	4-F	3-OCH_3	4-OCH_3	2-NO_2	3-NO_2	4-NO_2	H	-
IC_{50}(μM)	**0.91 ± 0.045**	85 ± 12	26 ± 5	23 ± 7	74 ± 11	42 ± 8	5.5 ± 0.7	72 ± 9	36 ± 5	59 ± 6	40 ± 4	9 ± 2	0.14 ± 0.03

peak of synthesized compounds was recorded in MS spectroscopy. Furthermore, $M^{+}+2$ was also reported for chlorinated compounds.

Anticholinesterase activity

According to Table 2, all compounds 4a-4l were tested against acetylcholinesterase and related IC_{50} ± SEM were calculated. Compound 4a with *ortho* chlorine substituent on phenyl ring was the most potent one in this series (IC_{50} = 0.91 ± 0.045 μM). *Para* position (compound 4c, IC_{50} = 26 ± 5 μM) was also favorable for anticholinesterase activity but on the other hands *meta* substitution of chlorine (compound 4b, IC_{50} = 85 ± 12 μM) led to the lowest inhibitory effect compared to other position for this moiety. Among compounds 4d-4f with fluorine moiety, compound 4d at position 2(*ortho*) showed the highest inhibitory property toward the acetylcholinesrase. Position 3(*meta*) was the worst position for fluorine and *para* substitution afforded an averaged potency in comparison with other positions. Compound 4g with *meta* substitution of methoxy substituent as electron donating group rendered a high potency derivative with IC_{50} = 5.5 ± 0.7 μM. A similar trend like chlorine and fluorine moieties was also observed for nitro group. Substitution of nitro group as electron withdrawing moiety at position 2(*ortho*) of the phenyl ring in compound 4i afforded the best effect. On the other hands, position 3(*meta*) was the worst position for nitro substituent (compound 4j). Insertion of nitro group at position 4(*para*) in compound 4k led to a moderate affinity for inhibition of acetylcholinesterase compared to positions 2 and 3. Compound 4l without any substituent on the phenyl ring was also one of the most potent inhibitor of acetylcholinesterase in this series. Totally, electron withdrawing moieties such as Cl, F and NO_2 at position 2(*ortho*) of the phenyl ring can enhance the potency of synthesized phthalimide derivatives. Electron donating group like methoxy at position 3 can also increase the enzyme inhibitory effects in these series.

Totally, electron withdrawing substituents are capable to enhance the anticholinestease activity of the phthalimide derivatives that synthesized in this research. Comparison of the different compounds with electron withdrawing moieties showed that *ortho* position is the best position for this type of substituents. Whereas, the *para* position was the worst position for all of the electron withdrawing moieties. Introducing of an electron donating group such as methoxy at *meta* position of the phenyl ring also led to the increasing of the potency. But, this change was not so effective like *ortho* substitution of chlorine atom. Absence of any moiety on the phenyl ring as observed about compound 4l could be an AChE inhibitor with an averaged potency. In fact, this compound exerted potency less than compound 4a with *ortho* chlorine as well as compound 4g with *meta* methoxy substituent.

Molecular modeling

All ligands 4a-4l were docked into the active site of acetylcholinesterase (PDB ID: 1EVE). For performing an accurate docking procedure, the binding site of donepezil was intended as probable binding site for all ligands especially for ligand 4a. Compound 4a as the best inhibitor of AChE *in vitro* was studied *in silico* to reveal the probable binding mode of synthesized compounds perfectly (Figure 3). Superimposed state for this ligand with donepezil was also explored. According to the Figure 4, a similar binding mode and conformation as observed for donepezil, was also seen for this ligand. In fact, the structure of synthesized compounds occupies a similar region like donepezil in the active site of AChE. As seen in Figure 4, phthalimide, piperazine and benzyl rings of compound **4a** adopt a same location like indanone, piperidine and benzyl rings of the donepezil respectively.

Conclusions

A new series of donepezil-like analogs were synthesized based on the phthalimide structure and anticholinesterase activity was assessed using Ellman test. All compounds exhibited a μM range in IC_{50} value (5.5-85 μM) for inhibition of AChE except for compound 4a that exhibited a nM range in IC_{50} value (0.91 μM). *In silico* study of compound 4a by docking method was also confirmed a similar binding mode like donepezil for this ligand.

Competing interests

The authors declare that they have no competing interests.

Acknowledgements

Authors are grateful from the research deputy of Kermanshah University of Medical Sciences for financial support. This work was performed in partial fulfillment of the requirement for PharmD of Mr. Aram Ahmadi.

Author details

[1]Department of Pharmacology, Toxicology and Medical Services, Faculty of Pharmacy, Kermanshah University of Medical Sciences, Kermanshah, Iran. [2]Students Research Committee, Kermanshah University of Medical Sciences, Kermanshah, Iran. [3]Neurobiomedical Research Center, Shahid Sadoughi University of Medical Sciences, Yazd, Iran. [4]Department of Medicinal

Chemistry, Faculty of Pharmacy, Kermanshah University of Medical Sciences, Kermanshah, Iran.

References

1. Sugimoto H, Yamanishi Y, Iimura Y, Kawakami Y: **Donepezil Hydrochloride (E2020) and Other Acetylcholinesterase Inhibitors.** *Curr Med Chem* 2000, **7**:303–339.
2. Mustazza C, Borioni A, Rosaria Del Giudice M, Gatta F, Ferretti R, *et al:* **Synthesis and cholinesterase activity of phenylcarbamates related to Rivastigmine, a therapeutic agent for Alzheimer's disease.** *Eur J Med Chem* 2002, **37**:91–109.
3. Maczurek A, Hager K, Kenklies M, Sharman M, Martins R, Engel J, *et al:* **Lipoic acid as an anti-inflammatory and neuroprotective treatment for Alzheimer's disease.** *Adv Drug Del Rev* 2008, **60**:1463–1470.
4. Scarpini E, Scheltens P, Feldman H: **Treatment of Alzheimer's disease: current status and new perspectives.** *Lancet Neurol* 2003, **2**:539–547.
5. Ucar G, Gokhan N, Yesilada A, Bilgin AA: **1-*N*-Substituted thiocarbamoyl-3 -phenyl-5-thienyl-2-pyrazolines: A novel cholinesterase and selective monoamine oxidase B inhibitors for the treatment of Parkinson's and Alzheimer's diseases.** *Neurosci Lett* 2005, **382**:327–331.
6. Vitorović-Todorović MD, Juranić IO, Mandić LM, Drakulic BJ: **4-Aryl-4-oxo-*N*-phenyl-2-aminylbutyramides as acetyl- and butyrylcholinesterase inhibitors. Preparation, anticholinesterase activity, docking study, and 3D structure–activity relationship based on molecular interaction fields.** *Bioorg Med Chem* 2010, **18**:1181–1193.
7. Araújo JQ, Araújo de Brito M, Bôas Hoelz LV, de Alencastro RB, Castro HC, Rodrigues C, *et al:* **Receptor-dependent (RD) 3D-QSAR approach of a series of benzylpiperidine inhibitors of human acetylcholinesterase (HuAChE).** *Eur J Med Chem* 2011, **46**:39–51.
8. Yu L, Cao R, Yi W, Yan Q, Chen C, Ma L, *et al:* **Synthesis of 4-[(diethylamino) methyl]-phenol derivatives as novel cholinesterase inhibitors with selectivity towards butyrylcholinesterase.** *Bioorg Med Chem Lett* 2010, **20**:3254–3258.
9. Trujillo-Ferrara J, Montoya Cano L, Espinoza-Fonseca M: **Synthesis, Anticholinesterase Activity and Structure-Activity Relationships of *m*-Aminobenzoic Acid Derivatives.** *Bioorg Med Chem Lett* 2003, **13**:1825–1827.
10. Weinstock M, Groner E: **Rational design of a drug for Alzheimer's disease with cholinesterase inhibitory and neuroprotective activity.** *Chem Biol Interact* 2008, **175**:216–221.
11. Liston DR, Nielsen JA, Villalobos A, Chapin D, Jones SB, Hubbard ST, *et al:* **Pharmacology of selective acetylcholinesterase inhibitors: implications for use in Alzheimer's disease.** *Eur J Pharmacol* 2004, **486**:9–17.
12. Racchi M, Mazzucchelli M, Porrello E, Lanni C, Govoni S: **Acetylcholinesterase inhibitors: novel activities of old molecules.** *Pharmacol Res* 2004, **50**:441–451.
13. Zhang J, Zhu D, Sheng R, Wu H, Hu Y, Wang F, *et al:* **BZYX, a novel acetylcholinesterase inhibitor, significantly improved chemicals-induced learning and memory impairments on rodents and protected PC12 cells from apoptosis induced by hydrogen peroxide.** *Eur J Pharmacol* 2009, **613**:1–9.
14. Hassan Khan MT: **Molecular interactions of cholinesterases inhibitors using *in silico* methods: current status and future prospects.** *New Biotechnol* 2009, **5**:331–346.
15. Silman L, Sussman JL: **Acetylcholinesterase: 'classical' and 'non-classical' functions and pharmacology.** *Curr Opin Pharmacol* 2005, **5**:293–302.
16. Kryger G, Silman I, Sussman JL: **Structure of acetylcholinesterase complexed with E2020 (Aricept®): implications for the design of new anti-Alzheimer drugs.** *Structure* 1999, **3**:297–307.
17. Nukoolkarn SV, Saen-oon S, Rungrotmongkol T, Hannongbua S, Ingkaninan K, Suwanborirux K: **Petrosamine, a potent anticholinesterase pyridoacridine alkaloid from a Thai marine sponge Petrosia n. sp.** *Bioorg Med Chem* 2008, **16**:6560–6567.
18. Mukherjee PK, Kumar V, Mal M, Houghton PJ: **Acetylcholinesterase inhibitors from plants.** *Phytomedicine* 2007, **14**:289–300.
19. Razavi SF, Khoobi M, Nadri H, Sakhteman A, Moradi A, Emami S: **Synthesis and evaluation of 4-substituted coumarins as novel acetylcholinesterase inhibitors.** *Eur J Med Chem* 2013, **46**:252–259.
20. Kapková P, Alptüzün V, Frey P, Erciyasb E, Holzgrabe U: **Search for dual function inhibitors for Alzheimer's disease: Synthesis and biological activity of acetylcholinesterase inhibitors of pyridinium-type and their Aβ fibril formation inhibition capacity.** *Bioorg Med Chem* 2006, **14**:472–478.
21. Alonso D, Dorronsoro I, Rubio L, Munoz P, García-Palomero E, Del Monte M, *et al:* **Donepezil-tacrine hybrid related derivatives as new dual binding site inhibitors of AChE.** *Bioorg Med Chem* 2005, **13**:6588–6597.
22. Mary A, Zafiarisoa Renko D, Guillou C, Thal C: **Potent Acetylcholinesterase Inhibitors: Design, Synthesis, and Structure-Activity Relationships of Bis-interacting Ligands in the Galanthamine Series.** *Bioorg Med Chem* 1998, **6**:1835–1850.
23. Zhao Q, Yang G, Mei X, Yuan H, Ning J: **Novel acetylcholinesterase inhibitors: Synthesis and structure-activity relationships of phthalimide alkyloxyphenyl N, N-dimethylcarbamate derivatives.** *Pestic Biochem Phys* 2009, **95**:131–134.
24. Sugimoto H, Iimura Y, Yamanishi Y, Yamatsu K: **Synthesis and Structure-Activity Relationships of Acetylcholinesterase Inhibitors: 1-Benzyl-4-[(5,6-dimethoxy-l-oxoindan-2 yl)methyl]piperidine Hydrochloride and Related Compounds.** *J Med Chem* 1996, **38**:4821–4829.
25. Kaur J, Zhang MQ: **Molecular modelling and QSAR of reversible acetylcholinesterase inhibitors.** *Curr Med Chem* 2000, **7**:273–294.
26. Nadri H, Pirali-Hamedani M, Moradi A, Sakhteman A, Vahidi A, Sheibani V: **5,6-Dimethoxybenzofuran-3-one derivatives: a novel series of dual Acetylcholinesterase/Butyrylcholinesterase inhibitors bearing benzyl pyridinium moiety.** *DARU: J Pharm Sci* 2013, **21**:15. doi:10.1186/2008-2231-21-15.
27. Alipour M, Khoobi M, Foroumadi A, Nadri H, Moradi A, Sakhteman A: **Novel coumarin derivatives bearing *N*-benzyl pyridinium moiety: Potent and dual binding site acetylcholinesterase inhibitors.** *Bioorg Med Chem* 2012, **20**:7214–7222.
28. Ragavendran JV, Sriram D, Patel SK, Reddy IV, Bharathwajan N, Stables J: **Design and synthesis of anticonvulsants from a combined phthalimide-GABA-anilide and hydrazone pharmacophore.** *Eur J Med Chem* 2007, **42**:146–151.
29. Li ZJ, Ren HY, Cui MC, Deuther-Conrad W, Tang RK, Steinbach J, *et al:* **Synthesis and biological evaluation of novel 4-benzylpiperazine ligands for sigma-1 receptor imaging.** *Bioorg Med Chem* 2011, **19**:2911–2917.
30. Nadri H, Pirali-Hamedani M, Shekarchi M, Abdollahi M, Sheibani V, Amanlou M, *et al:* **Design, Synthesis and anticholinesterase activity of a novel series of 1-benzyl-4-((6-alkoxy-3-oxobenzofuran-2(3H)-ylidin) methyl) pyridinum derivatives.** *Bioorg Med Chem* 2010, **18**:6360–6366.
31. ArgusLab 4.0 Mark A: *Thompson Planaria Software LLC.* Seattle, WA. http://www.arguslab.com.
32. Fernandez D, Aviles FX, Vendrell J: *Eur J Med Chem* 2009, **44**:3266–3271.
33. *Brookhaven protein databank.* http://RCSB.org.
34. *Molegro molecular viewer.* http://www.molegro.com.

Fabrication of docetaxel surfaced Fe_3O_4 magnetite nanoparticles and their cytotoxicity on 4 T1 breast cancer cells

MH Yazdi[1], Z Niazzadeh Najafi[1], MR Khorramizadeh[2], M Amini[3] and AR Shahverdi[1*]

Abstract

Background: In the recent years, there is an increasing attention to the using of Fe_3O_4 magnetite nanoparticles (MNPs) as drug delivery systems. Application of this nanoparticles could profit advantages of nanomedicine to enhance biological activity of pharmaceutical ingredients.

Methods: Fe_3O_4 MNPs were synthesised by a chemical method and characterized by transmission electron microscopy and energy-dispersive spectroscopy techniques. In the next step, docetaxel-coated Fe_3O_4 MNPs were prepared, using percipitation method. The surface chemistry of docetaxel-coated Fe_3O_4 MNPs as well as their thermal decomposition characteristics were examined using fourier transform infrared spectroscopy and thermogravimetric analyzer equipment, respectively. The cytotoxicity assay was conducted on 4 T1 breast cancer carsinoma by MTT assay to evaluate the possible *in vitro* antiproliferative effects of docetaxel-coated Fe_3O_4 MNPs.

Results: During precipitation process, docetaxel molecules were precipitated on the surface of Fe_3O_4 MNPs by the ratio of 3:100 w/w which indicates that each milligram of coated Fe_3O_4 MNPs averagely contained 30 μg pure docetaxel compound. Docetaxel showed aniproliferative effects against mentioned cell line. The higestest concentartion of docetaxel (80 μg/ml) caused about 80% cell death. However, the results demostarted that much lower amounts of docetaxel will be needed in combination of Fe_3O_4 MNPs to produce the potent antiproliferative effect compared to docetaxel alone. Dose response cytotoxicity assay of docetaxel-coated Fe_3O_4 MNPs against 4 T1 breast cancer cells showed that lower amount of docetaxel (0.6 μg/ml) can exhibit higher cytotoxic effect against this cancer cell line (90% cell death).

Keywords: Docetaxel, Fe_3O_4 magnetite nanoparticles, Antiproliferative effect, 4 T1 breast cancer cells

Introduction

Today, side effects of anti cancer drugs are still considered as a major problem in chemotherapy of cancer diseases (1). In the recent years, new drug delivery systems have been developed to reduce the side effects of these drugs (2–4). These systems mainly include nanotubes (5), liposomes (6), dendrimers (7) and nanoparticles (8). The potential biomedical applications of Fe_3O_4 magnetite nanoparticles (MNPs) are well discussed in the literature (9). Due to their magnetic properties, these nanomaretials have recieved particular attention as possible drug carriers (10). The conjugation of chemical or natural anticancer drugs to Fe_3O_4 magnetite nanoparticles (MNPs) can lead to increse the uptake of anticancer agents by targeted tumor and improve their therapeutic index (11). For example, a significant difference in antiproliferation effect of a natural product, umbelliprenin, and its Fe_3O_4 MNPs-conjugated form was observed *in vitro* model (12).

Docetaxel (Figure 1) is an insoluble semi-synthetic analogue of Taxol. Docetaxel leads to a significant decrease in free tubulin, required for microtubule formation, and results in inhibition of mitotic cell division between metaphase and anaphase, preventing further cancer cell progeny (13). In this study, docetaxel-coated Fe_3O_4 MNPs have been fabricated to determine the antiproliferative effect of this anticancer agent in combination with Fe_3O_4 MNPs against 4 T1 breast cancer cell line. The main hypothesis is

* Correspondence: shahverd@sina.tums.ac.ir
[1]Department of Pharmaceutical Biotechnology and Biotechnology Research Center, Faculty of Pharmacy, Tehran University of Medical Sciences, Tehran, Iran
Full list of author information is available at the end of the article

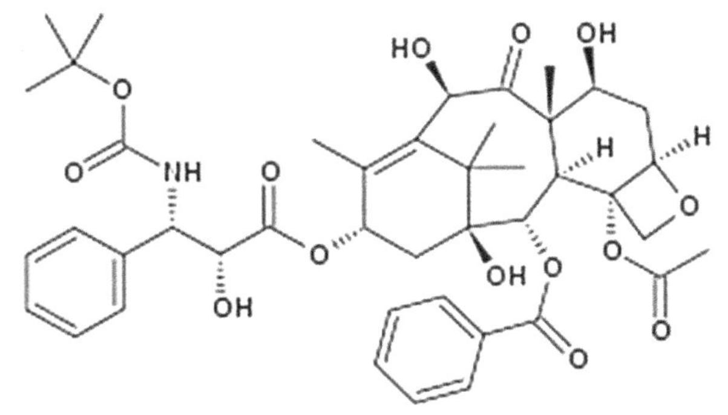

Figure 1 The structure of docetaxel.

evaluation of *in vitro* cytotoxicity of docetaxel in combination of Fe3O4 MNPs on 4 T1 breast cancer cells compared to the cytotoxicity of docetaxel alone.

Materials and methods

Synthesis of Fe_3O_4 magnetic nanoparticles and their characterization

A previously reported method was used for synthesis of Fe_3O_4 MNPs (14). Briefly, deionized water (200 ml) was deoxygenated by bubbling nitrogen gas for 1.5 h, then 50 ml of NH_4OH (1 M) was added and the mixture was stirred with mechanical agitation at 1000 rpm. Then, amounts of 6.76 g $FeCl_3.6H_2O$ (2.5 mmol) and 4.97 g $FeCl_2.4H_2O$ (2.5 mmol) were separately dissolved in 50 ml distilled water to make 0.5 M solutions. Subsequently, amounts of 10 ml ferrous chloride and 20 ml ferric chloride solutions were added to the ammonium hydroxide solution and the reaction mixture was stirred for 2.5 min at 1000 rpm. At this stage, a black precipitate formed which was washed four times with deionized water. Finally, using a magnet, the prepared Fe_3O_4 MNPs were separated from the solution. Freshly prepared Fe_3O_4 MNPs were characterized by transmission electron microscopy (model EM 208 Philips) and energy-dispersive spectroscopy (EDS).

Preparation of docetaxel-coated Fe_3O_4 nanoparticles and their surface characterization

In order to coat docetaxel on the surface of Fe_3O_4 MNPs, a simple precipitation method (Figure 2) was used as follows: A 2 mg/ml dichloromethane solution of docetaxel (Cipla, Mumbai, India) was prepared and reserved in a sealed container. Fe_3O_4 MNPs (100 mg) were dispersed in 5 ml distilled water. Thereafter, amount of 5 ml dichloromethane solution of docetaxel was added drop-by-drop to the suspension of Fe_3O_4 MNPs over a 15 min period under continuously stirring (300 rpm) condition, and using a laboratory magnetic stirrer. The resulting mixture was maintained in a static regime at 45°C for 24 hours. Docetaxel-coated Fe_3O_4 MNPs was separated from the solution by a magnet. Finally, the capped nanoparticles were washed three times with distilled water. A stock suspension of Fe_3O_4 MNPs and docetaxel-coated Fe_3O_4 MNPs were prepared (2 mg/ml) and used for antiproliferative bioassay. The surface chemistry of the docetaxel-coated Fe_3O_4 MNPs was studied using Fourier transform infrared spectroscopy (Nicolet Magna 550). Also thermal decomposition characteristics of docetaxel-coated Fe_3O_4 MNPs were determined using Thermogravimetric Analyzer *TGA* equipment as well.

Cell culture

The 4 T1 breast cancer cell line was obtained from the National Cell Bank of Iran (NCBI), Pasteur Institute of Iran, Tehran (Iran). The cells were cultured in a RPMI-1640 medium with 10% fetal calf serum, 100 u/ml penicillin and 100 μg/ml of streptomycin in 5% CO_2 at 37°C for one week and then used for cell proliferation assay.

Cell proliferation assay

Thiazolyl blue tetrazolium bromide assay (MTT) was performed to evaluate cell proliferation where 2×10^4 cells were seeded in 96 well plates and incubated with 0, 10, 20, 40 and 80 μg/ml of docetaxel-Fe_3O_4 MNPs, bared Fe_3O_4 MNPs or docetaxel alone for 24 hours. Then, 15 μl MTT (0.5 mg/ml) was added to each well, and the plates were incubated for 2 hrs. Then, the medium was replaced with 200 μl of DMSO and the absorbance was recorded at 570 nm (12). Each experiment was repeated three times and MTT assay was performed in 3 replicates for each experiments. The percentage of inhibition rate (IR) was measured using the following equation:

$$IR\,(\%) = [1 - ODexp/ODcon] \times 100$$

Where ODexp and ODcon were optical densities of treated and untreated cells, respectively. Finally, The percentage-inhibition curve was obtained by plotting "the percentage of inhibition" (i.e.[absorbance of test wells/absorbance of control wells]/100) against the concentration of cytotoxic compounds, compared to control (i.e. untreated) cells.

Results

Preparation and characterization of Fe_3O_4 MNPs

As mentioned earlier, Fe_3O_4 MNPs were chemically synthesized and their shape as well as size properties were confirmed by transmission electron microscopy. Upper illustration in Figure 3 demonstrates a representative TEM image of synthesized Fe_3O_4 MNPs. TEM image shows that the particles range in size below than 20 nm and possess an average size of 10 nm. The lower

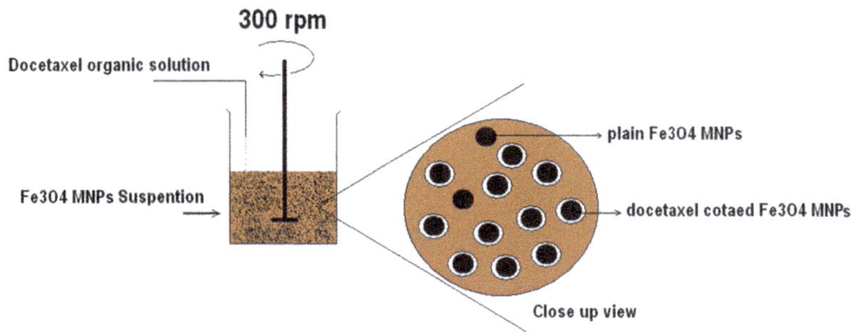

Figure 2 **Schematic presentation of the simple fabrication of docetaxel coated Fe_3O_4 MNPs used during study.**

illustration in Figure 3 depicts the energy dispersive spectrum of Fe_3O_4 MNPs revealed the presence of Fe and O elements peaks. These EDS peaks confirm the existence of iron-oxide nanoparticles. It should be mentioned that additional peaks, belonging to copper and carbon element are attributed to the grid used for TEM imaging.

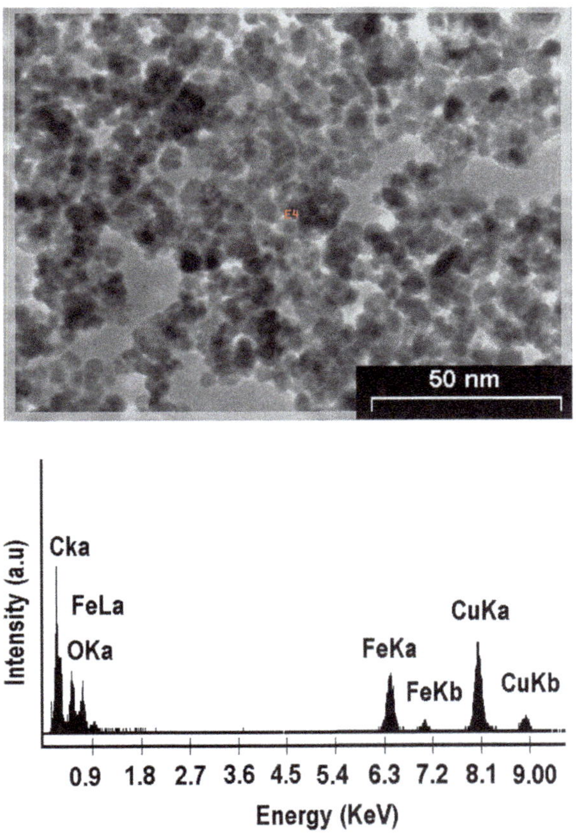

Figure 3 **TEM image of chemically-synthesized Fe_3O_4 MNPs (upper illustration) indicate that that Fe_3O_4 MNPs are well below 20 nm in size.** The magnetic forces between iron oxide particles -fortified by high surface area of nanoparticles- caused agglomeration among MNPs. Lower illustration shows energy dispersive spectrum (EDS) of Fe_3O_4 MNPs which confirms the presence of Fe and O atoms and the existence of iron-oxide nanoparticles. Additional peaks, of copper and carbon elements are attributed to the grid used for TEM imaging.

Preparation and surface characterization of docetaxel coated Fe_3O_4 MNPs

After drop-by-drop addition of the organic solution of docetaxel to Fe_3O_4 MNPs slurry, docetaxel molecules precipitated on the surface of the Fe_3O_4 nanoparticles by the ratio of about 3/100 w/w (it means that 1000 μg of coated Fe_3O_4 MNPs nanoparticles contained almost 30 μg docetaxel). This ratio was simply determined gravimetrically by weighing the coated Fe_3O_4 MNPs before and after it was washed with chloroform as solvent, for three times as well as the results obtained from thermogravimetric assay. Figure 4 demonstrates weight loss of docetaxel-coated Fe_3O_4 MNPs as a function of temperature which was determined using this method. This weight loss (%3) in the TGA curve indicated carbon oxidation which proved the presence of organic moieties

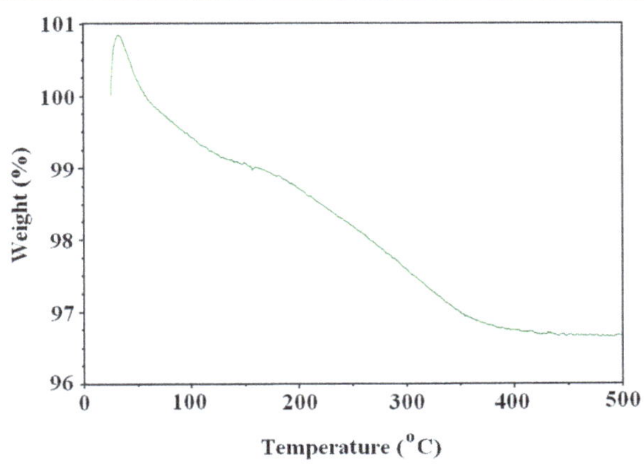

Figure 4 **Weight loss of docetaxel-coated Fe_3O_4 MNPs as a function of temperature which was determined using thermogravimetric method.** This weight loss in the TGA curve indicated carbon oxidation which proved the presence of organic moieties in the sample, thereby confirming that Fe_3O_4 MNPs are truly coated with docetaxel molecules.

Table 1 The FTIR spectroscopy data of Fe_3O_4 MNPs, docetaxel and docetaxel coated Fe_3O_4 MNPs

Sample	Main peaks wave numbers (cm^{-1})
Fe_3O_4 MNPs	584
docetaxel-coated Fe_3O_4 MNPs	2922, 2927, 1736, 1246, 1161, 1065
docetaxel alone	3487, 3377, 2937, 1735, 1712, 1246, 1169, 1072

Underlined data shows common corresponding peaks in FTIR spectra of docetaxel-coated Fe_3O_4 MNPs and docetaxel.

in sample, thereby confirming that Fe_3O_4 MNPs are truly coated with docetaxel molecules. The associated FTIR spectroscopic data of docetaxel-coated Fe_3O_4 MNPs, docetaxel-free Fe_3O_4 MNPs and docetaxel alone, are outlined in Table 1; which further confirmed the presence of docetaxel on the surface of synthesized Fe_3O_4 MNPs. In terms of chemical bonding, a main interaction is expected to occur between Fe_3O_4 MNPs and docetaxel: electrostatic bounds may form between carbonyl oxygen and hydroxyl groups of docetaxel with Fe chelating agent in Fe_3O_4 crystal (Table 1). This interaction lead to disappear of hydroxyl bands centered at 3487 and 3377 cm^{-1} in FTIR spectrum of docetaxel-coated Fe_3O_4 MNPs. It is possible that these interactions

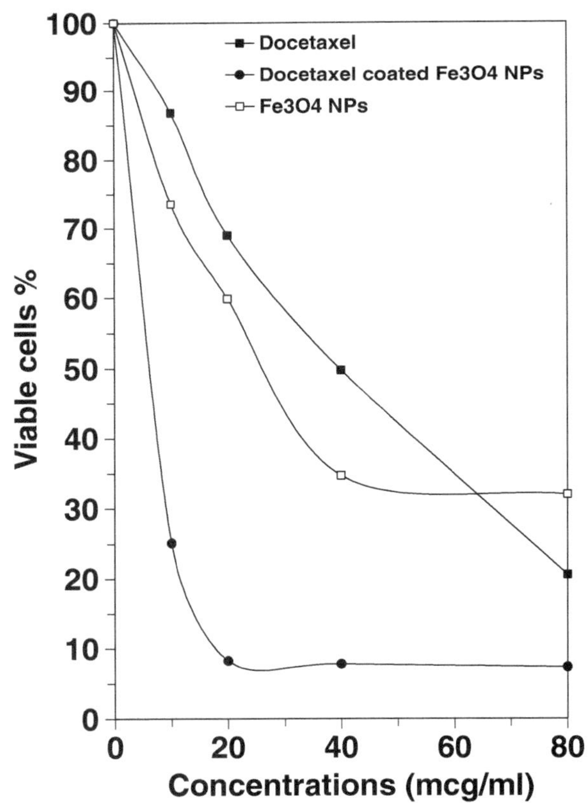

Figure 5 Antiproliferative effect of Fe_3O_4 MNPs, docetaxel and docetaxel-coated Fe_3O_4 MNPs against 4 T1 breast cancer.

make docetaxel -coated Fe_3O_4 MNPs a suitable carrier with bipolar properties which penetrates into both hydrophilic and hydrophobic (i.e. cell membrane) fluids at the same time.

Antiproliferative effects

Antiproliferative effects of docetaxel-coated Fe_3O_4 MNPs, docetaxel alone, and Fe_3O_4 MNPs alone were *in vitro* evaluated at different concentrations on 4 T1 breast cancer cells. Cytotoxicity analysis of samples suggested a direct dose–response relationship, in which cell proliferation decreased in higher concentrations (Figure 5). Samples were found to have different cytotoxicities on 4 T1 breast cancer cells, with docetaxel-coated nanoparticles being the most potent. The antiproliferative effect of test compounds increased in the following order: docetaxel < Fe_3O_4 MNPs < docetaxel-coated Fe_3O_4 MNPs. Moreover, the necessary concentrations to cause 50% cell death (IC_{50}) were more than 30 and 40 (μg/ml) in cells treated with Fe_3O_4 MNPs alone and docetaxel, respectively. Docetaxel-coated Fe_3O_4 MNPs could cause the same effect at 10 μg/ml concentration. In other words, the combination of docetaxel and Fe_3O_4 MNPs exhibited a much more potent antiproliferative activity than docetaxel and Fe_3O_4 MNPs alone. As clear in Figure 5, docetaxel at concentrations of 20 and 30 (μg/ml), moderately reduced the proportion of viable cells to 70% and 50%, respectively. The cytotoxicity curve for Fe_3O_4 MNPs alone followed almost similar pattern, though sharper. The percentage of viable cell number sharply decreased from 87% at the concentration of 10 μg/ml to 35% at 40 μg/ml concentration. In contrast, however, only the low concentration of 10 μg/ml docetaxel-coated Fe_3O_4 MNPs (equivalent to the concentration of approximately 0.3 μg/ml pure docetaxel), drastically reduced the proportion of viable cells by more than 70%. Also a considerable cytotoxicity (about 90%) was observed for 20 μg/ml docetaxel-coated Fe_3O_4 MNPs against 4 T1 breast cancer cells. In higher concentrations (>20 μg/ml), this proportion declined steadily, until it reached the remarkably-low amount of about 7% at 80 μg/ml concentration.

Discussion

Literature review shows that there are numerous reports on cytotoxicity of docetaxel in combination of different carrier (15,16). However, the efficiency of this compound in conjugation with Fe_3O_4 MNPs has not been yet investigated. Here, the antiproliferative effect of docetaxel enhanced in tumor cells when it was coated on the surface of Fe_3O_4 MNPs has been reported. As mentioned earlier, Fe_3O_4 MNPs, docetaxel and docetaxel-coated Fe_3O_4 MNPs, all showed antiproliferative effects on 4 T1 breast cancer cells, increasing in the order: docetaxel < Fe_3O_4 MNPs < docetaxel-coated Fe_3O_4 MNPs. It is noticeable that based on current study, docetaxel has considerable antiproliferative effect on 4 T1 breast cancer cells in concentrations of not below 10 μg/ml. However, obtained results demonstrated that when coated on Fe_3O_4 MNPs surface, docetaxel have antiproliferative effect, even at the low concentration of 0.3 μg/ml. This literally means that much lower amounts of docetaxel will be needed to produce the same antiproliferative effect as docetaxel alone. As described in above, during precipitation process, docetaxel molecules were precipitated on the surface of Fe_3O_4 MNPs by the ratio of 3/100 w/w which indicates that each milligram of coated Fe_3O_4 MNPs averagely contained 30 μg pure docetaxel compound. Therefore, it is deducible from Figure 5, that the concentration of 80 μg/ml docetaxel caused 79% cell death. However, when combined with Fe_3O_4 MNPs, the average concentration of 0.6 μg/ml docetaxel (which is equivalent to the concentration of about 20 μg/ml docetaxel- Fe_3O_4 MNPs) caused more than 90% cell death. Thus, it is concluded that by coating docetaxel on the surface of Fe_3O_4 MNPs, the required amount of docetaxel for showing a potent antiproliferative effects against 4 T1 breast cancer cells could be considerably lowered (more than 100 fold). As mentioned before, many pharmaceutical compounds have low solubility in biological fluids, which reduces their efficiency in *in vivo* models. Therefore, it is hypothesized that, Fe_3O_4 MNPs may be considered as efficient carriers for these insoluble compounds.

Conclusion

In this paper, the antiproliferative effect of docetaxel (IC_{50} =40 μg/ml) has been reported and the results revealed that the combination of Fe_3O_4 MNPs and docetaxel is significantly more cytotoxic (IC_{50} =10 μg/ml) than docetaxel alone. In conclusion, this result is of particular value since it demonstrates that by using metallic nanoparticles in combination therapy, lower amounts of these materials might be required, resulting in reduction of the potential hazards of docetaxel usage. Further investigations are needed to determine the antiproliferative effect of docetaxel-coated Fe_3O_4 MNPs in other cell lines. Moreover, studies on cytotoxic effects of docetaxel-coated Fe_3O_4 MNPs in animal models will be of great value.

Competing interests

The authors declare that they have no competing interest.

Authors' contibutions

MHY: Collaboration in proliferation assays. ZNN: Collaboration in fabrication of nanoparticles. MRK: Commented on cytotoxic assays. MA: Commented on surface chemistry analysis of the nanoparticles. ARS: Design of the project. All authors read and approved the final manuscript.

Acknowledgment

This study was supported by Deputy of Research, Tehran University of Medical Sciences, Tehran, Iran.

Author details

[1]Department of Pharmaceutical Biotechnology and Biotechnology Research Center, Faculty of Pharmacy, Tehran University of Medical Sciences, Tehran, Iran. [2]Department of Medical Biotechnology, School of Advanced Medical Technologies, Tehran University of Medical Sciences, Tehran, Iran. [3]Drug Design and Development Research Center, Faculty of Pharmacy, Tehran University of Medical Sciences, Tehran, Iran.

References

1. Carr C, Ng J, Wigmore T: **The side effects of chemotherapeutic agents.** *Curr Anaesth Crit Care* 2008, **19**:70–79.
2. Yoo HS, Park TG: **Folate-receptor-targeted delivery of doxorubicin nano-aggregates stabilized by doxorubicin-PEG-folate conjugate.** *J Control Release* 2004, **100**:247–256.
3. Li X, Li R, Qian X, Ding Y, Tu Y, Guo R, Hu Y, Jiang X, Guo W, Liu B: **Superior antitumor efficiency of cisplatin-loaded nanoparticles by intratumoral delivery with decreased tumor metabolism rate.** *Eur J Pharm Biopharm* 2008, **70**:726–734.
4. Cheung RY, Ying Y, Rauth AM, Marcon N, Wu XY: **Biodegradable dextran-based microspheres for delivery of anticancer drug mitomycin C.** *Biomaterials* 2005, **26**:5375–5385.
5. Liu Z, Chen K, Davis C, Sherlock S, Cao O, Chen X, Dai H: **Drug delivery with carbon nanotubes for in vivo cancer treatment.** *Cancer Res* 2008, **68**:6652–6660.
6. Lee RJ: **Liposomal delivery as a mechanism to enhance synergism between anticancer drugs.** *Mol Cancer Ther* 2006, **5**:1639–1640.
7. Cheng Y, Xu Z, Ma M, Xu T: **Dendrimers as drug carriers: applications in different routes of drug administration.** *J Pharm Sci* 2008, **97**:123–143.
8. Dubey M, Bhadauria S, Kushwah BS: **Green synthesis of nanosilver particles from extract of eucalyptus hybrida (saeda) leaf.** *Dig J Nanomater Bios* 2009, **4**:537–543.
9. Polyak B, Friedman G: **Magnetic targeting for site-specific drug delivery: applications and clinical potential.** *Expert Opin. Drug Del* 2009, **6**:53–70.
10. Bai Y, Teng B, Chen S, Chang Y, Li Z: **Preparation of magnetite nanoparticles coated with an amphiphilic block copolymer: A potential drug.** *Macromol. Rapid Commun* 2006, **27**:2107–2112.
11. Dinauer N, Balthasar S, Weber C, Kreuter J, Langer K, von Briesen H: **Selective targeting of antibody-conjugated nanoparticles to leukemic cells and primary T-lymphocytes.** *Biomaterials* 2005, **26**:5898–5906.
12. Khorramizadeh MR, Esmail-Nazari Z, Zarei-Ghaane Z, Shakibaie M, Mollazadeh-Moghaddam K, Iranshahi M, Shahverdi AR: **Umbelliprenin-coated Fe_3O_4 magnetite nanoparticles: Antiproliferation evaluation on human Fibrosarcoma cell line (HT-1080).** *Mater Sci Eng C* 2010, **30**:1038–1042.
13. Yvon AM, Wadsworth P, Jordan MA: **Taxol Suppresses Dynamics of Individual Microtubules in Living Human Tumor Cells.** *Mol Biol Cell* 1999, **10**:947–59.
14. Martínez-Mera I, Espinosa-Pesqueira ME, Pérez-Hernández R, Arenas-Alatorre J: **Synthesis of magnetite (Fe_3O_4) nanoparticles without surfactants at room temperature.** *Mater Lett* 2007, **61**:4447–4451.
15. Noori Koopaei M, Dinarvand R, Amini M, Rabbani H, Emami S, Ostad SN, Atyabi F: **Docetaxel immunonanocarriers as targeted delivery systems for HER2-positive tumor cells: preparation, characterization, and cytotoxicity studies.** *Int J Nanomed* 2011, **6**:1903–1912.
16. Saremi S, Atyabi F, Akhlaghi SP, Ostad SN, Dinarvand R: **Thiolated chitosan nanoparticles for enhancing oral absorption of docetaxel: preparation, in vitro and ex vivo evaluation.** *Int J Nanomed* 2011, **6**:119–128.

17

Synthesis, *in vitro* aerobic and hypoxic cytotoxicity and radiosensitizing activity of novel metronidazole tethered 5-fluorouracil

Khosrou Abdi[1,2], Ali Khalaj[2,4*], Seyed Nasser Ostad[3], Navid Lamei[4] and Mohammad Reza Khoshayand[5]

Abstract

Background and the purpose of the study: Several 2, 4-dinitrophenyl and 2,4-dinitrophenylamine tethered 5-FU (5-fluorouracil) compared to their components have shown minimal or no cytotoxicity to HT-29 cell line under aerobic conditions but high cytotoxicity and radiosensitizing effects under hypoxic conditions. In the present study the cytotoxicity and radiation potentiation of three novel analogues of these compounds by replacing 2,4-dinitrophenyl moiety with 2-methyl-5-nitroimidazole, a known radiosensitizer and cytotoxic agent was investigated.

Methods: Tethered compounds **7–9** were prepared by the reaction of 1-(*t*-butoxycarbonyl)-5-fluorouracil **6** with metronidazole esters **2–4** followed by removal of the *t*-butoxycarbonyl protecting group. Cytotoxicity of compounds in HT-29 cells with or without radiation were determined by 3-(4,5-Dimethylthiazol-2-yl)-2,5-diphenyltetrazolium bromide (MTT), propidium iodide (PI)-digitonin and clonogenic assays.

Results: Tethered compounds **7–9** induced time-and concentration–dependent cytotoxicity under hypoxia but had no significant effect under aerobic conditions. These compounds also showed selective and concentration- dependent radiosensitization effects under hypoxic conditions.

Conclusion: Tethered compounds **7–9** compared to 5-FU **5** showed minimal cytotoxicities under aerobic and selective radiosensitizing activities under hypoxic conditions. Also effects of these compounds were higher than those of metronidazole **1** which is a known cytotoxin and radiosensitizer under hypoxic conditions.

Keywords: Cytotoxicity, Radiosensitizing, Metronidazole, 5-Fluorouracil, MTT& PI-digitonin assays

Introduction

Oxygen as a radiosensitizer increases the effects of radiation by the formation of free radicals that damage DNA [1]. Electron affinic nitroaromatic and nitroheterocyclic compounds act like oxygen by formation of nitro radical anion through one electron reduction and are solid tumor targeting agents because of the presence of hypoxic cells in these tumors due to insufficient blood supply [2]. The cytotoxicity of these compounds under hypoxia has also been attributed to an increase in the oxidative damage of DNA, formation of hydroxyl compounds under deoxygenated conditions, and suppression of intracellular radioprotectors of sulfhydryl compounds [3]. Under aerobic conditions where the initially reduced species can be readily re-oxidized by molecular oxygen, the cytotoxicity of these compounds has been attributed to the parent nitro compounds, or bio-activation by NADPH: quinine oxido-reductase (DT diaphorase) which can act as an oxygen insensitive reductase [4].

Nitroimidazoles [1,2] specifically 2- and 5-nitro derivatives are known as cytotoxin and radiosensitizer toward hypoxic cells and have been subject of many clinical studies. However these compounds have shown limited therapeutic impact on radiotherapy due to clinical problems that includes dose-limiting side effects such as neurotoxicity [5]. Additionally several hybrid or dual functional agents have been described in which nitroimidazoles are attached through a linker unit to cytotoxic nitrogen mustards, [1,2,6] and aziridine moieties

* Correspondence: akhalaj@tums.ac.ir
[2]Department of Medicinal Chemistry, Tehran University of Medical Sciences, Tehran 14174, Iran
[4]Drug Design & Development Research Center, Tehran University of Medical Sciences, Tehran 14174, Iran
Full list of author information is available at the end of the article

[1,2,7] which have shown higher cytotoxicity and enhanced radiosensitizing activity than those of the corresponding counterparts in both aerobic and hypoxic cells. In these compounds cellular reduction of the nitro group to more electron donating species activate the nitrogen of the cytotoxic group by the release of electron through the aromatic ring and generate reactive alkylating species [7].

Previously, results of our study on *in vitro* aerobic cytotoxicity of 2, 4-dinitrophenylamine tethered 5-FU through three carbon atoms in HT-29 cell line with and without radiation showed that the compound unlike its components has no cytotoxicity but is radiosensitizer [8]. Since in the tested compound 5-FU is not a leaving group, it was reasoned that the aerobic cytotoxicity of the reported 2,4-dinitrophenylamine mustard [6] and 2,4-dinitrophenyl aziridine [7] are due to their alkylating moieties.

Also results of our investigations on 2,4-dinitrobenzyl, 2,4-dinitrobenzoyl, 3,5-dinitrobenzoyl and 2,4-dinitrophenacetyl derivatives of 5-FU showed that with exception of 3,5-dinitrobenzoyl derivatives other compounds have selective- cytotoxicity and radiosensitization effects under hypoxic conditions [9]. Since the IC_{50} values of compounds which showed selective cytotoxicity were not different significantly it was concluded that they have similar mechanism of action and might produce the same reactive species [9].

In continuation of our investigations on this type of bifunctional compounds [8-11] in the present study the cytotoxicity and radiosensitization effects of three novel analogues of these compounds by replacing 2,4-dinitrophenyl moiety with 2-methyl-5-nitroimidazole (metronidazole), a known radiosensitizer and cytotoxic agent [2,12] was investigated. This manuscript describes cytotoxicities and radiosensitizing activities of metronidazole tethered 5-FU through ethyl and labile ester groups which was hypothesized upon *in vivo* hydrolysis to generate active metabolites which might have synergistic actions.

Materials and methods

Chemistry

Metronidazole **1**, 5-FU **5**, di-*t*-butoxydicarbonate $(Boc)_2O$, triethylamine, sodium hydride and other chemicals and solvents not listed here were from Merck Chemical Co. (Merck, Germany). Thin layer chromatography was carried out using Kieselge l60, 230–400 mesh, (Merck, Germany) to monitor the progress of reactions. Melting points were determined on a MEL-270 Sibata melting point apparatus and are uncorrected. ^{1}HNMR spectra were recorded on 500 MHz a Bruker (Germany), using DMSO-d_6 or $CDCl_3$ as solvent. Chemical shifts (δ) are reported in ppm relative to TMS as internal standard. Mass spectra were obtained on a Finningan TSQ-70 (USA) instrument. Infrared spectra were recorded on a Nicolet Magna IR-550 (USA) spectrometer. All compounds were characterized by the above techniques. Analytical and spectroscopic data for the known compounds were consistent with the reported literature values and data only for new compounds are presented.

Synthesis of 2-(2-Methyl-5-nitro-1H-imidazole-1-yl) ethyl-2-chloroacetate (3)

To a solution of metronidazole **1** (3.9 g, 24 mmol) in 100 ml of anhydrous dichloromethane was added 1.9 ml (24 mmol) triethylamine at temperature below 5°C and after stirring for 30 min the solution was treated with 3.2 ml (40 mmol) of chloroacetyl chloride dropwise within 5 min and then the resulting solution was stirred at room temperature overnight. The mixture was filtered and the residue after evaporation of the solvent was subjected to flash chromatography using Pet-ether: EtOAC as eluting solvent (80:20) to give 7.9 g (64%) of the compound **3**. mp 80-82°C; ^{1}H NMR (DMSO-d_6): δ 8.01 (s, 1H-imidazole), 4.61 (t, J = 5.12 Hz, 2H, CH_2-O), 4.48 (t, J = 5.12Hz, 2H, CH_2-N), 4.35 (s, 2H, CH_2-Cl), 2.18 (s, 3H, CH_3); FT-IR (KBr): 1720 (C = O), 1546, 1350 (NO_2) cm^{-1}.

Synthesis of 2-(2-Methyl-5-nitro-1H-imidazole-1-yl) ethyl-3-chloropropanoate (4)

The reaction of metronidazole **1** (3.9 g, 24 mmol) with 3.85 ml (40 mmol) of 3-chloropropionyl chloride under above conditions for the preparation of the ester **3** but purification of the product by crystallization from Pet-ether: EtOAC instead of flash chromatography gave 4.1 g (71%) of the ester **4**. mp 89-93°C;^{1}H NMR (DMSO-d_6): δ 8.01 (s, 1H-imidazole), 4.58 (t, J = 5.10 Hz, 2H, CH_2-O), 4.40 (t, J = 5.10 Hz, 2H, CH_2-N), 3.7 (t, J = 5.3 Hz, 2H, CH_2-Cl), 2.5 (t, J = 5.3 Hz, 2H, CH_2-C = O), 2.18 (s, 3H, CH_3); FT-IR (KBr): 1729 (C = O), 1540, 1345 (NO_2) cm^{-1}.

General procedure for the synthesis of tethered compounds 7–9

To a stirred solution of 225 mg (1 mmol) of 1-(*t*-butoxycarbonyl)-5-FU **6** [13] in 10 ml of anhydrous DMF in a round bottom flask which was kept in an ice bath was added 30 mg (1.25 mmol) of sodium hydride within 10 min and after stirring for 30 min at 5°C the mixture was then treated with a solution of 1 mmol of metronidazole esters **2-4** in 10 ml of anhydrous DMF and the mixture stirred at room temperature for 18 h. The mixture was then diluted with the same volume of water, extracted with ethyl acetate (3×20 ml), and the organic layer was dehydrated using anhydrous sodium sulfate. Evaporation of ethyl acetate gave an oily residue which was dissolved in 10 ml of methanol, treated with 0.42 g potassium carbonate and the obtained mixture was stirred at room temperature for 1 h. After evaporation of the solvent under reduced pressure, the residue was dissolved in water-ethyl acetate mixture (1:1), the organic layer was separated and dehydrated using anhydrous sodium sulfate and then evaporated under reduced pressure. For the preparation of compound **7**, the residue after evaporation of the solvent was purified by flash chromatography using Pet-ether: EtOAC as eluting solvent (70:30) to give 100 mg (35%) of the product. For the preparation of compounds **8** and **9**, residues were crystallized from Hexan-EtOAC to give 310 mg (92%) and 330 mg (93%) of the pure products respectively.

5-fluoro-3-(2-(2-methyl-5-nitro-1H-imidazol-1-yl)ethyl) pyrimidine-2,4(1H,3H)-dione(7)

mp 185-189°C; ^{1}HNMR ($CDCl_3$): δ 7.9 (s, 1H-imidazol), 7.8 (d, 1H, CH = CF), 4.0 (t, CH_2), 3.9 (t, CH_2), 2.4 (s, 3H, CH_3); FT-IR (KBr): 3108 (NH), 1722, 1671 (C = O), 1550, 1350 (NO_2) cm^{-1}; MS: m/z 81(100%), 130 (78%), 238 (39%), 155(24%).

2-(2-methyl-5-nitro-1H-imidazol-1-yl)ethyl 2-(5-fluoro-2,6-dioxo-2,3-dihydropyrimidin-1(6H)-yl)-acetate(8)

mp 231–234°C; ^{1}H NMR (DMSO-d_6): δ 7.99 (s, 1H-imidazole), 7.93 (d, J = 8.5 Hz, 1H, CH = CF), 4.65 (t, J = 5.02 Hz, 2H, CH_2-O), 4.42 (s, 2H, CH_2-C = O), 3.98 (t, J = 5.02 Hz, 2H, CH_2-N), 2.42 (s, CH_3); FT-IR (KBr): 3131 (NH), 1725, 1656 (C = O), 1542, 1349 (NO_2) cm^{-1}; MS: m/z 341 (7%), 296 (23%), 212 (80%), 171(74%), 130 (100%), 126 (42%).

2-(2-methyl-5-nitro-1H-imidazol-1-yl) ethyl 2-(5-fluoro-2,6-dioxo-2,3-dihydropyrimidin-1(6H)-yl)-propanoate(9)

mp 247-250°C; ^{1}H NMR (DMSO-d_6): δ 8.01 (s, 1H-imidazole), 7.98 (d, J = 8.5Hz, 1H, CH = CF), 4.57 (t, J = 5.05 Hz, 2H, CH_2-O), 4.39 (t, J = 5.05 Hz, 2H, CH_2-N), 3.78 (t, J = 6.8 Hz, 2H, CH_2-N), 2.70 (t, J = 6.8 Hz, 2H, CH_2-C = O), 2.44 (s, CH_3); FT-IR (KBr): 3124 (NH), 1721, 1652 (C = O), 1547, 1350 (NO_2) cm^{-1}; MS: m/z 355 (5%), 309 (21%), 226 (86%), 185(75%), 171 (42%), 130 (100%), 126 (59%).

In vitro cytotoxicity

Materials HT-29 cells, originally derived from human colorectal carcinoma were obtained from Pasteur Institute (Tehran, Iran). Fetal Bovine Serum (FBS), Penicillin/Streptomycin 100X, Trypsin-EDTA 10X and Trypan blue were from Biosera (England). RPMI 1640 from Gibco (England), MTT and PI from Sigma (USA) and Digitonin from Merck (Germany) were used in this study.

Cell culture HT-29 cells were grown as an attached monolayer in RPMI 1640 supplemented with 10% fetal bovine serum, penicillin (50 unit/ml), and streptomycin (50 μg/ml). Cells were routinely grown in tissue culture flasks and kept in a humidified atmosphere of 5% CO_2 and 95% air at 37°C [14].

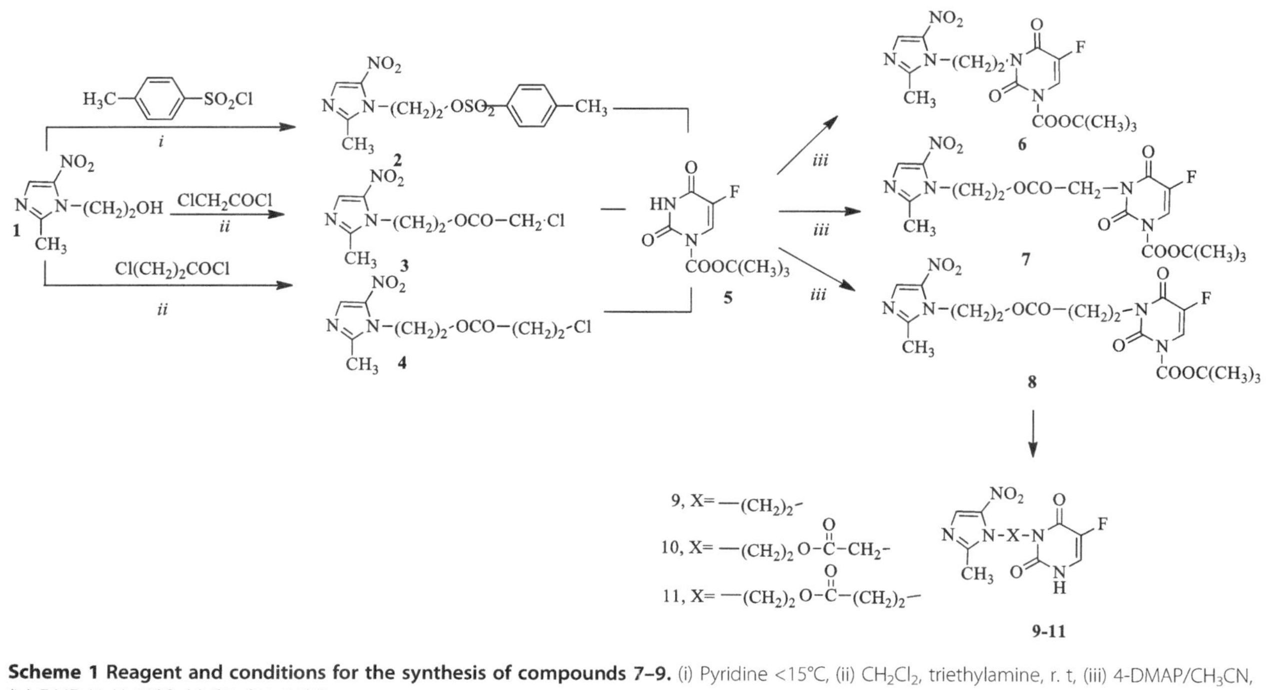

Scheme 1 Reagent and conditions for the synthesis of compounds 7–9. (i) Pyridine <15°C, (ii) CH_2Cl_2, triethylamine, r. t, (iii) 4-DMAP/CH_3CN, (iv) DMF, NaH, 80°C, (v) CH_3OH, K_2CO_3.

Methods of assay

Cytotoxicity of 5-FU**5**, metronidazole **1**, and tethered compounds **7–9** against HT-29 cells under both aerobic and hypoxic conditions were determined by measurement of the percentage of cell survivals using MTT [15] and PI-digitonin [16,17] and clonogenic forming assays [18]. Cells were seeded at the density of 10^4 cells/well in 96-well culture dishes and incubated for 4 h. Stock solutions of the tested compounds in DMSO at concentrations of 50 mmol which were prepared prior to the experiments diluted with culture media and at concentrations of 6.25-400 μmol/ml added to each well of plates. Cells in the control wells were treated with the same volume of medium which contained DMSO at concentration equal to those which were used in incubations treated with the tested compounds. Cell incubations were kept at 37°C under either air by purging with 95% nitrogen and 5% CO_2 or hypoxia in sealed GasPack jar by using Anoximat (Netherland) and an anaerobic chamber GasPak Jar (Merck, Germany) and GasPak pluss (Merck, Germany) [19] for 3 or 48 h. After removal of the supernatant of the culture medium, wells were washed with phosphate buffer saline (PBS), and the numbers of live cells were determined by following methods.

MTT assay

25 μl of the reagent (5 mg/ml in PBS) was added to each well, cell cultures were incubated for 4 h at 37°C and then the precipitated formazan was dissolved in 100 μl of DMSO and its absorbance was read in Elisa reader at 550 nm and a background wavelength of 690 nm. Survival was scored by the ratio of the absorbance of the treated cells to untreated cells with the tested compounds (control) and is expressed as percentage of the cell survival [15].

PI-digitonine assay

20 μl of a 1.53 mmol solution of PI in PBS for a final concentration of 30 μmol was added to each well, cell cultures were incubated for 60 min at 37°C and then the initial fluorescence intensity from the dead cells was measured in a multi-well plate reader, (BioTek, Synergy HT, USA) with 530-nm excitation and 645-nm emission filters. Then digitonin (600 nmol) was added to each well to permeabilize all cells and label all nuclei with PI and after 30 min incubation, the fluorescence intensity was measured again to obtain a value corresponding to the total number of cells. The percentage of dead cells was calculated as the proportion of fluorescence intensity of the dead cells to that of total cells multiplied by 100 and percentage of the cell viability was calculated by subtracting the percentage of dead cells from 100% [16].

The IC_{50} values for both MTT and PI-digitonine assays were determined from cell survival curves in which the percentages of cells that survived were plotted as a function of the concentration of the tested compounds.

Clonogenic forming assay

The medium of the cell cultures after treatment with the tested compounds and/or irradiation under aerobic or hypoxic conditions were first separated to remove the tested compounds, and washed with PBS. Cells were seeded in 6-well plates at concentration of 5×10^3 cells per well and maintained at 37°C for 14 days. The cells were then fixed in methanol, colonies which were formed stained with crystal violet and those containing more than 50 cells were scored. The number of colonies of treated and untreated dishes with the tested compounds were compared and expressed as the percentage of survival by clonogenic assay [18]. Clonogenic survival curves were constructed by plotting percent of survivals in response to different concentrations of the tested compounds.

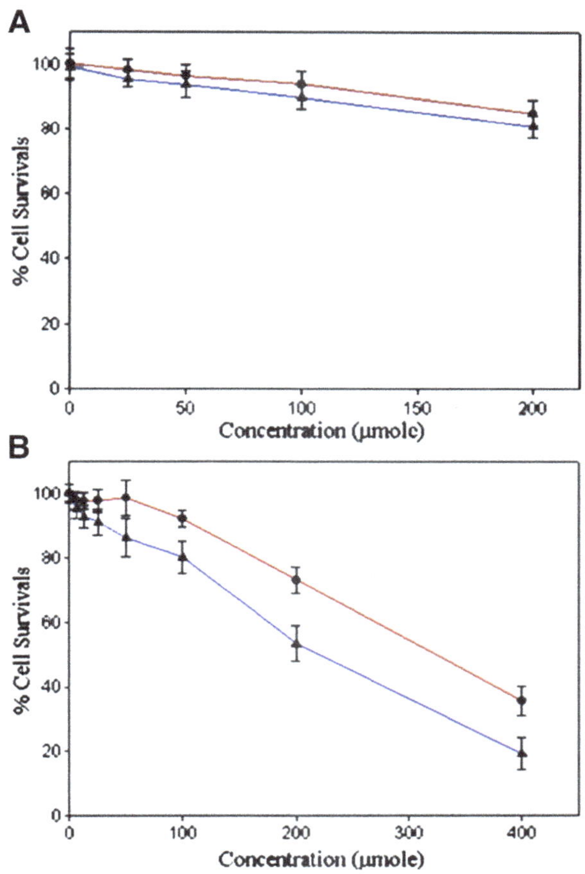

Figure 1 Clonogenic survival of incubation of HT-29 cell line with different concentration of compound 7 after 3 h (A) and 48 h (B) under aerobic (•) and hypoxic (▲) conditions. Data points were obtained from three independent experiments, and the standard deviations are given for each point. (Mean ± SD each set of experiments was performed in triplicates).

Table 1 Cytotoxicity and radiosensitization of metronidazole 1, 5-fluorouracil 5, and tethered compounds 7-9

Compound	IC_{50} (μmole)				SER					
	MTT assay[a]		PI assay[b]		Concentration (μmole)					
					25		50		100	
	Aerobic	Hypoxic	Aerobic	Hypoxic	Aerobic	Hypoxic	Aerobic	Hypoxic	Aerobic	Hypoxic
1	338 ± 12	265.9 ± 19	311 ± 16	250 ± 23	1.07 ± 0.06	1.26 ± 0.02	1.15 ± 0.09	1.69 ± 0.08	1.27 ± 0.02	2.06 ± 0.06
5	93 ± 9	89 ± 7	88 ± 7	84 ± 5	1.09 ± 0.06	1.04 ± 0.04	1.12 ± 0.09	1.18 ± 0.11	1.16 ± 0.11	1.12 ± 0.06
7	330 ± 16	240 ± 14	318 ± 20	230 ± 11	1.11 ± 0.11	1.41 ± 0.06	1.19 ± 0.05	1.85 ± 0.05	1.25 ± 0.010	2.17 ± 0.11
8	309 ± 25	232.1 ± 21	296 ± 18	229 ± 19	1.07 ± 0.03	1.51 ± 0.12	1.13 ± 0.08	1.95 ± 0.12	1.31 ± 0.12	2.26 ± 0.16
9	304 ± 18	234 ± 11	299 ± 14	224 ± 25	1.13 ± 0.06	1.43 ± 0.07	1.22 ± 0.10	1.79 ± 0.05	1.33 ± 0.05	2.13 ± 0.08

[a]3-(4,5-Dimethylthiazol-2-yl)-2,5-diphenyltetrazolium bromide.
[b]Propidium Iodide-Digitonin assay.

Radiosensitizing activity

Irradiation

HT-29 cells at 37°C under hypoxic or aerobic conditions were incubated with the tested compounds at concentrations of 25, 50, and 100 μmol for 3 h and then at room temperature were exposed to 4 different doses of radiation (2, 4, 8 and 12 Gy) at the dose rate of 1.67 Gy/min and Source Surface Distance (SSD) = 80 cm^2 by a ^{60}Co source (Theratron 780 MDS – Nordion).

Radiosensitivity measurement

Radiosensitivity of the tested compounds were determined through measurement of the cell growth inhibition using clonogenic assay [18]. Results are presented in terms of Sensitization Enhancement Ratio (SER) which were calculated from the equation SER = Do untreated cells/ Do treated cells, where Do values represent radiation dose that leads to 37% cell survival [20]. Do values were obtained from the survival curves of irradiation in the presence and absence of the tested compounds.

Statistical analyses

For the cell survival and cell death assays each experiment was repeated three times and results are mean ± SD of three independent experiments. Statistical analysis was performed using Sigmaplot 12 (Systat Software Inc.) for window and descriptive statistics are shown as arithmetic mean ± standard deviation. Independent samples' t-test was used to investigate the mean differences between irradiated and un-irradiated cells treated with the tested compounds and for comparison of more than two groups, Holm-Sidak multiple comparison test followed by one way analysis of variance (One way ANOVA) were performed and p value smaller than 0.05 was considered statistically significant.

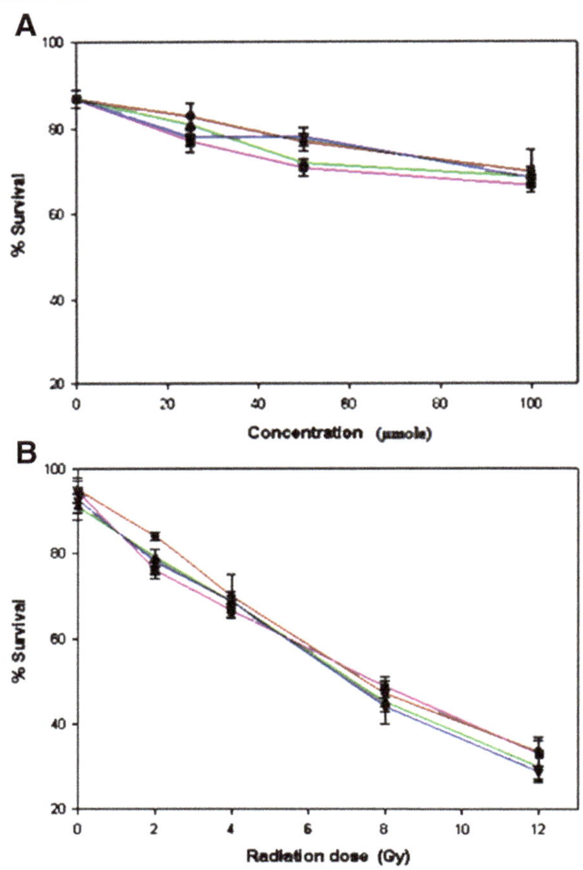

Figure 2 Clonogenic cell survival of HT-29 cells under aerobic conditions, (A): upon exposure to 4 Gy gamma-irradiation after incubation with different concentration (25, 50, 100 μmole) of metronidazole 1 and tethered compounds 7–9 for 3 h, (B): upon exposure to different doses (2, 4, 8 and 12 Gy) of radiation after incubation with 50 μmol of metronidazole 1 and tethered compounds 7–9 for 3 h. Each data points were obtained from three independent experiments, and the standard deviations are given for each point. (Mean ± SD).

Results and discussion

Tethered compounds **7–9** were prepared by the reaction of 1-(*t*-butoxycarbonyl)-5-FU **6** [13] with p-toluenesulfonic,

2-chloroacetic and 3-chloropropionic acid esters of metronidazole **1** (compounds **2–4**, Scheme 1) respectively in DMF in the presence of sodium hydride followed by removal of *t*-butoxycarbonyl group in methanolic potassium carbonate. Esters **3, 4** were obtained by the reported method for the preparation of the ester **2** [21] through the reaction of metronidazole **1** with 2-chloroacetyl chloride, and 3-chloropropionyl chloride respectively in pyridine.

Effects of different concentrations of 5FU **5**, metronidazole **1**, and tethered compounds **7–9** for different incubation periods on viability and proliferation of HT-29 cells were determined by MTT (15), PI-digitonin [16,17], and clonogenic assays (18). The tested compounds inhibited HT-29 cell proliferation in a time dependent manner and as it is shown for the compound **7** (Figure 1A) cell survival at 3 h after incubation were similar ($p > 0.05$) but after 48 h were significantly different ($p < 0.05$). IC_{50} values were assessed from cell survival curves in which the percentage of cells that survived after 48 h incubation were plotted as a function of the concentration of tested compounds (Table 1). Results of this study showed that IC_{50} values of each compound for the cell survival under aerobic or hypoxic conditions determined either by MTT or by PI-digitonin assays are not different significantly ($p > 0.05$) from each other and results of these tests which are seldom unanimous [12] were in good agreement.

While tethered compounds **7–9** under hypoxic conditions exhibited remarkable concentration–dependent cytotoxicity (Figure 1B), these compounds under aerobic conditions were not or were slightly cytotoxic whereas at concentrations up to 100 μmol could reduce viabilities of HT-29 cells only to less than 10% (Figure 1B). Consistent with these results the IC_{50} values of these compounds were significantly lower ($p < 0.05$) under hypoxic (232.1±21-240±14) compared to aerobic (304±18-330±16) conditions suggesting that compounds have hypoxia-selective cytotoxicity.

The radiosensitizing activities of all tested compounds were determined by measurement of the cell growth inhibition using a standard colony formation method following exposure of incubations with different concentrations of the tested compounds to different doses of the radiation [18]. Results are presented in term of Sensitization Enhancement Ratio (SER) which were obtained from the survival curves of irradiation in the presence and absence of the tested compounds for 37% survival respectively (20). The radiosensitization effects of compounds **7–9** at various concentrations under aerobic conditions were not different significantly ($p > 0.05$) (Figure 2A) and at a given concentration only increase in the dose of radiation resulted in decrease in the cell survival (Figure 2B). However under hypoxic conditions (Figures 3) radiosensitization effects of these compounds increased significantly with

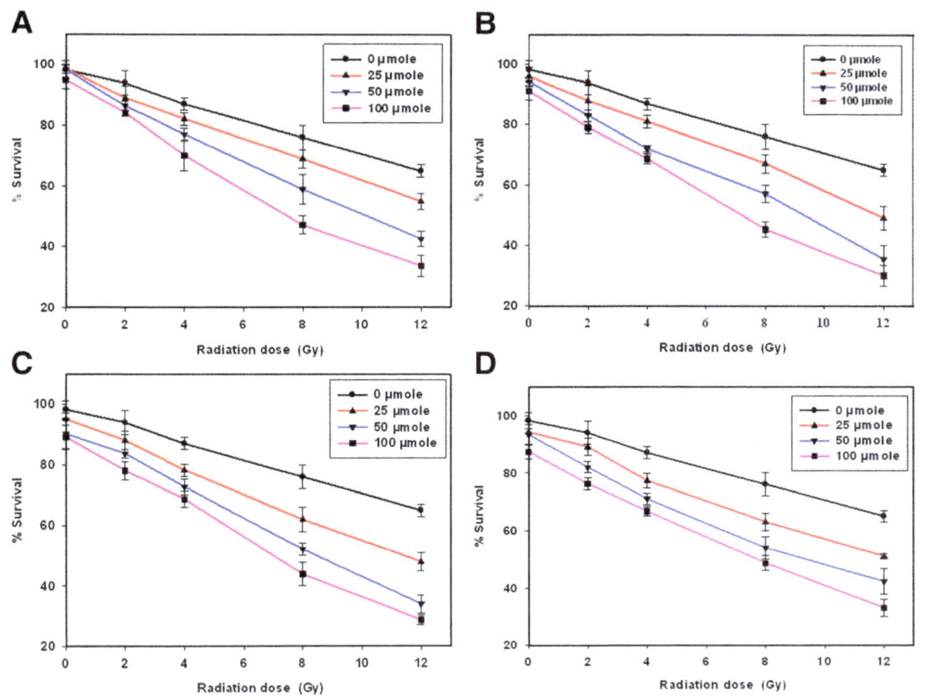

Figure 3 Clonogenic cell survival of HT-29 cells upon exposure to different doses of Gamma-radiation (2, 4, 6, 8 and 12 Gy) after incubation for 3 h with different concentrations (0, 25, 50 and 100 μmole) of metronidazole 1 and tethered compounds 7-9 under hypoxic conditions. Data points were obtained from three independent experiments, and the standard deviations are given for each point. (Mean ± SD, each set of experiments was performed in triplicates).

increase in their concentrations as well as the dose of radiation ($p < 0.05$) These results were further supported by their SER values (Table 1) which under hypoxic conditions were concentration- dependent and relative to aerobic conditions were significantly higher ($p < 0.05$). The SER values of tethered compound **7–9** under aerobic conditions at all concentrations were lower and under hypoxic conditions at concentrations of 50 and 100 μmol were higher than 1.6 which is the minimum required value [22] for an *in vitro* radiosensitizing activity, indicating that these compounds have hypoxia-selective radiosensitization effects. From the results of this study it appears that the functional groups and the length of the linker chain have no contribution on *in vitro* effects of tethered compounds **7–9** since cytotoxities and radiosensitizing activities of these compounds under either hypoxic or aerobic conditions were not significantly different from each other.

Conclusion

While the cytotoxicity of 5-FU **5** against HT-29 cell line under aerobic and hypoxic conditions were not different significantly and this compound at all concentrations showed no radiosensitizing activity, tethered compounds **7–9** showed higher cytotoxicities and selective radiosensitizing activities under hypoxic conditions. Also effects of these compounds relative to metronidazole **1** which is a known cytotoxin and radiosensitizer were comparable under aerobic but higher under hypoxic conditions. Further exploration of these compounds through modification of the linker chain might result in compounds which their uses in conjunction with tumor radiotherapy have greater toxicity to tumor than normal tissues.

Abbreviations

5 FU: 5- fluorouracil; MTT: 3-(4,5-Dimethylthiazol-2-yl)-2,5-diphenyltetrazolium bromide; PI: Propidium Iodide; SER: Sensitization enhancement ratio; PBS: Phosphate buffer saline; FBS: Fetal bovine serum.

Competing interests

The authors declare that they have no competing interests.

Authors' contributions

KA: Designer of the project, corresponding author of the manuscript. AK: Determination of cytotoxicity and radiosensitizing activity of the tested compounds. OS-N: Supervisor for the determination of the cytotoxocity and radiosensitizing activity of the tested compounds. LN: Synthesis of the tethered compounds. KMR: supervising statistical analyses. All authors read and approved the final manuscript.

Acknowledgements

This research was supported by deputy of research and drug design & development research center of Tehran University of Medical Sciences (TUMS).

Author details

[1]Department Radiopharmacy, Tehran University of Medical Sciences, Tehran 14174, Iran. [2]Department of Medicinal Chemistry, Tehran University of Medical Sciences, Tehran 14174, Iran. [3]Department of Toxicology & Pharmacology, Tehran University of Medical Sciences, Tehran 14174, Iran. [4]Drug Design & Development Research Center, Tehran University of Medical Sciences, Tehran 14174, Iran. [5]Department of Drug and Food Control, Faculty of Pharmacy, Tehran University of Medical Sciences, Tehran 14174, Iran.

References

1. Nagasawa H, Uto Y, Kirk KL, Hori H: **Design of hypoxia-targeting drugs as new cancer chemotherapeutics.** *Biol Pharm Bull* 2005, **29:**2335–2342.
2. Wardman P: **Chemical radiosensitizers for use in radiotherapy.** *Clin Oncol* 2007, **19:**397–417.
3. Tao C, Desai NP, Soon-Shiong P, Sandford PA: **Dual functional cytotoxic/radiosensitizer compounds and methods for the preparation thereof.** *PCT Int Appl WO 96 40,091. Chem Abstr* 1996, **126:**131664n.
4. Palmer BD, Wilson WR, Pullen SM, Denny WA: **Hypoxia-selective antitumor agents. 5. Synthesis of water-soluble nitroaniline mustards with selective cytotoxicity for hypoxic mammalian cells.** *J Med Chem* 1990, **35:**3214–3222.
5. Parrick J, Porssa P, Davies LK, Dennis MF, Patel KB, Stratford MRK, Wardman P: **Targeting radiosensitizers to DNA by minor groove binding: nitroarenes based on netropsin and distamycin.** *Bioorg Med Chem Lett* 1993, **3:**1697–1702.
6. Lee HH, Palmer BD, Wilson WR, Denny WA: **Synthesis and hypoxia-selective cytotoxicity of A 2-nitroimidazole mustard.** *Bioorg Med Chem Lett* 1998, **8:**1741–1744.
7. Ahmed L, Jenkins TC, Walling JM, Stratford IJ, Sheldon PW, Adams GE, Fielden EM: **Analogues of RSU-1069: radiosensitization and toxicity *in vitro* and *in vivo*.** *Int J Radiat Oncol* 1986, **12:**1079–1081.
8. Khalaj A, Doroudi AR, Ostad SN, Khoshayand MR, Babai M, Adibpour N: **Synthesis, aerobic cytotoxicity, and radiosensitizing activity of novel 2,4-dinitrophenylamine tethered 5-fluorouracil and hydroxyurea.** *Bioorg Med Chem Lett* 2006, **16:**6034–6038.
9. Abdi K, Khalaj A, Ostad SN, Khoshayand MR: **Cytotoxicity and radiosensitising activity of synthesized dinitrophenyl derivatives of 5-fluorouracil.** *DARU J Pharm Sci* 2012, **20:**1–9. Doi: 10.1186/1560-8115-20-3.
10. Abdi K, Nafisi S, Manouchehri F, Bonsaii M, Khalaj A: **Interaction of 5-Fluorouracil and its derivatives with bovine serum albumin.** *J Photochem Photobiol B* 2012, **107:**20–26.
11. Khalaj A, Abdi K, Ostad SN, Khoshayand MR, Lamei N, Nedaie HA: **Synthesis, *in vitro* cytotoxicity and radiosensitizing activity of novel 3-[(2,4-dinitrophenylamino)alkyl]derivatives of 5-fluorouracil.** *Chem Biol Drug Des*. in press.
12. Ramalho TC, Franca TCC, Cortopassi WA, Goncalves AS, da Saliva AWS, da Cunha EFF: **Topology and dynamics of the interaction between 5-nitroimidazole radiosensitizers and duplex DNA studied by a combination of docking, molecular dynamic simulations and NMR spectroscopy.** *J Mol Struct* 2011, **992:**65–71.
13. Jaime-Figueroa S, Zamilpa A, Guzman A, Morgans DJ: **N-3-Alkylation of uracil and derivatives via N-1-Boc protection.** *Synthetic Commun* 2001, **31:**3747–3757.
14. Freshney RI: *Culture of animal cells: a manual of basic technique.* 6th edition. New York: Wiley-Blackwell; 2010.
15. Mosmann T: **Rapid colorimetric assay for cellular growth and survival: application to proliferation and cytotoxicity assays.** *J Immunol Methods* 1983, **65:**55–63.
16. Puttonen KA, Lehtonen S, Lampela P, Mannisto PT, Raasmaja A: **Different viabilities and toxicity types after 6-OHDA and Ara-C exposure evaluated by four assays in five cell lines.** *Toxicol In Vitro* 2008, **22:**182–189.
17. Zhang L, Mizumoto K, Sato N, Ogawa T, Kusumoto M, Niiyama H, Tanaka M: **Quantitative determination of apoptotic death in cultured human pancreatic cancer cells by propodium iodide and digitonin.** *Cancer Lett* 1999, **142:**129–137.
18. Franken NP, Rodermond HM, Stap J, Haveman J, van Bree C: **Clonogenic assay of cells *in vitro*.** *Nat Protoc* 2006, **1:**2315–2319.
19. Naito M, Hashimoto C, Masui S, Tsuruo T: **Caspase-independent necrotic cell death induced by a radiosensitizer, 8-nitrocaffeine.** *Cancer Sci* 2004, **95:**361–366.
20. Cariveau MJ, Stackhouse M, Cui X, Tiwari K, Waud W, Secrist JA, Xu B: **Clofarabine acts as radiosensitizer *in vitro* and *in vivo* by interfering with DNA damage response.** *Int J Radiation Oncol Biol* 2008, **70:**213–220.

21. Trivedi MN, Gabhe SY, Vachhani UD, Patel RB, Shah CP: **Synthesis of some 2-methyl-5-nitroimidazole derivatives as potential antimicrobial agents.** *J Chem Pharm Res* 2011, **3**:313–319.
22. Nakae T, Uto Y, Tanaka M, Shibata H, Nakata E, Tominaga M, Maezawa H, Hashomoto T, Kirk KL, Nagasawa H, Hori H: **Design, synthesis, and radiosensitizing activities of sugar-hybrid hypoxic cell radiosensitizers.** *Bioorg Med Chem Lett* 2008, **16**:675–682.

Synthesis, analgesic and anti-inflammatory activities of new methyl-imidazolyl-1,3,4-oxadiazoles and 1,2,4-triazoles

Ali Almasirad[1*], Zahra Mousavi[2], Mohammad Tajik[3], Mohammad Javad Assarzadeh[1] and Abbas Shafiee[3]

Abstract

Background: Long-term clinical employment of nonsteroidal anti-inflammatory drugs (NSAIDs) is associated with significant side effects including gastrointestinal (GI) lesions and kidney toxicity. In this paper we designed and synthesized new imidazolyl-1,3,4-oxadiazoles and 1,2,4-triazoles by molecular hybridization of previously described anti-inflammatory compounds in the hope of obtaining new safer analgesic and anti-inflammatory agents.

Methods: The target structures were synthesized by preparation of 5-methyl-1H-imidazole-4-carboxylic acid ethyl ester 5. The reaction of hydrazine hydrate with this ester afforded the 5-methyl-1H-imidazole-4-carboxylic acid hydrazide 6 which was converted to target compounds 7-15 according to the known procedures. *In silico* toxicity risk assessment and drug likeness predictions were done, in order to consider the privileges of the synthesized structures as drug candidates.

Results and discussion: The analgesic and anti-inflammatory profile of the synthesized compounds were evaluated by writhing and carrageenan induced rat paw edema tests respectively. Compounds 8, 9 and 11-13 and 15 were active analgesic agents and compounds 8, 9 and 11-13 showed significant anti-inflammatory response in comparison with control. Compounds 11 and 13 were screened for their ulcerogenic activities and none of them showed significant ulcerogenic activity. The active Compounds 11 and 12 showed the highest drug likeness and drug score.

Conclusions: The analgesic and anti-inflammatory activities of title compounds were comparable to that of standard drug indomethacin with a safer profile of activity. The results revealed that both of oxadiazole and triazole scaffolds can be determined as pharmacophores. The *in silico* predictions and pharmacological evaluations showed that compounds 11 and 12 can be chosen as lead for further investigations.

Keywords: Analgesic, Anti-inflammatory, Non ulcerogenic, midazole, Oxadiazole, Triazole

Background

Cyclooxygenase (COX) and 5-Lipoxygenase (5-LO) are two key enzymes that play important roles in the metabolism of arachidonic acid (AA) to pro-inflammatory prostaglandins (PGs) and leukotrienes (LTs) respectively [1]. It has been pointed out that inhibiting COX enzyme could decrease cytoprotective PGs and increase the conversion of AA to LTs by 5-LO enzyme which are implicated in the ulceration induced by nonsteroidal anti-inflammatory drugs (NSAIDs) [2,3]. Conversion of AA to Leukotrien B_4 (LTB_4) leads to hyperalgesic response and related with rheumatoid arthritis and inflammatory bowel disease. However, dual inhibition of COX and 5-LO would provide an anti-inflammatory agent with better efficacy and fewer side effects [4-6]. During recent years, various structural families such as di-tert-butylphenols, thiophene and pyrazoline derivatives and modified NSAIDs have been investigated as dual COX/5-LO inhibitors [7-9]. Amongst them several 1,3,4-oxadiazole, 1,3,4-triazole and hydrazone derivatives, compounds 1 and 2 were dual COX, 5-LO inhibitors and anti-inflammatory agents (Figure 1) [7-12]. As a part of our ongoing research program to find novel anti-inflammatory and analgesic compounds, herein,we describe

* Correspondence: almasirad.a@iaups.ac.ir
[1]Department of Medicinal Chemistry, Pharmaceutical Sciences Branch, Islamic Azad University, Tehran, Iran
Full list of author information is available at the end of the article

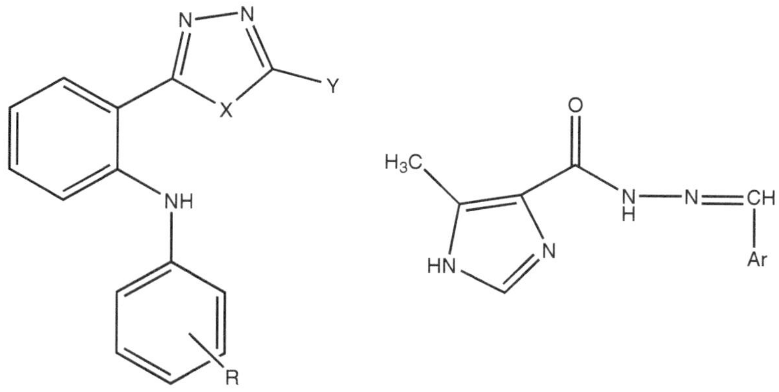

1 2

X= NR', Y= NH_2, OH, SH.....

Figure 1 Chemical structures of compounds 1 and 2 as dual COX/5-LO inhibitors and anti-inflammatory agents.

the synthesis of new imidazolyl-oxadiazole and triazole derivatives which were designed by molecular hybridization of previously described compounds, 1 and 2, in order to evaluate the plausible pharmacophoric contribution of the both imidazole and oxadiazole or triazole moieties in the pharmacological activities. *In silico* toxicity risk assessment and drug likeness predictions were done, in order to consider the privileges of the synthesized structures as drug candidates.

Methods

Chemistry

Chemicals were purchased from Merck Chemical Company (Tehran, Iran) and carrageenan was prepared from (Sigma-Aldrich, Dorset, UK). Melting points were taken on an electrothermal IA 9300 capillary melting-point apparatus (Ontario, Canada) and are uncorrected. ^{1}H-NMR spectra were obtained using a Bruker FT-400 spectrometer (Bruker, Rheinstetten, Germany). Tetramethyl silane was used as an internal standard. Mass spectra were obtained using a 5973 Network Mass Selective Detector at 70 eV (Agilent Technology). The FT-IR spectra were obtained using a Shimadzu FT-IR 8400S spectrographs (KBr disks).

5-Methyl-1H-Imidazole-4-carboxylic acid hydrazide (6)

To a stirring solution of ester 5 (10 g, 71.5 mmol) in 125 ml ethanol, at room temperature hydrazine hydrate (50 ml, 1000 mmol) was added and refluxed for 48 h. The resulting solution was concentrated, cooled and the precipitate was filtered, washed with dichloromethane and crystallized in ethanol to give 6.73 g (74%) of 6, mp 214-217°C. IR (KBr): υ cm^{-1} 3326, 3270 (NH_2, NH), 1656 (C = O). ^{1}H-NMR(DMSO-d6): δ(ppm) 11.95 (bs, 1H, NH), 8.61(bs, 1H, NH), 7.40(s, 1H, CH, imidazole), 4.09(bs, 2H, NH2), 2.51(s, 3H, CH3). MS: m/z (%) 140(M+, 100), 109(78), 54(20).

2-Amino-5-(5-methy-1H-imidazol-4-yl)-1,3,4-oxadiazole (7)

To a stirring suspension of hydrazide 6 (500 mg, 3.57 mmol) in dioxane (12 ml), sodium bicarbonate (300 mg) in water (1 ml) was added at room temperature. The mixture was stirred at room temperature for 5 min and cyanogen bromide (386 mg, 3.64 mmol) was added. After 24 h stirring at room temperature the solvent was evaporated and the resulting precipitate was purified by crystallization in methanol to give 400.7 mg(68%) of 7, mp 300-301°C. IR (KBr): υ cm^{-1} 3390, 3349 (NH_2, NH), 3135 (C-H). ^{1}H-NMR (DMSO-d_6): δ (ppm) 8.21 (bs, 1H, NH), 7.55(s, 1H, CH, imidazole), 6.85(bs, 2H, NH_2), 2.44(s, 3H, CH_3). MS: m/z (%) 165(M^+, 18), 69(58), 45(100).

5-(5-Methyl-1H-imidazol-4-yl)-1,3,4-oxadiazole-2(3H)-thione (8)

A mixtue of hyrazide 6 (500 mg, 3.57 mmol), potassium hydroxide (200 mg, 3.57 mmol), carbon disulfide (0.64 ml, 10.7 mmol) and ethanol (30 ml) was heated under reflux for 72 h. The solution was acidified with dilute hydrochloric acid. The resulting precipitate was removed by filtration and purified by crystallization in methanol to give 6.73 g (15%) of **8**, mp 261-262°C. IR (KBr): υ cm^{-1} 3477, 3281 (NH), 1626 (C = N), 1338 (C = S). ^{1}H-NMR (DMSO-d_6): δ (ppm) 13.97 (bs, 1H, NH), 8.20(bs, 1H, NH), 7.71 (s, 1H, CH, imidazole), 2.43(s, 3H, CH_3). MS: m/z (%) 182(M^+, 100), 122(87), 109(100).

5-(5-Methyl-1H-imidazol-4-yl)-1,3,4-oxadiazole-2(3H)-one (9)

To a solution of compound 6 (550 mg, 4 mmol) and triethyl amine (400 mg, 4 mmol) in DMF (50 ml), 1,1′-carbonyldiimidazole (0.84 g, 5.1 mmol) was added in one portion. The reaction mixture was refluxed for one week. The volatiles were removed in vacuo, and the residue was purified by TLC, eluting with ethyl acetate-petroleum ether (1:1) to provide 78.7 mg (11%) of **9**, mp 298-299°C. IR (KBr): υ cm^{-1} 3332(NH), 3206 (NH), 1714(C = O). ^{1}H-NMR (DMSO-d_6): δ (ppm) 9.1 (bs, 1H, NH), 8.1(bs, 1H,NH), 7.55(s, 1H, CH, imidazole), 2.43(s, 3H, CH_3). MS: m/z (%) 166(M^+, 10), 140(18), 109(100).

5-(5-Methyl-1H-imidazol-4-yl)-4H-1,2,4-triazole-3-thione (10)

A solution of hydrazide 6 (500 mg, 3.57 mmol), potassium thiocyanate (1 g, 10.71 mmol), concentrated hydrochloric acid (4 ml) and water 50 ml was stirred at room temperature for 24 h. To the resulting suspension, sodium hydroxide 4% (60 ml) was added and stirred for 24 h at 60-70°C.The resulting mixture was neutralized with hydrochloric acid and the resulting precipitate was filtered, washed with acetone and purified by two times crystallization in ethanol to give 219 mg (34%) of **10**, mp 225-227°C. IR (KBr): υ cm^{-1} 3400, 3134 (NH), 3114 (C-H), 1321 (C = S). ^{1}H-NMR (DMSO-d_6): δ (ppm) 13.87(bs, 1H, NH), 12.25(bs, 1H, NH), 9.1(bs, 1H, NH), 7.41(s, 1H, CH, imidazole), 2.31(s, 3H, CH_3). MS:m/z (%) 181(M^+, 13), 125(100), 107(90), 80(82), 67(58).

General procedures for the preparation of 4-substituted-5-(5-methyl-1H-imidazol-4-yl)-4H-1,2,4-triazole-3-thiones (11-15)

A mixture of compound 6 (500 mg, 3.57 mmol), corresponding isothiocyanate derivative (3.6 mmol) and absolute ethanol (5 ml) was stirred for 24 h. The resulting semicarbazide was filtered and washed with ether then added to 3% sodium hydroxide solution (50 ml) and refluxed for 24-48 h. The resulting solution was acidified with hydrochloric acid, the precipitate was filtered, dried and purified by crystallization.

4-Methyl-5-(5-methyl-1H-imidazol-4-yl)-4H-1,2,4-triazole-3-thione (11)

Yield 34%; mp 225-227°C (ethanol). IR (KBr): υ cm^{1-} 3376, 3149 (NH), 2526(weak, SH), 1337 (C = S). ^{1}H–NMR (DMSO-d_6): δ(ppm) 12.12(bs, 1H, NH), 8.25(bs, 1H, NH), 7.72(s, 1H, CH, imidazole), 3.74(s, 3H, CH3), 2.37 (s, 3H, CH_3). MS: m/z (%) 195(M^+, 100), 122(25), 108(30).

4-phenyl-5-(5-methyl-1H-imidazol-4-yl)-4H-1,2,4-triazole-3-thione (12)

Yield 13%; mp 275-277°C (THF/Water). IR (KBr): vcm^{1-} 3477(NH), 3410(NH), 3118(C-H, aromatic), 1326 (C = S). ^{1}H–NMR (DMSO-d_6): δ (ppm) 12.39 (bs, 1H, NH), 8.5 (bs, 1H, NH), 7.6-7.2(m, 6H, aromatic and CH, imidazole), 2.26 (s, 1H, CH_3). MS: m/z (%) 257(M^+, 100), 122(25), 108 (30).

5-(5-Methyl-1H-imidazol-4-yl)-4-(4-methylphenyl)-4H-1,2,4-triazole-3-thione (13)

Yield 24%; mp 268-270°C (Methanol). IR (KBr): υ cm^{-1} 3434(NH), 3210(NH), 3100(C-H,aromatic), 1340 (C = S). ^{1}H–NMR (DMSO-d_6): δ (ppm) 12.2(bs, 1H, NH), 8.5(bs, 1H, NH), 7.4(s, 1H, CH, imidazole), 7.3(d, J = 7.9Hz, 2H, aromatic), 7.1(d, J = 7.9 Hz, 2H, aromatic), 2.34(s, 1H, CH_3), 2.25(s, 3H, CH3). MS: m/z (%) 271(M^+, 20), 257 (100), 106(22), 77(30).

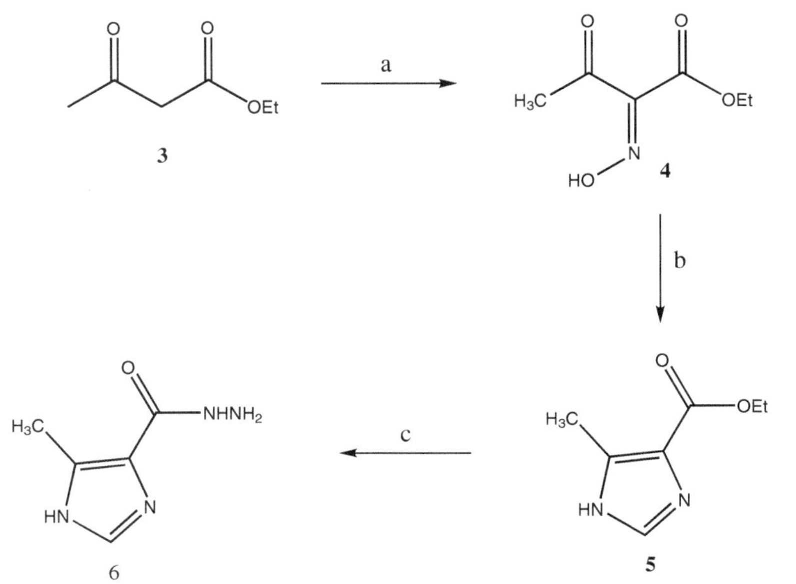

Scheme 1 Synthesis of hydrazide 6. (a) CH_3COOH, $NaNO_2$, 0°C; **(b)** HCHO, HCl, 0-5°C; NH_3, 70°C; **(c)** $NH_2NH_2.H_2O$, EtOH, reflux.

5-(5-Methyl-1H-imidazol-4-yl)-4-(4-methoxyphenyl)-4H-1,2,4-triazole-3-thione (14)

Yield 18%; mp 140-142°C (Ethylacetate/Acetone). IR (KBr): υ cm^{-1} 3430(NH), 3216(NH), 3144(C-H,aromatic), 1311(C = S). ^{1}H–NMR (DMSO-d_6): δ (ppm) 12.8(bs, 1H, NH), 8.5(bs, 1H, NH), 7.4(s, 1H, CH, imidazole), 7.2(d, J = 8.4Hz, 2H, aromatic), 6.9(d, J = 8.4Hz, 2H, aromatic), 3.76(s, 3H, OCH_3), 2.27(s, 3H, CH3). MS: m/z (%) 287(M^+, 100), 106(22), 77(30).

5-(5-Methyl-1H-imidazol-4-yl)-4-(4-fluorophenyl)-4H-1,2,4-triazole-3-thione (15)

Yield 20%; mp 150-152°C (Methanol). IR (KBr): υ cm^{-1} 3467 (NH), 3365 (NH), 3108(C-H, aromatic), 2520(weak, SH), 1321 (C = S). ^{1}H-NMR (DMSO-d_6): δ (ppm) 12.4 (bs, 1H, NH), 8.5 (bs, 1H, NH), 7.8-7.3 (m, 5H, aromatic and CH, imidazole), 2.25(s, 3H, CH_3). MS: m/z (%) 275 (M^+, 100), 106(22), 77(30).

Pharmacology

Male NMRI mice (20-25 g) and Wistar rats (100-150 g) were purchased from the animal breeding laboratories of Pasteur Institute (Karaj, Iran). Each group consisted of six animals. The animals were maintained in colony cages at 25 ± 2°C, relative humidity 45–55%, under a 12 h light-dark cycle; they were fed standard animal feed. All the animals were acclimatized for a week before use and all ethical manners for use of laboratory animals were considered carefully and the protocol was approved by Islamic Azad University of Pharmaceutical Sciences (IAUPS) ethical committee.

Analgesic activity evaluation

Acetic acid writhing test was performed on mice and indomethacin was used as standard drug [11]. Test compounds and the standard drug were administered intraperitoneally (ip) to the animals at the dose of 50 μmol/kg as

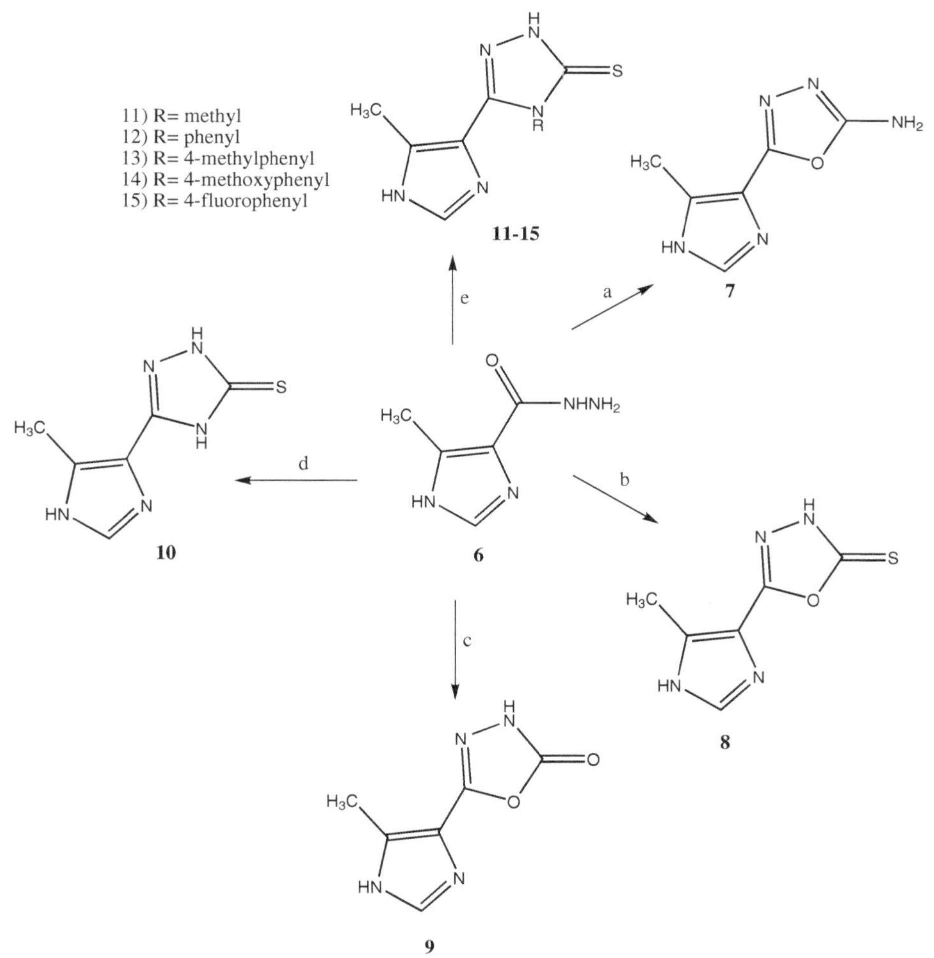

Scheme 2 Synthesis of target derivatives 7–15. (a) BrCN, Dioxane, rt; **(b)** CS_2, KOH, EtOH, reflux; **(c)** 1,1′-CDI, triethylamine, DMF, reflux; **(d)** (1) KSCN, HCl, H_2O, rt; (2) NaOH 3%, 60-70°C; **(e)** (1) Isothiocyanate derivatives, EtOH, rt; (2) NaOH, reflux.

suspension in saline and tween 80 (4% w/v). An acetic acid (0.6%, 0.1 ml/10 g) solution was administered ip 30 minutes after administration of compounds. The mean number of writhes for each experimental group and percentage decrease, compared with that of the control group were calculated during 30 minutes.

Anti-inflammatory activity against carrageenan induced rat paw edema

Effective compounds in analgesic test were screened for their anti-inflammatory activities using carrageenan induced paw edema on wistar male rats [13]. The standard and test groups received indomethacin as standard drug or target compounds, 50 μmol/kg body weight (ip) suspended in 4% tween in saline and the control animals received 4% tween in saline respectively. One hour after administration of drugs each rat received freshly prepared 0.1% w/v aqueous solution of carrageenan in the sub plantar region of right hind paw. The paw thickness was measured from the ventral to the dorsal surfaces using a dial caliper immediately prior to carrageenan injection and then at each hour, up to 5 h after the sub plantar injection. The edema was calculated as the thickness variation between the carrageenan and saline treated paw. Anti-inflammatory activity was expressed as the inhibition percent of the edema when compared with the control group.

Ulcerogenic activity

The ulcerogenic activity of newly synthesized compounds relative to known ulcerogenic drug, indomethacin was evaluated and scored by method of Cioli *et al.* [14]. Wistar rats (160-180 g) were fasted for 24 h before giving a single dose of each of vehicle, standard and test compounds (105 mg/kg in 0.5% v/v CMC suspension, peroral respectively and 17 h later, sacrificed under deep ether anesthesia and stomachs were removed and then examined by means of a magnifying glass to assess, the incidence of redness and spot ulcers. For each stomach, the mucosal damage was evaluated according to the following scoring system: 0.5: redness; 1.0: spot ulcers; 1.5: hemorrhagic streaks; 2.0: ulcers >3 but ≤5; 3.0: ulcers > 5. The mean score of each treated group minus the mean score of control group was regarded as gastric mucosal ulceration score.

In silico drug-score and toxicity assessments

Currently, there are several approaches to assess the drug-likeness of the drug candidates [15,16]. One such tool is the Osiris Property Explorer (OPE) a web based system which is able to calculate properties such as toxicity risk assessment and prediction of log p, solubility (log s), fragment-based drug-likeness and overall drug-score.

Results and discussion

Chemistry

The target compounds were prepared according to the Schemes 1 and 2. The ester 5 was synthesized as previously described method [17]. The key intermediate 6 was prepared from the reaction of hydrazine hydrate with ester 5. Reaction of hydrazide 6 with cyanogens bromide gave 2-amino-1,3,4-oxadiazole 7 [18]. The 1,3,4-oxadiazole-2-thone 8 and the 1,3,4-oxadiazole-2-one 9 were prepared by the reaction of hydrazide 6 with KOH and CS_2 or 1,1′-carbonyldiimidazole (1,1′-CDI) in the presence of triethylamine respectively [18,19]. The 1,2,4-triazole-3-thione 10 was synthesized via reaction of 6 with potassium thiocyanate and hydrochloric acid followed by cyclization of thiosemicarbazide intermediate with aqueous sodium hydroxide. Reaction of 6 with corresponding isothiocyanates yielded thiosemicarbazides as intermediate which were converted to 4-substituted-1,2,4-triazole-3-thiones **11-15** in aqueous sodium hydroxide [20-22]. The FCH group, Ukraine is the supplier of compound 11 and the synthesis of compound 12 has been previously reported [23].

Analgesic activity

The results of writhing test revealed that several synthesized compounds 8, 9, 11-13 and 15 as well as indomethacin showed significant antinociceptive effect in comparison with control (P < 0.001) (Table 1). In compounds 7-9, existence of a more lipophilic group on the position 2 of the oxadiazole ring lead to a more potent

Table 1 Effects of new imidazolyl oxadiazole and triazole derivatives, and Indomethacin in the inhibition of abdominal constrictions induced by acetic acid (%0.6) in Mice

Compound	Constriction no. (mean ± SEM)[1]	Inhibition (%)[2]	Relative activity[3]
Vehicle control	59.67 ± 6.8	-	-
Indomethacin	13.50 ± 2.9	77.37	1***
7	44.33 ± 8.1	25.70	0.33
8	18.00 ± 3.7	69.83	0.90***
9	24.67 ± 5.5	58.65	0.76***
10	44.67 ± 2.8	25.14	0.32
11	23.83 ± 4.8	60.06	0.77***
12	24.33 ± 3.3	59.22	0.76***
13	17.67 ± 2.9	70.39	0.91***
14	ND[4]	-	-
15	15.50 ± 3.9	74.02	0.96***

[1]All compounds were administered i.p. at the dose of 50 μmol/kg, number of animals in each group n = 6.
[2]% of inhibition obtained by comparison with vehicle control group.
[3]Analgesic activity relative to Indomethacin,***P < 0.001 significant as compared to control.
[4]Not determined.

Table 2 Effects of new imidazolyl, oxadiazole and triazole derivatives 50(μmol/kg), and Indomethacin in the Carrageenan-induced rat paw edema

Compound	Time (h)[1]	Volume variation (μL)[2,3]	% inhibition[4]
Vehicle control	1	1.53 ± 0.12	-
	2	1.84 ± 0.17	-
	3	2.22 ± 0.24	-
	4	2.44 ± 0.26	-
	5	2.11 ± 0.21	-
Indomethacin	1	1.17 ± 0.01	23.53
	2	1.35 ± 0.01	26.63
	3	1.14 ± 0.02	48.6**
	4	1.03 ± 0.02	57.79***
	5	0.89 ± 0.01	57.82***
8	1	1.60 ± 0.15	-4.60
	2	1.82 ± 0.16	1.10
	3	1.68 ± 0.18	24.32
	4	1.53 ± 0.21	37.30**
	5	1.19 ± 0.18	43.60**
9	1	1.78 ± 0.14	-16.34
	2	1.90 ± 0.14	-3.26
	3	1.96 ± 0.16	11.71
	4	1.78 ± 0.14	27.05
	5	1.32 ± 0.07	37.44*
11	1	1.95 ± 0.04	-27.45
	2	2.11 ± 0.06	-14.67
	3	1.82 ± 0.16	18.02
	4	1.67 ± 0.20	31.56*
	5	1.38 ± 0.22	34.60*
12	1	1.27 ± 0.04	16.99
	2	1.44 ± 0.06	21.74
	3	1.49 ± 0.04	32.88*
	4	1.45 ± 0.07	40.57*
	5	1.22 ± 0.08	42.18*
13	1	1.19 ± 0.16	22.22
	2	1.70 ± 0.15	7.60
	3	1.55 ± 0.12	30.2*
	4	1.66 ± 0.11	31.97*
	5	1.41 ± 0.10	33.17*
14	1	1.39 ± 0.07	9.15
	2	1.64 ± 0.10	10.87
	3	1.90 ± 0.14	14.41
	4	1.91 ± 0.11	21.72
	5	1.69 ± 0.12	19.90
15	1	1.46 ± 0.08	4.57
	2	1.78 ± 0.08	3.26
	3	1.96 ± 0.10	11.71
	4	2.02 ± 0.26	17.21
	5	1.98 ± 019	6.16

Table 2 Effects of new imidazolyl, oxadiazole and triazole derivatives 50(μmol/kg), and Indomethacin in the Carrageenan-induced rat paw edema *(Continued)*

[1]Time after carrageenan injection (0.1 mg/paw), number of animals in each group n = 6.
[2]All compounds were administered i.p, at the dose of 50 μmol/kg.
[3]Volume variation is the difference between the volumes of paw pre and post of Carrageenan injection.
[4]% of inhibition obtained by comparison with vehicle control group, $^{*}P < 0.05$, $^{**}p < 0.01$, $^{***}p < 0.001$ significant from control.

compound 8. In addition, bioisosteric replacement of oxygen atom in compound 8 with NH to give compound 10, decreased the activity. Replacement of hydrogen atom in 4th position of triazole ring with alkyl or aryl groups, compounds 11-15 caused a noticeable analgesic activity. The most potent analgesic derivative was 15 and it can be concluded that existence of both electron withdrawing and donating substituents on the para position of the phenyl moiety (compounds 13 and 15) could enhance the analgesic activity of triazole derivatives.

Anti-inflammatory activity

In vivo anti-inflammatory evaluation of target compounds is summarized in Table 2. Compounds 8-9 and 11-13 were active anti-inflammatory agents (33-43% inhibition) after 5 h in comparison with control and their activity was comparable to indomethacin. As shown in Table 2, there wasn't any significant difference between the activity of compounds 9, 11 and 13 and the most active derivatives were 8 and 12. Similar to analgesic activity results, it can be deduced by comparison of these data that the best substituent on position 2 of oxadiazole ring is a sufur moiety. In contrast to analgesic activity, the introduction of electron donating or withdrawing moieties on the para position of phenyl ring has a deleterious effect on the anti-inflammatory activity.

Ulcerogenic activity

The compounds 11 and 13 as two active derivatives, in anti-Inflammatory and analgesic tests respectively, were evaluated for their acute ulcerogenic activity. A significant

Table 3 Acute ulcerogenic activity of compounds (11 and 13) in the method of Cioli

Compound	Dose (mg/kg)[1]	Ulcerogenic activity (Severity index ± SEM)	P value
11	105	0.50 ± 0.01	p > 0.05
13	105	0.58 ± 0.08	p > 0.05
Indomethacin	105	1.67 ± 0.333	$P^{*} < 0.001$
Control	-	0.00 ± 0.00	-

[1]number of animals in each group n = 6, $^{*}p < 0.001$ significant from control.

Table 4 Drug-likeness of target compounds predicted by Osiris Property Explorer tool in comparison with indomethacin and celecoxib

Compound	Toxicity risk[1]				cLogP	Solubility	MW	Drug- likeness	Drug-score
	M[2]	T[3]	I[4]	R[5]					
7	-	-	-	-	0.06	-2.57	165	-1.88	0.54
8	-	-	-	-	0.92	-2.2	182	0.87	0.81
9	-	-	-	-	0.25	-2.12	166	-1.75	0.55
10	-	-	-	-	0.75	-2.06	181	1.39	0.86
11	-	-	-	-	1.04	-1.7	195	2.39	0.94
12	-	-	-	-	2.29	-3.55	257	2.46	0.82
13	-	-	-	-	2.61	-3.89	271	0.76	0.68
14	+	±	-	-	2.19	-3.56	287	0.7	0.34
15	-	-	-	-	2.35	-3.86	275	0.7	0.69
Indomethacin	-	-	-	-	3.83	-5.4	357	7.59	0.57
Celecoxib	-	-	-	-	2.27	-5.4	365	-9.50	0.31

[1]Ranked according to: (-) no bad effect, (±) medium bad effect, (+) bad effect; [2] M, Mutagenic effect; [3] T, Tumorgenic effect; [4]I, Irritating effect; [5]R, Reproductive effect.

reduction in ulcerogenic activity with the stomach ulceration score between 0.50 ± 0.01 and 0.58 ± 0.08.

was observed in the tested compounds. In fact, not only the standard drug, indomethacin showed a high score of 1.67 ± 0.33, but also none of these two evaluated derivatives induced significant ulceration in comparison to control (Table 3).

In silico drug-likeness and toxicity results

In this work, open-source program OPE was used to evaluate the fragment-based drug-likeness of title compounds and comparing them with indomethacin and celecoxib. The overall drug-score which was mentioned earlier combines drug-likeness, clogp, clogs, molecular weight and toxicity risk factors in one single value, where the occurrence frequency of each fragment is determined within the collection of approved drugs and within the supposedly non-drug like chemicals of fluka company. A positive drug-likeness value (0.1-10) states that a molecule contains fragments which are present in commercial drugs. The OPE study revealed that except compound 14 which showed high risk of mutagenic and medium risk of tumorgenic effects, all compounds, indomethacin and celecoxib are supposed to be non-mutagenic, non-tumorgenic, non-irritant with no reproductive effects. The *in silico* drug-relevant properties obtained by OPE are given in Table 4. The potential drug-likeness values of all designed compounds were significantly higher than that of celecoxib but this value for compounds 7 and 9 is negative so their similarity to commercial chemicals is more than traded drugs. Generally, the drug-score values of compounds 7-15 (0.34-0.94) were more than that of celecoxib (0.31) and these scores for compounds 8, 10-13 and 15 (0.68-0.94) were more than indomethacin and for compounds 7 and 9 comparable with indomethacin.

Conclusion

A series of new methyl-imidazolyl-1,3,4-oxadiazoles and 1,2,4-triazoles were designed and synthesized. The *in vivo* analgesic, anti-inflammatory and ulcerogenic evaluations, revealed that most of them were active in both tests without any ulcerogenic potential in comparison to control. The results revealed that both of oxadiazole and triazole scaffolds can be determined as pharmacophores. However, compounds 11 and 12 showed the highest values of drug-likeness and drug-score and acceptable pharmacological activity in both tests, so they could be selected as lead compounds for further modifications.

Statistics

Statistics were performed with one-way analysis of variance (ANOVA), which was followed by Tukey multi-comparison test. All data are presented as mean ± SEM, $p < 0.05$ was considered to be significant.

Competing interests

The authors declare that they have no competing interests.

Authors' contributions

AA: Design of target compounds, supervision of the synthetic part and manuscript preparation. ZM: Supervision of pharmacological part. MT: Synthesis of target compounds. MJA: Performed the pharmacological tests. AS: Collaboration in identifying of the structures of target compounds. All authors read and approved the final manuscript.

Acknowledgement

This work was supported by a grant from the vice chancellor for research of pharmaceutical sciences branch, Islamic Azad University (IAUPS).

Author details
[1]Department of Medicinal Chemistry, Pharmaceutical Sciences Branch, Islamic Azad University, Tehran, Iran. [2]Department of Toxicology and Pharmacology, Pharmaceutical Sciences Branch, Islamic Azad University, Tehran, Iran. [3]Department of Medicinal Chemistry, Faculty of Pharmacy and Pharmaceutical Sciences Research Center, Tehran University of Medical Sciences, Tehran, Iran.

References

1. Gonzalez-Periz A, Claria J: **New approaches to the modulation of the cyclooxygenase-2 and 5-lipoxygenase pathways.** *Curr Top Med Chem* 2007, **7**(3):297–309.
2. Pontiki E, Hadjipavlou-Litina D, Litinas K, Nicolotti O, Carotti A: **Design, synthesis and pharmacobiological evaluation of novel acrylic acid derivatives acting as lipoxygenase and cyclooxygenase-1 inhibitors with antioxidant and anti-inflammatory activities.** *EurJ Med Chem* 2011, **46**(1):191–200.
3. Eleftheriou P, Geronikaki A, Hadjipavlou-Litina D, Vicini P, Filz O, Filimonov D, Poroikov V, Shailendra S, Chaudhaery E, Roy KK, Saxena AK: **Fragment-based design, docking, synthesis, biological evaluation and structure–activity relationships of 2-benzo/benzisothiazolimino-5-aryliden-4-thiazolidinones as cycloxygenase/lipoxygenase inhibitors.** *Eur J Med Chem* 2012, **47**:111–124.
4. Geronikaki AA, Lagunin AA, Hadjipavlou-Litina DI, Eleftheriou PT, Filimonov DA, Poroikov VV, Alam I, Saxena AA: **Computer-aided discovery of anti-inflammatory thiazolidinones with dual cyclooxygenase/lipoxygenase inhibition.** *J Med Chem* 2008, **51**(6):1601–1609.
5. Celotti F, Laufer S: **Anti-inflammatory drugs: new multitarget compounds to face an old problem. The dual inhibition concept.** *Pharm Res* 2001, **43**(5):429–436.
6. Araico A, Terencio MC, Alcaraz MJ, Dominguez JN, Leon C, Ferrandiz ML: **Phenylsulfonyl urenyl chalcone derivatives as dual inhibitors of cyclo-oxygenase-2 and 5-lipoxygenase.** *Life Sci* 2006, **78**:2911–2918.
7. Charlier C, Michaux: **Dual inhibition of cyclooxygenase-2 (Cox-2) and lipoxygenase (5-Lox) as a new strategy to provide safer non-steroidal anti-inflammatory drugs.** *Eur J Med Chem* 2003, **38**:645–659.
8. Moreau A, Chen QH, Roa PNP, Knaus EE: **Design, synthesis and biological evaluation of (E)-3-(4-methanesulfonylphenyl)-2-(aryl)acrylic acids as dual inhibitors of cyclooxygenases and lipoxygenase.** *Bioorg Med Chem* 2006, **14**:7716–7727.
9. Rao PNP, Chen QH, Knaus EE: **Synthesis and biological evaluation of 1,3-diphenylprop-2-yn-1-ones as dual inhibitors of cyclooxygenase and lipoxygenase.** *Bioorg Med Chem Lett* 2005, **15**:4842–4845.
10. Leval XD, Julemont F, Delarge J, Pirotte B, Dogne JM: **New trends in dual 5-LOX/COX inhibition.** *Curr Med Chem* 2002, **9**(9):941–962.
11. Figueiredo JM, Câmara CA, Amarante EG, Miranda ALP, Santos FM, Rodrigues CR, Fraga CAM, Barreiro EJ: **Design and synthesis of novel potent antinociceptive agents: methyl-imidazolyl N-acylhydrazone derivatives.** *Bioorg Med Chem* 2000, **8**(9):2243–2248.
12. Moradi A, Navidpour L, Amini M, Sadeghian H, Shadnia H, Firouzi O, Miri R, Ebrahimi ES, Abdollahi M, Zahmatkesh MH, Shafiee A: **Design and Synthesis of 2-Phenoxynicotinic Acid Hydrazides as Anti-inflammatory and Analgesic Agents.** *Arch Pharm Chem Life Sci* 2010, **9**:509–518.
13. Panchaxari DM, Pampana S, Pal T, Devabhaktuni B, Aravapalli AK: **Design and characterization of diclofenac diethylamine transdermal patch using silicone and acrylic adhesives combination.** *DARU J Pharmaceut Sci* 2013, **21**(1):6.
14. Cioli V, Silvestrini B, Dordoni F: **Evaluation of potential of gastric ulceration after administration of certain drugs.** *Exp Mol Pathol* 1967, **6**:68–75.
15. *Organic Chemistry Portal*; 2013. Available at http://www.organic-chemistry.org/prog/peo/. Accessed September 3.
16. Ayati A, Falahati M, Irannejad H, Emami S: **Synthesis, in vitro antifungal evaluation and in silico study of 3-azolyl-4-chromanone phenylhydrazones.** *DARU J Pharmaceut Sci* 2012, **20**:46.
17. Graboyes H, Kasper TJ, Vaidya PD: **Process for preparating 5-methyl-4-imidazolecarboxylic acid esters.** In *European Patent No. EP 0049638.* Munich, Germany: European Patent Organization; 1987.
18. Amir M, Shikha K: **Synthesis and anti-inflammatory, analgesic, ulcerogenic and lipid peroxidation activities of some new 2-[(2,6-dichloroanilino) phenyl]acetic acid derivatives.** *Eur J Med Chem* 2004, **39**(6):535–545.
19. Gilani SJ, Khan SA, Siddiqui N: **Synthesis and pharmacological evaluation of condensed heterocyclic 6-substituted 1,2,4-triazolo-[3,4-b]-1,3,4-thiadiazole and 1,3,4-oxadiazole derivatives of isoniazid.** *Bioorg Med Chem Lett* 2010, **20**(16):4762–4765.
20. Almasirad A, Vousooghi N, Tabatabai SA, Kebriaeezadeh A, Shafiee A: **Synthesis, anticonvulsant and muscle relaxant activities of substituted 1,3,4-oxadiazole,1,3,4-thiadiazole and 1,2,4-triazole.** *Acta Chim Slov* 2007, **54**(2):317–324.
21. Almasirad A, Shafiee A, Abdollahi M, Noeparast A, Shahrokhinejad N, Vousooghi N, Tabatabai SA, Khorasani R: **Synthesis and analgesic activity of new 1, 3, 4-oxadiazoles and 1, 2, 4-triazoles.** *Med Chem Res* 2011, **20**(4):435–442.
22. Cretu OD, Barbuceanu SF, Saramet G, Draghici C: **Synthesis and characterization of some 1,2,4-triazole-3-thiones obtained from intramolecular cyclization of new 1-(4-(4-X-phenylsulfonyl)benzoyl)-4-(4-iodophenyl)-3-thiosemicarbazides.** *J Serb Chem Soc* 2010, **75**(11):1463–1471.
23. Siwek A, Wujec M, Dobosz M, Wawrzycka-Gorczyca I: **Study of direction of cyclization of 1-Azolil-4-Aryl/Alkyl-Thiosemicarbazides.** *Het Chem* 2010, **21**(7):521–532.

Synthesis and cytotoxic evaluation of some new [1,3]dioxolo[4,5-*g*]chromen-8-one derivatives

Eskandar Alipour[1], Zinatsadat Mousavi[1], Zahra Safaei[1], Mahboobeh Pordeli[2], Maliheh Safavi[3], Loghman Firoozpour[4], Negar Mohammadhosseini[5], Mina Saeedi[5], Sussan Kabudanian Ardestani[2], Abbas Shafiee[5] and Alireza Foroumadi[5*]

Abstract

Background: Homoisoflavonoids are naturally occurring compounds belong to flavonoid classes possessing various biological properties such as cytotoxicity. In this work, an efficient strategy for the synthesis of novel homoisoflavonoids, [1,3]dioxolo[4,5-*g*]chromen-8-ones, was developed and all compounds were evaluated for their cytotoxic activities on three breast cancer cell lines.

Methods: Our synthetic route started from benzo[*d*][1,3]dioxol-5-ol which was reacted with 3-bromopropanoic acid followed by the reaction of oxalyl chloride to afford 6,7-dihydro-8*H*-[1,3]dioxolo[4,5-*g*]chromen-8-one. The aldol condensation of the later compound with aromatic aldehydes led to the formation of the title compounds. Five novel derivatives **4a-e** were tested for their cytotoxic activity against three human breast cancer cell lines including MCF-7, T47D, and MDA-MB-231 using the MTT assay.

Results: Among the synthesized compounds, 7-benzylidene-6,7-dihydro-8*H*-[1,3]dioxolo[4,5-*g*]chromen-8-one (**4a**) exhibited the highest activity against three cell lines. Also the analysis of acridine orange/ethidium bromide staining results revealed that 7-benzylidene-6,7-dihydro-8*H*-[1,3]dioxolo[4,5-*g*]chromen-8-one (**4a**) and 7-(2-methoxybenzylidene)-6,7-dihydro-8*H*-[1,3]dioxolo[4,5-*g*]chromen-8-one (**4b**) induced apoptosis in T47D cell line.

Conclusion: Finally, the effect of methoxy group on the cytotoxicity of compounds **4b-4d** was investigated in and it was revealed that it did not improve the activity of [1,3]dioxolo[4,5-*g*]chromen-8-ones against MCF-7, T47D, and MDA-MB-231.

Keyword: Homoisoflavonoids, [1,3]dioxolo[4,5-*g*]chromen-8-one, Cancer, Cytotoxic activity

Background

Homoisoflavonoids, naturally occurring compounds belong to flavonoid classes and possess a wide spectrum of biological properties such as anti-inflammatory [1], antioxidant [2], antiproliferative [3], antifungal [4], antiviral [5], and antimutagenic activities [6]. They mainly include a chromanone, chromone, or chromane skeleton and are ubiquitous in plants such as *Ophiopogon* [7], *Polygonatum* [8], *Scilla* [9], *Eucomis* [10], and *Muscari* [11]. Recently, several homoisoflavonoids have been successfully isolated from plants and evaluated for their bioactivities [12,13].

Chalcones have been the center of attention owing to their significant biological activities [14-18]. Also they are the most important precursors for the formation of α, β-unsaturated carbonyl system in flavonoid classes. Homoisoflavonoids including chalcone system have shown selective biological activities [19]. The isolated natural homoisoflavonoids having 3-benzylidenechroman-4-one skeleton were found to be potent and selective MAO-B inhibitors. Compounds involving benzylidene chromanone have depicted significant medicinal properties such as antioxidant [20], anticancer [21], anti-inflammatory [22], anti-human-immune deficiency virus (HIV-I) activities [23].

Two naturally occurring homoisoflavonoids, bonducellin [24] **1** and eucomin [25] **2** (Figure 1), isolated from *Caesalpiniabonducella* and *Eucomis bicolor* BAK (Liliaceae) were

* Correspondence: aforoumadi@yahoo.com
[5]Department of Medicinal Chemistry, Faculty of Pharmacy and Pharmaceutical Sciences Research Center, Tehran University of Medical Sciences, Tehran, Iran
Full list of author information is available at the end of the article

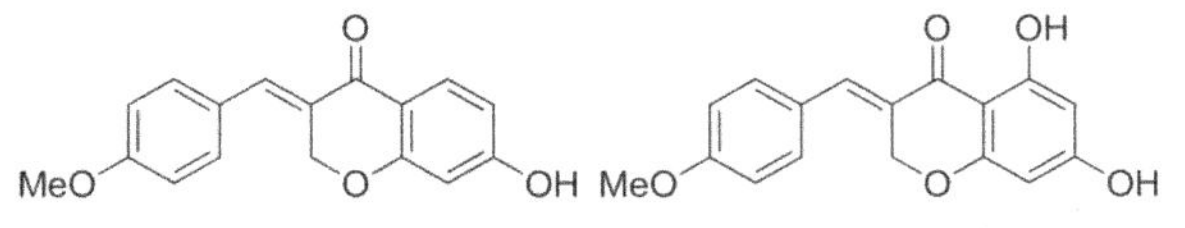

Bonducellin 1 Eucomin 2

Figure 1 Bonducellin 1 and Eucomin 2.

considered. These compounds and their synthetic analogues have shown important biological properties such as anti-tuberculosis activity [26] and inhibition of protein tyrosine kinase (PTK) [27].

On the synthesis of bioactiveheterocycles containing oxygen specially chalcones and homoisoflavonoids [9,21,28,29]; herein, we focused on new substituted [1,3]dioxolo[4,5-*g*] chromen-8-one derivatives **4** to profit from both chalcones and homoisoflavonoids (Scheme 1). Then, we evaluated their cytotoxic activities against three human breast cancer cell lines; MCF-7, T47D, and MDA-MB-231 using the MTT assay.

Methods

Chemistry

All starting materials, reagents, and solvents were prepared from Merck (Germany). Melting points were determined on a Kofler hot stage apparatus (Vienna, Austria) and are uncorrected. ^{1}H-NMR spectra were recorded using a Bruker 400 spectrometer (Bruker, Rheinstatten, Germany), and chemical shifts are expressed as δ (ppm) with tetramethylsilane (TMS) as internal standard. The IR spectra were obtained on a Nicolet Magna FT-IR 550 spectrophotometer (potassium bromide disks).

General procedure for the synthesis of [1,3]dioxolo[4,5-g] chromen-8-one derivatives 4

3-(Benzo[*d*][1,3]dioxol-5-yloxy)propanoic acid **2** and 6,7-dihydro-8*H*-[1,3]dioxolo[4,5-*g*]chromen-8-one **3** prepared according to [30] (Scheme 1).

Dry hydrogen chloride gas was passed through an ice-cold solution of 6,7-dihydro-8*H*-[1,3]dioxolo[4,5-*g*]chromen-8-one **3** (0.5 mmol) and benzaldehyde derivative (0.7 mol) in absolute EtOH (3 mL) for 2 min. The reaction mixture was allowed to stand at room temperature for 48 h. The precipitated product was filtered off, dried, and recrystallized from ethanol and water.

7-Benzylidene-6,7-dihydro-8H-[1,3]dioxolo[4,5-g]chromen-8-one (4a)

Yield: 48%, mp 141–144°C. IR (KBr): 1664 (C = O) cm^{-1}. ^{1}H-NMR ($CDCl_3$, 400 MHz) δ: 7.83 (s, 1H, benzylidene), 7.43 (s, 1H, H_9), 7.42-7.25 (m, 5H, Ph), 6.41 (s, 1H, H_4), 6.00 (s, 2H, H_1, CH_2), 5.29 (s, 2H, CH_2). Anal. Calcd. for $C_{17}H_{12}O_4$: C, 72.85; H, 4.32. Found: C, 72.68; H, 4.18.

7-(2-Methoxybenzylidene)-6,7-dihydro-8H-[1,3]dioxolo[4,5-g] chromen-8-one (4b)

Yield: 31%, mp 160–163°C. IR (KBr): 1660 (C = O) cm^{-1}. ^{1}H-NMR ($CDCl_3$, 400 MHz) δ: 7.961 (s, 1H, benzylidene), 7.39 (s, 1H, H_9), 7.04-6.94 (m, 4H, $H_{3'}$, $H_{4'}$, $H_{5'}$, $H_{6'}$), 6.40 (s, 1H, H_4), 6.00 (s, 2H, H_1, CH_2), 5.17 (s, 2H, CH_2), 3.86 (s, 3H, OCH_3). Anal. Calcd. for $C_{18}H_{14}O_5$: C, 69.67; H, 4.55. Found: C, 69.52; H, 4.41.

7-(3-Methoxybenzylidene)-6,7-dihydro-8H-[1,3]dioxolo[4,5-g] chromen-8-one (4c)

Yield: 42%, mp 161–163°C. IR (KBr): 1662 (C = O) cm^{-1}. ^{1}H-NMR ($CDCl_3$, 400 MHz) δ: 7.79 (s, 1H, benzylidene), 7.38 (s, 1H, H_9), 7.04-6.93 (m, 4H, $H_{2'}$, $H_{4'}$, $H_{5'}$, $H_{6'}$), 6.41 (s, 1H, H_4), 6.00 (s, 2H, H_1, CH_2), 5.29 (s, 2H, CH_2), 3.84 (s, 3H, OCH_3). Anal. Calcd. for $C_{18}H_{14}O_5$: C, 69.67; H, 4.55. Found: C, 69.83; H, 4.72.

7-(4-Methoxybenzylidene)-6,7-dihydro-8H-[1,3]dioxolo[4,5-g] chromen-8-one (4d)

Yield: 31%, mp 169–172°C. IR (KBr): 1665 (C = O) cm^{-1}. ^{1}H-NMR ($CDCl_3$, 400 MHz) δ: 7.79 (s, 1H, benzylidene), 7.38 (s, 1H, H_9), 7.26 (d, J = 8.4 Hz, 2H, $H_{2'}$, $H_{6'}$), 6.96 (d, J = 8.4 Hz, 2H, $H_{3'}$, $H_{5'}$), 6.42 (s, 1H, H_4), 6.00 (s, 2H, H_1, CH_2), 5.32 (s, 2H, CH_2), 3.86 (s, 3H, OCH_3). Anal. Calcd. for $C_{18}H_{14}O_5$: C, 69.67; H, 4.55. Found: C, 69.53; H, 4.82.

7-(Benzo[d][1,3]dioxol-5-ylmethylene)-6,7-dihydro-8H-[1,3] dioxolo[4,5-g]chromen-8-one (4e)

Yield: 42%, mp 198–200°C. IR (KBr): 1667 (C = O) cm^{-1}. ^{1}H-NMR ($CDCl_3$, 400 MHz) δ: 7.73 (s, 1H, benzylidene), 7.37 (s, 1H, H_9), 6.86-6.67 (m, 3H, $H_{3'}$, $H_{4'}$, $H_{6'}$), 6.41 (s, 1H, H_4), 6.03 (s, 2H, $H_{1'}$,CH_2), 6.00 (s, 2H, H_1, CH_2), 5.29 (s, 2H, CH_2). Anal. Calcd. for $C_{18}H_{12}O_6$: C, 66.67; H, 3.73. Found: C, 66.48; H, 3.55.

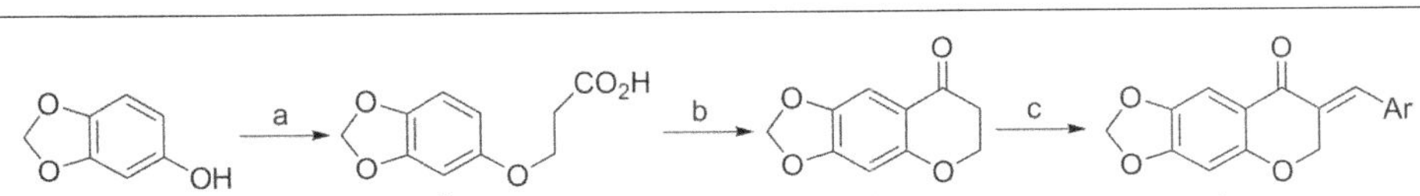

Scheme 1 Synthesis of [1,3]dioxolo[4,5-*g*]chromen-8-ones 4. (a) NaOH, Na_2CO_3, $Br(CH_2)_2COOH$, H_2O, reflux, **(b)** oxalyl chloride, $SnCl_4$, benzene, **(c)** aromatic aldehydes, HCl (g), 0°C.

Biological assay

Cell lines and cell culture

Human breast cancer cell lines including MDA-MB231, MCF-7 and T47D cells were obtained from the National Cell Bank of Iran, Pasteur Institute, Tehran, Iran. Cancer cell lines were grown in RPMI-1640 medium supplemented with 10% heat-inactivated fetal calf serum, 100 μg/ml streptomycin and 100 U/ml penicillin at 37°C in a humidified atmosphere with 5% CO_2.

In vitro cytotoxicity assay

The in vitro cytotoxic activity of [1,3]dioxolo[4,5-*g*]chromen-8-ones **4a-e** was achieved using MTT colorimetric assay. The *in-vitro* cytotoxic activity of all synthesized compounds were evaluated against three human breast cancer cell lines including MCF-7, T47D and MDA-MB-231 using MTT colorimetric assay according to the method of Mosman [31]. Cancer cell lines were grown in RPMI-1640 medium supplemented with 10% heat-inactivated fetal calf serum (Gibco BRL), 100 μg/ml streptomycin and 100 U/ml penicillin at 37°C in a humidified atmosphere with 5% CO_2.

Briefly, cultures in the exponential growth phase were trypsinized and diluted in complete growth medium to give a total cell count of 5×10^4 cells/ml. 195 μl of the cell suspension was seeded into the wells of 96-well plates (Nunc, Denmark). The plates were incubated overnight in a humidified air atmosphere at 37°C with 5% CO_2. After overnight incubation, 5 μl of the media containing various concentrations of the compounds was added per well in triplicate (final concentration 1, 5, 10 and 20 μg/ml). The plates were incubated for further 72 h. The final concentration of DMSO in the highest concentration of the applied compounds was 0.1%. In each plate, there were three control wells (cells without test compounds) and three blank wells (the medium with 0.1% DMSO) for cell viability. Etoposide and doxorubicine were used as positive controls for cytotoxicity. After treatment, the medium was removed and 200 μl phenol red-free medium containing MTT (1 mg/ml), was added to wells, followed by 4 h incubation. After incubation, the culture medium was then replaced with 100 μl of DMSO and the absorbance of each well was measured by using a microplate reader at 492 nm. For each compound, the concentration causing 50% cell growth inhibition (IC_{50}) compared with the control was calculated from concentration response curves by regression analysis.

Fluorescence microscopy evaluation

Acridine orange/ethidium bromide (AO/EB) double staining [32] was applied to observe the morphological changes in cell death induced by the most potent compounds **4a** and **4b**. Acridine orange is taken up by both viable and dead cells and emitting green fluorescence if intercalated into double stranded nucleic acid (DNA) or red fluorescence if bound to single stranded nucleic acid (RNA) due to its accumulation in lysosomes. Ethidium bromide is taken up only by cells with an altered cell membrane and emits red fluorescence by intercalation into DNA. Cells were seeded in 6-well plates (4×10^5 cell/well) for 24 h. Then, cells were treated with IC_{50} concentration of test compounds for 24 h at 37°C with 5% CO_2. After treatment, cells were washed twice with phosphate buffer saline (PBS) and then 1 μl of dye mixture (100 μg/ml AO and 100 μg/ml EB in PBS were mixed with 25 μl of cell suspension (0.4×10^6 cells/well) on a clean microscope slide. The suspension was immediately examined by Axoscope 2 plus fluorescence micro- scope from Zeiss (Germany) at 40× magnification.

Results and discussions

Benzo[*d*][1,3]dioxol-5-ol **1** (Scheme 1) was converted to 3-(benzo[d][1,3]dioxol-5-yloxy)propanoic acid **2** and subsequently to 6,7-dihydro-8*H*-[1,3]dioxolo[4,5-*g*]chromen-8-one **3** according to the procedure [30]. In the next step, we investigated the reaction of 6,7-dihydro-8*H*-[1,3]dioxolo[4,5-*g*]chromen-8-one **3** and 4-methoxybenzaldehyde to obtain the corresponding product, 7-(4-methoxybenzylidene)-6,7-dihydro-8*H*-[1,3]dioxolo[4,5-*g*]chromen-8-one (**4d**) (Table 1).

To run successful aldol condensation reaction, acid-catalyzed and base-catalyzed approaches were investigated using various conventional acids and base in different solvents. It was found that the aldol condensation was conducted in better yield in the presence of HCl (g).

Then, various derivatives including 7-(2-methoxybenzylidene)-6,7-dihydro-8*H*-[1,3]dioxolo[4,5-*g*]chromen-8-one (**4b**) and 7-(3-methoxybenzylidene)-6,7-dihydro-8*H*-[1,3]dioxolo[4,5-*g*]chromen-8-one (**4c**) possessing methoxy (OMe) group at ortho and meta positions were prepared to compare their bioactivities against the studied cell lines with that of the control. Also other two derivatives, 7-benzylidene-6,7-dihydro-8*H*-[1,3]dioxolo[4,5-*g*]

Table 1 Chemical structures and *in vitro* cytotoxic activity (IC_{50} , μg/ml)[a] of compounds 4a-4e against breast cancer cell lines

Entry	Compound	MCF-7	T47D	MDA-MB-231
1		6.2 ± 0.1	4.6 ± 0.1	9.3 ± 2.1
2		> 100	5.7 ± 0.07	27.3 ± 7.1
3		> 100	18.8 ± 2.3	29.05 ± 1.7
4		> 100	9.2 ± 2.9	> 100
5		> 100	> 100	> 100
6	Doxorubicin	0.002 ± 0.002	0.03 ± 0.002	0.006 ± 0.004
7	Etoposide	7.5 ± 0.32	7.9 ± 0.45	11.9 ± 0.87

[a]The IC_{50} values represent an average of three independent experiments (mean ± SD).

chromen-8-one (**4a**) and 7-(benzo[*d*][1,3]dioxol-5-ylmethylene)-6,7-dihydro-8*H*-[1,3]dioxolo[4,5-*g*]chromen-8-one (**4e**) were prepared to investigate the effect of methxoy substituent on the cytotoxicity (Table 1).

The *in vitro* cytotoxic activity of [1,3]dioxolo[4,5-*g*] chromen-8-one derivatives **4**, were tested against three human breast cancer cell lines including MCF-7, T47D, and MDA-MB-231. The 50% growth inhibitory concentration (IC_{50}) for all derivatives were calculated and depicted in Table 1.

According to MTT assay results in Table 1, 7-benzylidene-6,7-dihydro-8*H*-[1,3]dioxolo[4,5-*g*]chromen-8-one (**4a**) showed the highest activity against MCF-7, T47D, and MDA-MB-231 cell lines with IC_{50} values of 6.2 ± 0.1, 4.6 ± 0.1, and 9.3 ± 2.1 μg/ml, respectively. In contrast, 7-(benzo[*d*][1,3]dioxol-5-ylmethylene)-6,7-dihydro-8*H*-[1,3]dioxolo[4,5-*g*]chromen-8-one (**4e**) did not show any cytotoxicity at the concentrations used. It seems that the presence of benzo[*d*][1,3]dioxole in benzylidene moiety decreases the cytotoxic activity of the corresponding compound. As can be seen in Table 1 (Entries 2–4), by introduction of OMe into the ortho, meta or para positions of benzylidenemoiety (compounds **4b**, **4c**, and **4d**), different results were observed. All of them were inactive against MCF-7 cell line (IC_{50} > 100 μg/ml), whereas they exhibited good activity against T47D cell line with IC_{50} values of 5.7 ± 0.07, 18.8 ± 2.3, and 9.2 ± 2.9 μg/ml, respectively. It should be noted that compounds **4b** and **4c** were active against MDA-MB-231 cell line and **4d** did not show any activity in this cell line. Presence of OMe in benzylidene moiety did not play crucial role on the improvement of cytotoxicity effects.

To study the effect of our synthetic compounds on cell lines, acridine orange/ethidium bromide double staining technique was used to evaluate the occurrence of apoptosis in cells. Analysis of the acridine orange/ethidium bromide staining results showed that 7-benzylidene-6,7-dihydro-8*H*-[1,3]dioxolo[4,5-*g*]chromen-8-one (**4a**) and 7-(2-methoxybenzylidene)-6,7-dihydro-8*H*-[1,3]dioxolo [4,5-*g*]chromen-8-one (**4b**) induced apoptosis in T47D cell line (Figure 2). The cells treated with the most potent compounds increased the extent of apoptosis relative to untreated control cells. As shown in Figure 2, the non-apoptotic control cells were stained green and the apoptotic cells had orange particles in their nuclei due to nuclear DNA fragmentation.

Conclusion

In conclusion, novel [1,3]dioxolo[4,5-*g*]chromen-8-one derivatives were synthesized and tested for their cytotoxic activity against three human breast cancer cell lines including MCF-7, T47D, and MDA-MB-231 using the MTT assay. 7-Benzylidene-6,7-dihydro-8*H*-[1,3]dioxolo [4,5-*g*]chromen-8-one (**4a**) showed the highest activity

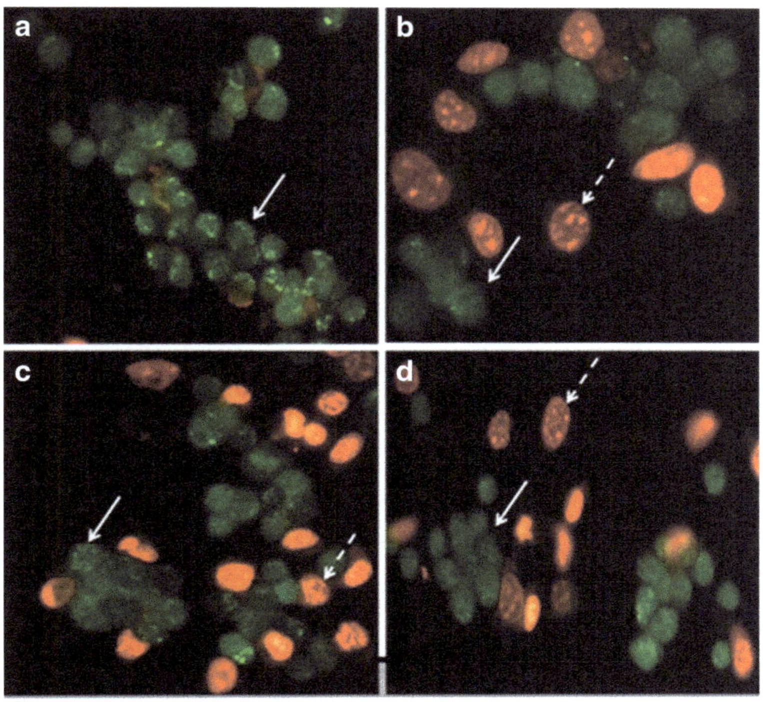

Figure 2 Morphological analysis of T47D cells treated with 4a and 4b by acridine orange/ethidium bromide double staining method. **a)** DMSO 1% as control, **b)** etoposide as positive control, **c)** cells treatedwith 4a for 24 h. **d)** cells treatedwith 4b for 24 h. White arrow indicates live cells, dashed arrow shows apoptotic cells. The images of cells were taken with a fluorescence microscope at 400 × magnification.

against the three studied cell lines. Also the analysis of acridine orange/ethidium bromide staining results revealed that the cytotoxic effect of 7-benzylidene-6,7-dihydro-8*H*-[1,3]dioxolo[4,5-*g*]chromen-8-one (**4a**) and 7-(2-methoxybenzylidene)-6,7-dihydro-8H-[1,3]dioxolo [4,5-g]chromen-8-one (**4b**) may be due to inducing apoptosis in cancer cell lines.

Competing interests

The authors declare that they have no competing interests.

Authors' contributions

EA: Supervision of the synthetic part. ZM: Synthesis of the title compounds. ZS: Synthesis of the title compounds. MP: Performed the cytotoxic tests. MS: Performed the cytotoxic tests and collaborated in manuscript preparation. LF: Design of target compounds. NM: Synthesis of the title compounds. MS: collaborated in manuscript preparation. SKA: Supervision of the cytotoxic tests. AS: Collaboration in identifying the structures of target compounds. AF: Design of target compounds and supervision of the synthetic and pharmacological parts. All authors read and approved the final manuscript.

Acknowledgements

The authors are thankful for financial support from the Research Council of Islamic Azad University and Iran National Elite Foundation (INEF).

Author details

[1]Department of Chemistry, Islamic Azad University, Tehran-North Branch, Zafar St, Tehran, Iran. [2]Department of Biochemistry, Institute of Biochemistry and Biophysics, University of Tehran, Tehran, Iran. [3]Biotechnology Department, Iranian Research Organization for Science and Technology, Tehran, Iran. [4]Drug Design and Development Research Center, Tehran University of Medicinal Sciences, Tehran, Iran. [5]Department of Medicinal Chemistry, Faculty of Pharmacy and Pharmaceutical Sciences Research Center, Tehran University of Medical Sciences, Tehran, Iran.

References

1. Hung TM, Thu CV, Dat NT, Ryoo SW, Lee JH, Kim JC, Na M, Jung HJ, Bae K, Min BS: **Homoisoflavonoid derivatives from the roots of Ophiopogon japonicus and their in vitro anti-inflammation activity.** *Bioorg Med Chem Lett* 2010, **20:**2412–2416.
2. Siddaiah V, Maheswara M, Rao CV, Venkateswarlu S, Subbaraju GV: **Synthesis, structural revision, and antioxidant activities of antimutagenic homoisoflavonoids from Hoffmanosseggiaintricata.** *Bioorg Med Chem Lett* 2007, **17:**1288–1290.
3. Perjési P, Das U, De Clercq E, Balzarini J, Kawase M, Sakagami H, Stables JP, Lorand T, Rozmer Z, Dimmock JR: **Design, synthesis and antiproliferative activity of some 3-benzylidene-2,3-dihydro-1-benzopyran-4-ones which display selective toxicity for malignant cells.** *Eur J Med Chem* 2008, **43:**839–845.
4. Al Nakib T, Bezjak V, Meegan MJ, Chandy R: **Synthesis and antifungal activity of some 3-benzylidenechroman-4-ones, 3-benzylidenethiochroman-4-ones and 2-benzylidene-1-tetralones.** *Eur J Med Chem* 1990, **25:**455–462.
5. Tait S, Salvati AL, Desideri N, Fiore L: **Antiviral activity of substituted homoisoflavonoids on enteroviruses.** *Antiviral Res* 2006, **72:**252–255.
6. Miadokova E, Masterova I, Vlckova V, Duhova V, Toth J: **Antimutagenic potential of homoisoflavonoids from Muscari racemosum.** *J Ethnopharmacol* 2002, **81:**381–386.
7. Li N, Zhang JY, Zeng KW, Zhang L, Che YY, Tu PF: **Anti-inflammatory homoisoflavonoids from the tuberous roots of *Ophiopogon japonicus*.** *Fitoterapia* 2012, **83:**1042–10455.
8. Guo H, Zhao H, Kanno Y, Li W, Mu Y, Kuang X, Inouye Y, Koike K, Jiang H, Bai H: **A dihydrochalcone and several homoisoflavonoids from *Polygonatum odoratum* are activators of adenosine monophosphate-activated protein kinase.** *Bioorg Med Chem Lett* 2013, **23:**3137–3139.
9. Bezabih M, Famuyiwa SO, Abegaz BM: **HPLC analysis and NMR identification of homoisoflavonoids and stilbenoids from the inter-bulb surfaces of Scilla nervosa.** *Nat Prod Commun* 2009, **4:**1367–1370.
10. Koorbanally C, Crouch NR, Langlois A, Du Toit K, Mulholland DA, Drewes SE: **Homoisoflavanones and spirocyclic nortriterpenoids from three Eucomis species: E. comosa, E. schijffii and E. pallidiflora subsp. pole-evansii (Hyacinthaceae).** *S Afr J Bot* 2006, **72:**428–433.
11. Urbancíková M, Masterová I, Tóth J: **Estrogenic/antiestrogenic activity of homoisoflavonoids from bulbs of Muscari racemosum (L.) Miller.** *Fitoterapia* 2002, **73:**724–726.
12. Mutanyatta J, Matapa BG, Shushu DD, Abegaz BM: **Homoisoflavonoids and xanthones from the tubers of wild and in vitro regenerated Ledebouria graminifolia and cytotoxic activities of some of the homoisoflavonoids.** *Phytochemistry* 2003, **62:**797–804.
13. Qi J, Xu D, Zhou YF, Qin MJ, Yu BY: **New features on the fragmentation patterns of homoisoflavonoids in Ophiopogon japonicus by high-performance liquid chromatography/diode-array detection/electrospray ionization with multi-stage tandem mass spectrometry.** *Rapid Commun Mass Spectrum* 2010, **24:**2193–2206.
14. Hsieh HK, Tsao LT, Wang JP, Lin CN: **Synthesis and anti-inflammatory effect of chalcones.** *J Pharm Pharmacol* 2000, **52:**163–171.
15. Domínguez JN, León C, Rodrigues J, de Domínguez NG, Gut J, Rosenthal PJ: **Synthesis and evaluation of new antimalarial phenylurenylchalcone derivatives.** *J Med Chem* 2005, **48:**3654–3658.
16. Nielsen SF, Larsen M, Boesen T, Schønning K, Kromann H: **Cationic chalcone antibiotics. design, synthesis, and mechanism of action.** *J Med Chem* 2005, **48:**2667–2677.
17. Qiao Z, Wang Q, Zhang F, Wang Z, Bowling T, Nare B, Jacobs RT, Zhang J, Ding D, Liu Y, Zhou H: **Chalcone–Benzoxaborole hybrid molecules as potent antitrypanosomal agents.** *J Med Chem* 2012, **55:**3553–3557.
18. Lorenzo P, Alvarez R, Ortiz MA, Alvarez S, Piedrafita FJ, de Lera AR: **Inhibition of IκB kinase-β and anticancer activities of novel chalcone adamantyl arotinoids.** *J MedChem* 2008, **51:**5431–5440.
19. Desideri N, Bolasco A, Fioravanti R, Monaco LP, Orallo F, Yáñez M, Ortuso F, Alcaro S: **Homoisoflavonoids: natural scaffolds with potent and selective monoamine oxidase-B inhibition properties.** *J Med Chem* 2011, **54:**2155–2164.
20. Foroumadi A, Samzadeh-Kermani A, Emami S, Dehghan G, Sorkhi M, Arabsorkhi F, Heidari MR, Abdollahi M, Shafiee A: **Synthesis and antioxidant properties of substituted 3-benzylidene-7-alkoxychroman-4-ones.** *Bioorg Med Chem Lett* 2007, **17:**6764–6769.
21. Noushini S, Alipour E, Emami S, Safavi M, Ardestani SK, Gohari AR, Shafiee A, Foroumadi A: **Synthesis and cytotoxic properties of novel (E)-3-benzylidene-7-methoxychroman-4-one derivatives.** *DARU J Pharm Sci* 2013, **21:**31.
22. Shaikh MM, Kruger HG, Bodenstein J, Smith P, du Toit K: **Anti-inflammatory activities of selected synthetic homoisoflavanones.** *Nat Prod Res* 2012, **26:**1473–1482.
23. Xu ZQ, Bucheit RW, Stup TL, Flavin MT, Khilevich A, Rezzo JD, Lin L, Zembower DE: **In vitro anti-human immunodeficiency virus (HIV) activity of the chromanone derivative, 12-oxocalanolide A, a novel NNRTI.** *Bioorg Med Chem Lett* 1998, **8:**2179–2184.
24. Purushothaman KK, Kalyani K, Subramaniam K: **Structure of bonducellin: a new homoisoflavonoids from Caesalpinia bonducella.** *India J Chem Sect B: Org Chem Incl Med Chem* 1982, **21:**383–386.
25. Heller W, Andermatt P, Schaad WA, Tamm E: **Homoisoflavonone IV. Neue inhaltsstoffe der eucomin-reihe von Eucomis bicolor.** *HelV Chim Acta* 1976, **59:**2048–2058.
26. Yempala T, Sriram D, Yogeeswari P, Kantevari S: **Molecular hybridization of bioactives: synthesis and antitubercular evaluation of novel dibenzofuran embodied homoisoflavonoids via Baylis–Hillman reaction.** *Bioorg Med ChemLett* 2012, **22:**7426–7430.
27. Lin LG, Xie H, Li HL, Tong LJ, Tang CP, Ke CQ, Liu QF, Lin LP, Geng MY, Jiang H, Zhao WM, Ding J, Ye Y: **Naturally occurring homoisoflavonoids function as potent protein tyrosine kinase inhibitors by c-Src-based high-throughput screening.** *J Med Chem* 2008, **51:**4419–4429.
28. Nakhjiri M, Safavi M, Alipour E, Emami S, Atash AF, Jafari-Zavareh M, Ardestani SK, Khoshneviszadeh M, Foroumadi A, Shafiee A: **Asymmetrical 2,6-bis (benzylidene)cyclohexanones: synthesis, cytotoxic activity and QSAR study.** *Eur J Med Chem* 2012, **50:**113–123.

29. Vosooghi M, Yahyavi H, Divsalar K, Shamsa H, Kheirollahi A, Safavi M, Ardestani SK, Sadeghi-Neshat S, Mohammadhosseini N, Edraki N, Khoshneviszadeh M, Shafiee A, Foroumadi A: **Synthesis and In vitro cytotoxic activity evaluation of (E)-16-(substituted benzylidene) derivatives of dehydroepiandrosterone.** *DARU J Pharm Sci* 2013, **21**:34.
30. Cueva JP, Giorgioni G, Grubbs RA, Chemel RB, Watts VJ, Nichols DE: **Trans-2,3-Dihydroxy-6a,7,8,12b-tetrahydro-6H-chromeno[3,4-c] isoquinoline: synthesis, resolution, and preliminary pharmacological characterization of a new dopamine D1 receptor full agonist.** *J Med Chem* 2006, **49:**6848–6857.
31. Mosmann T: **Rapid colorimetric assay for cellular growth and survival: application to proliferation and cytotoxicity assays.** *J Immunol Methods* 1983, **65:**55–63.
32. Baskic D, Popovic S, Ristic P, Arsenijevic NN: **Analysis of cycloheximide-induced apoptosis in human leukocytes: fluorescence microscopy using annexin V/propidium iodide versus acridin orange/ethidium bromide.** *Cell BiolInt* 2006, **30:**924–932.

Synthesis and anti-proliferative activity evaluation of *N*3-acyl-*N*5-aryl-3,5-diaminoindazole analogues as anti-head and neck cancer agent

Jinho Lee[1*], Jina Kim[1], Victor Sukbong Hong[1] and Jong-Wook Park[2]

Abstract

Background: Head and neck squamous cell carcinoma (HNSCC) is the 11th leading cancer by incidence worldwide. Surgery and radiotherapy have been the major treatment for patients with HNSCC while chemotherapy has become an important treatment option for locally advanced HNSCC. Understanding of the molecular mechanisms underlying HNSCC impelled the development of targeted therapeutic agents. The development and combinations of targeted therapies in different cellular pathways may be needed to fulfill the unmet needs of current HNSCC chemotherapy.

Results: A series of *N*3-acyl-*N*5-aryl-3,5-diaminoindazoles were synthesized and their anti-proliferative activities were evaluated against human cancer cell lines, Caki, A549, AMC-HN1, AMC-HN3, AMC-HN4, AMC-HN6, and SNU449. The cellular selectivity of compound was obtained by the modification of substituent at *N*5-aryl group of 3,5-diaminoindazole. Compound 9a and 9b showed more than 7-fold selectivity for AMC-HN4 and AMC-HN3, respectively.

Conclusions: *N*3-acyl-*N*5-aryl-3,5-diaminoindazole analogues can be used as hits in the development of anticancer drug for HNSCC.

Keywords: Indazole, 3,5-diaminoindazole, Anticancer, HNSCC

Background

Head and neck squamous cell carcinoma (HNSCC) is the 11th leading cancer by incidence worldwide [1]. The 5-year survival for all stages combined on the basis of Surveillance Epidemiology and End Results (SEER) data is about 60% [2]. The primary risk factors are smoking, smokeless tobacco product, alcohol consumption, and the infection with human papillomavirus (HPV) [3].

Surgery and radiotherapy have been the major treatment for patients with HNSCC. Surgery is a standard treatment but is frequently limited by resectability of tumor and desire for organ preservation. Radiotherapy is used as a single treatment option in early-stage cancers and as an adjuvant treatment. A combination of radiotherapy and chemotherapy has increasingly been used for the treatment of HNSCC. Ten year follow up study of the Head and Neck trials showed that the concomitant non-platinum chemotherapy and radiotherapy reduce recurrences, new tumors, and deaths in patients who have not undergone previous surgery [4]. Chemotherapy has become an important treatment option for locally advanced HNSCC. Bleomycin, taxanes, cisplatin, carboplatin, methotrexate, and 5-fluorouracil (5-FU) are used as chemotherapy regimen in patients with recurrent or metastatic HNSCC and produce response rates from 10% to 40% [2].

Advances in molecular biology increased the knowledge about molecular mechanisms underlying HNSCC and led to the development of targeted therapeutics. Increased EGFR protein expression is observed over 90% of HNSCC. Overexpression of EGFR has been associated with disease recurrence and poor prognosis [5]. Along with the approval of cetuximab (BMS and Merck), monoclonal antibody that blocks the EGFR signaling, clinical trials using small molecular EGFR tyrosine kinase inhibitors have actively been performed. Gefitinib (AstraZeneca) showed a response rate of 10.6% in a phase II study for recurrent/metastatic HNSCC while erlotinib (Roche) demonstrated

* Correspondence: jinho@kmu.ac.kr
[1]Department of Chemistry, Keimyung University, Daegu 704-701, Korea
Full list of author information is available at the end of the article

a response rate of 4.3% in patients with recurrent/metastatic HNSCC. Lapatinib (GSK) in combination with concurrent radiation and cisplatin showed increased complete response rate in phase II/III studies [6]. Lessons learned from clinical studies of EGFR inhibitors suggested the direction for the development of targeted agents for HNSCC. Inhibition of a single growth signaling pathway may not be enough to provide a clinically significant response for HNSCC. Therefore, development and combinations of targeted therapies in different cellular pathways may be needed to fulfill the unmet needs of current HNSCC chemotherapy.

In addition to EGFR overexpression, cyclin D1 overexpression and p53 mutation are frequently occurred in HNSCC. This abnormality may provide cancer cells with limitless replicative potential. Mutations in PI3K-PTEN-AKT signaling pathways are also found in about 10-20% of HNSCC. Activating mutations in PI3K and inactivating mutations of PTEN activate downstream signaling molecules such as Akt/protein kinase B (PKB), mammalian target of rapamycin (mTOR) and ribosomal protein S6 kinase (S6K). It was reported that AKT activation causes reduction of apoptosis as well as increased migration and invasion [7]. Therefore, new therapeutic agents targeting these pathways may provide synergistic effect with clinically advanced EGFR inhibitors when used in combination.

3-Aminoindazole-based small molecular inhibitors showed strong inhibitory activities against several kinases including CDK1 & 2 [8], KDR, cKIT, FLT3 [9], PDK1 [10] and exhibited potent anti-cancer activity [11]. The structures of representative compound are shown in Figure 1.

Previously, we reported that the treatment of HNSCC cell lines, AMC-HN4 and AMC-HN6, with compound B induced apoptosis in association with growth inhibition, cell cycle arrest, caspase-3 activation, and cytochrome C release [12]. While the compound B showed strong inhibitory effects on cancer cell growth, it had low selectivity, which may pose potential toxicity in *in vivo* studies. As part of our ongoing effort to discover potent and selective kinase inhibitors as potential anticancer agents, a series of 3-aminoindazole derivatives were synthesized and tested for their cancer cell line selectivity.

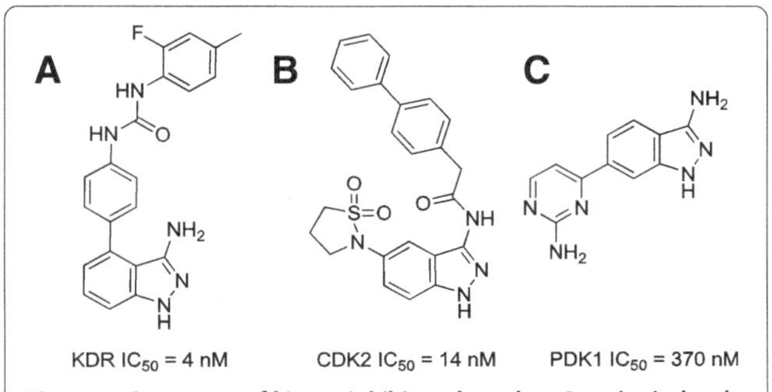

Figure 1 Structures of kinase inhibitors based on 3-aminoindazole. **A**: ABT-869, multitargeted RTK inhibitor such as KDR, cKIT, and FLT3 [9]. **B**: CDK1 and CDK2 inhibitor [8]. **C**: PDK1, Aurora A, CDK2, and IKK1 inhibitor [10].

Methods

Chemistry

^{1}H- NMR and ^{13}C-NMR spectra were recorded on a Bruker AVANEC 400 (400 MHz) spectrometer and chemical shifts (δ) are reported in ppm using tetramethylsilane (TMS) as an internal standard. Mass spectra were obtained using Waters ACQUITY UPLC, Micromass Quattro microTM API. TLC was performed on E. Merck silica gel 60 F254 plates (0.25mm). Silica gel column chromatography was performed using Merck silica gel 60 (230-400 mesh). Unless otherwise noted, all starting materials were obtained from commercially available sources and they were used without further purification. Tetrahydrofuran (THF) was freshly distilled from sodium and benzophenone. All reactions were performed under a nitrogen atmosphere.

5-Bromo-1H-indazol-3-ylamine (2)

To a solution of 5-bromo-2-fluorobenzonitrile (3.0 g, 15 mmol) in *n*-butanol (20 mL) was added hydrazine (4.7 mL, 150 mmol). The reaction mixture was refluxed for 6 h. *n*-Butanol was then evaporated, and the residue was dissolved in ethyl acetate. The resulting solution was washed with saturated aqueous Na_2CO_3 solution and dried over $MgSO_4$. Removal of solvent gave the title compound (2.97 g, 93.4%). ^{1}H NMR (DMSO-d_6, 400 MHz) δ 11.58 (s, 1H, $NH_{indazole}$), 7.92 (s, 1H, H_{phenyl}), 7.30 (d, J = 8.8 Hz, 1H, H_{phenyl}), 7.20 (d, J = 8.8 Hz, 1H, H_{phenyl}), 5.44 (s, 2H, $NH_{2\ indazole}$).

N-(5-Bromo-1 H-indazol-3-yl)-2-(4-ethoxyphenyl)acetamide (3b)

To a solution of compound **2** (0.80 g, 3.8 mmol) in THF (10 mL) was added 4-ethoxyphenylacetyl chloride (1.9 g, 9.5 mmol). The reaction mixture was refluxed for 10 h under N_2 atmosphere. After cooled to room temperature, 1N NaOH (14 mL) was added and the reaction mixture was stirred for 2 h. The precipitate formed during evaporation of solvent was collected by filtration and washed with H_2O. The product was dried in vacuo and obtained 1.2 g in 84.4% yield: ^{1}H NMR (DMSO-d_6, 400 MHz) δ 12.88 (s, 1H, $NH_{indazole}$), 10.70 (s, 1H, NH_{amide}), 7.97 (s, 1H, H_{phenyl}), 7.42 (s, 2H, H_{phenyl}), 7.28 (d, J = 8.4 Hz, 2H, H_{phenyl}), 6.89 (d, J = 8.4 Hz, 2H, H_{phenyl}), 4.00 (q, J = 6.8 Hz, 2H, CH_2-O), 3.64 (s, 2H, CH_2), 1.32 (t, J =6.8 Hz, 3H, CH_3CH_2-O).

N-(5-Bromo-1-trityl-1H-indazol-3-yl)-2-(4-ethoxyphenyl) acetamide (4b)

To a solution of compound **3a** (0.070 g, 0.19 mmol) in CH_3CN (20 mL) were added K_2CO_3 (0.040 g, 0.28 mmol) and trityl chloride (0.080 g, 0.28 mmol) and the reaction mixture was refluxed for 12 h. Acetonitrile was then evaporated, and the residue was dissolved in ethyl acetate. The resulting solution was washed with brine and dried over $MgSO_4$. The crude product was purified by flash chromatography with a hexane:ethyl acetate (3:1) mixture to provide the title compound (0.060 g, 51%). ^{1}H NMR ($CDCl_3$, 400 MHz) δ 8.16 (s, 1H, NH_{amide}), 7.71 (s, 1H, H_{phenyl}), 7.26-7.15 (m, 17H, H_{phenyl}), 7.01 (d, $J = 9.2$ Hz, 1H), 6.89 (d, $J = 8.4$ Hz, 2H, H_{phenyl}), 6.21 (d, $J = 9.2$ Hz, 1H, H_{phenyl}), 4.07 (q, $J = 6.8$ Hz, 2H, CH_2-O), 3.67 (s, 2H, CH_2), 1.41 (t, $J = 6.8$ Hz, 3H, CH_3CH_2-O).

2-(4-Ethoxyphenyl)-N-[5-(2-fluorophenylamino)-1-trityl-1H-indazol-3-yl]acetamide (5b)

To a solution of compound **4a** (0.040 g, 0.065 mmol) in toluene (2 mL) were added 2-fluoroaniline (0.008 mL, 0.08 mmol), sodium *tert*-butoxide (0.013 g, 0.14 mmol), $Pd_2(dba)_3$ (0.001 g, 0.001 mmol), and (R)-BINAP (0.0015 g, 0.0023 mmol). The reaction mixture was refluxed for 4 h under N_2 atmosphere. Solvents were evaporated, and the residue was treated with ethyl acetate. The resulting mixture was washed with brine and dried over $MgSO_4$. The crude product was purified by flash chromatography with a hexane:ethyl acetate (3:1) mixture to provide the title compound (0.016 g, 38%). ^{1}H NMR ($CDCl_3$, 400 MHz) δ 7.93 (d, $J = 7.6$ Hz, 1H, H_{phenyl}), 7.82 (s, 1H, H_{phenyl}), 7.23-7.20 (m, 19H, H_{phenyl}), 7.00-6.94 (m, 2H, H_{phenyl}), 6.87 (d, $J = 6.8$ Hz, 2H, H_{phenyl}), 6.36 (d, $J = 8.4$ Hz, 1H, H_{phenyl}), 4.01 (q, $J = 6.8$ Hz, 2H, CH_2-O), 3.66 (s, 2H, CH_2), 1.42 (t, $J = 6.8$ Hz, 3H, CH_3CH_2-O).

2-(4-Ethoxyphenyl)-N-[5-(2-fluorophenylamino)-1H-indazol-3-yl] acetamide (6b)

To a solution of compound **5a** (0.040 g, 0.062 mmol) in CH_2Cl_2 (5 mL) were added trifluoroacetic acid (0.16 mL), phenol (0.013 mL), water (0.014 mL), and triisopropylsilane (0.007 mL) and the reaction mixture was stirred for 4 h at room temperature. Solvents were then evaporated, and the residue was dissolved in ethyl acetate. The resulting solution was washed with saturated aqueous Na_2CO_3 solution and dried over $MgSO_4$. The crude product was purified by flash chromatography with a dichloromethane: methanol (95:5) mixture to provide the title compound (0.01 g, 40 %). ^{1}H NMR ($CDCl_3$, 400 MHz) δ 7.77 (s, 1H, H_{phenyl}), 7.66 (s, 1H, H_{phenyl}), 7.28-7.23 (m, 2H, H_{phenyl}), 7.13-7.04 (m, 2H, H_{phenyl}), 6.97 (t, $J =$ 7.2 Hz, 1H, H_{phenyl}), 6.90 (d, $J = 7.6$ Hz, 2H, H_{phenyl}), 6.77 (m, 1H, H_{phenyl}), 5.87 (s, 1H, H_{phenyl}), 4.02 (q, $J = 6.8$ Hz, 2H, CH_2-O), 3.75 (s, 2H, CH_2), 1.42 (t, $J = 6.8$ Hz, 3H, CH_3CH_2-O); ^{13}C NMR ($CDCl_3$, 100 MHz) δ 169.9 (CO), 158.6 (C_{phenyl}), 151.0 (C_{phenyl}), 140.3 (C_{phenyl}), 138.8 (C_{phenyl}), 134.8 (C_{phenyl}), 130.7 (CH_{phenyl}), 127.6 (C_{phenyl}), 126.0 (C_{phenyl}), 124.4 (CH_{phenyl}), 124.2 (CH_{phenyl}), 119.2 (CH_{phenyl}), 119.1 (CH_{phenyl}), 116.9 (C_{phenyl}), 115.3 (CH_{phenyl}), 115.1 (CH_{phenyl}), 113.3 (CH_{phenyl}), 110.6 (CH_{phenyl}), 63.5 (CH_2-O), 43.2 (CH_2), 14.8 (CH_3).

2-(1,1'-Biphenyl-4-yl)-N-(5-(2-fluorophenylamino)-1H-indazol-3-yl)acetamide (6a)

The title compound was synthesized using the same procedure used for the synthesis of **6b**.

^{1}H NMR (DMSO-d_6, 400 MHz) δ 12.17(s, 1H, $NH_{indazole}$), 10.58 (s, 1H, NH_{amide}), 8.10 (s, 1H, H_{phenyl}), 7.66-7.59 (m, 4H, H_{phenyl}), 7.47-7.43 (m, 4H, H_{phenyl}), 7.36-7.32 (m, 2H, H_{phenyl}), 7.25-7.20 (m, 1H, H_{phenyl}), 7.11 (t, $J =$ 7.6 Hz, 1H, H_{phenyl}), 6.99-6.94 (m, 1H, H_{phenyl}), 6.79-6.76 (m, 2H, H_{phenyl}), 3.74 (s, 1H, CH_2); ^{13}C NMR (DMSO-d_6, 100 MHz): δ 169.4 (CO), 169.3 (C_{phenyl}), 155.7 (C_{phenyl}), 153.3 (C_{phenyl}), 143.2 (C_{phenyl}), 143.1 (C_{phenyl}), 140.8 (C_{phenyl}), 140.6 (CH_{phenyl}), 138.9 (CH_{phenyl}), 136.0 (CH_{phenyl}), 131.2 (C_{phenyl}), 130.2 (CH_{phenyl}), 129.4 (CH_{phenyl}), 127.8 (CH_{phenyl}), 127.1 (CH_{phenyl}), 125.3 (CH_{phenyl}), 123.5 (CH_{phenyl}), 122.7 (C_{phenyl}), 121.3 (CH_{phenyl}), 116.6 (CH_{phenyl}), 113.3 (CH_{phenyl}), 111.0 (C_{phenyl}), 93.8 (C_{phenyl}), 42.4 (CH_2).

General procedure for the synthesis of compound **9a** to **9h**.

5-Nitro-1H-indazol-3-ylamine

To a solution of 2-fluoro-5-nitrobenzonitrile (5 g, 30.1 mmol) in *n*-butanol (20 mL) was added hydrazine (2.8 mL, 90 mmol). The reaction mixture was refluxed for 4 h, and *n*-butanol was evaporated. The precipitate formed during evaporation was collected by filtration and washed with H_2O. The product was dried in vacuo and obtained 5.0 g in 93.2 % yield. ^{1}H NMR (DMSO-d_6, 400 MHz) δ 12.18 (s, 1H, $NH_{indazole}$), 8.90 (s, 1H, H_{phenyl}), 8.05 (d, $J = 9.0$ Hz, 1H, H_{phenyl}), 7.34 (d, $J = 9.0$ Hz, 1H, H_{phenyl}), 6.01 (s, 2H, $NH_{2\ indazole}$).

2-(4-Ethoxyphenyl)-N-(5-nitro-1H-indazol-3-yl)acetamide

To a solution of 5-nitro-1H-indazol-3-ylamine (5.0 g, 28 mmol) in THF (20 mL) was added 4-ethoxyphenylacetyl chloride (11.1 g, 56 mmol). The reaction mixture was refluxed for 5 h under N_2 atmosphere. After cooled to room temperature, 2N NaOH (40 mL) was added and the reaction mixture was stirred for 2 h. The precipitate formed during evaporation was collected by filtration and washed with H_2O. The product was dried in vacuo and obtained 7.2 g in 75.6% yield. ^{1}H NMR (DMSO-d_6, 400 MHz) δ 11.05 (s, 1H, $NH_{indazole}$), 9.00 (d, $J = 2.2$ Hz, 1H, H_{phenyl}), 8.14 (dd, $J = 2.2$, 9.2 Hz, 1H, H_{phenyl}), 7.60 (d, $J = 9.2$ Hz, 1H, H_{phenyl}), 7.29 (d, $J = 8.4$ Hz, 2H,

H_{phenyl}), 6.89 (d, $J = 8.4$ Hz, 2H, H_{phenyl}), 3.99 (q, $J = 6.8$ Hz, 2H, CH_2-O), 3.70 (s, 2H, CH_2), 1.31 (t, $J = 6.8$ Hz, 3H, CH_3CH_2-O).

2-(4-Ethoxyphenyl)-N-(5-nitro-1-trityl-1H-indazol-3-yl) acetamide

To a solution of 2-(4-ethoxyphenyl)-N-(5-nitro-1H-indazol-3-yl)acetamide (7.2 g, 21 mmol) in CH_3CN (100 mL) were added triethylamine (8.8 mL, 63 mmol) and trityl chloride (8.8 g, 32 mmol). The resulting mixture was heated to reflux for 3 h. The precipitate formed during evaporation of solvent was collected. The crude product was purified by recrystallization using a mixture of dichloromethane and hexane to provide the title compound (9.18 g, 75%). ^1H NMR ($CDCl_3$, 400 MHz) δ 7.90 (s, 1H, H_{phenyl}), 7.80 (dd, $J = 2$, 9.5 Hz, 1H, H_{phenyl}), 7.31-7.13 (m, 17H, H_{phenyl}), 6.90 (d, $J = 8$ Hz, 2H, H_{phenyl}), 6.37 (d, $J = 9.5$ Hz, 1H, H_{phenyl}), 4.03 (q, $J = 6.8$ Hz, 2H, CH_2-O), 3.73 (s, 2H, CH_2), 1.26 (t, $J = 6.8$ Hz, 3H, CH_3CH_2-O).

N-(5-Amino-1-trityl-1H-indazol-3-yl)-2-(4-ethoxyphenyl) acetamide (7)

To a solution of 2-(4-Ethoxyphenyl)-N-(5-nitro-1-trityl-1H-indazol-3-yl)acetamide (3.45 g, 5.9 mmol) in methanol:dichloromethane (7:1) mixture was added catalytic amount of Pd/C. The resulting mixture was stirred for 12 h under H_2 atmosphere. The reaction mixture was filtered through a plug of celite and purified by flash chromatography with hexane:ethyl acetate (1:1) mixture to provide the title compound (2.2 g, 67.5%). ^1H NMR ($CDCl_3$, 400 MHz) δ 7.25-7.18 (m, 17H, H_{phenyl}), 7.09 (d, $J = 1.8$ Hz, 1H, H_{phenyl}), 6.87 (d, $J = 8.8$ Hz, 2H, H_{phenyl}), 6.42 (dd, $J = 1.8$, 9.1 Hz, 1H, H_{phenyl}), 6.15 (d, $J = 9.1$ Hz, 1H, H_{phenyl}), 4.02 (q, $J = 7.0$ Hz, 2H, CH_2-O), 3.65 (s, 2H, CH_2), 1.41 (t, $J = 7.0$ Hz, 3H, CH_3CH_2-O).

4-{3-[2-(4-Ethoxyphenyl)acetylamino]-1-trityl-1H-indazol-5-ylamino}-3-fluorobenzoic acid ethyl ester

To a solution of compound **7** (2.0 g, 3.6 mmol) in toluene (10 mL) were added ethyl 4-bromo-3-fluorobenzoate (1.34 g, 5.4 mmol), sodium *tert*-butoxide (0.70 g, 7.2 mmol), $Pd_2(dba)_3$ (0.10 g, 0.11 mmol), and (R)-BINAP (0.10 g, 0.16 mmol). The reaction mixture was refluxed for 6 h under N_2 atmosphere. Solvents were evaporated, and the crude product was purified by flash chromatography with a hexane:ethyl acetate (3:1) mixture to provide the title compound (1.57 g, 60.3%). ^1H NMR ($CDCl_3$, 400 MHz): δ 7.80 (s, 1H, H_{phenyl}), 7.68-7.63 (m, 2H, H_{phenyl}), 7.17-7.15 (m, 15H, H_{phenyl}), 7.02 (d, $J = 8.2$ Hz, 2H, H_{phenyl}), 6.83 (d, $J = 9.0$ Hz, 1H, H_{phenyl}), 6.70 (d, $J = 8.2$ Hz, 2H, H_{phenyl}), 6.36 (d, $J = 9.0$ Hz, 1H, H_{phenyl}), 6.31 (s, 1H, H_{phenyl}), 4.27 (q, $J = 6.8$ Hz, 2H, CH_2-OCO), 3.83 (q, $J = 6.8$ Hz, 2H, CH_2-O), 3.31 (s, 2H, CH_2), 1.31 (t, $J = 6.8$ Hz, 6H, CH_3CH_2-O).

4-{3-[2-(4-Ethoxyphenyl)acetylamido]-1-trityl-1H-indazol-5-ylamino}-3-fluorobenzoic acid (8)

To a solution of 4-{3-[2-(4-Ethoxyphenyl)acetylamido]-1-trityl-1H-indazol-5-ylamino}-3-fluorobenzoic acid ethyl ester (1.3 g, 1.8 mmol) in THF:methanol:H_2O (3:1:1) mixture was added $LiOH \cdot H_2O$ (0.4 g, 10 mmol). The resulting mixture was refluxed for 2 hr. Solvents were evaporated and the crude product was purified by flash chromatography with hexane:ethyl acetate(1:2) mixture to provide the title compound (0.89 g, 71.6%). ^1H NMR ($CDCl_3$, 400 MHz) δ 7.74 (s, 1H, H_{phenyl}), 7.68-7.65 (m, 2H, H_{phenyl}), 7.24-7.20 (m, 17H, H_{phenyl}), 7.04 (t, $J = 8.4$ Hz, 1H, H_{phenyl}), 6.89 (dd, $J = 1.6$, 9.2 Hz, 1H, H_{phenyl}), 6.83 (d, $J = 8.4$ Hz, 2H, H_{phenyl}), 6.38 (d, $J = 9.2$ Hz, 1H, H_{phenyl}), 3.97 (q, $J = 6.8$ Hz, 2H, CH_2-O), 3.59 (s, 2H, CH_2), 1.37 (t, $J = 6.8$ Hz, 3H, CH_3CH_2-O).

2-(4-Ethoxyphenyl)-N-{5-[2-fluoro-4-(morpholine-4-carbonyl) phenylamino]-1-trityl-1H-indazol-3-yl}acetamide

To a solution of compound **8** (0.1 g, 0.15 mmol) in DMF (10 mL) were added morpholine (0.015 mL, 0.17 mmol), EDC (0.058 g, 0.3 mmol), and HOBt (0.041 g, 0.3 mmol). The resulting solution was stirred for 9 h at room temperature. Solvents were then evaporated, and the residue was dissolved in ethyl acetate. The resulting solution was washed with saturated aqueous Na_2CO_3 solution and dried over $MgSO_4$. The crude product was purified by flash chromatography with a dichloromethane:methanol (95:5) mixture to provide the title compound (0.10 g, 88 %). ^1H NMR ($CDCl_3$, 400 MHz): δ 8.35 (s, 1H, H_{phenyl}), 7.73 (s, 1H, H_{phenyl}), 7.20-7.17 (m, 15H, H_{phenyl}), 7.12 (d, J = 8.8 Hz, 2H, H_{phenyl}), 7.05-7.01 (m, 1H, H_{phenyl}), 6.83 (dd, J = 2.4, 9.2 Hz, 1H, H_{phenyl}), 6.78 (d, J = 8.4 Hz, 2H, H_{phenyl}), 6.32 (d, J = 9.2 Hz, 1H, H_{phenyl}), 6.06 (d, J = 2.4 Hz, 1H, H_{phenyl}), 3.93 (q, J = 7.2 Hz, 2H, CH_2-O), 3.65-3.60 (m, 8H, $CH_{2\ morpholine}$), 3.47 (s, 2H, CH_2), 1.36 (t, J = 6.8 Hz, 3H, CH_3CH_2-O).

2-(4-Ethoxyphenyl)-N-{5-[2-fluoro-4-(morpholine-4-carbonyl) phenylamino]-1H-indazol-3-yl}acetamide (9a)

Trityl protecting group was removed using the method which was used for the synthesis of compound **6b**. The product was obtained in 73% yield (0.050 g). ^1H NMR ($CDCl_3 + CD_3OD$, 400 MHz) δ 7.49 (s, 1H, H_{phenyl}), 7.41 (d, $J = 8.8$ Hz, 1H, H_{phenyl}), 7.27 (d, $J = 8.8$ Hz, 2H, H_{phenyl}), 7.25-7.18 (m, 2H, H_{phenyl}), 7.11 (t, $J = 8.4$ Hz, 1H, H_{phenyl}), 7.04 (d, $J = 8.4$ Hz, 1H, H_{phenyl}), 6.82 (d, $J = 8.4$ Hz, aromatic, 2H, H_{phenyl}), 3.96 (q, $J = 6.8$ Hz, 2H, CH_2-O), 3.64 (m, 10H, CH_2, $CH_{2\ morpholine}$), 1.34 (t, $J = 6.8$ Hz, 3H, CH_3CH_2-O); ^{13}C NMR ($CDCl_3 + CD_3OD$, 100 MHz) δ 172.1 (CONH), 170.4 (COmorpholine), 158.1 (C_{phenyl}), 152.3 (C_{phenyl}), 149.9 (C_{phenyl}), 139.3 (C_{phenyl}), 138.7 (C_{phenyl}), 136.5 (C_{phenyl}), 133.8 (C_{phenyl}), 129.8 (CH_{phenyl}), 127.1

(CH_{phenyl}), 124.1 (CH_{phenyl}), 123.7 (C_{phenyl}), 116.9 (C_{phenyl}), 114.6 (CH_{phenyl}), 114.3 (CH_{phenyl}), 113.3 (CH_{phenyl}), 112.3 (CH_{phenyl}), 110.9 (CH_{phenyl}), 66.4 (O-CH_2 $_{morpholine}$), 63.1 (CH_2-O), 48.5 (CH_2), 41.6 (N-CH_2 $_{morpholine}$), 13.8 (CH_3); ESI MS: m/z = 518 $[M + H]^+$.

2-(4-Ethoxyphenyl)-N-{5-[2-fluoro-4-(4-methylpiperazine-1-carbonyl)phenylamino]-1H-indazol-3-yl}acetamide (9b)
^{1}H NMR ($CDCl_3$ + CD_3OD, 400 MHz) δ 7.49 (s, 1H, H_{phenyl}), 7.42 (d, *J* = 8.8 Hz, 1H, H_{phenyl}), 7.28 (d, *J* = 8.6 Hz, 2H, H_{phenyl}), 7.25 (dd, *J* = 1.6, 8.4 Hz, 1H, H_{phenyl}), 7.19 (dd, *J* = 1.2, 8.8 Hz, 1H, H_{phenyl}), 7.12 (t, *J* = 8.4 Hz, 1H, H_{phenyl}), 7.05 (dd, *J* = 1.6, 8.4 Hz, 1H, H_{phenyl}), 6.84 (d, *J* = 8.6 Hz, 2H, H_{phenyl}), 3.98 (q, *J* = 7.2 Hz, 2H, CH_2-O), 3.67-3.65 (m, 6H, CH_2), 2.45 (s, 4H, CH_2), 2.31 (s, 3H, CH_3-N), 1.35 (t, *J* = 7.2 Hz, 3H, CH_3CH_2-O); ^{13}C NMR ($CDCl_3$ + CD_3OD, 100 MHz) δ 172.1 (CONH), 170.3 (COmorpholine), 158.1 (C_{phenyl}), 152.3 (C_{phenyl}), 149.9 (C_{phenyl}), 139.3 (C_{phenyl}), 138.7 (C_{phenyl}), 136.5 (C_{phenyl}), 133.9 (C_{phenyl}), 130.3 (CH_{phenyl}), 129.3 (CH_{phenyl}), 127.2 (CH_{phenyl}), 124.6 (CH_{phenyl}), 123.8 (CH_{phenyl}), 116.9 (CH_{phenyl}), 114.4 (CH_{phenyl}), 112.8 (CH_{phenyl}), 111.6 (C_{phenyl}), 110.31 (C_{phenyl}), 63.1 (CH_2-O), 54.4 (CH_2-N), 48.8 (CH_2-N), 44.6 (CH_3-N), 41.6 (CH_2), 13.8 (CH_3); ESI MS: m/z = 531 $[M + H]^+$.

N-(2-Dimethylaminoethyl)-4-{3-[2-(4-ethoxyphenyl)acetylamido]-1H-indazol-5-ylamino}-3-fluorobenzamide (9c)
^{1}H NMR(CD_3OD, 400 MHz) δ 7.58 (d, *J* = 12.8 Hz, 1H, H_{phenyl}), 7.50 (s, 1H, H_{phenyl}), 7.47 (d, *J* = 10 Hz, 1H, H_{phenyl}), 7.43 (d, *J* = 8.8 Hz, 1H, H_{phenyl}), 7.29 (d, *J* = 8.6 Hz, 2H, H_{phenyl}), 7.26 (d, *J* = 10 Hz, 1H, H_{phenyl}), 7.08 (t, *J* = 8.4 Hz, 1H, H_{phenyl}), 6.83 (d, *J* = 8.6 Hz, 2H, H_{phenyl}), 3.95 (q, *J* = 6.8 Hz, 2H, CH_2-O), 3.68 (s, methylenic, 2H, CH_2), 3.50 (t, *J* = 6.8 Hz, 2H, CH_2-N), 2.59 (t, *J* = 6.8 Hz, 2H, CH_2-N), 2,33 (s, 6H, CH_3-N), 1.34 (t, *J* = 6.8 Hz, 3H, CH_3CH_2-O); ^{13}C NMR(CD_3OD, 100 MHz) δ 172.2 (CONH), 167.5 (CONH), 158.1 (C_{phenyl}), 152.3 (C_{phenyl}), 150.0 (C_{phenyl}), 139.3 (C_{phenyl}), 138.8 (C_{phenyl}), 137.6 (C_{phenyl}), 133.7 (C_{phenyl}), 130.3 (CH_{phenyl}), 129.3 (CH_{phenyl}), 127.1 (CH_{phenyl}), 124.2 (C_{phenyl}), 123.2 (CH_{phenyl}), 116.9 (CH_{phenyl}), 114.3 (CH_{phenyl}), 113.2 (CH_{phenyl}), 111.4 (CH_{phenyl}), 110.4 (C_{phenyl}), 63.0 (CH_2-O), 57.9 (CH_2-N), 44.0 (CH_2-N), 41.6 (CH_2), 37.0 (CH_3-N), 13.8 (CH_3); ESI MS: m/z = 519 $[M + H]^+$.

N-(2-Diethylaminoethyl)-4-{3-[2-(4-ethoxyphenyl)acetylamido]-1H-indazol-5-ylamino}-3-fluorobenzamide (9d)
^{1}H NMR (CD_3OD, 400 MHz) δ 7.57 (d, *J* = 12.8 Hz, 1H, H_{phenyl}), 7.50 (s, 1H, H_{phenyl}), 7.47 (d, *J* = 9.2 Hz, 1H, H_{phenyl}), 7.44 (d, *J* = 8.8 Hz, 1H, H_{phenyl}), 7.31-7.25 (m, 3H, H_{phenyl}), 7.10 (t, *J* = 8.8 Hz, 1H, H_{phenyl}), 6.84 (d, *J* = 8.4 Hz, 2H, H_{phenyl}), 3.97 (q, *J* = 6.8 Hz, 2H, CH_2-O), 3.69 (s, 2H, CH_2), 3.49 (t, *J* = 7.2 Hz, 2H, CH_2-NCO), 2.75-2.66 (m, 6H, CH_2-N), 1.35 (t, *J* = 6.8 Hz, 3H, CH_3CH_2-O), 1.11 (t, *J* = 7.2 Hz, 6H, CH_3CH_2-N); ^{13}C NMR (CD_3OD, 100 MHz) δ 172.2 (CONH), 167.5 (CONH), 158.1 (C_{phenyl}), 152.3 (C_{phenyl}), 149.9 (C_{phenyl}), 139.3 (C_{phenyl}), 138.8 (C_{phenyl}), 137.6 (C_{phenyl}), 133.6 (C_{phenyl}), 130.3 (CH_{phenyl}), 129.3 (CH_{phenyl}), 127.1 (CH_{phenyl}), 124.2 (C_{phenyl}), 123.1 (CH_{phenyl}), 116.9 (CH_{phenyl}), 114.7 (CH_{phenyl}), 113.3 (CH_{phenyl}), 110.4 (CH_{phenyl}), 110.3 (C_{phenyl}), 63.0 (CH_2-O), 51.3 (CH_2-N), 46.2 (CH_2-N), 41.6 (CH_2), 36.7 (CH_2-N), 13.8 (CH_3), 10.0 (CH_3); ESI MS: m/z = 547 $[M + H]^+$.

4-{3-[2-(4-Ethoxyphenyl)acetylamido]-1H-indazol-5-ylamino}-3-fluoro-N-(2-morpholin-4-yl-ethyl)benzamide (9e)
^{1}H NMR (CD_3OD, 400 MHz) δ 7.56 (d, *J* = 12.4 Hz, 1H, H_{phenyl}), 7.51 (s, 1H, H_{phenyl}), 7.44 (d, *J* = 8.8 Hz, 1H, H_{phenyl}), 7.40 (d, *J* = 9.2 Hz, 1H, H_{phenyl}), 7.27-7.22 (m, 3H, H_{phenyl}), 7.07 (t, *J* = 8.4 Hz, 1H, H_{phenyl}), 6.79 (d, *J* = 8.4 Hz, 2H, H_{phenyl}), 3.91 (q, *J* = 6.8 Hz, 2H, CH_2-O), 3.68-3.66 (m, 6H, CH_2), 3.48 (t, *J* = 6.8 Hz, 2H, CH_2), 2.54 (t, *J* = 6.8 Hz, 2H, CH_2), 2.49 (s, 4H, CH_2), 1.31 (t, *J* = 6.8 Hz, 3H, CH_3CH_2-O); ^{13}C NMR (CD_3OD, 100 MHz) δ 172.2 (CONH), 167.5 (CONH), 158.1 (C_{phenyl}), 152.3 (C_{phenyl}), 149.9 (C_{phenyl}), 139.6 (C_{phenyl}), 137.6 (C_{phenyl}), 133.6 (CH_{phenyl}), 129.8 (CH_{phenyl}), 128.2 (C_{phenyl}), 127.1 (CH_{phenyl}), 124.2 (CH_{phenyl}), 123.7 (CH_{phenyl}), 123.2 (C_{phenyl}), 116.9 (C_{phenyl}), 114.3 (CH_{phenyl}), 113.4 (C_{phenyl}), 112.7 (CH_{phenyl}), 110.9 (CH_{phenyl}), 67.3 (CH_2-$O_{morpholine}$), 63.0 (CH_2-O), 57.4 (CH_2-$N_{morpholine}$), 53.3 (CH_2-N), 41.6 (CH_2), 36.23 (CH_2-NCO), 13.8(CH_3); ESI MS: m/z = 561 $[M + H]^+$.

N-(3-Dimethylaminopropyl)-4-{3-[2-(4-ethoxyphenyl)acetylamido]-1H-indazol-5-ylamino}-3-fluorobenzamide (9f)
^{1}H NMR (CD_3OD, 400 MHz) δ 7.56 (dd, *J* = 2.0, 12.6 Hz, 1H, H_{phenyl}), 7.55 (d, *J* = 1.6 Hz, 1H, H_{phenyl}), 7.45 (dd, *J* = 1.6, 8.4 Hz, 1H, H_{phenyl}), 7.41 (d, *J* = 9.2 Hz, 1H, H_{phenyl}), 7.27 (d, *J* = 8.4 Hz, 2H, H_{phenyl}), 7.26-7.23 (m, 1H, H_{phenyl}), 7.08 (t, *J* = 8.8 Hz, 1H, H_{phenyl}), 6.81 (d, *J* = 8.8 Hz, 2H, H_{phenyl}), 3.93 (q, *J* = 7.2 Hz, 2H, CH_2-O), 3.67 (s, 2H, CH_2), 3.36 (t, *J* = 6.8 Hz, 2H, CH_2), 2.44 (t, *J* = 7.2 Hz, 2H, CH_2), 2.28 (s, 6H, CH_3-N), 1.78 (m, 2H, CH_2), 1.33 (t, *J* = 7.2 Hz, 3H, CH_3CH_2-O); ^{13}C NMR (CD_3OD, 100 MHz) δ 172.2 (CONH), 167.4 (CONH), 158.1 (C_{phenyl}), 152.3 (C_{phenyl}), 149.9 (C_{phenyl}), 139.3 (C_{phenyl}), 138.8 (C_{phenyl}), 137.6 (C_{phenyl}), 133.6 (C_{phenyl}), 130.3 (CH_{phenyl}), 129.3 (CH_{phenyl}), 127.1 (CH_{phenyl}), 124.2 (C_{phenyl}), 123.3 (CH_{phenyl}), 116.9 (CH_{phenyl}), 114.3 (CH_{phenyl}), 113.3 (CH_{phenyl}), 111.4 (CH_{phenyl}), 110.4 (C_{phenyl}), 63.0 (CH_2-O), 56.8 (CH_2), 43.9 (CH_2), 41.6 (CH_2), 37.7 (CH_2), 26.7 (CH_3), 13.8 (CH_3); ESI MS: m/z = 533 $[M + H]^+$.

***N*-(3-Diethylaminopropyl)-4-{3-[2-(4-ethoxyphenyl) acetylamido]-1*H*-indazol-5-ylamino}-3-fluorobenzamide (9g)**

^{1}H NMR (CD_3OD, 400 MHz) δ 7.56 (dd, *J* = 2.0, 12.6 Hz, 1H, H_{phenyl}), 7.50 (s, 1H, H_{phenyl}), 7.45 (d, *J* = 8.4 Hz, 1H, H_{phenyl}), 7.42 (d, *J* = 9.2 Hz, 1H, H_{phenyl}), 7.28-7.23 (m, 3H, H_{phenyl}), 7.09 (t, *J* = 8.4 Hz, 1H, H_{phenyl}), 6.81 (d, *J* = 8.8 Hz, 2H, H_{phenyl}), 3.94 (q, *J* = 7.2 Hz, 2H, CH_2-O), 3.67 (s, 2H, CH_2), 3.37-3.35 (m, 2H, CH_2), 2.61-2.55 (m, 6H, CH_2), 1.77 (m, 2H, CH_2), 1.33 (t, *J* = 7.2 Hz, 3H, CH_3CH_2-O), 1.04 (t, *J* = 7.2 Hz, 6H, CH_3); ^{13}C NMR (CD_3OD, 100 MHz) δ 172.2 (CONH), 167.4 (CONH), 158.1 (C_{phenyl}), 152.3 (C_{phenyl}), 149.9 (C_{phenyl}), 139.3 (C_{phenyl}), 138.8 (C_{phenyl}), 137.6 (C_{phenyl}), 133.6 (C_{phenyl}), 130.3 (CH_{phenyl}), 129.3 (CH_{phenyl}), 127.1 (CH_{phenyl}), 124.2 (C_{phenyl}), 123.3 (CH_{phenyl}), 116.9 (CH_{phenyl}), 114.5 (CH_{phenyl}), 113.2 (CH_{phenyl}), 111.4 (CH_{phenyl}), 110.3 (C_{phenyl}), 63.0 (CH_2-O), 50.0 (CH_2), 46.3 (CH_2), 41.6 (CH_2), 38.1 (CH_2), 25.5 (CH_2), 13.3 (CH_3), 9.8(CH_3); ESI MS: m/z = 561 $[M + H]^+$.

***N*-(3-Dimethylaminopropyl)-4-{3-[2-(4-ethoxyphenyl) acetylamido]-1*H*-indazol-5-ylamino}-3-fluoro-*N*-methylbenzamide (9h)**

^{1}H NMR (CD_3OD, 400 MHz) δ 7.49 (s, 1H, H_{phenyl}), 7.43 (d, *J* = 8.8 Hz, 1H, H_{phenyl}), 7.29 (d, *J* = 8.4 Hz, 2H, H_{phenyl}), 7.26 (d, *J* = 10.4 Hz, 1H, H_{phenyl}), 7.19 (d, *J* = 12.4 Hz, 1H, H_{phenyl}), 7.13 (t, *J* = 8.4 Hz, 1H, H_{phenyl}), 7.07 (m, 1H, H_{phenyl}), 6.85 (d, *J* = 8.4 Hz, 2H, H_{phenyl}), 3.99 (q, *J* = 7.0 Hz, 2H, CH_2-O), 3.68(s, 2H, CH_2), 3.06 (s, 3H, CH_3), 2.30-2.15 (m, 8H, CH_2, CH_3), 1.83 (m, 2H, CH_2), 1.35 (t, *J* = 7.0 Hz, 3H, CH_3CH_2-O), 1.28 (s, 2H, CH_2); ^{13}C NMR (CD_3OD, 100 MHz) δ 170.0 (CONH), 157.7 (CONH), 152.3 (C_{phenyl}), 149.9 (C_{phenyl}), 140.1 (C_{phenyl}), 138.6 (C_{phenyl}), 135.5 (C_{phenyl}), 133.8 (CH_{phenyl}), 131.0 (CH_{phenyl}), 130.0 (CH_{phenyl}), 128.3 (CH_{phenyl}), 126.5 (C_{phenyl}), 124.1 (C_{phenyl}), 117.1 (CH_{phenyl}), 115.1 (CH_{phenyl}), 114.2 (CH_{phenyl}), 113.4 (C_{phenyl}), 111.8 (CH_{phenyl}), 110.8 (C_{phenyl}), 63.4 (CH_2-O), 56.7 (CH_2-N), 46.3 (CH_2-NCO), 45.7 (CH_3-N), 45.2 (CH_2), 41.8 (CH_3-NCO), 15.5 (CH_2), 14.8 (CH_3); ESI MS: m/z = 547 $[M + H]^+$.

Biological assay

Cell growth inhibition assay (SRB assay)

The sulforhodamine B (SRB) assay was carried out as previously described [13]. Briefly, the cells were plated in 96-well culture plates at a density of 3,000 cells/well in phenol red free-medium and allowed to attach for 10 h. After 24 h or 48 h treatment of compounds, culture media were removed. 0.07 mL of 0.4% (w/v) SRB (Sigma) in 1% acetic acid solution were added to each well and left at room temperature for 20 min. SRB was removed and the plates washed 5 times with 1% acetic acid before air drying. Bound SRB was solubilized with 0.2 mL of 10 mM unbuffered Tris-base solution (Sigma) and plates were left on a plate shaker for at least 10 min. Absorbance was read in a 96-well plate reader at 492 nm subtracting the background measurement at 620 nm. The test optical density (OD) value was defined as the absorbance of each individual well, minus the blank value ('blank' is the mean OD of the background control wells).

Results and discussion

*N*3-Acyl-*N*5-aryl-3,5-diaminoindazole derivatives were synthesized using two different procedures (Figures 2 and 3). Figure 2 was used to synthesize compound **6a** and **6b** which had no additional substitution at 2-fluoroaniline ring. 3-Amino-5-bromoindazole was synthesized from 5-bromo-2-fluoronitrile and hydrazine. Mono-acylation

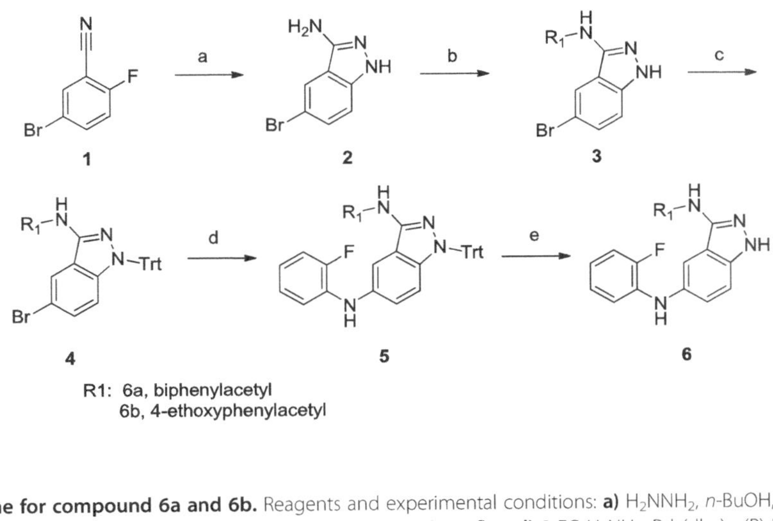

Figure 2 Synthetic scheme for compound 6a and 6b. Reagents and experimental conditions: **a)** H_2NNH_2, *n*-BuOH, reflux, **b)** i) 4-$C_2H_5OC_6H_4$ CH_2COCl (or 4-$PhC_6H_4CH_2COCl$), THF, reflux, ii) 2N NaOH, **c)** TrtCl, K_2CO_3, CH_3CN, reflux, **d)** 2-$FC_6H_4NH_2$, $Pd_2(dba)_3$, (R)-BINAP, NaOBu-*t*, toluene, reflux, **e)** TFA:Phenol:H_2O:TIPS (88:5:5:2), DCM.

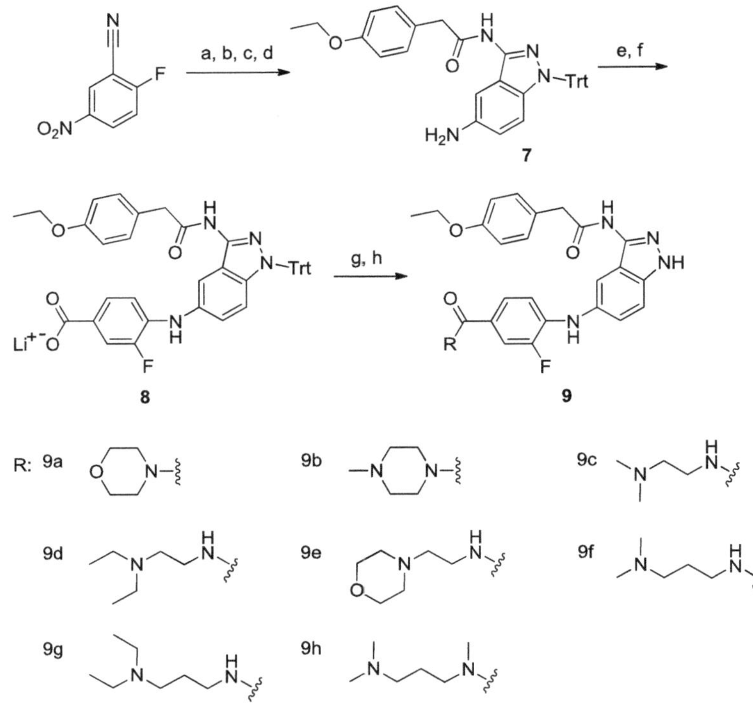

Figure 3 Synthetic scheme for compound 9a to 9h. Reagents and experimental conditions: **a)** H_2NNH_2, *n*-BuOH, reflux, **b)** i) *p*-$C_2H_5OC_6H_4CH_2COCl$, THF, reflux, ii) 2N NaOH **c)** TrtCl, Et_3N, CH_3CN, reflux, **d)** Pd/C, H_2, MeOH/DCM, **e)** 2-F-4-$EtO_2CC_6H_3Br$, $Pd_2(dba)_3$, (R)-BINAP, NaOBu-*t*, toluene, reflux, **f)** LiOH, THF:H_2O:MeOH (3:1:1), reflux, **g)** RH, EDC, HOBT, DMF, **h)** TFA, DCM.

at 3-amino position of indazole was performed by consecutive diacylation and deacylation reaction. Buchwald-Hartwig palladium catalyzed amination and deprotection provided 3,5-diaminoindazole **6a, b**.

Syntheses of indazole substituted with 4-amino-3-fluorobenzamide derivatives were carried out with 2-fluoro-5-nitrobenzonitrile as shown in Figure 3. Various amines were introduced to 3-fluorobenzoic acid moiety which is at *N*5 position of 3,5-diaminoindazole while keeping 4-ethoxyphenylacetyl group at *N*3 position. After Buchwald-Hartwig palladium catalyzed amination with ethyl 4-bromo-3-fluorobenzoate, derivatized compound was obtained by ester hydrolysis followed by amide coupling. The structures of the synthesized compounds were characterized by ^1H NMR, ^{13}C NMR and ESI-MS [See Additional file 1].

The *in vitro* anti-proliferative activities of the synthesized compounds were evaluated by SRB assay [13] against human cancer cell lines and the results are shown in Table 1.

Modification of substituent at 5-position of indazole was performed based on the previous results that substituent structure at 3-position of indazole influenced on the potency but not the selectivity between cancer cell lines

Table 1 Anti-proliferative activity of the synthesized compounds against human cancer cell lines

	IC_{50} (μM)[a]			
	AMC-HN4	A549	Caki	SNU-449
Compd B[b]	93%	91%	81%	-
Adriamycin[b]	89%	52%	65%	-
5-FU	>10	4.9 ± 1.5	>10	>10
6a	0.37 ± 0.10	1.0 ± 0.1	7.2 ± 1.4	1.7 ± 0.5
6b	0.71 ± 0.17	1.3 ± 0.2	>10	3.8 ± 1.0
9a	0.21 ± 0.04	1.5 ± 0.2	11.0 ± 0.1	3.1 ± 1.3
9b	2.5 ± 0.3	>10	> > 10[c]	>10
9c	2.9 ± 0.6	>10	> > 10[c]	> > 10[c]
9d	2.6 ± 0.4	>10	> > 10[c]	> > 10[c]
9e	>10	> > 10[c]	> > 10[c]	>10
9f	>10	> > 10[c]	> > 10[c]	> > 10[c]
9g	5.5 ± 1.3	> > 10[c]	> > 10[c]	> > 10[c]
9h	2.0 ± 0.5	> > 10[c]	> > 10[c]	>10

[a]Data are mean of three independent experiments ± standard deviation.
[b]% inhibition at 0.75 μM.
[c]No inhibition up to 10 μM.

[8]. As a first step, 2-fluoroaniline was introduced instead of 1λ^6-isothiazolidine-1,1-dione at 5-position of indazole. This approach improved the cell selectivity but resulted in reduction of inhibitory activity, (**B** vs. **6a**). When 1,1′-biphenyl group was replaced with 4-ethoxyphenyl group, the selectivity over Caki cell was enhanced, (**6a** vs. **6b**).

A good dependency between the structure and selectivity was obtained by changing the substituent on 2-fluoroaniline. Also, subtle structural differences in carboxamide at 2-fluoroaniline brought a significant change on the growth inhibitory activity. The compound with morpholine **9a** showed high potency on AMC-HN4 with more than 7-fold selectivity over other cancer cells. AMC-HN4 was known less sensitive to 5-FU which is widely used for the treatment of HNSCC, while a little prone to Adriamycin.

Though the activity was dropped by an order of magnitude by switching morpholine to 4-methylpiperazine, the selectivity for AMC-HN4 was not diminished, (**9a** vs. **9b**). Structurally similar substituents such as 2-(dimethylamino)ethylamine **9c** and 2-(diethylamino) ethylamine **9d** showed similar activity and selectivity while 2-molpholinoethylamine **9e** resulted in drastic loss of activity. The activity difference between 3-(dimethylamino) propylamine **9f**, 3-(diethylamino)propylamine **9g** and 3-(dimethylamino)propyl(methyl)amine **9h** may be understood as the target and its structural information are elucidated. Compounds **6b**, **9a**, and **9b** showed the growth inhibition of other HNSCCs (Table 2). Even though both **9a** and **9b** showed similar potency to AMC-HN3, only **9b** showed high selectivity to AMC-HN3 compared to other cancer cell lines.

The alterations in the function of Epidermal Growth Factor Receptor (EGFR) have been linked to tumor development and progression. Numerous EGFR inhibitors are currently in clinical trials based on the previous studies that EGFR overexpression is detected in 40% ~ 90% of HNSCCs [6]. Phase II trials of gefitinib, selective EGFR tyrosine kinase inhibitor, for recurrent/metastatic HNSCC have shown antineoplastic activity. However, in a phase III study, gefitinib did not improve the response rates or overall survival. The resistance of the EGFR-targeted therapy with gefitinib had been linked with the overexpression of cyclin D1 [14]. It was suggested that the combination of CDK inhibitors with EGFR inhibitors might be a useful therapeutic strategy for HNSCC. Both AMC-HN3 and AMC-HN4 cell have mutations delivering inactivation of p16 and overexpression of cyclin D1 [15]. As a result, the compound showing selective potency to either AMC-HN3 or AMC-HN4 has high potential to show synergistic effect with EGFR inhibitors.

Table 2 Anti-proliferative activity of the synthesized compounds against HNSCC

	IC_{50} (μM)[a]		
	AMC-HN1	AMC-HN3	AMC-HN6
6b	0.63 ± 0.04	0.58 ± 0.04	3.6 ± 1.1
9a	0.19 ± 0.03	0.23 ± 0.04	2.8 ± 0.9
9b	1.3 ± 1.0	0.34 ± 0.12	> > 10[b]

[a]Data are mean of three independent experiments ± standard deviation.
[b]No inhibition up to 10 μM.

Small molecular drugs that have been used in HNSCC therapy or clinical trial have relatively low cellular potency. For example, 5-FU has $IC_{50} > 10$ μM (Table 1) while *cis*-platin has IC_{50} values between 2.7 to 36.7 μM [16]. The IC_{50} values of gefitinib are in the range of 0.4 and 14.4 μM [14]. A series of compounds tested in this research displayed comparable AMC-HN4 cellular activity to 5-FU, *cis*-platin and gefitinib. They also have a high level of AMC-HN3 selectivity over other cancer cell lines.

Conclusions

In summary, we have designed and synthesized a series of *N*3-acyl-*N*5-aryl-3,5-diaminoindazole derivatives, and evaluated their anti-proliferative activity against human cancer cell lines, Caki, A549, AMC-HN1, 3, 4, and 6, and SNU449. The study of structure and activity relationship showed that the selectivity against cell lines could be achieved by modification of substituents at N5-aryl group of 3,5-diaminoindazole. Compound **9a** was the most potent compound with about 7-fold selectivity against cancer cell lines tested. Other compounds such as **9b, c**, **d**, and **h** showed lower potency but increased selectivity. For example, **9b** was very selective for AMC-HN3. It is notable that *N*3-acyl-*N*5-aryl-3,5-diaminoindazole analogues can be used as hits in the development of anticancer drug for HNSCC.

Additional file

Additional file 1: Supporting Information.

Competing interests

The authors declare that they have no competing interests.

Authors' contributions

JL: Design of target compounds and supervision of the synthetic and pharmacological parts. JK: Design and synthesis of target compounds. VH: collaboration in manuscript preparation. JP: Supervision of biological tests. All authors read and approved the final manuscript.

Author details

[1]Department of Chemistry, Keimyung University, Daegu 704-701, Korea.
[2]Department of Immunology, Keimyung University School of Medicine, Daegu 704-701, Korea.

References

1. Jemal A, Bray F, Center MM, Ferlay J, Ward E, Forman D: **Global cancer statistics.** *CA Cancer J Clin* 2011, **61:**69–90.

2. Argiris A, Karamouzis MV, Raben D, Ferris RL: **Head and neck cancer.** *Lancet* 2008, **371**:1695–1709.
3. Molinolo AA, Amornphimoltham P, Squarize CH, Castilho RM, Patel V, Gutkind JS: **Dysregulated molecular networks in head and neck carcinogenesis.** *Oral Oncol* 2009, **45**:324–334.
4. Tobias JS, Monson K, Gupta N, MacDougall H, Glaholm J, Hutchison I, Kadalayil L, Hackshaw A: **Chemoradiotherapy for locally advanced head and neck cancer: 10-year follow-up of the UK Head and Neck (UKHAN1) trial.** *Lancet Oncol* 2010, **11**:66–74.
5. Le Tourneau C, Faivre S, Siu LL: **Molecular targeted therapy of head and neck cancer: review and clinical development challenges.** *Eur J Cancer* 2007, **43**:2457–2466.
6. Rao SD, Fury MG, Pfister DG: **Molecular-targeted therapies in head and neck cancer.** *Semin Radiat Oncol* 2012, **22**:207–213.
7. Leemans CR, Braakhuis BJM, Brakenhoff RH: **The molecular biology of head and neck cancer.** *Nat Rev Cancer* 2011, **11**:9–22.
8. Lee J, Choi H, Kim K-H, Jeong S, Park J-W, Baek C-S, Lee S-H: **Synthesis and biological evaluation of 3,5-diaminoindazoles as cyclin-dependent kinase inhibitors.** *Bioorg Med Chem Lett* 2008, **18**:2292–2295.
9. Dai Y, Hartandi K, Ji Z, Ahmed AA, Albert DH, Bauch JL, Bouska JJ, Bousquet PF, Cunha GA, Glaser KB, *et al*: **Discovery of N-(4-(3-amino-1H-indazol-4-yl) phenyl)-N'-(2-fluoro-5-methylphenyl)urea (ABT-869), a 3-aminoindazole-based orally active multitargeted receptor tyrosine kinase inhibitor.** *J Med Chem* 2007, **50**:1584–1597.
10. Medina JR, Blackledge CW, Heerding DA, Campobasso N, Ward P, Briand J, Wright L, Axten JM: **Aminoindazole PDK1 inhibitors: a case study in fragment-based drug discovery.** *ACS Med Chem Lett* 2010, **1**:439–442.
11. Raffa D, Maggio B, Cascioferro S, Raimondi MV, Schillaci D, Gallo G, Daidone G, Plescia S, Meneghetti F, Bombieri G, *et al*: **Synthesis and antiproliferative activity of 3-amino-N-phenyl-1H-indazole-1-carboxamides.** *Eur J Med Chem* 2009, **44**:165–178.
12. Shin HC, Song DW, Baek WK, Lee SR, Kwon TK, Lee J, Park SH, Jang BC, Park JW: **Anticancer activity and differentially expressed genes in head and neck cancer cells treated with a novel cyclin-dependent kinase inhibitor.** *Chemotherapy* 2009, **55**:353–362.
13. Papazisis KT, Geromichalos GD, Dimitriadis KA, Kortsaris AH: **Optimization of the sulforhodamine B colorimetric assay.** *J Immunol Methods* 1997, **208**:151–158.
14. Kalish LH, Kwong RA, Cole IE, Gallagher RM, Sutherland RL, Musgrove EA: **Deregulated cyclin D1 expression is associated with decreased efficacy of the selective epidermal growth factor receptor tyrosine kinase inhibitor gefitinib in head and neck squamous cell carcinoma cell lines.** *Clin Cancer Res* 2004, **10**:7764–7774.
15. Park HW, Song SY, Lee TJ, Jeong D, Lee TY: **Abrogation of the p16-retinoblastoma-cyclin D1 pathway in head and neck squamous cell carcinomas.** *Oncol Rep* 2007, **18**:267–272.
16. Åkervall J, Kurnit DM, Adams M, Zhu S, Fisher SG, Bradford CR, Carey TE: **Overexpression of cyclin D1 correlates with sensitivity to cisplatin in squamous cell carcinoma cell lines of the head and neck.** *Acta Otolaryngol (Stockh)* 2004, **124**:851–857.

Potential therapeutic effect of *Allium cepa* L. and quercetin in a murine model of *Blomia tropicalis* induced asthma

Tatiane Teixeira Oliveira[1], Keina Maciele Campos[1], Ana Tereza Cerqueira-Lima[1], Tamires Cana Brasil Carneiro[1], Eudes da Silva Velozo[2], Ingrid Christie Alexandrino Ribeiro Melo[3], Eugênia Abrantes Figueiredo[3], Eduardo de Jesus Oliveira[3], Darizy Flávia Silva Amorim de Vasconcelos[1], Lain Carlos Pontes-de-Carvalho[4], Neuza Maria Alcântara-Neves[1] and Camila Alexandrina Figueiredo[1*]

Abstract

Background: Asthma is an inflammatory condition characterized by airway hyperresponsiveness and chronic inflammation. The resolution of inflammation is an essential process to treat this condition. In this study we investigated the effect of *Allium cepa* L. extract (AcE) and quercetin (Qt) on cytokine and on smooth muscle contraction *in vitro* and its therapeutic potential in a murine model of asthma.

Methods: AcE was obtained by maceration of *Allium cepa* L. and it was standardized in terms of quercetin concentration using high performance liquid chromatography (HPLC). *In vitro*, using AcE 10, 100 or 1000 μg/ml or Qt 3.5, 7.5, 15 μg/ml, we measured the concentration of cytokines in spleen cell culture supernatants, and the ability to relax tracheal smooth muscle from A/J mice. *In vivo*, *Blomia tropicalis* (BT)-sensitized A/J mice were treated with AcE 100, 1000 mg/kg or 30 mg/kg Qt. We measured cell influx in bronchoalveolar lavage (BAL), eosinophil peroxidase (EPO) in lungs, serum levels of Bt-specific IgE, cytokines levels in BAL, and lung histology.

Results: We observed a reduction in the production of inflammatory cytokines, a relaxation of tracheal rings, and a reduction in total number of cells in BAL and EPO in lungs by treatment with AcE or Qt.

Conclusion: AcE and Qt have potential as antiasthmatic drugs, as they possess both immunomodulatory and bronchodilatory properties.

Keywords: Natural product, Asthma, *Blomia tropicalis*, *Allium* cepa L., Quercetin

Background

Asthma is an inflammatory condition characterized by airway hyperresponsiveness, mucus cell hyperplasia, inflammatory cell infiltration and reversible bronchoconstriction, which may progress to airway remodeling with fibrosis and an increase in smooth muscle reactivity [1-4]. In allergic asthma, exposure to allergens causes an imbalance between the T helper type (Th) 1 and Th2 responses. Cytokines produced by the Th2-type CD4 + T cells (interleukin (IL-4, IL-5, IL-13) in asthma have a central role in orchestrating the inflammatory response. Strong support for this T-cell-centric paradigm has been enriched by the identification of Treg cells with the capacity to control both Th1 and Th2 responses [5]. The synthesis and release of IL-4 (which stimulates B cells to synthesize IgE), IL-13 (which stimulates mucus production) and IL-5 (which is necessary for eosinophilic infiltration to the lung tissue) increase vascular permeability and chemotaxis, which amplify the inflammatory response. Additionally, activated mast cells are able during an allergen challenge to release several inflammatory and bronchoconstrictor mediators [6,7].

The prevalence of asthma continues to rise worldwide [8], and treatment of asthma faces many challenges, including under diagnosis, access to care, ability of healthcare workers to manage asthma, education of healthcare

* Correspondence: cavfigueiredo@gmail.com
[1]Instituto de Ciências da Saúde, Universidade Federal da Bahia, Salvador, Bahia, Brazil
Full list of author information is available at the end of the article

providers and patients, and availability and affordability of inhaled therapy [9]. Treatment with inhaled steroids and bronchodilators often results in good control of symptoms [10]. However, the treatment for patients with severe asthma with uncontrolled and frequent exacerbations still contributes to morbidity and mortality of asthma in all age groups and remains a challenge [11,12]. The safety concerns and the obstacles for the asthmatic patients justify continued efforts to find new alternative therapies [13].

Historically, herbal medicine has been studied in asthma treatment, and some of the drugs currently used to treat this disease such as the inhaled corticosteroids, sympathomimetics, anti-cholinergics, methylxanthines and cromones have origins in herbal treatments [14]. Thus, our group performed an ethnopharmacological survey [15], and one of the herbs described was *Allium cepa* L., commonly used to treat inflammatory conditions such as asthma [16,17].

Several plant-derived secondary metabolites have been shown to interfere directly with molecules and mechanisms, such as the mediation of inflammatory responses and activity of second messengers, as well as the expression of transcription factors and key pro-inflammatory molecules [18]. The main compounds found in *Allium cepa* L. extract (AcE) are the flavonoids such as quercetin, which are natural phenolic compounds present in fruits and vegetables, exhibiting many pharmacological properties such as its anti-inflammatory and antioxidant effects [17,19-21]. Along with flavanols, the major bioactive constituents in *Allium cepa* L. are sulfurous compounds. In previous studies, using mass spectrometry for direct analysis of volatile sulfurous compounds has described the presence of propanethiol, dipropyl disulfide and thiosulfinates [22-24]. The sulfoxides, which are responsible for the onion flavor and odor, might also be responsible in part for the onion biological activity of different *Allium* spp. species. The propanethiol is suggested to be the main source of the characteristic onion odor [23,24].

In previous studies, the anti-allergic potential of the extracts of *Allium cepa* L. [16,17] and its flavonoid quercetin [18,19,25] has been reported using a mouse model of ovalbumin (OVA)-induced asthma. This study is the first which was conducted using extracts of *Allium cepa* L. (AcE) and quercetin treatment in murine model of allergic airway disease induced by the sensitization to the clinically relevant aeroallergen *Blomia tropicalis* mite. This mite is a major house dust mite in dust worldwide [26]. In addition, it has been shown that flavonoids, typically found in *Allium cepa,* have a relaxing effect on the smooth muscle of isolated trachea and may have bronchodilator effect [25,27,28].

Thus, the objective of this study was to assess the therapeutic potential (anti-inflammatory and bronchodilator) of the methanolic extract of *Allium cepa* L. (AcE) and its flavonoid quercetin (Qt) in a murine model of respiratory allergy to *Blomia tropicalis* mite.

Methods

Animals

A/J mice aged 5–7 weeks (20–25 g), females, were from the Fundação Oswaldo Cruz, Bahia, Brazil. Five animals per group were used in each experiment. Mice were housed in controlled temperature and humidity environment with 12-hour light–dark cycles, and had free access to food and water. The experimental procedures were approved by the Ethical Committee for Use of Experimental Animals of the Faculdade de Odontologia, Universidade Federal da Bahia, Brazil (protocol number: 02/09).

Sensitization and challenge of mice with *Blomia tropicalis* (Bt-sensitized mice)

A *B. tropicalis* extract was obtained as previously described [15]. The experimental model of allergy to *B. tropicalis* (Bt) dust mite was used as previously described [29]. The animals were sensitized with subcutaneous injections of Bt (100 µg of protein) adsorbed to 4 mg/ml of $Al(OH)_3$ in saline on days 0 and 7, and 1 day after the last sensitization the animals received four intranasal challenges with Bt (10 µg/instilation) every other day. Animals were euthanized with intraperitoneal injections of xilazine and ketamine (40 mg/kg/body weight), 24 hours after the last challenge. A schematic diagram of the sensitization and allergen challenge schedule is shown in Figure 1.

Preparation of the *Allium cepa* L. extract and obtaining of quercetin

A methanolic extract was obtained by maceration of *Allium cepa* L. previously peeled and cut in a closed container containing 1000 ml of 99.8% methyl alcohol (CH_3OH) during 7 days at room temperature. Subsequently, we proceeded to filtration of the extractive liquid, which then was rota-evaporated at a temperature of 60–70°C in a thermostatic bath. This concentration process was repeated three times. The AcE was dried in the oven and then maintained at -20°C until use.

The flavonoid quercetin [2-(3, 4-dihydroxyphenyl)-3, 5, 7-trihydroxy-4H-1-benzopyran-4-one, 3, 3′, 4′, 5, 6 -entahydroxyflavone] was obtained commercially (98% purity) from Sigma-Aldrich® (St. Louis, MA, USA).

In vitro, different concentrations of AcE—10 µg/ml (AcE_{10}), 100 µg/ml (AcE_{100}), or 1000 µg/ml (AcE_{1000}), and Qt—3.5 µg/ml ($Qt_{3.5}$), 7.5 µg/ml ($Qt_{7.5}$) or 15 µg/ml (Qt_{15}) were tested. *In vivo,* the tested groups were animals sensitized to Bt and daily treated orally with AcE containing 100 mg/kg (AcE_{100}) and 1000 mg/kg (AcE_{1000}) or 30 mg/kg Qt (Qt_{30}) dissolved in saline (vehicle) from the 8th to the 14th day of the experimental

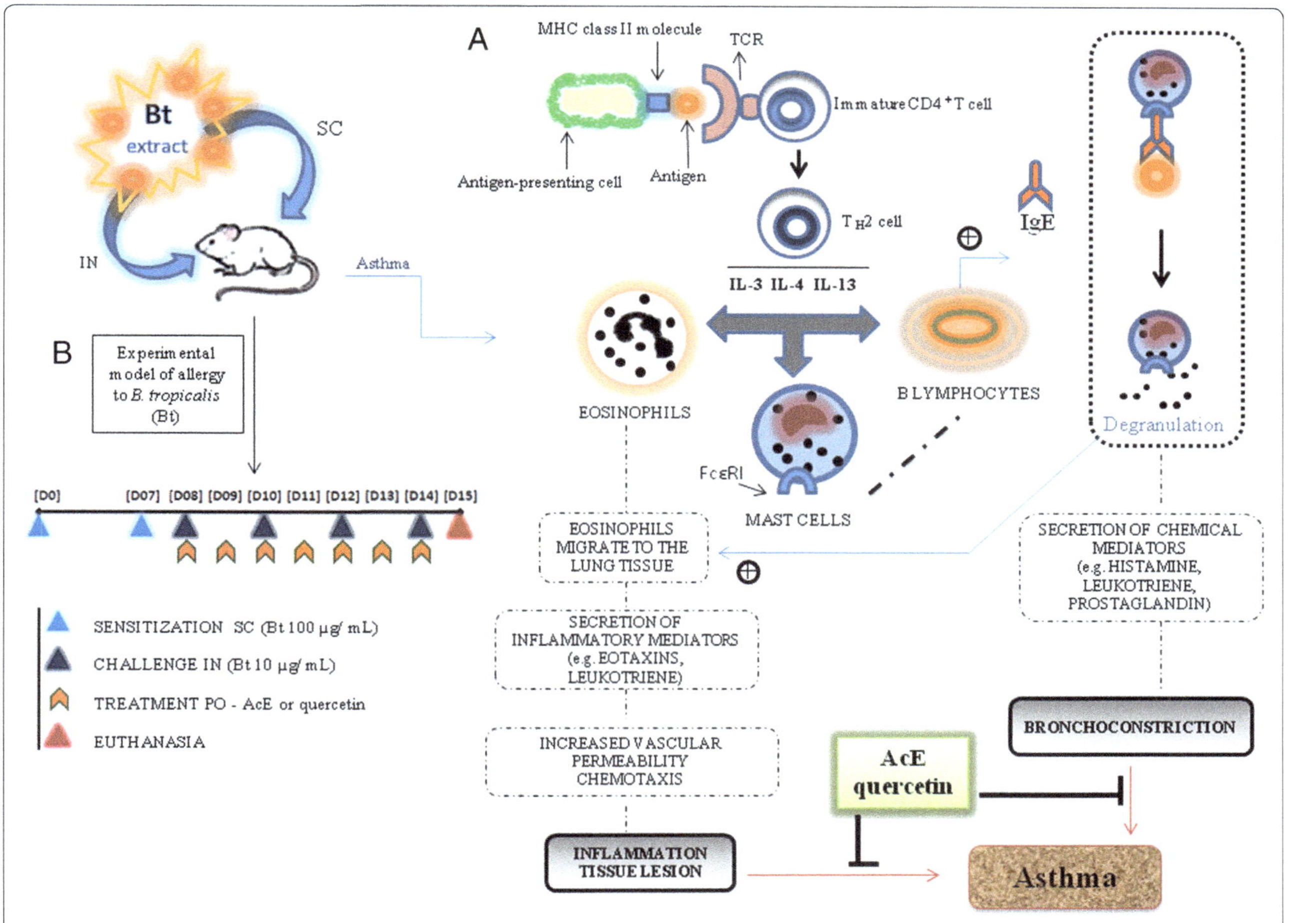

Figure 1 Representation of the asthmatic response (A) and experimental design of allergy to *B. tropicalis* (Bt) in B.

protocol and one hour after the intranasal challenges with Bt. Mice receiving the following treatments were studied: non-sensitized and vehicle-treated mice (negative control group); Bt, Bt-sensitized mice and vehicle-treated mice (positive control group); Bt/AcE_{100}, Bt-sensitized and AcE_{100}-treated mice; Bt/AcE_{1000}, Bt-sensitized and AcE_{1000}-treated mice; Bt/Qt, Bt-sensitized and Qt_{30}-treated mice (tested groups).

Standardization of *Allium cepa* L. extract

The major flavonoid found in *Allium cepa* L. is quercetin [30,31]. The AcE was standardized in terms of quercetin concentration by high performance liquid chromatography, with ultraviolet light detection at 250 nm, using a C-18 column (150 × 4.6 mm ID, 5 µm particle size, Thermo Scientific) and a C-18 pre-column (Phenomenex, Torrance, USA). The mobile phase consisted of 0.1% aqueous formic acid (A) and methanol (B) at a flow rate of 1.0 ml/min. The following gradient elution method was used for separation: 5% to 90% of B in A in 30 min. The injection volume was 20 µL and quercetin calibration curves were in the range of 5 to 100 µg/ml.

Cell viability assay

Cell viability after *in vitro* exposure to AcE and Qt was determined using the MTT assay. Spleen cells were seeded at a density of 5×10^5 cells/well in 96-well plate and were then exposed to AcE and Qt diluted in RPMI. After 48 hours of incubation, the viability of the cells was evaluated by using FCS-free medium containing 1 mg/ml of 3-[4, 5-dimethylthiazol-2-yl]-2, 5 diphenyltetrazoliumbromide (MTT, Sigma). After 4 hours of incubation at 37°C, the medium was discarded and the formazan blue dissolved with DMSO. The optical density (OD) was measured at 540 nm. The percentage of viable cells was calculated by defining the cell viability without treatment as 100%.

In vitro cytokine production by spleen cells

Levels of IL-4, IL-5 and IL-13 T-helper (Th) type 2 cytokines in splenocytes cultures were evaluated. According to the method described by Bezerra-Santos [32], splenocytes from Bt-sensitized mice were washed twice in RPMI medium by centrifugation at 200 × g for 10 min. The obtained pellet was resuspended in RPMI medium supplemented with 200 mM l-glutamine, 100 units/ml penicillin, 100 μg/ml streptomycin, 5β-mercaptoethanol and 10% fetal calf serum (Gibco, Pisley, UK). Viable cells number was determined in a hemocytometer by exclusion using trypan blue. The spleen cells were plated in 96-well flat-bottomed tissue culture plates (Costar, Cambridge, MA, USA) at a density of 5×10^5 cells/well. The cells were treated with non-cytotoxic concentrations of AcE or Qt and stimulated with 5 μg/ml of pokeweed (PWM) (Sigma Aldrich, Saint Louis, MA, USA). The cells were incubated at 37°C in a humidified atmosphere of 5% CO_2 for 48 hours. Supernatants of the cell cultures were collected and analyzed by enzyme-linked immunosorbent assay (ELISA) for IL-4, IL-5 and IL-13 cytokine concentrations (BD Pharmingen, San Diego, CA, USA).

In vitro airway smooth muscle relaxation

AJ mice were euthanized and the trachea was rapidly removed. The trachea was cleared of loose connective tissue and divided into 2 rings of 2 mm, containing on average three to four cartilage bands. The rings were suspended on metal rods, attached to a force transducer (FORT10 WPI, Sarasota, USA) and placed in tanks for isolated organ with Krebs-bicarbonate solution (composition in mM: NaCl 119, $NaHCO_3$ 25, $CaCl_2 \times H_2O$ 1.6, KCl 4.7, KH_2PO_4 1.2, $MgSO_4 \times 7H_2O$ 1.2 and glucose 11.1), aerated with a carbogen mixture (95% O_2 and 5% CO_2) and maintained at 37°C. After the stabilization period (1 hour at 0.5 g), the rings were contracted with 10 μM of carbachol (Cch; Sigma, St Louis, MA, USA) to assess the contractile state of the tissue and to evaluate the presence of functional epithelium. The rings, after reaching a plateau of contractile state, were stimulated with bradykinin (Bk; Sigma, St Louis, MA, USA) (10^{-6} M). The rings were again contracted with Cch (10 μM) and cumulatively increasing concentrations of AcE or Qt were added. Concentration response curve was constructed and data were analyzed. Additionally, the tracheal rings were previously exposed to IL-13 in culture as described previously [33] to evaluate the effects of AcE or Qt on the hyper-responsive airway smooth muscle. The rings were placed individually in each well of a 48-well plate and incubated at 37°C in the presence or absence of IL-13 (10 ng/ml, 24 hours; BD Pharmingen, San Diego, CA, USA) in supplemented Dulbecco's modified Eagle's medium (containing 25 mM D-glucose, 1 mM sodium pyruvate, 100 U/ml penicillin, 100 μg/ml streptomycin, 0.2 M L-glutamine, 2.5 μg/ml Fungizone, and 0.1% w/v bovine serum albumin) (Sigma, St Louis, MA, USA) for 24 hours. Cumulative concentration-response curves to Cch after incubation in the absence or presence of IL-13 was built to analyze the hyper-reactivity of smooth muscle. After that, concentration-response curved for AcE or Qt was built.

Collection of bronchoalveolar lavage (BAL) fluid and cell counting

The trachea of the euthanized mice were canulated and BAL fluid was obtained by three successive aspirations (total volume 1.5 ml) via tracheal cannulation of phosphate buffered saline, pH 7.4 (PBS) containing 1% of bovine serum albumin (Sigma-Aldrich St. Louis, MA, USA). Total number of leukocytes in the BAL was determined using Trypan blue and differential cell counts for eosinophils were performed by using Wright-stained cytospin preparations. Differential counts of eosinophils of at least 100 cells were made in a blind fashion in accordance with standard morphologic protocol. The concentrations of IL-4, IL-5 and IL-13 in BAL were quantified by ELISA, as recommended by the manufacturer (BD Pharmingen, San Diego, CA, USA).

Eosinophil peroxidase (EPO) activity in lung

The cell suspensions from mouse lungs were frozen and thawed three times in liquid nitrogen. After centrifugation at 4°C for 10 min at 1000 g, the cell lysates were placed into wells of 96-well plates, followed by the addition of the chromogen and substrate solution (1.5 mmol/L of o-phenylenediamine and 6.6 mmol/L of H_2O_2 in 0.05 mol/L Tris–HCl, pH 8.0). After 30 minutes room temperature, the reaction was stopped with the addition of 0.2 mol/L citric acid, and the absorbance of the sample determined at 492 nm in an ELISA reader.

Measurement of serum levels of Bt-specific IgE

Anti-Bt IgE antibody levels from mice were determined by indirect ELISA. 96-well micro titer high-binding plate (Costar, Cambridge, MA, USA) were coated with Bt (100 μg/well) overnight (at 4°C). The serum samples were added and the plates were incubated again. Biotin-conjugated IgE anti-mouse (BD Pharmingen, San Diego, CA, USA) were added to the wells and incubated during 1 hour at room temperature (RT). A solution of avidin-horseradish peroxidase (BD Pharmingen, San Diego, CA, USA) was then added to each well for 30 minutes. After that, a solution containing 3, 3′, 5, 5′-tetramethylbenzidine and hydrogen peroxide (BD Pharmingen, San Diego, CA, USA) was added and incubated during additional 30 minutes (at RT). The reaction was stopped with 4 M sulfuric acid. Between all steps the wells were washed 3 times with PBS containing 0.05% Tween 20 (PBS-T). The absorbance of each sample was determined at 492 nm in an ELISA reader.

Lung histology

The analyses the histopathological changes and the degree of inflammation in peribronchiolar and perivascular regions were performed. The lungs were perfused, via the heart right ventricle, to remove residual blood, and immersed in 10% (v/v) formaldehyde (Sigma-Aldrich St. Louis, MA, USA). The tissue was dehydrated, embedded in paraffin and cut in 5 μm sections. The slides were stained with hematoxylin-eosin (HE) for inflammatory cell infiltration and were then stained with periodic acid-Schiff (PAS) for the evaluation of mucus production, under light microscopy with 40× magnification.

Statistical analysis

Multiple comparisons were performed by one-way analysis of variance (ANOVA) and Tukey's post-test (for data with normal distribution). Data were expressed as mean ± standard error of the mean. Differences in p values ≤0.05 were considered statistically significant. Each experiment was repeated at least twice.

Results

Quercetin is present in the methanolic extract of *Allium cepa* L

The chromatogram of the methanolic extract of AcE (Figure 2A) and a quercetin standard solution (Figure 2B) demonstrated the separation of a compound in the methanolic extract with the same retention time of Qt in the standard sample (Figure 2A and B). The calculated average percentage of Qt in the AcE extract is 2.5% (based on peak area).

Effect of AcE and Qt on cell viability and cytokine levels in spleen cells culture

The non-cytotoxic concentrations of AcE and Qt used were determined by MTT assay. As can be seen in Figure 3A, none of the evaluated concentrations were toxic for spleen cells (AcE: 1000–10 μg/ml and Qt: 15–3.75 μg/ml). The production of Th2 cytokines, including IL-4, IL-5, and IL-13 by PWM-stimulated splenocytes from Bt-sensitized mice was increased in comparison to that by PWM-non-stimulated splenocytes from Bt-sensitized mice ($p < 0.001$). IL-4 (Figure 3B), IL-5 (Figure 3C), and IL-13 (Figure 3D) levels were significantly lower in the culture supernatants

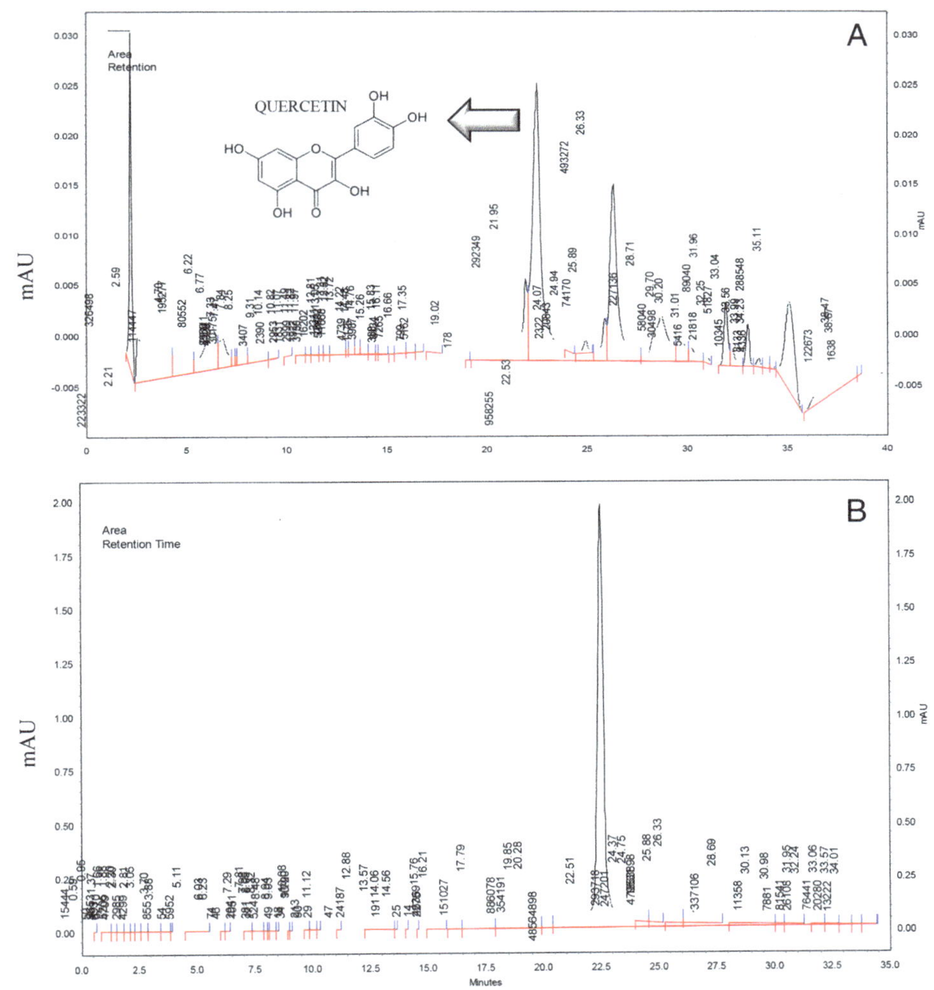

Figure 2 Chromatogram of samples subjected to high performance liquid chromatography. (A) Chromatogram of *Allium cepa* L. methanol extract. **(B)** Chromatogram of quercetin. Retention times of 22.51 minutes are shown above peaks in **(A)** and **(B)**.

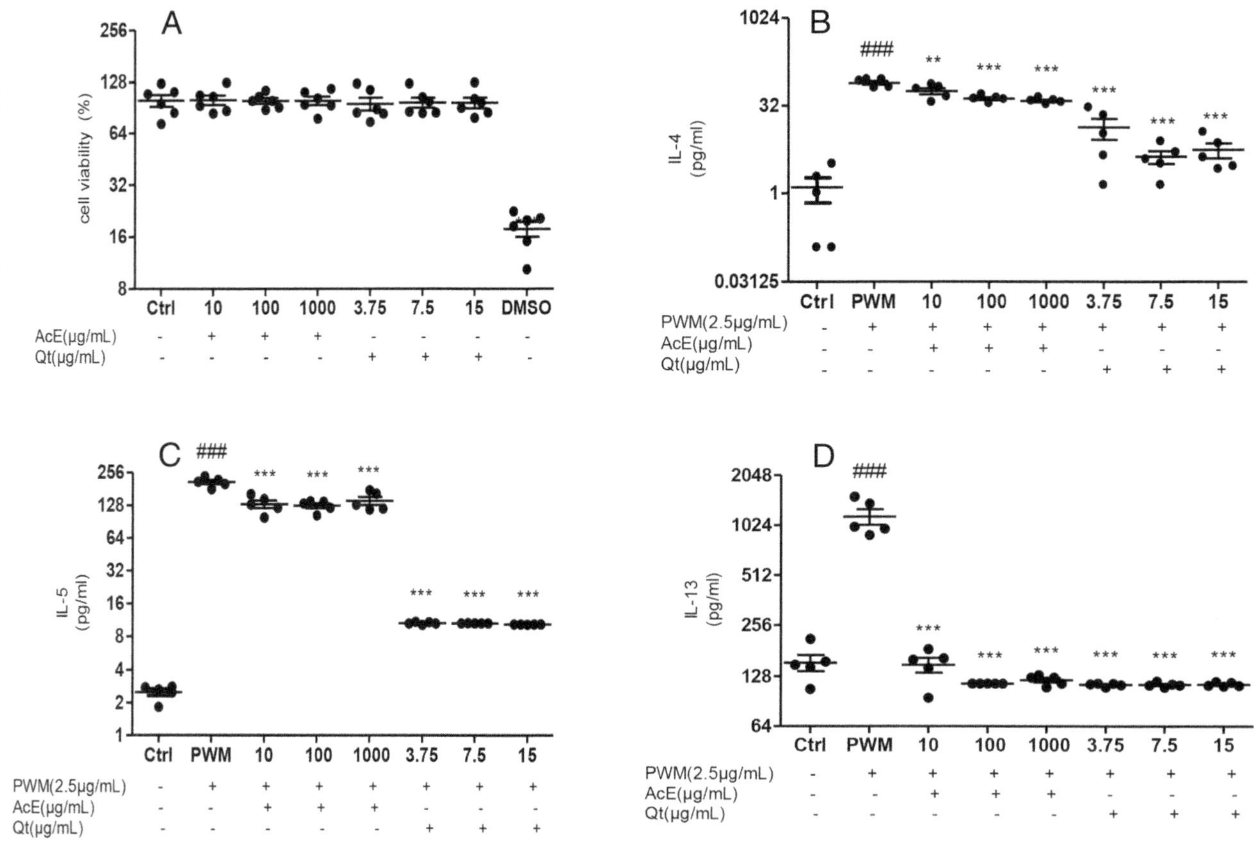

Figure 3 Effect of the in vitro treatment with AcE or Qt on cell viability (A) and on the levels of IL-4 (B), IL-5 (C) and IL-13 (D). The following groups were presented: splenocytes supernatant from animals Bt-sensitized without stimulation (control), stimulated with PWM (PWM) and stimulated with PWM and exposed to different concentrations of AcE (10 μg/ml, 100 μg/ml or 1000 μg/ml) or Qt (3.75 μg/ml, 7.5 μg/ml, or 15 μg/ml). Values represent mean ± SEM (n = 5, per group). ###p < 0.001 vs. control, and ***p < 0.001, **p < 0.01 vs. PWM group (one-way ANOVA followed by Tukey's test).

of splenocytes from PWM-stimulated mice that had been treated with AcE or Qt, when compared to the control group.

Effect of AcE and Qt on airway smooth muscle contractility

As can be seen in Figure 4(A and C), the cumulative addition of AcE (1, 3, 10, 30, 10^2, and 3×10^2 μg/ml) and Qt (10^{-8}, 10^{-7}, 10^{-6}, 10^{-5}, 10^{-4}, and 10^{-3} M), respectively, induced a transient relaxing effect, in a concentration-dependent manner, with the values of CE50 = 7.1 (1.8 – 27.4) mg/ml and CE50 = 8.9 (4.8 – 16.2) × 10^{-5} M for AcE and Qt, respectively. The data set may be seen in Figure 4 (B and D), which shows an ACE concentration-response curve. The percentage of the maximum relaxation (Emax) induced by AcE was Emax = 47.2 ± 7.0 (%), and induced by Qt was Emax = 84.0 ± 13.1 (%).

Additionally, in our in vitro model of hyper-reactivity using IL-13, murine tracheal rings that were incubated overnight with IL-13 (10 ng/ml) increased the constrictor responses to Cch but without changes in pharmacological potency (Emax = 0.84 ± 0.08 (%); pD2 = 6.8 ± 0.1091) when compared with non-treated rings Emax = 0.55 ± 0.04 (%); pD2 = 6.4 ± 0.1887 (Figure 4E). Moreover, a reduction in intensity of smooth muscle contraction in the absence or presence of IL-13 with different concentrations of AcE (CE50 = 0.075 (0.011-0.5) Emax = 25.14 ± 5.52 (%)) or Qt (pD2 = 4.6 ± 0.07 Emax = 104.42 ± 2.94 (%) was observed (Figure 4F and G). However, the efficacy and potency of the tested drugs in hyper-reactive tracheal rings (sensitized with IL-13) were not altered when the drugs were tested in normal rings, not sensitized with IL-13.

Effect of AcE or Qt on cell influx in BAL fluid and on EPO levels in lungs

We examined changes in total cell numbers in the BAL fluid to determine the effects of AcE or Qt on experimental respiratory allergy. The BAL cellularity was estimated by counting the cells recruited to the BAL fluid 48 h after the last challenge. In relation to the control group, Bt-sensitized mice displayed a significant increase in total cell numbers ($p < 0.01$). However, in Bt-sensitized mice, the

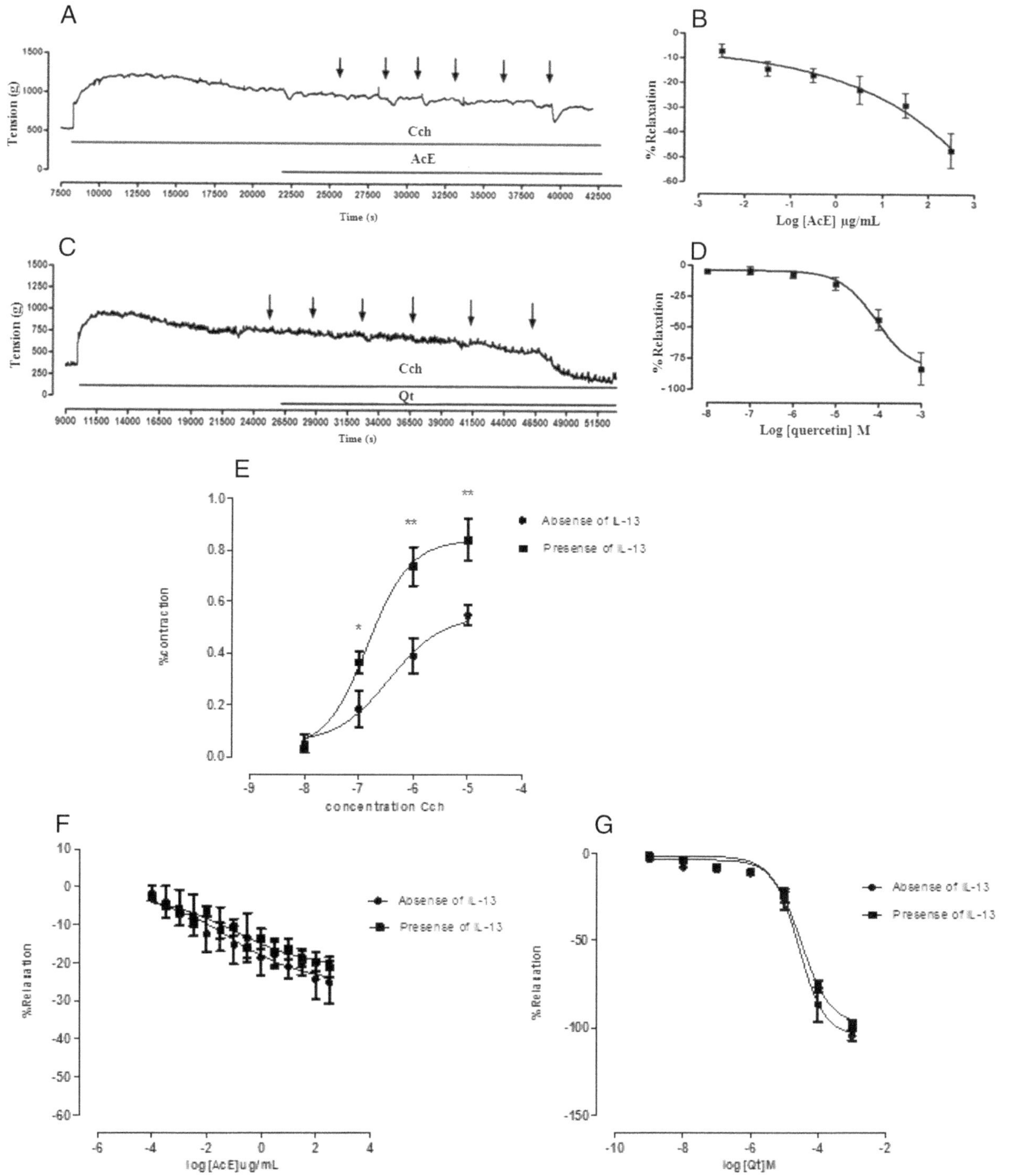

Figure 4 Effect of AcE or Qt in mice airway smooth muscle. A and C) The original record, the arrows indicate the time of addition of AcE (1, 3, 10, 30, 102 and 3×10^{2} /ml, cumulatively) and Qt (10^{-8}, 10^{-7}, 10^{-6}, 10^{-5}, 10^{-4} and 10^{-3} M). **B and D)** Logarithmic concentration–response curve of relaxant response of AcE (Emax = 47.2 ± 7.0 (%) EC50 = 7.1 (1.8-27.4) mg /ml) and Qt (Emax = 84.0 ± 13.1 (%), EC50 = 8.9 (4.8 to 16.2) × 10^{-5} M) on tracheal rings pre-contracted with 1 µM carbachol, in the absence of functional epithelium (n = 6). **E)** Concentration-response curve of tracheas isolated from AJ mice without epithelium pre-treated with IL-13 (■) or absence of IL-13 (•) and pre-contracted with Cch (10^{-9} M - 10^{-4} M). The concentration-response curve was significantly higher in rings pretreated with IL-13 compared with absence of IL-13. Values are expressed as means ± SEM. $^{*}p < 0.05$ and $^{**}p < 0.01$ vs. tracheas absence of IL-13. The data were examined using unpaired Student's t-tests. **F and G)** Concentration-response curves showing the relaxant effect of AcE and Qt in tracheas rings denuded epithelium pre-contracted or not with IL-13 (n = 6).

treatment with AcE_{100} ($p < 0.05$), AcE_{1000} ($p < 0.01$) or Qt_{30} ($p < 0.05$) decreased the total number of cells in relation to untreated Bt-sensitized mice (Figure 5A). Additionally, the lung tissue was collected 48 hours after the final Bt challenge and EPO activity were measured. The EPO levels from lung tissue of Bt-sensitized mice were increased in relation to control group ($p < 0.001$). The mice from Bt-sensitized group and treated with AcE_{100} ($p < 0.001$) or AcE_{1000} ($p < 0.001$) had significantly lower EPO levels after respiratory allergy induction. No effect in EPO levels was observed in mice treated with Qt_{30} (Figure 5B).

Effect of treatment with AcE or Qt on inflammatory cell infiltration and amount of mucus in lungs

Because AcE or Qt inhibits inflammatory cell recruitment into the lung tissue and EPO levels in lungs, we examined the histology of lung tissue. In Bt-induced asthmatic lung tissue, we observed a marked infiltration of inflammatory cells into the perivascular and the peribronchiolar regions (Figure 6A-E), and airway mucus hypersecretion (Figure 6F-J) compared with the normal tissue. Cell infiltration and mucus hypersecretion in lungs of Bt-sensitized were attenuated by treatment with AcE when compared with the level seen in Bt-sensitized mice, as shown in Figure 6.

Effect of treatment with AcE or Qt on cytokine levels in BAL fluid

To determine whether AcE or Qt influenced the generation of a Th2-type immune response, cytokine concentrations in BAL fluid (IL-4, IL-5 and IL-13) were measured by ELISA 24 hours after the last challenge. As shown in Figure 7, Bt-sensitized animals had significantly higher IL-4 ($p < 0.01$), IL-5 ($p < 0.01$) and IL-13 ($p < 0.05$) levels in the BAL fluid than control mice. In Bt-sensitized mice the treatment with AcE or Qt significantly decreased IL-4 and IL-5 levels ($p < 0.05$) when compared with the levels seen in the Bt-sensitized group. The oral treatment with AcE did not affect the levels of IL-13 in the BAL of Bt-sensitized mice.

Effect of treatment with AcE or Qt on serum levels of Bt-specific IgE antibodies

The cross-linking of allergen-specific IgE on the surface of mast cells upon allergen challenge is relevant to the initiation of the early asthmatic reaction. The serum levels of Bt-specific IgE were measured 24 hours after the last challenge. We observed that sensitization and challenge with Bt resulted in increased serum levels of Bt-specific IgE when compared with non-sensitized animals ($p < 0.001$). The treatment of sensitized mice with AcE or Qt did not reduce significantly Bt-specific IgE (Figure 8).

Discussion

The chronic inflammatory response to allergens on allergic asthma is characterized by eosinophilia, airway hyperresponsiveness (AHR) and increased mucus production. The actions of inflammatory cells in airways are tightly regulated by a network of Th2 cytokines, such as IL (interleukin)-4, IL-5, and IL-13 [34]. The present study was conducted using a murine model of allergic airway disease induced by *Blomia tropicalis* mite that was previously characterized by our research group [29]. Previous studies show that once Bt sensitization induced cells infiltration to the lungs, increased EPO activity and high amounts of Bt-specific IgE were obsrved. All these were associated to a Th2-type cytokine profile (with the production of IL-5, IL-13 and IL-4), which is important for the development and maintenance of the Th2 response characteristic of asthma [29,15]. The resolution of inflammation is fundamental to the return of normal physiological parameters. In this study we observed that *Allium cepa* L. and quercetin were associated to anti-inflammatory and bronchodilator activities in an airway inflammation murine model of asthma. As previously described [29], the total BAL cell numbers were increased in Bt-sensitized mice.

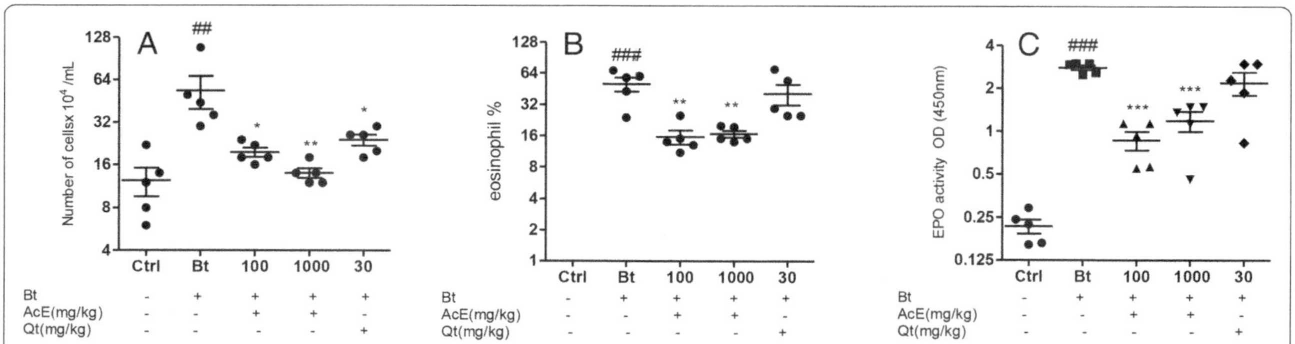

Figure 5 Effect of AcE or Qt on the levels of total cells in the BAL and on EPO in lungs. Effect of the treatment with AcE or Qt on the level of **A)** total cells counting **B)** eosinophilia in the BAL and **C)** eosinophil peroxidase (EPO) activity in lung tissue. Control (Ctrl); Bt-sensitized animals (Bt); and Bt-sensitized, AcE (100 or 1000 mg/kg) or Qt (30 mg/kg) treated mice. Values represent mean ± SEM (n = 5, per group). ##$p < 0.01$; ###$p < 0.001$ vs. control; *$p < 0.05$; **$p < 0.01$; ***$p < 0.001$ vs. Bt group (one-way ANOVA followed by Tukey's test).

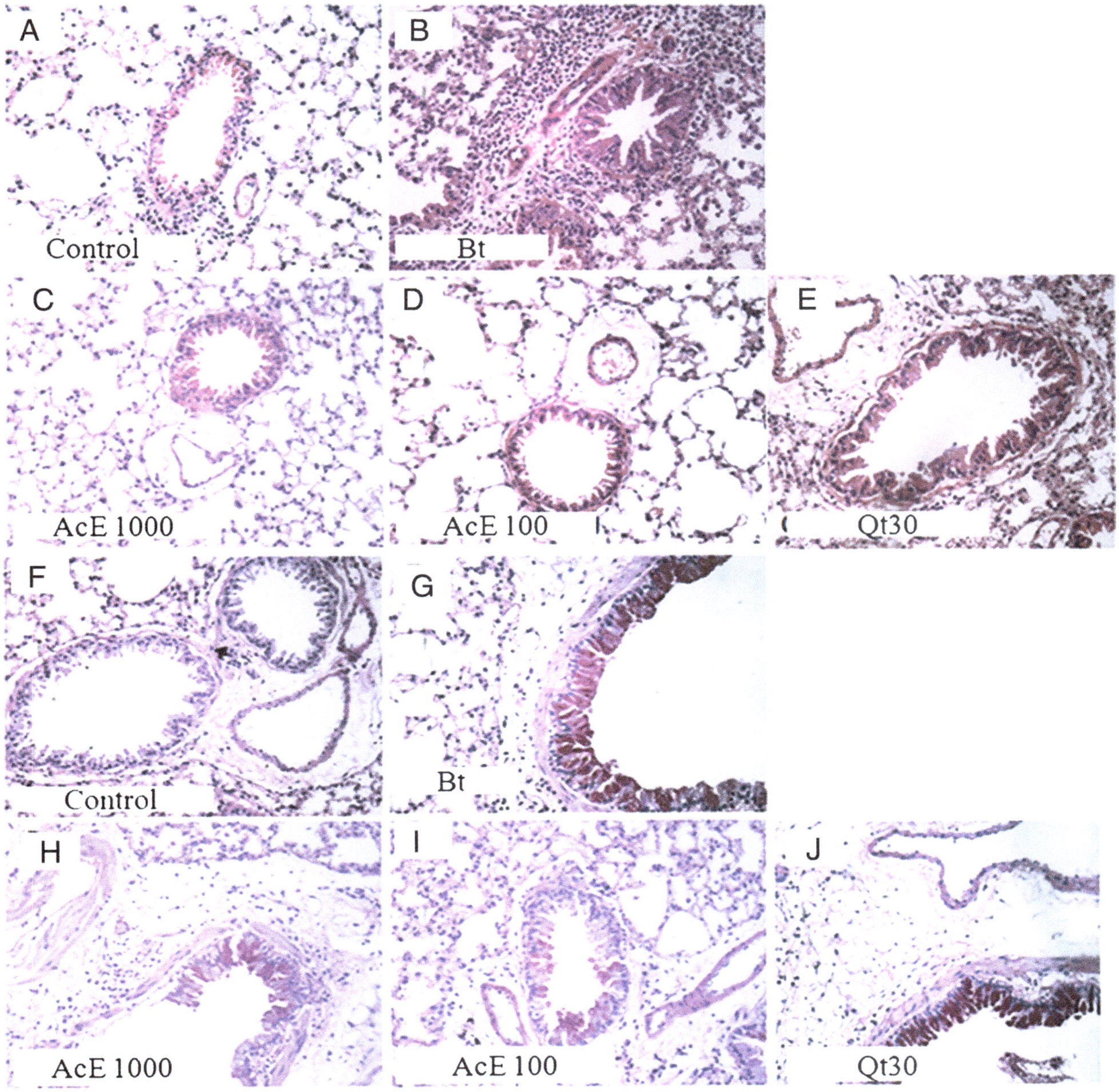

Figure 6 Effect of the treatment with AcE or Qt on celular infiltration and mucus production in lung tissues. Sections were stained with hematoxylin-eosin (magnification × 400) **(A-E)** and sections were stained with periodic acid-Schiff (magnification × 400) **(F-J)**. **(A and F)** Lung section from a control, saline-treated mice; **(B and G)** Lung section from a Bt-sensitized, saline-treated mice; **(C and H)** Lung section from a Bt-sensitized, AcE 100 mg/kg treated mice; **(D and I)** Lung section from a Bt-sensitized, AcE 1000 mg/kg treated mice; **(E and J)** Lung section from a Bt-sensitized, Qt 30 mg/kg treated mice.

Additionally, there was a statistically significant decrease in total cell numbers in the groups of Bt-sensitized animals treated with AcE_{10}, AcE_{1000}, or Qt_{30}. Drugs that modulate the recruitment of eosinophils and their activation may be important in reducing lung inflammation in asthma [35,29,36]. AcE and Qt when administered to allergic mice induce a decrease in total cellularity in BAL, a parameter required to suppress eosinophil degranulation. Despite the fact that Qt_{30} did not significantly modulate EPO in the lung, the Bt-sensitized mice treated with AcE_{100} or AcE_{1000} had significantly lower EPO levels than untreated Bt-sensitized control mice, suggesting that a substance other than Qt is mediating this effect in AcE.

Previous studies in humans have shown that the addition of anti-IL-5 monoclonal antibody on asthma therapy significantly accelerated apoptosis of eosinophils, thereby

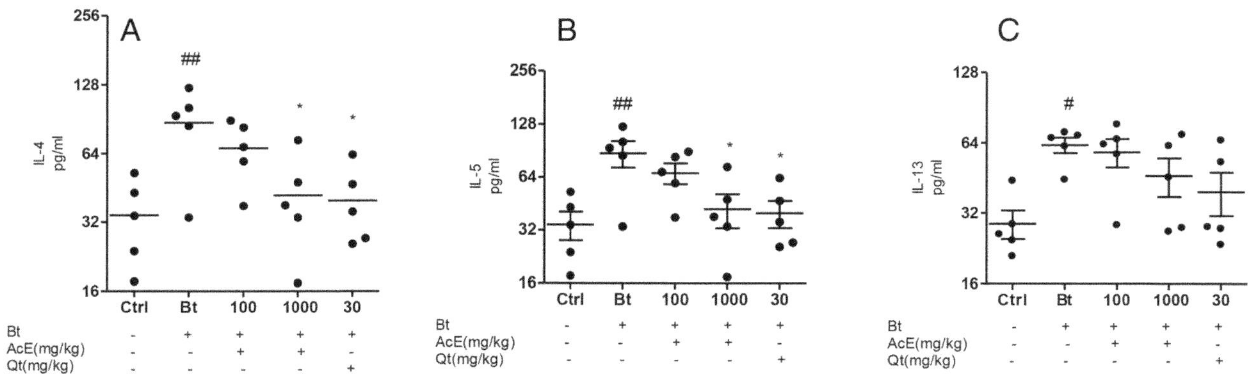

Figure 7 Effect of AcE or Qt on cytokine levels in BAL fluid. Effect of the treatment with AcE or Qt on the levels of **A)** IL-4 and **B)** IL-10 **C)** IL-13 in the BAL of Control (Ctrl); Bt-sensitized animals (Bt); and Bt-sensitized, AcE (100 or 1000 mg/kg) or Qt (30 mg/kg) treated mice. Values represent mean ± SEM (n = 5, per group). $^{\#}p < 0.05$ vs. control; $^{\#\#\#}p < 0.001$ vs. control; $^{**}p < 0.01$ vs. Bt group and $^{***}p < 0.001$ vs. Bt group (one-way ANOVA followed by Tukey's test).

decreasing pulmonary eosinophilia [37]. In this study, we could observe a significant reduction of IL-5, accompanied by a significant decrease in eosinophil peroxidase in the lungs of sensitized mice treated with Bt and AcE.

AcE and Qt had a statistically significant inhibitory effect on IL-4 and IL-5 levels in the BAL fluid of mice treated with AcE_{100} and Qt_{30}. Despite the modulation of IL-13 *in vitro*, a similar effect could not be observed *in vivo*. AcE and Qt suppressed the secretion of IL-4, IL-5 and IL-13 by spleen cells stimulated with PWM. This fact reinforces the importance of *in vivo* studies to elucidate the mechanisms involved in drug activities.

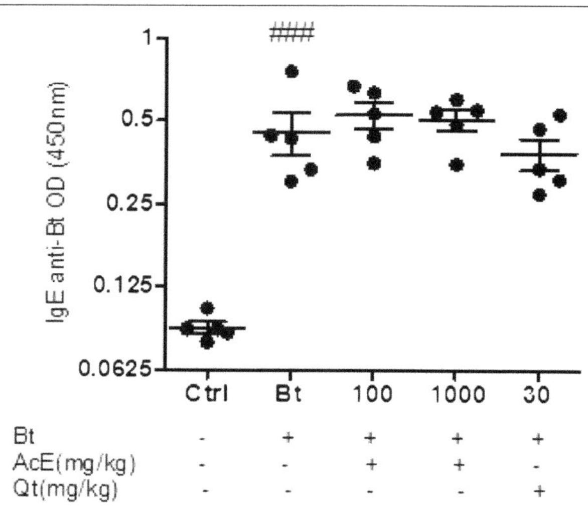

Figure 8 Effect of AcE or Qt on the levels of IgE anti-Bt. Effect of the treatment with AcE or Qt on the level of IgE in control (Ctrl); Bt-sensitized animals (Bt); and Bt-sensitized, AcE (100 or 1000 mg/kg) or Qt (30 mg/kg) treated mice. Antibody levels were measured by indirect ELISA. Values represent mean ± SEM (n = 5, per group). $^{\#\#\#}p < 0.001$ vs. control (one-way ANOVA followed by Tukey's test).

IL-4 along with IL-5 modulates eosinophil activation to stimulate B cells, IgE production, and mast cell degranulation [38] and their reduction, has been shown in this study, could be involved in the modulation of symptoms of allergic disease.

IL-13 also plays important role in allergic asthma [33,34], such as eosinophilic lung infiltration and mucus hypersecretion [39,40], which could be observed in our allergic mice. As there was no significant modulation of IL −13 by the tested drugs, we believe that in this work, as well as in other prior work, mucus is strongly connected to increased levels of IL-13 on asthmatic mice [40]. Nevertheless, AcE (AcE_{100}) was able to decrease the amount of mucus in the lungs of treated and Bt-sensitized mice. This effect was not observed with Qt_{30}.

Regarding IgE levels, no reduction on antibody titers were observed. These results may be related to the lack of a modulating effect on IL-13, which in addition to IL-4, is an important regulator of IgE production. Another hypothesis to explain the absence of effect on IgE levels is related to the short duration of our acute model, which may not be suitable for evaluating humoral responses, considering the necessary time for the variation in certain cytokine levels to reflect on serum antibody concentrations.

The interaction between the allergen and IgE present on mast cells plays a critical role in allergic inflammation. IgE cross-linking on mast cells leads to the release of histamine, prostaglandin (PG) D2 and leukotrienes, which results in smooth muscle contraction, mucous secretion and vasodilatation [41,42]. In previous studies [25,27,28], the therapeutic potential of flavonoids in isolated trachea was investigated. In this study it was observed that both AcE and Qt exerted a relaxing activity on the smooth muscle of isolated murine trachea precontracted with Cch. Additionally, our study supports the findings that interleukin-13 has been implicated as a key cytokine in smooth muscle hyperreactivity on asthma, since we demonstrated an increased contractility in response to Cch in airway smooth muscle induced by IL-13 [33]. Significant changes in Emax were observed, indicating that IL-13 seemed to increase smooth muscle contractility and cause hyperreactivity at the level of contractions. However the bronchodilatory potential of AcE or Qt is not selective for IL-13-induced hyperactivity pathway, as there was no difference between their effect on hyperreactive smooth muscle (IL-13- sensitized) and their effect on normal smooth muscle.

This study corroborates other previous studies on the anti-inflammatory and antiallergic properties of *Allium cepa* L. and quercetin [16-19,25], which might be linked to the ability of AcE an quercetin in down-modulate inflammatory processes through different signaling pathways such as NF-κB [43-45]. On the other hand, some authors discuss allergic reaction to onion. In such previous studies regarding onion hypersensitivity, authors reported patients producing IgE as well as cell-mediated mechanisms against plant lipid transfer proteins (LTPs) [46]. These are a group of highly-conserved proteins found in higher plant tissues [47]. The hypersensitivity to onion has been described as a cause of asthma induced by handling of onions. However, few publications in the literature report allergic reactions due to onion ingestion despite its wide use [48]. No toxic effect was found in animals exposed to AcE in the present study (data not shown).

AcE displayed a greater efficacy when compared to Qt, as it was able to regulate a greater amount of the parameters evaluated. This research corroborates with previous studies of natural products, which state that better biological responses can be achieved by the additive or synergistic effects of different compounds from an extract [49]. However, further studies are required in order to elucidate the cellular and molecular mechanisms by which AcE performs its action and to determine what substances are present in AcE in addition to quercetin, that contribute to the observed biological responses.

Conclusions

The results obtained in this work provide the first evidence that *Allium cepa* L. may have an anti-allergic effect more intense than Qt, and may be a future target for new molecules to treat allergic asthma. Our work may also validate and explain the long-held traditional use of this species by folk Brazilian medicine to treat asthma. This work also opens new perspectives in the context of elucidating the cellular and molecular mechanisms involved in the mechanism of action of *Allium cepa* L. as a way to enable clinical trials to evaluate its efficacy in humans.

Competing interests

The authors declare that they have no competing interests.

Authors' contributions

TTO- Collaboration in vitro and vivo experiments, statistical analysis, interpretation of data, draft of the manuscript and revising. KMC- Collaboration in *in vitro* and *in vivo* experiments, statistical analysis, interpretation of data, draft of the manuscript. ANCL- Collaboration in *in vivo* experiments and revising the manuscript. TCBC- Collaboration in *in vitro* experiments and revising the manuscript. ESV- study design and AcE supervised the extract production. ICARM and EAF- standardization of the extract in terms of quercetin concentration by high performance liquid chromatography (HPLC). EJO- Study design, standardization of the extract in terms of quercetin concentration by high performance liquid chromatography (HPLC), draft of the manuscript and final review. DFSAV-Collaboration in *in vitro* experiments, draft of the manuscript and revising the manuscript. LPC- study design, draft of the manuscript and revising the manuscript. NMAN- study design, draft the manuscript and revising the manuscript. CAF- study design, interpretation of data, draft the manuscript and revising the manuscript. All authors read and approved the final manuscript.

Acknowledgments

The authors want to thank the Brazilian agencies FAPESB, CNPq and CAPES for financial support.

Author details

[1]Instituto de Ciências da Saúde, Universidade Federal da Bahia, Salvador, Bahia, Brazil. [2]Faculdade de Farmácia, Universidade Federal da Bahia, Salvador, Bahia, Brazil. [3]Centro de Biotecnologia, Universidade Federal da Paraíba, João Pessoa, Paraíba, Brazil. [4]Centro de Pesquisas Gonçalo Moniz, Fundação Oswaldo Cruz, Salvador, Bahia, Brazil.

References

1. Hogg JC. Pathology of asthma. J Allergy Clin Immunol. 1993;92:1–5.
2. Holgate S, Smith N, Massanari M, Jimenez P. Effects of omalizumab on markers of inflammation in patients with allergic asthma. Allergy. 2009;64(12):1728–36.
3. Lougheed MD, Olajos-Clow JG. Asthma care pathways in the emergency department. Curr Opin Allergy Clin Immunol. 2010;10(3):181–7.
4. Deckers J, Branco Madeira F, Hammad H. Innate immune cells in asthma. Trends Immunol. 2013;34(11):540–7.
5. Illi S, Depner M, Genuneit J, Horak E, Loss G, Strunz-Lehner C, et al. Protection from childhood asthma and allergy in Alpine farm environments-the GABRIEL Advanced Studies. J Allergy Clin Immunol. 2012;129:1470–7.
6. Barnes PJ. Theophylline: new perspectives for an old drug. Am J Respir Crit Care Med. 2003;167(6):813–8.
7. Nauta AJ, Engels F, Knippels LM, Garssen J, Nijkamp FP, Redegeld FA. Mechanisms of allergy and asthma. Eur J Pharmacol. 2008;585(2–3):354–60.
8. Lee SI. Prevalence of childhood asthma in Korea: international study of asthma and allergies in childhood. Allergy Asthma Immunol Res. 2010;2(2):61–4.
9. Zar HJ, Levin ME. Challenges in treating pediatric asthma in developing countries. Paediatr Drugs. 2012;14:353–9.
10. Kew KM, Karner C, Mindus SM, Ferrara G. Combination formoterol and budesonide as maintenance and reliever therapy versus combination inhaler maintenance for chronic asthma in adults and children. Cochrane Database Syst Rev. 2013;12:CD009019.
11. Hashimoto S, Bel EH. Current treatment of severe asthma. Clin Exp Allergy. 2012;42(5):693–705.
12. Busse W. Asthma diagnosis and treatment: filling in the information gaps. J Allergy Clin Immunol. 2011;128:740–50.
13. Martinez FD, Vercelli D. Asthma. Lancet. 2013;382(9901):1360–72.
14. Mullane K. The increasing challenge of discovering asthma drugs. Biochem Pharmacol. 2011;82(6):586–99.
15. Costa RS, Brasil TC, Santos CJ, Santos DB, Barreto ML, Alcântara-Neves NM, et al. Natural products used for asthma treatment in children living in Salvador-BA, Brazil. Rev Bras Farmacogn. 2010;20:594–9.
16. Dorsch W, Wagner H, Bayer T, Fessler B, Hein G, Ring J, et al. Anti-asthmatic effects of onions. Alk(en)ylsulfinothioic acid alk(en)yl-esters inhibit histamine release, leukotriene and thromboxane biosynthesis in vitro and counteract PAF and allergen-induced bronchial obstruction *in vivo*. Biochem Pharmacol. 1988;1;37(23):4479–86.

17. Kaiser P, Youssouf MS, Tasduq SA, Singh S, Sharma SC, Singh GD, et al. Anti-allergic effects of herbal product from *Allium cepa* (bulb). J Med Food. 2009;12(2):374–82.
18. Rogerio AP, Kanashiro A, Fontanari C, da Silva EV, Lucisano-Valim YM, Soares EG, et al. Anti-inflammatory activity of quercetin and isoquercitrin in experimental murine allergic asthma. Inflamm Res. 2007;56(10):402–8.
19. Park HJ, Lee CM, Jung ID, Lee JS, Jeong YI, Chang JH, et al. Quercetin regulates Th1/Th2 balance in a murine model of asthma. Int Immunopharmacol. 2009;9(3):261–7.
20. Elberry AA, Mufti S, Al-Maghrabi J, Abdel Sattar E, Ghareib SA, Mosli HA, et al. Immunomodulatory effect of red onion (Allium cepa Linn) scale extract on experimentally induced atypical prostatic hyperplasia in Wistar rats. Mediators Inflamm. 2014;2014:640746.
21. Guo C, Hou GQ, Li XD, Xia X, Liu DX, Huang DY, et al. Quercetin triggers apoptosis of lipopolysaccharide (LPS)- induced osteoclast and inhibits bone resorption in RAW 264.7 cells. Cell Physiol Biochem. 2012;30(1):123–36.
22. Kubec R, Cody RB, Dane AJ, Musah RA, Schraml J, Vattekkatte A, et al. Applications of direct analysis in real time-mass spectrometry (DART-MS) in Allium chemistry. (Z)-butanethial S-oxide and 1-butenyl thiosulfinates and their S-(E)-1-butenylcysteine S-oxide precursor from Allium siculum. J Agric Food Chem. 2010;58(2):121–8.
23. Løkke MM, Edelenbos M, Larsen E, Feilberg A. Investigation of volatiles emitted from freshly cut onions (Allium cepa L.) by real time proton-transfer reaction-mass spectrometry (PTR-MS. Sensors (Basel). 2012;12(12):16060–76.
24. Colina-Coca C, González-Peña D, Vega E, de Ancos B, Sánchez-Moreno C. Novel approach for the determination of volatile compounds in processed onion by headspace gas chromatography–mass spectrometry (HS GC-MS). Talanta. 2013;103:137–44.
25. Joskova M, Franova S, Sadlonova V. Acute bronchodilator effect of quercetin in experimental allergic asthma. Bratisl Lek Listy. 2011;112(1):9–12.
26. Fernández-Caldas E, Puerta L, Caraballo L. Mites and allergy. Chem Immunol Allergy. 2014;100:234–42.
27. Capasso R, Aviello G, Romano B, Atorino G, Pagano E, Borrelli F. Inhibitory effect of quercetin on rat trachea contractility in vitro. J Pharm Pharmacol. 2009;61(1):115–9.
28. Fernandez J, Reyes R, Ponce H, Oropeza M, Vancalsteren MR, Jankowski C, et al. Isoquercitrin from Argemone platyceras inhibits carbachol and leukotriene D4-induced contraction in guinea-pig airways. Eur J Pharmacol. 2005;522(1–3):108–15.
29. Baqueiro T, Russo M, Silva VM, Meirelles T, Oliveira PR, Gomes E, et al. Respiratory allergy to Blomia tropicalis: immune response in four syngeneic mouse strains and assessment of a low allergen-dose, short-term experimental model. Respir Res. 2010;1:11:51.
30. Ly TN, Hazama C, Shimoyamada M, Ando H, Kato K, Yamauchi R. Antioxidative compounds from the outer scales of onion. J Agric Food Chem. 2005;53(21):8183–9.
31. Lee J, Mitchell AE. Quercetin and isorhamnetin glycosides in onion (*Allium cepa* L.): varietal comparison, physical distribution, coproduct evaluation, and long-term storage stability. J Agric Food Chem. 2011;59(3):857–63.
32. Bezerra-Santos CR, Balestiari FM, Rossi-Bergmann B, Peçanha LM, Piuvezam MR. Cissampelos sympodialis Eichl. (Menispermaceae): oral treatment decreases IgE levels and induces a Th1-skewed cytokine production in ovalbumin-sensitized mice. J Ethnopharmaco. 2004;95(2–3):191–7.
33. Farghaly HS, Blagbrough IS, Medina-Tato DA, Watson ML. Interleukin13 increases contractility of murine tracheal smooth muscle by a phosphoinositide 3-kinase p110 delta-dependent mechanism. Mol Pharmacol. 2008;73(5):1530–7.
34. Walter DM, McIntire JJ, Berry G, McKenzie AN, Donaldson DD, DeKruyff RH, et al. Critical role for IL-13 in the development of allergen-induced airway hyperreactivity. J Immunol. 2001;167(8):4668–75.
35. Baatjes AJ, Sehmi R, Saito H, Cyr MM, Dorman SC, Inman MD, et al. Anti-allergic therapies: effects on eosinophil progenitors. Pharmacol Ther. 2002;95(1):63–72.
36. Cerqueira-Lima AT, Alcântara-Neves NM, de-Carvalho LC, Costa RS, Barbosa-Filho JM, Piuvezam M, et al. Effects of Cissampelos sympodialis Eichl. and its alkaloid, warifteine, in an experimental model of respiratory allergy to Blomia tropicalis. Curr Drug Targets. 2010;11(11):1458–67.
37. Simon HU, Yousefi S, Schranz C, Schapowal A, Bachert C, Blaser K. Direct demonstration of delayed eosinophil apoptosis as a mechanism causing tissue eosinophilia. J Immunol. 1997;158(8):3902–8.
38. Galli SJ, Tsai M. IgE and mast cells in allergic disease. Nat Med. 2012;18(5):693–704.
39. Wynn TA. IL-13 effector functions. Annu Rev Immunol. 2013;21:425–56.
40. Kibe A, Inoue H, Fukuyama S, Machida K, Matsumoto K, Koto H, et al. Differential regulation by glucocorticoid of interleukin-13-induced eosinophilia, hyperresponsiveness, and goblet cell hyperplasia in mouse airways. Am J Respir Crit Care Med. 2003;167(1):50–6.
41. Bateman ED, Hurd SS, Barnes PJ, Bousquet J, Drazen JM, FitzGerald M, et al. Global strategy for asthma management and prevention: GINA executive summary. Eur Respir J. 2008;31(1):143–78.
42. Hamid Q, Tulic M. Immunobiology of asthma. Annu Rev Physiol. 2009;71:489–507.
43. Yamaguchi M, Weitzmann MN. Quercetin, a potent suppressor of NF-κB and Smad activation in osteoblasts. Int J Mol Med. 2011;28(4):521–5.
44. Tang CH, Huang TH, Chang CS, Fu WM, Yang RS. Water solution of onion crude powder inhibits RANKL-induced osteoclastogenesis through ERK, p38 and NF-kappab pathways. Osteoporos Int. 2009;20(1):93–103.
45. Wattel A, Kamel S, Prouillet C, Petit JP, Lorget F, Offord E, et al. Flavonoid quercetin decreases osteoclastic differentiation induced by RANKL via a mechanism involving NF kappa B and AP-1. J Cell Biochem. 2004;92(2):285–95.
46. Valdivieso R, Subiza J, Varela-Losada S, Subiza JL, Narganes MJ, Martinez-Cocera C, et al. Bronchial asthma, rhinoconjunctivitis, and contact dermatitis caused by onion. J Allergy Clin Immunol. 1994;94(5):928–30.
47. Asero R, Mistrello G, Roncarolo D, Amato S. Relationship between peach lipid transfer protein specific IgE levels and hypersensitivity to non-Roseaceae vegetable foods in patients allergic to lipid transfer protein. Ann Allergy Asthma Immunol. 2004;92(2):268–72.
48. Enrique E, Malek T, De Mateo JA, Castelló J, Lombardero M, Barber D, et al. Involvement of lipid transfer protein in onion allergy. Ann Allergy Asthma Immunol. 2007;98(2):202.
49. Jaki BU, Franzblau SG, Chadwick LR, Lankin DC, Zhang F, Wang Y, et al. Purity-activity relationships of natural products: the case of anti-TB active ursolic acid. J Nat Prod. 2008;71(10):1742–8.

Tacrolimus ameliorates functional disturbances and oxidative stress in isoproterenol-induced myocardial infarction

Arash Khorrami[1,2], Mojtaba Hammami[2], Mehraveh Garjani[2], Nasrin Maleki-Dizaji[1] and Alireza Garjani[1*]

Abstract

Background: The inflammatory responses play a major role in the pathogenesis of acute myocardial infarction (MI). Early inhibition of inflammation may improve post MI cardiac function. The aim of this study was to investigate the effects of tacrolimus on cardiac function, hemodynamic parameters as well as histopathologic and electrocardiographic changes in isoproterenol-induced myocardial infarction.

Methods: Male Wistar rats were randomly divided into six groups of control, isoproterenol alone, tacrolimus alone, and isoproterenol plus tacrolimus (0.5, 1 and 2 mg/kg). Isoproterenol (100 mg/kg) was injected subcutaneously for two consecutive days to induce myocardial infarction, and simultaneously tacrolimus was administered orally twice a day for three days.

Results and conclusions: Administration of isoproterenol resulted in myocardial edema and necrosis as well as a marked reduction in the left ventricular systolic pressure (LVSP), left ventricular contractility ($LVdP/dt_{max}$) and relaxation ($LVdP/dt_{min}$) along with a severe elevation in left ventricular end-diastolic pressure (LVEDP). Isoproterenol also elevated the ST-segment and suppressed the R-amplitude and R-R interval on ECG. It was found that all doses of tacrolimus could amend the ECG pattern and ameliorated the isoproterenol induced disturbances in cardiac function. Acute and short term treatment with tacrolimus at dose of 2 mg/kg significantly ($P < 0.001$) improved $LVdP/dt_{max}$ from 2712 ± 82 in myocardial infarcted rats to 4592 ± 149 mmHg/sec. Similarly, tacrolimus lowered LVEDP from 17.6 ± 0.68 in MI group to the value of 5.6 ± 0.22 mmHg ($P < 0.001$). Furthermore, tacrolimus was found to reduce malondialdehyde concentration in serum and myocardium by 50-70% ($P < 0.001$).
The results of this study showed that acute treatment with tacrolimus, coincided with the occurrence of myocardial infarction, strongly protected the myocardium against the isoproterenol-induced myocardial infarction; where this might be due to the anti-inflammatory properties of tacrolimus.

Keywords: Tacrolimus, Myocardial infarction, Isoproterenol, Electrocardiography

Background

Cardiovascular disease (CVD), predominantly myocardial infarction, is the leading cause of death worldwide [1,2]. Reductions in the myocardial blood flow due to the coronary artery occlusion can considerably compromise the energy metabolism. Coronary artery occlusion, only as short as 5 minutes, can lead to oxidative stress and then functional abnormalities of the myocardium that persist up to 24–48 hours after reperfusion [3-5].

* Correspondence: garjania2002@yahoo.com
[1]Department of Pharmacology and Toxicology, Faculty of Pharmacy, Tabriz University of Medical Sciences, Tabriz, Iran
Full list of author information is available at the end of the article

The existing therapeutic approaches are designed to reduce the myocardial necrosis and also amendment of cardiac function after a myocardial infarction. Several studies have shown that consecutive vigorous inflammatory and immune reactions increases the generation of cytokines and oxidative stress, recruits inflammatory and T cells, and initiates the complement cascade [6,7]. The inflammatory responses induced by myocardial ischemia play a major role in the pathogenesis of acute myocardial infarction (AMI). In addition, recent studies have demonstrated that myocardial necrosis and subsequent oxidative stress trigger a cytokine cascade initiated by Tumor Necrosis Factor (TNF)-α. These inflammatory responses are found to exacerbate myocardial injury and remodeling after AMI [1,6,8], which lead to a progressive and irreversible myocardial damage. One of the principal interventions that exist for AMI is early inhibition of the inflammatory cycle and thus achieves a better recovery of the myocardium.

Tacrolimus (FK506) is a macrolide produced by the bacteria *Streptomyces tsukubaensis*. It is an immunosuppressant mainly used in organ transplantation in order to reduce the risk of graft rejection. Activation of T cells by allogenic antigens in transplanted tissue increases intracellular calcium concentration that contributes to the calcium-calmodulin complex formation. Calcium-calmodulin complex, in turn, activates calcineurin, a crucial phosphatase for T cell signaling [9,10]. Tacrolimus binding to the FK506 binding protein (FKBP), a respective cytoplasmic receptor, inactivates calcineurin, thereby the inflammatory response. FKBP is present in most tissues, including the myocardium. In addition to the anti-inflammatory effects of FK506-FKBP complex, it plays a critical role in modulating myocardial calcium homeostasis and rhythm regulation by stabilizing Ryanodine receptors [7,11]. The complex of FK506-FKBP inhibits the phosphatase activity of calcineurin and the calcium-dependent inflammatory responses. Moreover, some experimental studies have revealed that tacrolimus can effectively inhibit MAPK and PI3K-Akt signaling pathways in various inflammatory diseases [7].

Isoproterenol (ISO) is a synthetic beta-adernoceptor agonist and its subcutaneous injection induces irreversible cellular damage and ultimately myocardial infarction in rats. The acute hemodynamic and electrocardiographic changes in isoproterenol induced myocardial infarction resemble closely to those occurring in patients with myocardial infarction [12]. Therefore, the rat model of isoproterenol induced myocardial infarction offers a reliable non-invasive technique for studying the effects of various potentially cardioprotective agents [13].

The aim of the present study was to investigate the potential cardioprotective effects of tacrolimus on acute heart remodeling, hemodynamic, electrocardiographic, and biochemical changes in isoproterenol-induced myocardial infarction in rats.

Materials and methods

Animals

Male albino Wistar rats weighing between 260 and 280 g were used in the present study. The animals were housed in standard polypropylene cages (six per cage) under a 12/12 h light/dark cycle at a constant temperature of 20 ± 1.8°C and ambient humidity of 50 ± 10%. The rats were given food and water freely. This study was performed in accordance with the Guide for the Care and Use of Laboratory Animals of Tabriz University of Medical Sciences, Tabriz-Iran (National Institutes of Health publication No 85–23, revised 1985).

Induction of acute myocardial infarction

Isoproterenol (Sigma Co; USA) was dissolved in normal saline and injected subcutaneously to rats (100 mg/kg) for two consecutive days at an interval of 24 hours to induce acute myocardial infarction. Animals were sacrificed 48 hours after the first injection of isoproterenol [13].

Experimental protocol

The animals were randomly divided into six groups consisting of six rats each. Rats in group1 (normal control) received a subcutaneous injection of normal saline (0.5 ml) and were left untreated for the entire experimental period. Rats in group 2 (sham) were received an oral administration of tacrolimus (2 mg/kg; twice daily) for two consecutive days and were subcutaneously injected with normal saline. To induce myocardial infarction, rats in group 3 (MI control; ISO) were subcutaneously (SC) injected with isoproterenol (100 mg/kg) dissolved in normal saline as a vehicle (0.5 ml) for two consecutive days at an interval of 24 h. Rats in groups 4 to 6 were orally treated with tacrolimus at 0.5, 1 and 2 mg/kg twice daily. The treatment was started immediately prior to induction of MI (SC injection of isoproterenol) for the ensuing 2 days.

Hemodynamic measurements

About 24 to 48 hours after the last administration of drug, the animals were anesthetized by the intraperitoneal injection of a mixture of ketamine (50 mg/kg), xylazine (30 mg/kg), and acepromazine (20 mg/kg). When rats did not respond to noxious stimuli, a standard limb lead (II) observed constantly during the experimental period and any changes in ECG pattern were documented. To observe the hemodynamic parameters, a ventral midline skin incision was made from the lower mandible posteriorly to the sternum (~3 cm) and the left common carotid artery was isolated. The artery was temporary occluded toward the heart using a dieffenbach serrefines clamp (Elcon; Germany). Vannas micro iris scissors (Medi Plus; USA) was used to make a tiny incision on the carotid artery. A polyethylene cannula (Protex; OD 0.98 mm, ID 0.58 mm), coupled to a pressure transducer (Powerlab system; AD Instruments, Australia), was inserted into the artery for the recording systemic arterial blood pressure. The mean arterial blood pressure was calculated from the systolic and diastolic blood pressure traces. To assess the cardiac left ventricular function, a Mikro-Tip® catheter transducer (Millar Instruments, INC) was inserted to the lumen of the left ventricle. This helped to measure the left ventricular systolic pressure (LVSP), left ventricular end-diastolic pressure (LVEDP), maximum and minimum rates of developed left ventricular pressure ($LVdP/dt_{max}$ and $LVdP/dt_{min}$

respectively) and the rate of pressure change at a fixed left ventricular pressure (LVdP/dt/P). All the parameters were continuously recorded using a Powerlab system (AD Instruments, Australia) [14].

Tissue weights

Subsequent to hemodynamic measurements, the animals were euthanized, the hearts were removed, weighed, and histological examinations were done. The wet heart weight to body weight ratio was calculated to assess the degree of myocardial weight gain.

Determination of lipid peroxidation in serum and myocardium

Malondialdehyde (MDA), a thiobarbiturate reactive substance, was measured as a marker for oxidative stress in serum and myocardial homogenates using a method prescribed by Satoh [15]. To prepare the homogenates, another set of experiment (n = 6) including all groups was repeated and 500 mg of heart tissues from apex were homogenized in a ratio of 1:10 in 0.15% KCl by means of a homogenizer. Consequently the homogenates were centrifuged at 4 000 rpm at 4°C for 10 min. Then 3 mL of phosphoric acid and 1 mL of TBA 0.67% were added to 250 μL of supernatant of each homogenate to analyze the MDA level in tissue samples. After addition of 3 mL of n-Butanol to each sample, they heated in a water bath for 40 min and the absorbance of MDA was measured spectrophotometrically. The lipid peroxidation level expressed as nanomole MDA production per gram myocardium and nonomole per milliliter serum.

Histopathological examination

The hearts were fixed in 10% buffered formalin. The heart tissues were embedded in paraffin, sectioned at 5 μm, and stained with hematoxylin and eosin (H&E) for histologic evaluation and observed microscopically. Myocardial necrosis and edematous were evaluated in each of the four quadrants of the left ventricular cross section in each heart in the zone lying within 1.5 mm of the ventricular endocardium, using a morphometric point-counting procedure [16]. Two persons graded the histopathological changes as 1, 2, 3, and 4 for low, moderate (focal myocyte damage or small multifocal degeneration with slight degree of inflammation), high (extensive myofibrillar degeneration and/or diffuse inflammatory process), and intensive (necrosis with diffuse inflammatory process) pathological changes, respectively.

Measurements of serum TNF-α level by ELISA

The serum level of TNF-α was determined using an enzyme-linked immunosorbent assay (ELISA) (Rat TNF-α, IBL, Hamburg, Germany) according to the manufacture's instruction. Briefly, the samples were homogenized or mixed in an ice-cold solution containing 50 mM Tris–HCl, 150 mM NaCl, 5 mM Sodium Pyrophosphate (NaPPi), 50 mM NaF, 1 mM EDTA, 1 mM.

dithiothreitol (DTT), 0.1%SDS (w/v), 1% TXT-100 (v/v), and protease inhibitor cocktail (Roche, Mannheim, Germany). The samples were then centrifuged twice at 10,000 (rpm) for 10 min at 4°C. The resulting supernatants were used for assay. The concentration of the cytokines was expressed as pg/ml of serum.

Statistics

Data were presented as mean ± SEM. One-way ANOVA was used to make comparisons between the groups. If the ANOVA analysis indicated significant differences, Student–Newman–Keuls post test was employed to compare the mean values between the treatment groups and the control. Differences between the groups were considered significant if $P < 0.05$.

Results

Effects of tacrolimus on electrocardiogram

The Lead II electrocardiograms obtained from animals were shown in Figure 1. The rats were received tacrolimus alone (sham) showed normal patterns of ECG, while the rats treated with isoproterenol alone (MI group) demonstrated significant changes in ECG pattern. The changes included a marked elevation of ST segment from 95 ± 5.2 μv in control group to 194 ± 14.2 μv in ISO-treated group ($P < 0.001$), and a reduction in R wave amplitude from 448 ± 27 μv in control group to 267 ± 15 μv in ISO-treated group ($P < 0.001$) which both are indicative of myocardial infarction (Figure 2). Oral treatment with tacrolimus at doses of 0.5, 1 and 2 mg/kg significantly suppressed the isoproterenol-induced ST-segment elevation from 194 ± 14.2 μv in ISO-treated group to 169 ± 12.7, 113 ± 8.4 and 121 ± 11 μv in tacrolimus-treated groups, respectively.

Furthermore, treatment with all doses of tacrolimus resulted in a significant increase in the R-amplitude ($P < 0.001$) as compared to the rats treated with isoproterenol alone (Figure 2).

Effects of tacrolimus on hemodynamic responses

The mean arterial pressure (MAP) was significantly decreased from 79.5 ± 1.78 mmHg in control group to 37 ± 1 mmHg in isoproterenol-treated group ($P < 0.001$; Table 1). There was a significant increase in the mean arterial pressure to the value of 52 ± 1.12, 79 ± 1.86 and 78.2 ± 2 mmHg, respectively, after administration of 0.5, 1 and 2 mg/kg tacrolimus.

The intraventricular pressure was measured to determine the degree of left ventricular response to isoproterenol. Isoproterenol reduced the LVSP from 112.8 ± 2.71 mmHg in the control group to 72.8 ± 1.38 mmHg ($P < 0.001$).

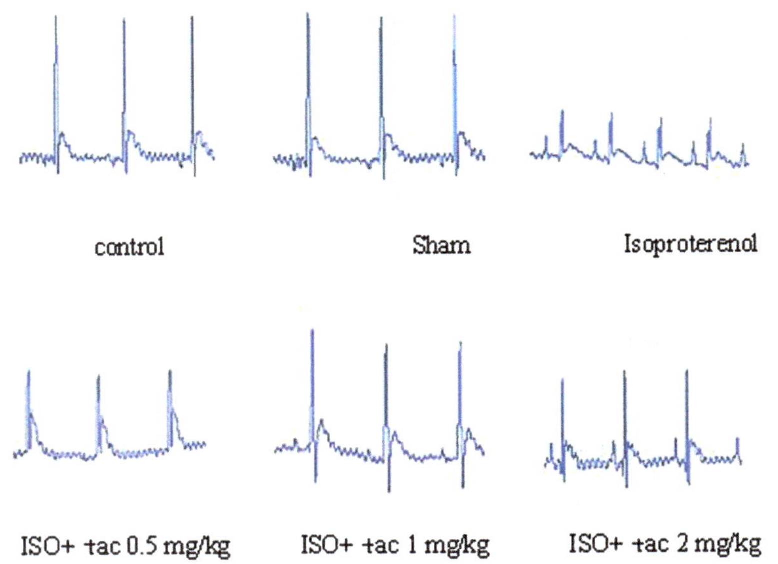

Figure 1 Effect of tacrolimus on electrocardiographic patterns and changes (recorded from limb lead II) in normal control, tacrolimus alone treated group (Sham), isoproterenol alone injected (ISO), and rats treated with tacrolimus (Tac: 0.5, 1, 2 mg/kg).

Tacrolimus was found to increase the LVSP toward the normal value in a dose-dependent manner.

Furthermore, isoproterenol treatment leads to almost a three-fold elevation in LVEDP, which was indicative of left ventricular dysfunction. All three doses of tacrolimus remarkably ($P < 0.01$) improved the left ventricular function by lowering LVEDP from 17.6 ± 0.68 mmHg in isoproterenol-treated rats to 10.2 ± 0.45, 6 ± 0.24 and 5.6 ± 0.22, respectively (Table 1).

Compared with the control group, the rats with left ventricular dysfunction (MI group) demonstrated a reduction in the value of left ventricular maximal and minimal rates of pressure (LV dP/dt_{max}; LV dP/dt_{min}; $P < 0.01$; Figure 3) as well as a lower rate of pressure change at a fixed ventricular pressure (LV dP/dt/P; $P < 0.05$; Table 1). The mentioned indices of myocardial contractility, along with LVSP, were considerably improved by administration of all three doses of tacrolimus (Figure 3). In this regard, tacrolimus at doses of 0.5, 1 and 2 mg/kg significantly increased LV dP/dt_{Max} to 3702 ± 308 ($P < 0.05$), 4484 ± 318 ($P < 0.001$) and 4592 ± 333 mmHg/s ($P < 0.001$), respectively, from 2712 ± 181 mmHg/s in isoproterenol alone treated group. Tacrolimus had a similar effect on LV dP/dt_{Min}.

Effects of tacrolimus on the heart weight to body weight ratio

The heart weight to body weight ratio (mg/kg) was determined to evaluate the amount of heart weight gain developed by the injection of isoproterenol (Figure 4). Isoproterenol injection significantly increased the ratio from 2.58 ± 0.22 in control group to 3.94 ± 0.14 ($P < 0.01$). Acute treatment with 1 mg/kg of tacrolimus resulted in a substantial ($P < 0.01$) reduction in the heart to body weight ratio in comparison to the isoproterenol alone treated rats.

Effects of tacrolimus on lipid peroxidation

To determine the lipid peroxidation, MDA levels were measured in serum and myocardial homogenates. Both serum and heart MDA levels were considerably increased ($P < 0.001$) in isoproterenol alone treated rats in comparison with normal control group (Table 2). However, treatment with tacrolimus significantly suppressed the rise of MDA levels of serum and myocardium ($P < 0.001$; Table 2).

Histopathological examination of the cardiac tissue

In the control group, myocardial fibers were arranged regularly with clear striations, without any damage or necrosis in the tissue (Figure 5). Histopathological sections of the isoproterenol alone treated hearts displayed extensive hypertrophy, necrosis and increased edematous inter muscular space. Scoring the necrosis showed that all three doses of tacrolimus significantly prevented inflammatory responses. Tacrolimus at doses of 0.5, 1 and 2 mg/kg reduced isoproterenol-induced edema and necrosis by 28% ($P < 0.05$), 35% ($P < 0.01$) and 24% ($P < 0.05$), respectively (Figure 6).

Effects of tacrolimus on the level of TNF-α in serum after myocardial infarction

In the present study, the effects of tacrolimus on the concentration of TNF-α in serum of rats with isoproterenol

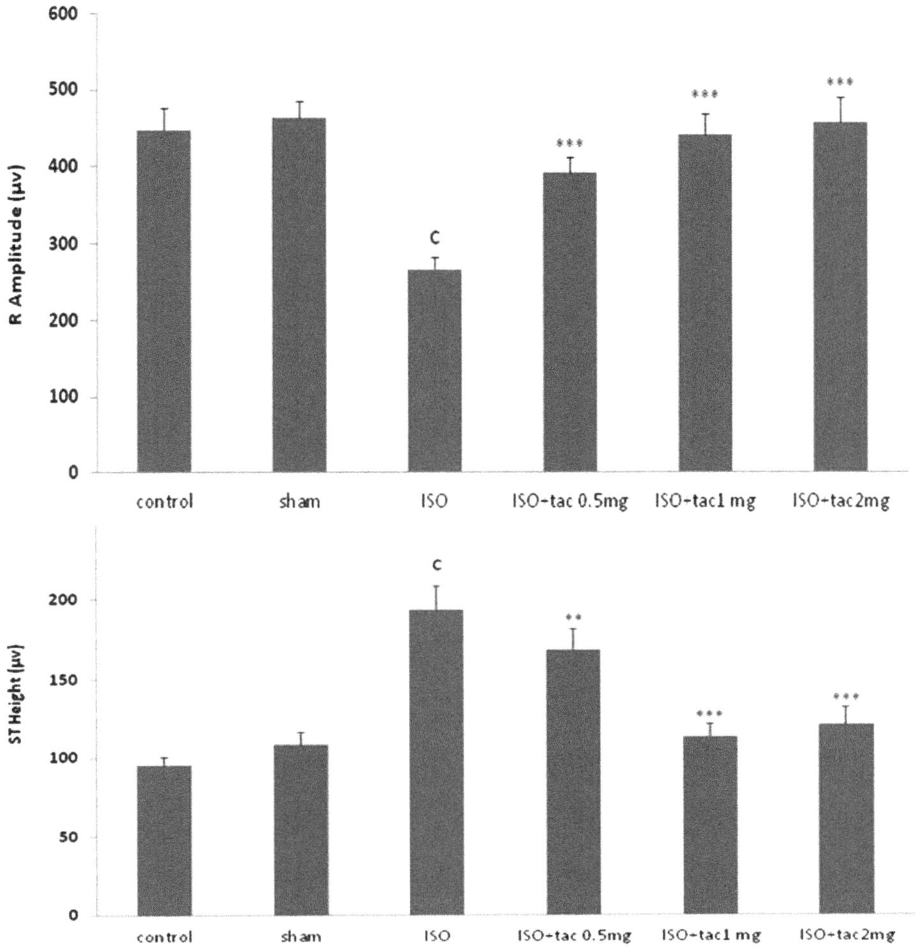

Figure 2 Effects of oral administration of tacrolimus (tac) on ST segment and R-amplitude (recorded from limb lead II). [c]P < 0.001 compared to normal controls. **P < 0.01 and ***P < 0.001 as compared to the ISO-treated group. Data are reported as mean ± SEM (n = 6).

induced MI were also investigated in order to determine whether inflammatory condition in myocardium are associated with the level of pro-inflammatory cytokines. It was found that the level of TNF-α was profoundly increased in the isoproterenol group in comparison to the control group (P < 0.001) in serum (Figure 7). It was observed that tacrolimus alone (100 mg/kg/12 h) in the sham group had no effect on the level of TNF-α in serum. The increased level of TNF-α by isoproterenol was markedly decreased by treatment with tacrolimus serum. The maximal effect

Table 1 Effects of short term oral administration of tacrolimus (tac) on hemodynamic parameters in normal and isoproterenol (ISO) induced myocardial infarction rats

Groups	MAP ± SEM (mmHg)	HR ± SEM (bpm)	LVSP ± SEM (mmHg)	LVEDP ± SEM (mmHg)	LVdp/dt/p ± SEM (1/sec)
Control	79.5 ± 1.78	197.8 ± 3.05	112.8 ± 2.71	6.3 ± 0.21	85.2 ± 1.49
Sham	80.4 ± 2.52	216.4 ± 6.21	117.6 ± 4.03	5.4 ± 0.36	85.6 ± 1.52
ISO	37 ± 1.05[c]	290 ± 7.9[c]	72.8 ± 1.389[c]	17.6 ± 0.68[c]	53.4 ± 1.07[a]
ISO + tac 0.5 mg	52 ± 1.12*	247 ± 7.35*	83.4 ± 1.57	10.2 ± 0.45***	65 ± 1.96*
ISO + tac 1 mg	79.8 ± 1.86***	200.2 ± 4.84***	120.6 ± 3.76***	6 ± 0.24***	86.6 ± 2.07***
ISO + tac 2 mg	78.2 ± 2.06***	212.8 ± 5.43***	117.8 ± 3.24***	5.6 ± 0.22***	83.4 ± 1.95***

[a]P < 0.05, [c]P < 0.001 compared to normal control group. *P < 0.05 and ***P < 0.001 as compared to the ISO-treated group. Mean arterial pressure (MAP), heart rate (HR), left ventricular systolic pressure (LVSP), left ventricular end diastolic pressure (LVEDP), left ventricular pressure changes at a fixed pressure (LV dP/dt/P). Data are shown as mean ± SEM (n = 6).

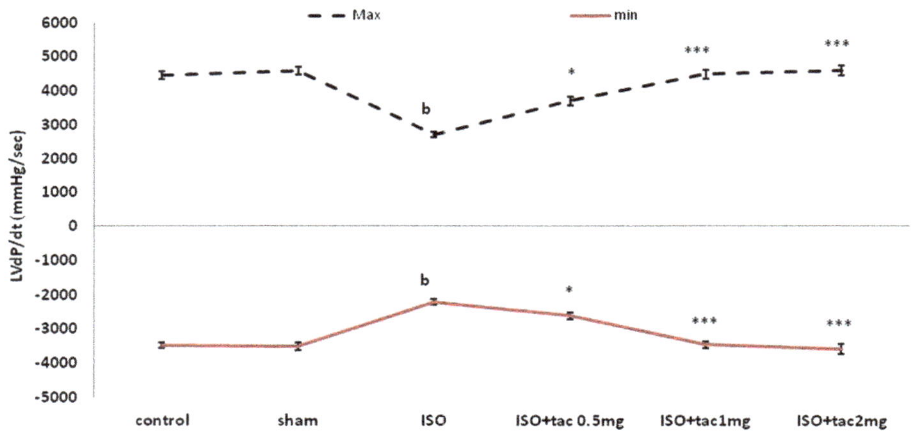

Figure 3 The effect of oral administration of tacrolimus (tac) on the minimum and maximum left ventricular pressure ($LVdP/dt_{Max}$, $LVdP/dt_{Min}$). [c]P < 0.001 as compared to the normal control group, *P < 0.05 and ***P < 0.001 as compared to the ISO-treated group. Data are reported as mean ± SEM (n = 6).

was seen by 1 mg/kg of tacrolimus, where the concentration of TNF-α was significantly reduced from 410 ± 22 pg/mL of serum to 160 ± 14 pg/mL (P < 0.001) (Figure 7).

Discussion

Electrocardiogram (ECG) is considered the most important clinical tool for the diagnosis of many types of myocardial infarction, especially for detection of ST segment elevation myocardial infarction (STEMI). Subcutaneous injection of isoproterenol (100 mg/kg) for two consecutive days caused ST- segment elevation and R-amplitude depression. The elevated ST-segment implies the loss of cell membrane function and the consequent potential difference between the ischemic and non-ischemic regions and the depressed R-amplitude might be due to the isoproterenol-induced myocardial edema [14]. Tacrolimus administration significantly amended the ECG pattern, indicating its protective effects on cell membrane function and electrical discharges.

Isoproterenol injection was followed by a significant decrease in arterial pressure indices, including ventricular contractility ($LVdP/dt_{max}$) and relaxation ($LVdP/dt_{min}$), as well as an increase in the left ventricular end-diastolic pressure (LVEDP). These disturbances were compatible with the hemodynamic changes occurring in the acute myocardial infarction.

The principal goal of post-MI therapy is to preserve the contractility of the heart ($LVdP/dt_{max}$ and $LVdP/dt_{min}$) and to decrease the elevated LVEDP. Lower values of LVEDP result in improved blood flow to the subendocardial tissue, which is greatly susceptible to ischemic necrosis.

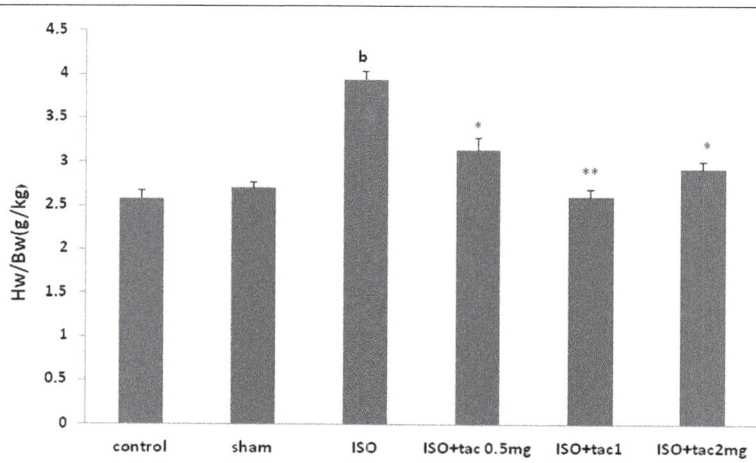

Figure 4 Effects of isoproterenol (ISO) injection as well as tacrolimus (tac) on heart weight (HW) to body weight (BW) ratio as an index of tissue edemathose in different groups. [b]P < 0.01 compared to respective group in healthy animals, *P < 0.05 and **P < 0.01 as compared to isoproterenol (ISO) treated group. Data are reported as mean ± SEM (n = 6).

Table 2 The effects of acute treatment with tacrolimus (tac) on malondialdehyde (MDA) levels in the serum and heart tissue of control and rats with myocardial infarction

Groups (n = 6)	MDA (nmol/mL serum)	MDA (nmol/g tissue)
Control	5.4 ± 0.48	2.7 ± 0.08
sham	4.9 ± 0.3	2.4 ± 0.09
Isoproterenol (Iso)	13.7 ± 0.2[a]	5.78 ± 0.17[c]
Iso + tac (0.5 mg/kg)	7.8 ± 1.7***	4.54 ± 0.12**
Iso + tac (1 mg/kg)	7.2 ± 0.6***	2.9 ± 0.06***
Iso + tac (2 mg/kg)	4.2 ± 0.5***	2.5 ± 0.09***

[a]P < 0.001, [c]P < 0.01 from respective control value; *P < 0.05, **P < 0.01 and ***P < 0.001 as compared with ISO-treated group. Data are expressed as mean ± SEM (n = 6).

The results of the present study clearly demonstrated the beneficial effects of acute treatment with tacrolimus, administered concurrently with the induction of myocardial infarction, on various parameters of cardiac function. Tacrolimus was found to effectively raise the arterial blood pressure and myocardial contractility, along with decreasing the left ventricular end diastolic pressure.

Tacrolimus had more significant protective effects on the left ventricular function at the low dose of 1 mg/kg compared with the dose of 2 mg/kg. This might be due to the paradoxical effects of the high dose of tacrolimus on inflammatory process and on intracellular calcium homestasis. Tacrolimus binds to FKBP and suppresses inflammatory responses. On the other hand, since FKBP plays a critical role in modulating myocardial calcium homeostasis by stabilizing ryanodine receptors, the binding may disturbs the calcium homeostasis and therefore, reverse the protective effects of the drug [7,11]. It seems

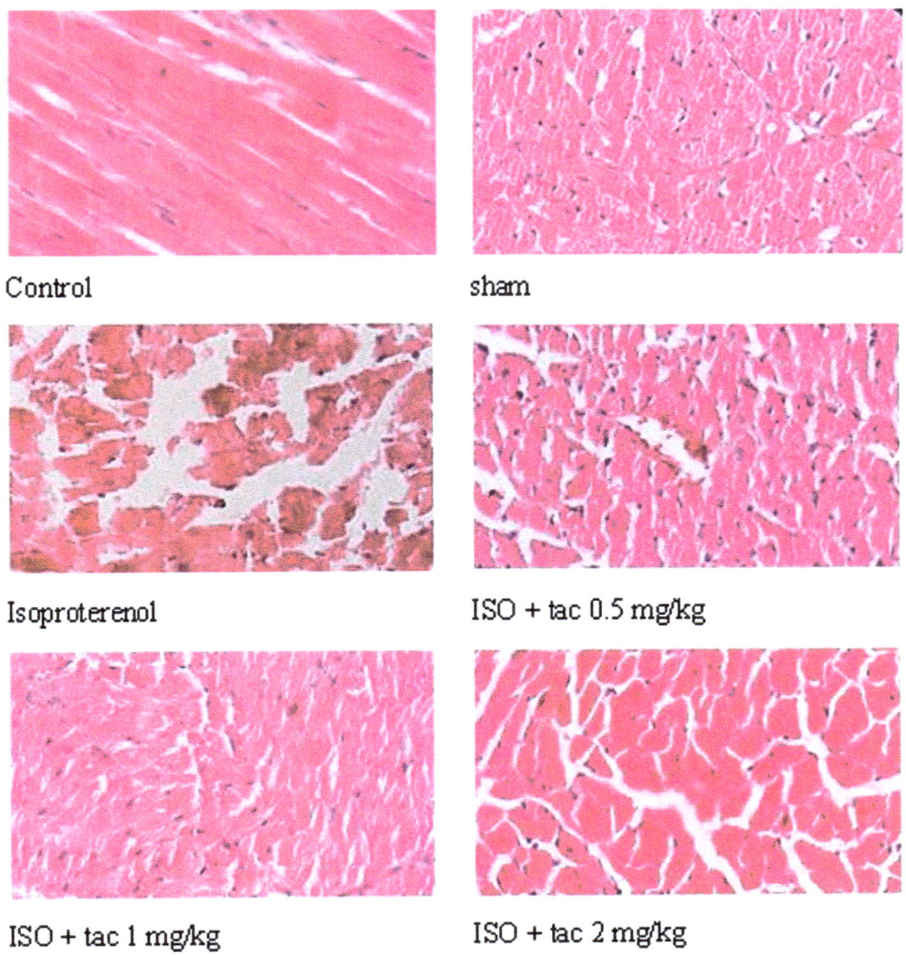

Figure 5 Photomicrographs of sections of rat cardiac apexes. Heart tissue of a rat treated with isoproterenol (ISO) showed intensive cardiomyocyte necrosis and increased edematous intramuscular space. Acute treatment with tacrolimus (tac) demonstrated a marked improvement. H&E (40' magnification).

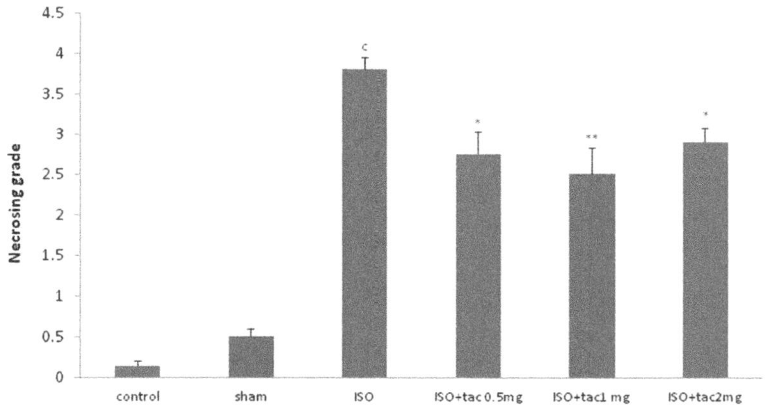

Figure 6 Grading of histopathological changes in the rat's cardiac apex tissues. Grades 1, 2, 3, and 4 showed low, moderate, high and intensive pathological changes, respectively. $^{c}P < 0.001$ compared to respective group in healthy animals, $^{*}P < 0.05$ and $^{**}P < 0.01$ as compared to isoproterenol treated group. Data are reported as mean ± SEM (n = 6).

that the high dose of the drug reduces remodeling by suppressing inflammatory responses and meanwhile, it inhibits the stabilizing effects of FKBP on ryanodine receptors by binding to it [17].

The importance of oxidative stress is implicated in the pathology of myocardial infarction. There is appreciable evidence validating the direct toxic effects of free radicals on heart tissue [18]. In fact, one of the mechanisms of isoproterenol-induced myocardial infarction is to generate highly cytotoxic free radicals, as superoxide. Malondialdehyde, a product of the oxidative degradation of unsaturated fatty acids, is a biomarker of oxidative stress, and the concentration increases in response to the free radical production in myocardial infarction, and decreases by antioxidant systems [19,20]. The results of the present study suggest that tacrolimus possesses an in vivo antioxidant activity. Tacrolimus administration substantially reduced peroxylipid levels by 50 - 70% in isoproterenol-induced myocardial infarction. This reduction may relate to blunted polymorphonuclear leukocyte accumulation [21]. Tacrolimus treatment ameliorates oxidative stress augmentation which plays a pivotal role in the myocardial infarction pathology.

Histopathological examination of infarcted myocardial tissue elucidated extensive hypertrophy, subendocardial necrosis, and edema. All three doses of tacrolimus considerably attenuated the edema and necrosis in the isoproterenol-treated heart.

The heart to body weight ratio was significantly increased following isoproterenol injection. The heart weight gain might be due to water absorption and increase in protein content of muscular cells. Cardiac hypertrophy is due to increased cardiac performance. Treatment with all doses of tacrolimus markedly reduced the heart to body weight ratio. However, the drug was very effective at the low dose of 1 mg/kg.

Conclusions

Limited data are available on the cardioprotective effects of tacrolimus. However, our study finds that administration of tacrolimus, simultaneous to the myocardial infarction incidence, has a remarkable protective potential

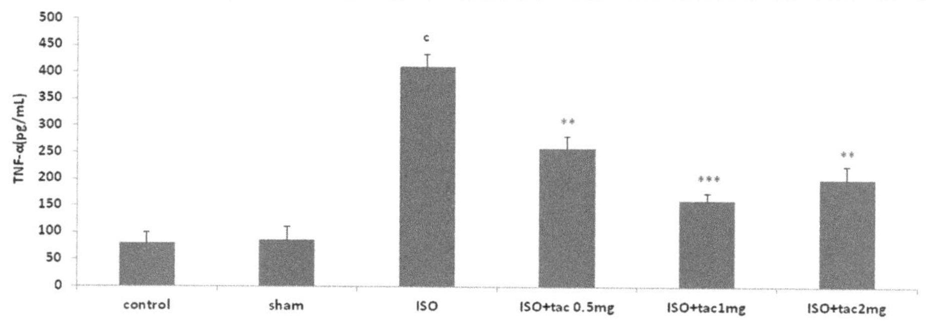

Figure 7 The effect of acute and short term treatment with tacrolimus (tac) at the doses of 0.5, 1 and 2 mg/kg/12 h on TNFα concentration in serum. $^{c}P < 0.001$ from respective control value; $^{**}P < 0.01$ and $^{***}P < 0.001$ as compared with isoproterenol (ISO) injected group. Data are reported as mean ± SEM (n = 6).

against damages caused by isoproterenol-induced myocardial infarction. The cardioprotective effects of acute treatment with tacrolimus are confirmed by amending electrocardiographic pattern, improvement of hemodynamic and left ventricular functions, and less histopathological damage following isoproterenol-induced myocardial infarction. It is proposed that tacrolimus exerts this cardioprotective effects through its anti-inflammatory and antioxidant properties. Although this study has provided a possible new therapeutic tool for myocardial infarction, more studies are required to elucidate the precise mechanism of tacrolimus in reversing the pathogenesis of myocardial infarction.

Competing interests

The authors declare that they have no competing interests.

Authors' contribution

MH Carried out animals grouping and handling and the biochemical experiments. AK Carried out the hemodynamic experiments. MG Accompanied Mojtaba Hammami in MI induction and helped in preparing manuscript. NM Histopathological works and interpretations. AG Supervising and directing the project carried out the data analysis and interpretations and prepared the manuscript. All authors read and approved the final manuscript.

Acknowledgments

The present study was supported by a grant from the Research Vice Chancellors of Tabriz University of Medical Sciences; Tabriz, Iran. This article is based on a thesis submitted for PharmD degree (No: 5/4/3419) in Faculty of Pharmacy, Tabriz University of Medical Sciences, Tabriz, Iran.

Author details

[1]Department of Pharmacology and Toxicology, Faculty of Pharmacy, Tabriz University of Medical Sciences, Tabriz, Iran. [2]Student Research Committee, Tabriz University of Medical Sciences, Tabriz, Iran.

References

1. Xie N, Zhang W, Li J, Liang H, Zhou H, Duan W, Xu X, Yu S, Zhang H, Yi D: **α-linolenic acid intake attenuates myocardial ischemia/reperfusion injury through anti-inflammatory and anti-oxidative stress effects in diabetic but not normal rats.** *Arch Med Res* 2011, **42**:171–181.
2. Colditz GA, Rimm EB, Giovannucci E, Stampfer MJ, Rosner B, Willett WC: **A prospective study of parental history off myocardial infarction and coronary artery disease in men.** *Am J Cardiol* 1991, **67**:933–938.
3. Neumar RW, Browns CG, Robitaille P-ML, Altschul RA: **Myocardial high energy phosphate metabolism during ventricular fibrillation with total circulatory arrest.** *Resuscitation* 1990, **19**:199–226.
4. Ivan Hall R, Amos Moffitt E: **The effects of anaesthetics on coronary artery blood flow and myocardial metabolism: a review of studies in animals and man.** *Baillières Clin Anaesthesiol* 1989, **3**:27–46.
5. Bodi V, Sanchis J, Morales JM, Marrachelli VG, Nunez J, Forteza MJ, Chaustre F, Gomez C, Mainar L, Minana G, Rumiz E, Husser O, Noguera I, Diaz A, Moratal D, Carratala A, Bosch X, Llacer A, Chorro FJ, Viña JR, Monleon D: **Metabolomic profile of human myocardial ischemia by nuclear magnetic resonance spectroscopy of peripheral blood serum: a translational study based on transient coronary occlusion models.** *J Am Coll Cardiol* 2012, **59**:1629–1641.
6. Maekawa N, Wada H, Kanda T, Niwa T, Yamada Y, Saito K, Fujiwara H, Sekikawa K, Seishima M: **Improved myocardial ischemia/reperfusion injury in mice lacking tumor necrosis factor-α.** *J Am Coll Cardiol* 2002, **39**:1229–1235.
7. Yang CH, Sheu JJ, Tsai TH, Chua S, Chang LT, Chang HW, Lee FY, Chen YL, Chung SY, Sun CK, Leu S, Yen CH, Yip HK: **Effect of tacrolimus on myocardial infarction is associated with inflammation, ROS, MAP kinase and Akt pathways in mini-pigs.** *J Atheroscler Thromb* 2013, **20**:9–22.
8. Mazzone A, Cusa C, Mazzucchelli I, Vezzoli M, Ottini E, Pacifici R, Zuccaro P, Falcone C: **Increased production of inflammatory cytokines in patients with silent myocardial ischemia.** *J Am Coll Cardiol* 2001, **38**:1895–1901.
9. Van Rossum H, Romijn F, Smit N, de Fijter J, Van Pelt J: **Everolimus and sirolimus antagonize tacrolimus based calcineurin inhibition via competition for FK-binding protein 12.** *Biochem Pharmacol* 2009, **77**:1206–1212.
10. Chua S, Leu S, Sheu JJ, Lin YC, Chang LT, Kao YH, Yen CH, Tsai TH, Chen YL, Chang HW, Sun CK, Yip HK: **Intra-coronary administration of tacrolimus markedly attenuates infarct size and preserves heart function in porcine myocardial infarction.** *J Inflamm* 2012, **9**:21–33.
11. Su Z, Sugishita K, Li F, Ritter M, Barry W: **Effects of FK506 on [Ca2+]i differ in mouse and rabbit ventricular myocytes.** *J Pharmacol Exp Ther* 2003, **304**:334–341.
12. Yousefi K, Soraya H, Fathiazad F, Khorrami A, Hamedeyazdan S, Maleki-Dizaji N, Garjani A: **Cardioprotective effect of methanolic extract of Marrubium vulgare L. on isoproterenol-induced acute myocardial infarction in rats.** *Indian J Exp Biol* 2013, **51**:653–660.
13. Fathiazad F, Matlobi A, Khorrami A, Hamedeyazdan S, Soraya H, Hammami M, Maleki-Dizaji N, Garjani A: **Phytochemical screening and evaluation of cardioprotective activity of ethanolic extract of Ocimum basilicum L. (basil) against isoproterenol induced myocardial infarction in rats.** *DARU J Pharm Sci* 2012, **20**:87–97.
14. Garjani A, Andalib S, Biabani S, Soraya H, Doustar Y, Garjani A, Maleki-Dizaji N: **Combined atorvastatin and coenzyme Q10 improve the left ventricular function in isoproterenol-induced heart failure in rat.** *Eur J Pharmacol* 2011, **666**:135–141.
15. Satoh K: **Serum lipid peroxide in cerebrovascular disorders determined by a new colorimetric method.** *Clinica Chimica Acta* 1978, **90**:37–43.
16. Benjamin IJ, Jalil JE, Tan LB, Cho K, Weber KT, Clark WA: **Isoproterenol-induced myocardial fibrosis in relation to myocyte necrosis.** *Circ Res* 1989, **65**:657–670.
17. Shawn D, St. P, Adyr AM, David CM: **Effects of tacrolimus on ischemia-reperfusion injury.** *Liver Transpl* 2003, **9**:105–116.
18. Rona G: **Catecholamine cardiotoxicity.** *J Mol Cell Cardiol* 1985, **7**:291–306.
19. Radovanovic S, Savic-Radojevic A, Pljesa-Ercegovac M, Djukic T, Suvakov S, Krotin M, Simic DV, Matic M, Radojicic Z, Pekmezovic T, Simic T: **Markers of oxidative damage and antioxidant enzyme activities as predictors of morbidity and mortality in patients with chronic heart failure.** *J Card Fail* 2012, **18**:493–501.
20. Ho E, Karimi Galougahi K, Liu C-C, Bhindi R, Figtree GA: **Biological markers of oxidative stress: applications to cardiovascular research and practice.** *Redox Biol* 2013, **1**:483–491.
21. Squadrito F, Altavilla D, Squadrito G, Saitta A, Deodato B, Arlotta M, Minutoli L, Quartarone C, Ferlito M, Caputi AP: **Tacrolimus limits polymorphonuclear leucocyte accumulation and protects against myocardial ischaemia–reperfusion injury.** *J Mol Cell Cardiol* 2000, **32**:429–440.

The immunological benefit of higher dose N-acetyl cysteine following mechanical ventilation in critically ill patients

Atabak Najafi[1], Mojtaba Mojtahedzadeh[1,2,3], Keyvan Haji Ahmadi[2], Mohammad Abdollahi[3], Maryam Mousavi[4], Legese Chelkeba[2,3], Farhad Najmeddin[2] and Arezoo Ahmadi[1*]

Abstract

Background: Sepsis complication is a major cause of death in multiple trauma critically ill patients. Defensin (cysteine rich anti-microbial peptides), as an important component of immune system, might play an important role in this process. There is also rising data on immunological effects of N-acetyl-cysteine (NAC), a commonly used anti-oxidant in oxidative stress conditions and glutathione (GSH) deficiencies. The aim of the present study was to evaluate the potential beneficial effects of NAC administration on multiple trauma patients with sepsis.

Methods: In a prospective, randomized controlled study, 44 multiple trauma critically ill patients who were mechanically ventilated and met the criteria of sepsis and admitted to the intensive care unit (ICU) were randomized into two groups . Control group received all standard ICU therapies and NAC group received intravenous NAC 3 gr every 6 hours for 72 hours in addition to standard therapies. Acute Physiology and Chronic Health Evaluation II (APACHE II) and Sequential Organ Failure Assessment (SOFA) scores, length of ICU stay, ICU mortality were recorded. Levels of serum Immunoglobulin M (IgM), Human β-Defensin 2 (HβD2) and GSH were assessed at baseline and 24, 72, 120 hours after intervention.

Results: During a period of 13-month screening, 44 patients underwent randomization but 5 patients had to be excluded. 21 patients in NAC group and 18 patients in control group completed the study. For both groups the length of ICU stay, SOFA score and systemic oxygenation were similar. Mortality rate (40% vs. 22% respectively, $p = 0.209$) and ventilator days (Mean ± SD 19.82 ± 19.55 days vs. 13.82 ± 11.89 days respectively, $p = 0.266$) were slightly higher for NAC group. IgM and GSH levels were similar between two groups ($p = 0.325$, 0.125 respectively), HβD2 levels were higher for NAC group (at day 3).

Conclusion: High dose of NAC administration not only did not improve patients' outcome, but also raised the risk of inflammation and was associated with increased serum creatinine.

Keywords: N-Acetyl, Cysteine (NAC), Glutathione (GSH), Human β Defensin 2 (HβD2), Immunoglobulin M (IgM), Multiple trauma, Sepsis

Background

Multiple trauma, a complex syndrome of injuries to various anatomical regions with defined intensity and subsequent systemic reactions [1]. Trauma is the major cause of death before the age of 45 in developed countries [2,3], claiming over 6 million kills annually around the world which is preventable in approximately 20% of cases [4,5]. Three pre-eminent causes of death in this patients are head trauma, hemorrhage and sepsis/Multi Organ Failure (MOF) [6]. Tissue ischemia induces Reactive Oxygen Species (ROS) production which in turn activates neutrophils and attracts them to the injury site. Extensive progression of this and other similar processes following trauma insult enhance the local inflammatory response to remote organs, resulting in the development of Systemic Inflammatory Response Syndrome (SIRS) [7-12]. In sepsis,

* Correspondence: aarezoo24@gmail.com
[1]Department of Anesthesiology and Critical Care Medicine, Sina Hospital, Faculty of Medicine, Tehran University of Medical Sciences, Tehran, Iran
Full list of author information is available at the end of the article

acute immunologic response and excessive release of pro-inflammatory cytokines [Interleukin 1(IL-1), Tumor Necrosis Factor α (TNF-α)] trigger target cells (leukocytes, endothelial cells, hepatocytes, lung and intestine epithelium) and induce cytokine, chemokine, ROS and proteolytic enzymes production [13-16].

It is obvious that patients with sepsis or multiple trauma require mechanical ventilation support. Due to the high concentration of inspired oxygen used, the probability of alveolar epithelial damage is high as the result of formation of free oxygen radicals. Some studies have suggested that the use of high doses of antioxidants in these patients could be beneficial [7].

Defensins are cysteine rich endogenous antimicrobial peptides which consist of to approximately 5% of total granulocyte proteins, following infection their levels in systemic circulation increases, defensins have a significant effect on a wide spectrum of microorganisms [17-19] and beyond that they also act as immunologic mediators [20]. Human β Defensin 2 (HβD2) is an inducible defensin, whose induction is impaired during sepsis [20,21].

NAC is a well-known anti-oxidant which is administered in various conditions where oxidative stress is present [22-24]. NAC is thiol containing compound that in addition to direct radical scavenging properties is a precursor for glutathione (GSH) synthesis [23,24]. NAC seems to have immunological effects (doses higher than 12 gram/day) that can affect different cytokines (IL-2, IL-4, IL-6, IL-10, TNF-α, NF-κB) [25,26] and phagocytic function [27]. NAC has received so much credit for its nephro-protective properties when used prior to radio-contrast media administration. The ischemia compounded by increased medullary O_2consumption may somewhat resemble ischemic acute tubular necrosis (ATN) in trauma and sepsis. Although near 10 Meta-Analyses has been published to justify its use many of these studies have significant pitfalls [25-27].

To our knowledge there are no studies about the effect of NAC as an antioxidant and/or immunomodulator in patients with SIRS/sepsis criteria following multiple trauma. Therefore, this study aimed to investigate HβD2 levels in multiple trauma patients with SIRS/sepsis and its potential correlation with progress and outcome of therapy, and to evaluate the effects of high dose NAC administration, in the early onset of sepsis during first hours to days after trauma, on immunologic responses and overall outcome. Furthermore, this study sought to examine the hypothesis that NAC administration can alter HβD2 levels either by immuno-modulatory activity or as a cysteine source.

Methods

Study design and patient population

Between March 2011 to April 2012, this prospective randomized clinical trial was conducted in general ICU of "Sina"and "Imam Khomeini" Hospital of Tehran University of Medical Sciences (TUMS), Iran. In all cases, informed consents were received from their legal guardian. The study protocol was approved by the ethical committee of TUMS. Our clinical trial was registered in Iranian Registry of Clinical Trial with code number of (IRCT 2014010716120 N1).

All the patients enrolled in the study had multiple trauma. The inclusion criteria were age older than 18 years, mechanical ventilation with FiO_2 more than 50%, an Acute Physiology and Chronic Health Evaluation (APACHE) II score greater than 15, suspected infection and at least two Systemic Inflammatory Response (SIRS) criteria (defined as the following conditions: body temperature > 38°C or < 36°C, heart rate > 90 beats/min, respiratory rate > 20 breath/min or $Paco_2 < 32$ mmHg, WBC >12,000 cells/mm^3, or < 4000 cells/mm^3, or > 10% immature [band] cells) diagnosed during the first 24 hours of ICU admission. Exclusion criteria for all patients were ages below 18 years, pregnancy, breast feeding, beyond 24 hours of sepsis diagnosis, Central Venous Pressure (CVP) > 18 mmHg, Systolic Blood Pressure < 90 mmHg or Mean Arterial Pressure (MAP) < 60 mmHg, Serum Creatinine ≥ 2 mg/dl, liver dysfunction (defined as the presence of hepatic cirrhosis or concentration of serum transaminases greater than third times the upper limit of normal range), history of myocardial infarction or heart failure (EF < 40%) and those received N-acetyl Cysteine (NAC) before initiation of study.

Patients were randomized via block randomization to receive one of the following treatments: standard treatment for sepsis (control group) and standard treatment plus NAC (intervention group) for 72 hours. Standard treatments for sepsis were implemented as following: early resuscitation within the first 6 hours of admission, appropriate diagnostic studies to ascertain causative organisms before starting antibiotics, early administration of broad-spectrum antibiotic therapy, reassessment of antibiotic therapy with microbiology and clinical data to narrow coverage, appropriate Volume resuscitation or vasopressor therapy, Mechanical ventilation adjusted to maintain $SaO_2 > 95\%$, $PaO_2 > 90$ mmHg and $PaCO_2$ between 38 and 42 mmHg, appropriate analgesia and sedation provided for all patients, insulin treatment was administered to maintain glucose at < 200 mg/dl and appropriate prophylactic measures for deep vein thrombosis (DVT) and stress-related mucosal damage (SRMD). Patients in intervention group received intravenous NAC (Exir Pharmaceutical company, Tehran, Iran) 3gr in 250 ml 5% dextrose over 30 min every 6 hours for the first 72 hours of admission (Figure 1).

Demographic data and clinical information were obtained at the beginning. Monitoring parameters including MAP, heart rate, respiratory rate and CVP of each patient were recorded in the ICU flow sheets every

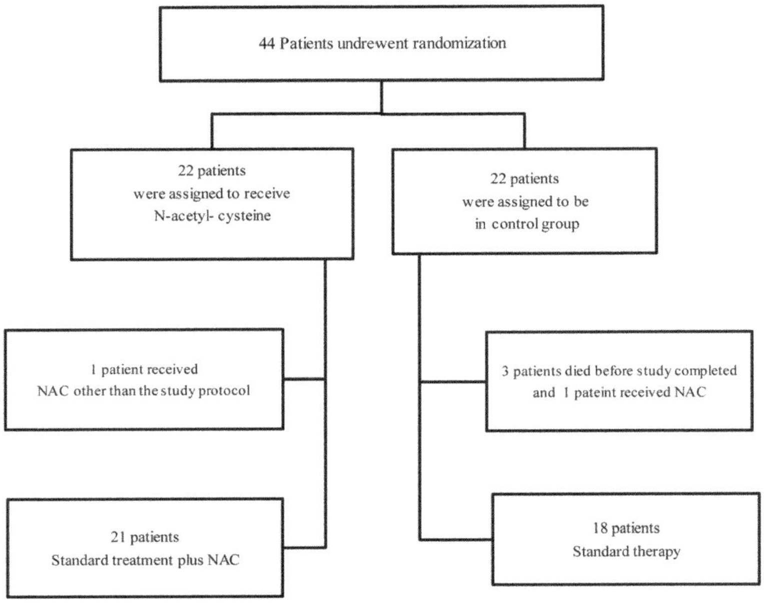

Figure 1 Enrollment and protocol study.

3 hours. Laboratory data including serum creatinine, Blood Urea Nitrogen (BUN), hemoglobin, platelet and white blood cell (WBC) counts, albumin, sodium and potassium were also collected daily during 5 days of study period.

Measurements

All patients had central venous catheter and arterial catheter for blood sampling. For all patients there were four scheduled time points to assess the level of IgM, GSH and HβD2. Blood samples were collected at baseline and 24, 72 and 120 hours after intervention and centrifuged at 3000 × g for 15 minutes to remove cells and cellular debris. The plasma stored at −80°C until the time of analysis. Levels of IgM, GSH and HβD2 were measured by commercially available enzyme-linked immunosorbent assay (ELISA) kits (CUSABIO® biotech co LTD, Wuhan Hubei, China) according to manufacturer instruction.

APACHE score was measured at the beginning and Sequential organ failure assessment (SOFA) score was calculated daily for 5 days. Length of ICU stay, ICU mortality and ventilator free days were recorded for all patients.

Statistical Analysis

All data were expressed as Mean ± SD. The unpaired *t* test for parametric data and Mann–Whitney test for nonparametric data were used to compare the differences between the treatment groups at each time point. Comparisons of the differences between the time points in each treatment group, repeated-measure one-way analysis of variance and nonparametric analysis of variance (Friedman test) were performed to analyze changes in levels of the biomarkers. The paired *t* test for parametric data and Wilcoxon rank sum test for nonparametric data were done to analyze changes in variables with 2 time points (at baseline and 24 hours after). P values less than 0.05 were considered statistically significant.

Results

Between March 2011 to April 2012, 44 consecutive patients who met the inclusion criteria were enrolled in the study. Five patients excluded from the study, three of them died before the end of the study and the other 2 patients received NAC dosage other than the study protocol. The remaining 39 patients were randomly assigned to NAC group and control group, each with 21 and 18 patients respectively. Demographic and baseline values for APACHE and SOFA scores have been summarized in Table 1. The differences in age and sex were not significant between two groups. ($p = 0.450$ and 0.204 respectively). Differences in baseline values for APACHE and SOFA scores were not statistically significant either (Table 1). Also the patients in each group were similar at baseline regarding to heart rate, MAP, temperature and Pao_2/Fio_2 (Table 1).

In comparison between two groups, in NAC group, ventilator days were longer (19.82 ± 19.55 vs. 13.82 ± 11.69 days), length of ICU stay was shorter (21.2 ± 20.71 vs. 27.72 ± 39.46 days) and mortality rate was higher (40% versus 22%), although the differences in ventilator days, length of ICU stay and mortality rate were not statistically significant ($p = 0.266$, $p = 0.545$, $p = 0.209$

Table 1 Demographic and baseline clinical characteristic of patients

	Control group	NAC group	P value
Age (years)	44.44 ± 17.684	40.14 ± 17.828	0.450
Male number	15	20	0.204
APACHE II	20.06 ± 5.162	21.05 ± 512	0.476
SOFA	7.28 ± 2.109	6.86 ± 1.457	0.468
GCS	7.28 ± 1.934	6.55 ± 1.143	0.145
MAP(mmHg)	92.72 ± 17.376	93.39 ± 14.467	0.899
HR(beat/min)	89.94 ± 18.005	97.09 ± 19.079	0.234
Temperature(°C)	37.339 ± 1.01	37.145 ± 0.965	0.536
PaO2/FiO2	196.607 ± 105.504	219.594 ± 123.307	0.529
SCr(mg/dl)	1.046±	1.053 ± 0.373	0.945

NAC: N-Acetylcysteine, APACHE: Acute Physiology and Chronic Health Evaluation, SOFA: Sequential Organ Failure Assessment, GCS: Glasgow Coma Scale, MAP: Mean Arterial Pressure, HR: Heart Rate.
Data shown as Mean ± SD. P values <0.05 consired significant.

respectively). Moreover, SOFA scores are associated with a trend towards a reduction in NAC group specially on day 3 but the trend was not statistically significant (Figure 2).

Pao_2:Fio_2 ratio improved in both groups (specially in the NAC group on day 3), although the difference was not significant (p = 0.567) (Figure 3). An upward trend in MAP, heart rate, WBC counts and Absolute Neutrophil Count (ANC) were shown in NAC group on day 1 through 5 after the start of NAC (Table 2). By means of paired *t*-test (before-after analysis) method, we had a significant decline in mean serum creatinine level between 1–3 days in control group (1.04 ± 0.25 versus 0.891 ± 0.253 p = 0.019). The mean serum creatinine level rose on day 1 through 3 in NAC group, however; this increase was not statistically significant (1.05 ± 0.373 versus 1.48 ± 2.87, p = 0.514). On day 5, creatinine levels reached similar levels in both groups (0.851 ± 0.205 Control group versus 0.920 ± 0.385 NAC group p = 0.502).

Furthermore the changes in the level of IgM (p = 0.325) and GSH (p = 0.125) were not significant among two groups but the mean serum levels of GSH were higher in NAC group (Table 3). Despite a non significant difference in HβD2 levels between two groups (p = 0.463), HβD2 levels are associated with a trend towards an increase in NAC group specially on day 3 (Figure 4).

Discussion

The aim of the current study was to focus on potential immunological effects of NAC administration in critical illness, we have also reassessed the antioxidant properties which had already been well established. In previous study, immunological effects of NAC were seen with doses relatively higher than usual dosage for antioxidant effects (higher than 9 gram/day) [25-27]. So we have administered 12 gram/day of NAC in our study. The previous study [24] reviewed the effects of NAC in a condition of GSH deficiency such as pulmonary disease and oxidative stress, they concluded that oral administration of NAC was a safe and beneficial supplement in setting of GSH deficiency. In other study conducted on piglets, it was observed that NAC has no significant effect on the total GSH level [28]. Another study investigated the effects of NAC (150 mg/kg bolus and then 12 mg/kg/day as continuous infusion for 3–5 days) on total antioxidant potential in 60 critically ill patients [29]. The need for inotropic support and mechanical ventilation and ICU stay did not vary significantly between NAC and placebo group. Also levels of total antioxidant potential remain unchanged during intervention. Other study evaluates the effects of NAC (150 mg/kg bolus followed by a continuous infusion of 12 mg/kg/hr from a minimum of 3 days up to a maximum of 5 days) for prevention of multisystem organ failure [30]. The mortality, the required days of inotropic support, mechanical ventilation, and intensive care did not significantly change between two groups.

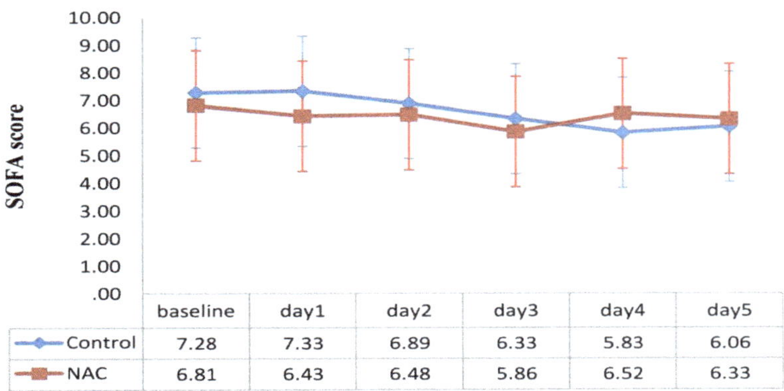

Figure 2 Changes of patients SOFA score in different days of study. Difference between two groups is not significant (P=0.708). Figure shows mean SOFA score±SE.

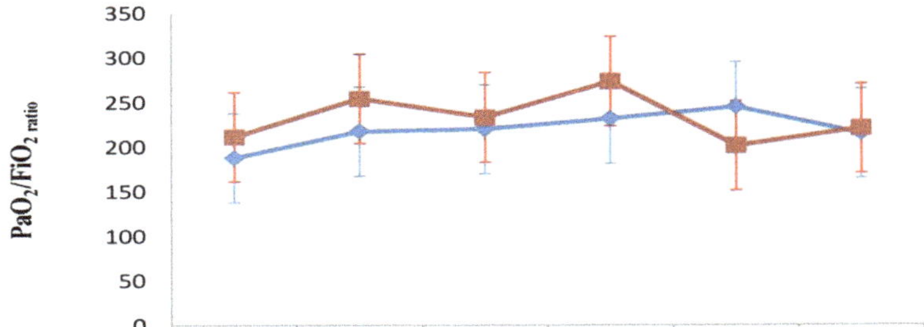

	Baseline	day1	day2	day3	day4	day5
Control	187.23	216.79	219.42	230.93	243.89	214.09
NAC	210.62	253.29	232.27	272.55	200.39	219.59

Figure 3 Changes of Pao_2/Fio_2 ratio in patients in different days of study. Difference between two groups is not significant (P = 0.567). Figure shows mean ±SE.

Furthermore, patients admitted after 24 hrs of hospital admission had a significantly worse mortality in the NAC group as well. Indeed, during 10 years ago several clinical randomized trials suggested that the beneficial impact of NAC were achieved if given early, due to attenuating inflammatory response by free radical scavenging effects, but if commenced in a later phase of sepsis, it may also worsen outcome, as a result of the impaired granulocyte – dependent bacterial killing [30-32]. Nevertheless, prophylactic NAC treatment failed to prevent postoperative organ dysfunction following major abdominal surgery [33].

The results of this study show that high doses of NAC (12 gram/day) for the first 72 hours in mechanically ventilated multiple trauma patients with sepsis patients (patients with sepsis diagnosis over 24 hour was excluded), do not significantly change in the total serum GSH level. Meanwhile in NAC group, the mean level of GSH is higher than control group, it is not along with any improvement in outcome. The ventilator day and mortality rate are higher in NAC group and it shows a negative impact on HR and MAP as well. Our data suggests reconsideration and conducts large sized trials in order to evaluate the efficacy of NAC as an anti-oxidant and a thiol group supplement for GSH deficiency. Further studies are recommended to conduct with focus on commencing NAC treatment in an earlier phase of sepsis, dosage and safety issues. In our study we have observed that NAC, which is often considered as a safe and well tolerated entity, is not as safe. Furthermore, in some circumstances its indication is questionable and present data are not satisfactory.

We have assessed systemic oxygenation and respiratory functions in terms of changes in PaO_2/FiO_2 ratio and the number of ventilator days. In other study administered 190 mg/kg/day NAC as continuous infusion for 3 days in 42 patients with established Acute Respiratory Distress Syndrome (ARDS) and compared it with placebo [34]. The mortality rate, the need for ventilator support and ICU stay and PaO2/FiO2 ratio did not differ significantly between both groups. In another randomized double-blind, placebo controlled clinical trial by Bernard et al. NAC 70 mg/kg every 8 hours was administered for ARDS patients for 10 days [35]. The number of days of acute lung injury decreased in NAC group, yet mortality rate did not change significantly between groups. In our study we encounter similar results. The analyses show no significant difference on day 1 through 5. Improvement in Pao2/Fio2 ratio is seen on day 5 in both groups. The number of ventilator days is longer for

Table 2 Changes of patients HR, MAP, WBC count, ANC in different days of study

		Base line	Day 1	Day 2	Day 3	Day 4	Day 5	P. value
HR	Control	89.94	90.67	87.89	84.67	86.56	89.00	0.040
	Intervention	96.43	97.19	97.81	100.86	97.67	94.19	
MAP	Control	91.18	80.29	87.47	85.12	83.71	82.53	0.042
	Intervention	94.48	89.29	92.05	94.33	90.95	89.95	
WBC count	Control	11726	10597	8930	7890	8117	89	0.06
	Intervention	13094	11791	10165	10874	11087	11191	
ANC	Control	10306.07	7737.73	7425.16	5804.00	5569.42	6732.95	0.001
	Intervention	10261.22	9507.84	8468.47	9800.79	9754.49		

MAP: Mean Arterial Pressure, HR: Heart Rate, ANC: Absolute Neutrophil Count.

Table 3 Changes of patients IgM and GSH level in different days of study

		Base line	Day1	Day3	Day5
IgM(mg/dl)	Control	35.28 ± 8.67	34.59 ± 8.87	32.00 ± 2.69	34.43 ± 5.69
	NAC	34.22 ± 6.38	33.35 ± 6.80	32.18 ± 6.28	31.64 ± 3.93
GSH(μg/dl)	Control	11.89 ± 8.95	11.05 ± 9.52	10.99 ± 7.20	9.26 ± 6.76
	NAC	15.9 ± 9.55	14.79 ± 12.89	15.35 ± 9.51	13.51 ± 6.76

NAC: N-AcetylCysteine, IgM: Immunoglobulin M, GSH: Gluthathione, Data are shown as Mean ± SD.

NAC group although the difference is not statistically significant. We can suggest that routine administration high dose of NAC has no effect on ventilator days and can be harmful.

Various studies have investigated the potential effect of NAC on immune system function in different setting (animal and human studies) and focused on diverse pathological conditions (ARDS, SIRS or sepsis, hepatic injury and etc.). For instance, in other study in critically ill patients with SIRS or sepsis noticed that, high doses of NAC (12, 18 gram/day) resulted in significantly improved phagocytic activity of neutrophils as compared with low doses of NAC. In contrast, they found that high dose NAC decreases respiratory burst and leads to impaired clearance of microorganisms [27].

Santiago and co-workers investigated NAC's effects on inflammatory response and reported that plasma IL-4 and IL-10 (anti-inflammatory cytokines) levels were higher in NAC treated group with respect to time of hepatic reperfusion, indicating a positive modulation effect of NAC on the anti inflammatory response mediated by this cytokines [25]. In in-vitro settings, NAC with similar concentrations above 25 mmol/L completely inhibited NF-κB signal. The trend was the same in in-vivo part of the study, Paterson and colleagues reported. A significant decrease in IL-8 levels in severe sepsis patients treated with NAC, while NAC had no effect on IL-6 levels as reported in that study [26]. Several studies evaluated the immune-modulating effects of NAC and its usage in sepsis, but the results were contradictory. Considerable amount of evidence showed that NAC administration suppressed neutrophils and macrophages activation, attenuating leukocyte–endothelial cell adhesion and inhibited TNF-α and IL-8 release [26,36-38]. Emet and co-workers reported that early NAC administration in severe sepsis did not affect cytokine levels [38,39].

In the current study, immune-modulating effect is evaluated by white blood cell count, absolute neutrophil count and serum IgM levels. In NAC group, WBC count and subsequently ANC are higher than control group which would be indicated more extensive inflammatory condition. The consistent tachycardia, elevated serum creatinine levels and higher 28 days mortality rate have observed in NAC group allegedly support these findings. IgM levels decrease from1 day through 5 in both groups. All patients are IgM deficient and NAC administration neither increase nor decrease IgM levels and it seems that no immune modulation properties are found in high doses of NAC.

Cysteine rich endogenous anti-microbial peptide HβD2 is an important component of immune system (Innate and adaptive) [20,40-43]. This study attempt to investigate whether HβD2 level can be accounted as a marker of SIRS or sepsis. In addition, the study also investigate whether NAC administration (as a cysteine source with probable immune-modulating properties) can elevate HβD2 levels

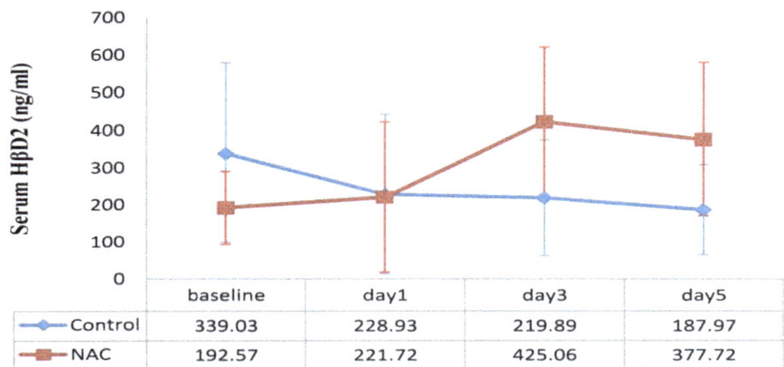

Figure 4 Changes in Serum HβD$_2$ in different days of study. Difference between two groups is not significant (P = 0.463). Figure shows mean±SE.

(HβD2 is known as an inducible one [44,45] among other defensins). Attributed roles to HβD2 in immune system are controversial, yet it is not clear whether HβD2 is an anti-inflammatory protective mediator during sepsis or vice versa. In other study, no difference was observed between survivors and non-survivors of severe sepsis and critical illness in terms of HβD2 levels. Ex-vivo inducible expression of HβD2 by peripheral blood cells was impaired in samples from patients with severe sepsis but this was not along with low levels of HβD2, interestingly HβD2 levels were significantly higher in patients with severe sepsis compared to non-septic critically ill and healthy controls. Which according to Chen et al., NF-κB was as crucial factor for activation of HβD2 gene. In conclusion Book and coworkers noted that up-regulation of HβD2 in sepsis occurred as a result of elevated pro-inflammatory cytokines (such as IL-1 and TNF) [46,47] and was an indicator of higher activity of inflammation and the availability of sources other than peripheral blood cells for HβD2 [21].

Circulating defensins were increased in non-neutropenic children with systemic infection and sepsis. Neutrophils were the major source of defensins, they served as a specific marker for PMN activation. Defensins were not associated with organ failure or poor outcome during sepsis, defensins released into systemic circulation is an indicator of host response to sepsis. These were observations from Thomas and colleagues in a study on levels of HβD2 and lactoferrin in children with severe sepsis, the reported range by them was 450 ng/ml (median) and 194–1032 (25%-75% range) for day 1, and 300 nano-gram/ml (median) and 75–681 (25%-75% range) [41].

We hypothesized that NAC as a cysteine rich source could increase HβD2 levels and our result has confirmed this hypothesis. According to the results of our study, HβD2 levels are associated with an upward trend in NAC and a downward trend in control group. The difference between means of the two groups, however were only noteworthy on day 3. Results indicate that NAC administration with such dosage may have induced HβD2 expression. Regarding the previous discussion on immune-modulating effect of NAC, the elevated HβD2 levels in response to NAC administration appears to be the consequence of profound cysteine source. In our survey, despite higher level of HβD2 in SIRS and sepsis, no potential benefits were found concerning SOFA score and outcome (evaluated based on 28 days mortality rate and ICU length of stay). In accordance with our results supposedly considered as a marker of inflammation in patients with sepsis, however, due to limitations of our study regarding sample size, difficulties in measuring other defensin subtypes with corresponding structure and lack of data on important cytokines like IL-1 and TNF, further studies are necessary in order to clarify HβD2 and other defensin activities and characterization of potential therapeutic or diagnostic targets.

One of the possible protective effects of NAC as a preventive in contrast induced nephropathy still remains undetermined. Based on various studies and meta -analyses NAC administration decreases the risk of contrast induced nephropathy [48-52]. In addition NAC may attenuate contrast induced nephropathy, as defined by albumin excretion, and seems to be independent of any effect on creatinine (NAC dosage: 500 mg IV prior to cardiac catheterization) [53].

Marenzi et al. suggested that NAC should have a protective effect solely when oxidative stress, induced by ischemia and reperfusion, is present (NAC dosage: 600 mg intravenous bolus before primary angioplasty and 600 mg orally twice daily for the 48 hours after angioplasty) [54]. Carbonell et al. found NAC's protect in the prevention of contrast induced nephropathy is based on reducing serum creatinine (SrCr) levels. The incidence of contrast induced nephropathy was significantly lower in NAC group but this effect was only valuable in high risk patients considering similar results that normal saline hydration produced in patients with normal renal function [55,56]. In conclusion Carbonell and coworkers recommend intravenous NAC prior to coronary angioplasty in high risk patients with SrCr ≥1.4 mg/dl, especially when hydration is impossible (NAC dosage: 600 mg every 12 hours IV) [56]. Macedo et al. in a study with focus on acute renal failure (ARF) associated with elective aortic aneurysm repair surgery, did not observe a change in ARF incidence and SrCr peak by NAC administration, in summary the study implied that potential beneficial effects of NAC in prevention of radiocontrast induced nephropathy should not be generalized to other insults applied to kidneys (NAC dosage: 1200 mg orally twice daily 24 hours before and 600 mg IV twice daily for 48 hours after) [57].

In chronic kidney disease (CKD) patients, some benefits has been observed by NAC, NAC reduces cardiovascular events in patients with stage 5 CKD and improves nitric oxide bioavailability (NAC dosage: Tepel et al., 600 mg Twice daily orally, Efrati et al. 1gr IV twice daily, 24 hours before and after angiography) [58,59]. Wittstock et al. demonstrated administration of NAC during dialysis session significantly improved arterial vascular reactivity in end stage CKD patients (NAC dosage: 5 gram IV during dialysis session) [60]. Contrary to that Renke et al. had reported, NAC had no effect on proteinuria and markers of tubular and renal fibrosis in non-diabetic CKD patients (NAC dosage: 1200 mg/day orally) [61].

In a study by Rosato and coworkers who evaluated the NAC effects on vascular system function in Systemic

Sclerosis patients, authors concluded that NAC improved vascular renal function in patients with low severity of disease (NAC dosage: 15 mg/kg/hour for 5 hours) [62].

Our study was not designed to assess how NAC affects the kidneys function, not to mention the fact that the dosage of NAC administered in this study was higher than dosages administered in studies on nephro-protective properties. Considering that rising in SrCr levels is noticeable. Using paired *t*-test (before after analysis) statistical method shows a significant increase in the mean of SrCr level in NAC group while at the same time the mean level of SrCr in control group is reduced. The mean level of SrCr during NAC administration have reached 1.48 mg/dl on day 3 and interestingly SrCr levels after discontinuation of NAC (on day 3) is decreased to its baseline (as low as 0.92 mg/dl). This may partially declare that high doses NAC administration is associated with progression towards acute kidney injury.

Conclusion

Considering adverse reactions observed in our study in terms of tachycardia, high blood pressure, leukocytosis and prolonged ventilator days and regarding the fact that no signs of improvement were observed in terms of mortality rate which was slightly higher for NAC group, high dosage of NAC is not recommended in critically ill patients with sepsis. NAC usage, even low dose, shall be administered with great caution in critically ill patients. Further studies on dosage and possible ceiling effect for NAC and re-evaluating safety of that, being conducted along with increased risk and extent of inflammatory profile. In this study no immuno-modulating effect associated with NAC was detected. According to SrCr variations during our study, we recommend to conduct further studies with adequate sample size to evaluate nephro-protective effects of NAC.

Competing interests

The authors declare that they have no competing interests.

Authors' contributions

MM: study design, patient selection, sample collection and handling, statistical analysis, analysis and interpretation of data, draft the manuscript and revising. KHA: study design, patient selection, sample collection and handling, analysis and interpretation of data, draft the manuscript and revising. MA: study design, sample analyzing via commercially available enzyme-linked immunosorbent assay kit, revised the manuscript. AN: study design, patient selection, sample collection and handling, draft the manuscript and revising. MM: study design. LCK: draft the manuscript and revising. FN: interpretation of data, revising the manuscript. AA: study design, patient selection, sample collection and handling, statistical analysis, analysis and interpretation of data, draft the manuscript and revising. All authors read and approved the final manuscript.

Acknowledgements

This work was supported by a grant from TUMS, Tehran, Iran. We thank Exir® pharmaceutical company for providing the drug. We also thank Dr. Alireza Ahmadvand and Maryam Baeeri for participating in this research.

Author details

[1]Department of Anesthesiology and Critical Care Medicine, Sina Hospital, Faculty of Medicine, Tehran University of Medical Sciences, Tehran, Iran. [2]Department of Clinical Pharmacy, Faculty of Pharmacy, Tehran University of Medical Sciences, Tehran, Iran. [3]Faculty of Pharmacy and Pharmaceutical Sciences Research Center, Tehran University of Medical Sciences, Tehran, Iran. [4]Department of Clinical Pharmacy, Faculty of Pharmacy, Mashhad University of Medical sciences, Mashhad, Iran.

References

1. Ertel W, Trentz O: **Polytrauma and multi-organ failure syndrome. Definition-pathophysiology-therapy.** *Zentralbl Chir* 1994, **119**:159.
2. Vyrostek SB, Annest JL, Ryan GW: **Surveillance for fatal and nonfatal injuries-United States, 2001.** *MMWR Surveill Summ* 2004, **53**:1–57.
3. Bardenheuer M, Obertacke U, Waydhas C, Nast-Kolb D: **Epidemiology of the severe multiple trauma-a prospective registration of preclinical and clinical supply.** *J Orthop Trauma* 2000, **14**:453.
4. Esposito TJ, Sanddal TL, Reynolds SA, Sanddal ND: **Effect of a voluntary trauma system on preventable death and inappropriate care in a rural state.** *J Trauma and Acute Care Surgery* 2003, **54**:663–670.
5. Brohi K, Singh J, Heron M, Coats T: **Acute traumatic coagulopathy.** *J Trauma* 2003, **54**:1127.
6. Homer T, Peter C, Frederick B: **Causes of death following multiple trauma.** *Curr Orthop* 2004, **18**:304–310.
7. Swain SD, Rohn TT, Quinn MT: **Neutrophil priming in host defense: role of oxidants as priming agents.** *Antioxid Redox Signal* 2002, **4**:69–83.
8. Martin P, D'Souza D, Martin J: **Wound healing in the PU. 1 null mouse—tissue repair is not dependent on inflammatory cells.** *Curr Biol* 2003, **13**:1122–1128.
9. Hietbrink F, Koenderman L, Rijkers G, Trauma L: **The role of the innate immune system.** *World J Emergency Surgery* 2006, **1**:15.
10. Power CP, Wang JH, Manning B: **Bacterial lipoprotein delays apoptosis in human neutrophils through inhibition of caspase-3 activity: regulatory roles for CD14 and TLR-2.** *J Immunol* 2004, **173**:5229–5237.
11. Echtenacher B, Hultner L, Mannel DN: **Cellular and molecular mechanisms of TNF protection in septic peritonitis.** *J Inflamm* 1996, **47**:85–89.
12. Cobb JP, O'Keefe GE: **Injury research in the genomic era.** *Lancet* 2004, **363**:2076–2083.
13. Vincent J-L, Sakr Y, Sprung CL: **Sepsis in European intensive care units: results of the SOAP study*.** *Crit Care Med* 2006, **34**:344–353.
14. Silva E, Pedro MA, Sogayar A: **Brazilian sepsis epidemiological study (BASES study).** *Crit Care* 2004, **8**:R251–R260.
15. Martin GS, Mannino DM, Eaton S, Moss M: **The epidemiology of sepsis in the United States from 1979 through 2000.** *N Engl J Med* 2003, **348**:1546–1554.
16. Angus DC, Pereira C, Silva E: **Epidemiology of severe sepsis around the world.** *Endocr Metab Immune Disord Drug Targets* 2006, **6**:207.
17. Milner SM, Bhat S, Buja M, Gulati S, Poindexter BJ, Bick RJ: **Expression of human β defensin 2 in thermal injury.** *Burns* 2004, **30**:649–654.
18. Burd RS, Furrer JL, Sullivan J, Smith AL: **Murine [BETA]-defensin-3 is an inducible peptide with limited tissue expression and broad-spectrum antimicrobial activity.** *Shock* 2002, **18**:461–464.
19. Ganz T, Lehrer RI: **Defensins.** *Pharmacol Ther* 1995, **66**:191–205.
20. Röhrl J, Yang D, Oppenheim JJ, Hehlgans T: **Human β-defensin 2 and 3 and their mouse orthologs induce chemotaxis through interaction with CCR2.** *J Immunol* 2010, **184**:6688–6694.
21. Book M, Chen Q, Lehmann LE: **Inducibility of the endogenous antibiotic peptide β-defensin 2 is impaired in patients with severe sepsis.** *Crit Care* 2007, **11**:R19.
22. Millea PJ: **N-acetylcysteine: multiple clinical applications.** *Am Fam Physician* 2009, **80**:265–269.
23. Kelly GS: **Clinical applications of N-acetylcysteine. Alternative medicine review.** *J Clinical Therapeutic* 1998, **3**:114.
24. Atkuri KR, Mantovani JJ, Herzenberg LA: **N-Acetylcysteine-a safe antidote for cysteine/glutathione deficiency.** *Curr Opin Pharmacol* 2007, **7**:355–359.
25. Santiago F, Bueno P, Olmedo C: **Effect of n-Acetylcysteine administration on intraoperative plasma levels of interleukin-4 and interleukin-10 in liver transplant recipients.** *Transplant Proc* 2008, **40**:2978–2980.
26. Paterson RL, Galley HF, Webster NR: **The effect of N-acetylcysteine on nuclear factor-[kappa] B activation, interleukin-6, interleukin-8, and**

intercellular adhesion molecule-1 expression in patients with sepsis*. *Crit Care Med* 2003, **31**:2574–2578.

27. Heller AR, Groth G, Heller SC: **N-acetylcysteine reduces respiratory burst but augments neutrophil phagocytosis in intensive care unit patients.** *Crit Care Med* 2001, **29**:272–276.
28. Lee TF, Jantzie LL, Todd KG, Cheung PY: **Postresuscitation N-acetylcysteine treatment reduces cerebral hydrogen peroxide in the hypoxic piglet brain.** *Intensive Care Med* 2008, **34**:190–197.
29. Molnar Z, MacKinnon K, Shearer E, Lowe D, Watson I: **The effect of N-acetylcysteine on total serum anti-oxidant potential and urinary albumin excretion in critically ill patients.** *Intensive Care Med* 1998, **24**:230–235.
30. Molnar Z, Shearer E, Lowe D: **N-Acetylcysteine treatment to prevent the progression of multisystem organ failure: A prospective, randomized, placebo-controlled study.** *Crit Care Med* 1999, **27**:1100–1104.
31. Spies CD, Reinhart K, Witt I: **Influence of N-acetlcycteine on direct indicators of tissue oxygenation in septicshock patients: Results from a prospective, randomized, double-blind study.** *Crit Care Med* 1994, **22**:1738–1746.
32. Ortolani O, Conti A, De Gaudio AR: **Protective effects of N-acetlcycteine and rutin on the lipid peroxidation of the lung epithelium during the adult respiratory syndrome.** *Shock* 2000, **13**:14–18.
33. Szakmany T, Marton S, Molnar Z: **Lack of effect of prophylactic N-acetlcycteine on postopertavie organdysfunction following major abdominal tumour surgery.** *Anaesth Intensive Care* 2003, **31**:267–271.
34. Domenighetti G, Suter PM, Schaller MD, Ritz R, Perret C: **Treatment with N -acetylcysteine during acute respiratory distress syndrome: a randomized, double-blind, placebo-controlled clinical study.** *J Crit Care* 1997, **12**:177–182.
35. Bernard GR, Wheeler AP, Arons MM: **A trial of antioxidants N-acetylcysteine and procysteine in ARDS.** *Chest* 1997, **112**:164–172.
36. Spapen H: **N-acetylcysteine in clinical sepsis: a difficult marriage.** *Crit Care* 2004, **8**:229–230.
37. Schmidt H, Schmidt W, Muller T, Bohrer H, Gebhard MM, Martin E: **N-acetylcysteine attenuates endotoxin-induced leukocyte-endothelial cell adhesion and macromolecular leakage in vivo.** *Crit Care Med* 1997, **25**:858–863.
38. Kharazmi A, Nielsen H, Schiøtz P: **N-acetylcysteine inhibits human neutrophil and monocyte chemotaxis and oxidative metabolism.** *Int J Immuno Pharmacology* 1988, **10**:39–46.
39. Emet S, Memis D, Pamukçu Z: **The influence of N-acetyl-L-cystein infusion on cytokine levels and gastric intramucosal pH during severe sepsis.** *Crit Care* 2004, **8**:229–230.
40. Yamaguchi Y, Ouchi Y: **Antimicrobial peptide defensin: Identification of novel isoforms and the characterization of their physiological roles and their significance in the pathogenesis of diseases.** *Proc Jpn Acad Ser B Phys Biol Sci* 2012, **88**:152.
41. Thomas NJ, Carcillo JA, Doughty LA, Sasser H, Heine RP: **Plasma concentrations of defensins and lactoferrin in children with severe sepsis.** *Pediatr Infect Dis J* 2002, **21**:34–38.
42. Shi Z, Zhao Z, Shu Q: **Protective effect of recombinant beta-defensin-2 on acute lung injury induced by sepsis in rats.** *Zhejiang da xue xue bao Yi xue ban J Zhejiang University Medical sciences* 2006, **35**:605.
43. Krisanaprakornkit S, Kimball JR, Weinberg A, Darveau RP, Bainbridge BW, Dale BA: **Inducible expression of human β-defensin 2 byFusobacterium nucleatum in oral epithelial cells: multiple signaling pathways and role of commensal bacteria in innate immunity and the epithelial barrier.** *Infect Immun* 2000, **68**:2907–2915.
44. Harder J, Bartels J, Christophers E, Schroder J: **A peptide antibiotic from human skin.** *Nature* 1997, **387**:861–61.
45. Liu K-X, Chen S-Q, Zhang H, Guo J-y, Li Y-S, Huang W-Q: **Intestinal ischaemia/reperfusion upregulates β-defensin-2 expression and causes acute lung injury in the rat.** *Injury* 2009, **40**:950–955.
46. Tsutsumi-Ishii Y, Nagaoka I: **Modulation of human β-defensin-2 transcription in pulmonary epithelial cells by lipopolysaccharide-stimulated mononuclear phagocytes via proinflammatory cytokine production.** *J Immunol* 2003, **170**:4226–4236.
47. Liu L, Roberts AA, Ganz T: **By IL-1 signaling, monocyte-derived cells dramatically enhance the epidermal antimicrobial response to lipopolysaccharide.** *J Immunol* 2003, **170**:575–580.
48. Tepel M, Van Der Giet M, Schwarzfeld C, Laufer U, Liermann D, Zidek W: **Prevention of radiographic-contrast-agent–induced reductions in renal function by acetylcysteine.** *N Engl J Med* 2000, **343**:180–184.
49. Kay J, Chow WH, Chan TM: **Acetylcysteine for prevention of acute deterioration of renal function following elective coronary angiography and intervention.** *JAMA* 2003, **289**:553–558.
50. Durham JD, Caputo C, Dokko J: **A randomized controlled trial of N-acetylcysteine to prevent contrast nephropathy in cardiac angiography.** *Kidney Int* 2002, **62**:2202–2207.
51. Duong MH, MacKenzie TA, Malenka D: **N-acetylcysteine prophylaxis significantly reduces the risk of radiocontrast-induced nephropathy: comprehensive meta-analysis.** *Catheter Cardiovasc Interv* 2005, **64**:471–479.
52. Birck R, Krzossok S, Markowetz F, Schnülle P, Van Der Woude FJ, Braun C: **Acetylcysteine for prevention of contrast nephropathy: meta-analysis.** *Lancet* 2003, **362**:598–603.
53. Levin A, Pate GE, Shalansky S: **N-acetylcysteine reduces urinary albumin excretion following contrast administration: evidence of biological effect.** *Nephrol Dial Transplant* 2007, **22**:2520–2524.
54. Marenzi G, Assanelli E, Marana I: **N-acetylcysteine and contrast-induced nephropathy in primary angioplasty.** *N Engl J Med* 2006, **354**:2773–2782.
55. Miner SE, Dzavik V, Nguyen-Ho P: **N-acetylcysteine reduces contrast-associated nephropathy but not clinical events during long-term follow-up.** *Am Heart J* 2004, **148**:690–695.
56. Carbonell N, Sanjuán R, Blasco M, Jordá Á, Miguel A: **N-acetylcysteine: short-term clinical benefits after coronary angiography in high-risk renal patients.** *Rev Esp Cardiol* 2010, **63**:12–19.
57. Macedo E, Abdulkader R, Castro I, Sobrinho AC, Yu L, Vieira JM: **Lack of protection of N-acetylcysteine (NAC) in acute renal failure related to elective aortic aneurysm repair-a randomized controlled trial.** *Nephrol Dial Transplant* 2006, **21**:1863–1869.
58. Tepel M, van der Giet M, Statz M, Jankowski J, Zidek W: **The antioxidant acetylcysteine reduces cardiovascular events in patients with End-stage renal failure a randomized, controlled trial.** *Circulation* 2003, **107**:992–995.
59. Efrati S, Dishy V, Averbukh M: **The effect of N-acetylcysteine on renal function, nitric oxide, and oxidative stress after angiography.** *Kidney Int* 2003, **64**:2182–2187.
60. Wittstock A, Burkert M, Zidek W, Tepel M, Scholze A: **N-acetylcysteine improves arterial vascular reactivity in patients with chronic kidney disease.** *Nephron Clin Pract* 2009, **112**:c184–c189.
61. Renke M, Tylicki L, Rutkowski P: **The effect of N-acetylcysteine on proteinuria and markers of tubular injury in Non-diabetic patients with chronic kidney disease.** *Kidney Blood Press Res* 2008, **31**:404–410.
62. Rosato E, Cianci R, Barbano B: **N-acetylcysteine infusion reduces the resistance index of renal artery in the early stage of systemic sclerosis.** *Acta Pharmacol Sin* 2009, **30**:1283–1288.

Formulation of inhalable lipid-based salbutamol sulfate microparticles by spray drying technique

Zahra Daman[1], Kambiz Gilani[1,2*], Abdolhossein Rouholamini Najafabadi[1], Hamid Reza Eftekhari[1] and Mohammad Ali Barghi[3]

Abstract

Background: The aim of this work was to develop dry powder inhaler (DPI) formulations of salbutamol sulfate (SS) by the aid of solid lipid microparticles (SLmPs), composed of biocompatible phospholipids or cholesterol.

Methods: The SLmPs were prepared by using two different solvent systems (ethanol and water-ethanol) and lipid carriers (dipalmitoylphosphatidylcholine (DPPC) and cholesterol) with/without L-leucine in the spray drying process. The spray-dried microparticles were physically-mixed with coarse lactose monohydrate in order to make our final DPI formulations and were investigated in terms of physical characteristics as well as in vitro drug release profile and aerosolization behavior.

Results: We observed significant differences in the sizes, morphologies, and in vitro pulmonary depositions between the formulations. In particular, the SS-containing SLmPs prepared with water-ethanol (30:70 v/v) solution of DPPC and L-leucine which had then been blended with coarse lactose (1:9 w/w) exhibited the highest emitted dose (87.9%) and fine particle fraction (42.7%) among the formulations. In vitro drug release study indicated that despite of having a significant initial burst release for both cholesterol and DPPC-based microparticles, the remained drug released more slowly than the pure drug.

Conclusion: This study demonstrated the potential of using lipid carriers as well as L-leucine in DPI formulations of SS to improve its aerosolization behavior and retard the release profile of the drug.

Keywords: Dry powder inhalation, Spray drying, Salbutamol sulfate, Solid lipid microparticles, Particle engineering, L-leucine

Background

Local administration of drugs to the lungs presents several advantages, especially, in patients with specific pulmonary diseases, such as asthma, pulmonary infections or lung cancer. The advantages include reduction in systemic side effects, elevated drug concentration at the site of action, and reduction in amount of drug administered to the patient compared to traditional routs [1-3]. In this regard, the area of particle engineering is becoming increasingly attractive for the development of more efficient inhaled therapeutics.

One of the attractive applications of particle engineering is to develop a sustained release (SR) formulation by using suitable carriers, a kind of formulation that has not been marketed yet, despite active research conducted on this subject. A SR formulation will provide the active drug over an extended duration of time, and therefore may improve therapy by enhancing the compliance of the patients. In such formulations, it is expected that the overall amount of drug and the side effects will be reduced [4-6]. However, the efforts for finding suitable, non-toxic excipients, which can produce a desired drug release profile and improve the respirable fraction of the inhaled particles to maximize drug deposition into smaller airways are continuous and extensive.

One approach to SR delivery to the respiratory tract utilizes liposomal formulations. Liposomes are promising vehicles for pulmonary drug delivery owing to their

* Correspondence: gilani@tums.ac.ir
[1]Aerosol Research Laboratory, Department of Pharmaceutics, School of Pharmacy, Tehran University of Medical Sciences, Tehran, Iran
[2]Medicinal Plants Research Center, Tehran University of Medical Sciences, Tehran, Iran
Full list of author information is available at the end of the article

capacity to increase drug retention time and reduce the toxicity of drugs after administration [7,8]. Several factors such as the composition of lipids and the size of liposomes can affect the performance of the system [9-11]. Many studies have shown the applicability of liposomes in lung delivery of a large variety of drugs such as cytotoxic agents, anti-asthma drugs, antimicrobial agents, and drugs for systemic action like insulin and other proteins [4,10]. However, there are some disadvantages about liposomal vehicles that limits their application as commercial formulations such as high production cost and instability during storage even at low temperatures [12], and nebulization [13,14] that can cause premature release of the entrapped drug. The latter problem has been reported even about the dry powder formulations prepared by jet milling micronization of lyophilized liposomes, which deleteriously affected their integrity [15].

Another approach for development of an inhalable SR formulation is to produce solid lipid microparticles (SLmPs). It has been suggested that SLmPs offer high tolerability in the pulmonary tract, as they are mainly made of biocompatible and biodegradable materials [16,17]. Moreover, they possess several other advantages compared to traditional vehicles such as polymeric drug carriers, micelles or liposomes, including more physiochemical stability, incorporation of both lipophilic and hydrophilic drugs, low large-scale production cost and having no significant biotoxicity [16-19]. Phospholipids and cholesterol have been previously used in inhalation formulations as solid lipid carriers or fillers to improve drug targeting to the lung. The prepared SLmPs presented spherical shapes, reduced agglomeration tendency and high fine particle fraction (FPF) [17,20].

Spray drying is an attractive solidification technique in the field of respiratory drug delivery, with respect to its relative simplicity, availability of large-scale equipment, capability to produce homogenous particle size distribution, and ability to control various parameters that optimize the particulate product characteristics such as size, size distribution, shape, morphology and density [21-23]. Therefore, it can be used as a suitable technology to produce dry powder inhaler (DPI) products, which possess several advantages over pressurized metered dose inhalers (pMDI), such as being breath-activated and having no requirement of any propellant [24].

Thus, the aim of this study was to design SLmPs using cholesterol or dipalmitoylphosphatidylcholine (DPPC) by spray drying method. The idea was emerged from the potential ability of these excipients to entrap both water-soluble and water-insoluble drugs, as well as providing a prolonged local drug release [6,16]. Moreover, the safety issue of these SLmPs over other vehicles was a key consideration in our design process, since they are mainly made from endogenous materials [25,26]. For this purpose, we chose to work with SS, a short acting beta2-adrenoceptor stimulant with plasma half-life of 4–6 hours, which requires frequent dosing for daily management of asthma. A SR preparation of this agent is desirable approach to improve therapy of asthma, especially in non-compliant patients and also for covering the nocturnal decline of the drug [27], when administered at the bed time.

Aside from SR properties, an effective DPI formulation should offer optimum particle characteristics to achieve high FPF and reduce the central deposition in pulmonary airways. In other words, a suitable DPI formulation should have the ability to reach deep lung regions and disperse adequately within the airflow of the patient. Indeed, decreasing of both particle size and density can be achieved by spray drying technique in order to generate particles with satisfactory respirable fraction [23]. However, the dispersibility of the particles is another factor that has to be taken into consideration. The particle aggregation associated with cohesive forces between them can be regulated using excipients such as coarse crystalline lactose, which is currently serving as the drug carrier and also the bulking agent in most available DPI products [23]. Usually, drug particles and such excipients are combined in a physical blending process during which the microparticles are attached to the surface of the carrier. Therefore, our final DPI formulations consisted of physically-mixed SLmPs with large coarse lactose carrier particles. To aid dispersibility, it has been also proven that co-spray drying of simple amino acids, especially the hydrophobic ones such as L-leucine, can improve dispersion of the powder and may enhance the fraction of respirable particles [28]. Thus, we used this amino acid in our spray drying process to evaluate its effects on the aerodynamic performance of the resultant DPI formulation.

In the present study, the obtained SLmPs were further characterized for their physical properties, in vitro aerosolization behavior, and their potential of being a SR delivery system.

Methods

Materials

SS was supplied as micronized powder from Darupakhsh (Iran). Cholesterol was purchased from Merck (Germany), and the phospholipid, DPPC, was supplied from Lipoid (Germany). Inhalation grade lactose (Pharmatose 325 M) with D50% of about 60 μm was obtained from DMV Internationals (The Netherlands). Other chemical reagents and solvents including the HPLC grade ones were purchased from either Merck or Sigma. L-Leucine was also supplied from Merck (Germany).

Preparation of the lipid-based microparticles

The SLmPs were prepared, at laboratory scale, by spray drying method using a Büchi Minispray dryer B-191-a from Büchi Laboratory-Technique (Switzerland). In this study, we decided to improve the drying efficiency of the lipid excipients by using a jacketed cyclone with cold-water circulation, to cool down the cyclone separator wall and thus decrease the lipid particles' adhesion and agglomeration.

Two different types of formulations were spray dried for the preparation of SLmPs. The first type was prepared by dispersing the SS microparticles within an ethanol solution of the hydrophobic excipients, cholesterol or DPPC. The suspensions were sonicated for 10 min before spray drying to ensure the adequate dispersion of the drug. The second type of formulations was obtained from spray drying of water-ethanol (30:70 v/v) solution of the drug and the lipid materials. Details are shown in Table 1.

The spray drying conditions were as following: Solid content, 5% w/v; Nozzle size, 0.5 mm; Inlet temperature, 80/100°C (depending on the solvent system); Outlet temperature, 54/65°C (depending on the inlet temperature); Spraying air flow rate, 800 L/h; Feed rate, 0.2 g/min; Cold water circulation in the jacketed cyclone, 0°C.

Furthermore, as shown in Table 1, L-leucine was co-spray dried at the amount of 10% w/w with respect to the solid content with water-ethanol solution of DPPC and SS. Finally, all the obtained formulations were physically blended with inhalation grade lactose monohydrate (Pharmatose® 325 M) at a ratio of 1:9 w/w in a Turbula mixer from Dorsa Novin (Iran) for 60 min at a low speed (46 rpm).

Determination of SS content

Quantification of CIP was conducted by HPLC using a mobile phase consisting of water, methanol and phosphate buffer (pH 2.8) in the ratio of 60:20:20 at a flow rate of 1 mL/min. The phosphate buffer was prepared by dissolving 2.625 g ammonium phosphate in 50 mL purified deionized water, adding 2.8 mL of phosphoric acid (85%) and diluting to 100 mL with purified deionized water. The HPLC system consisted of a pump (Waters 600E, Millipore, USA), a C18 Tracer Excel column (15 × 0.46 cm, 5 μm, Spain) and a UV detector (Waters 486, USA) at 276 nm. Bamethan sulfate (to final concentration of 10 μg/mL) was added as the internal standard to each sample just before analysis. From the relative area under the peak, linearity (R2 = 0.999) was achieved using standard aqueous solutions of SS between 0.5 and 50 μg/mL.

For all the prepared DPI formulations, the content uniformity was evaluated by taking 10 random samples, each weighing 10 mg powder which were subjected to lipid extraction by adding 1.5 mL chloroform to each one and centrifugation at 37565 × g for 20 min. The recovered drug was diluted with mobile phase before being subjected to HPLC analysis. Mixtures with relative standard deviation values of less than 10%, as recommended by The United States Pharmacopeia, were considered to be satisfactorily mixed.

Particle size measurement

The size distribution of the microparticles was determined by laser diffraction method using Malvern Mastersizer X (UK) after the formulations had been dispersed in appropriate medium (saturated solution of SS in water) and sonicated for 2 min. The geometrical diameter was expressed as volume median diameter (D50%). Also the Span values of formulations were defined as $\frac{D90\%-D10\%}{D50\%}$, which represents the breadth of the particle distribution. Each measurement was repeated in triplicate.

Scanning electron microscopy

Particle morphology was observed by scanning electron microscopy (SEM) using Philips XL30 equipment (The Netherlands). The samples were coated with gold under relative vacuum by means of Bal-Tec/SCDOOS sputter coater (Switzerland) and were examined under an accelerating voltage of 25 kv.

Determination of true density

The density was assessed with Quantachrome helium pycnometer (USA). The basis of this method is on putting the sample of known mass into a cell of known volume. Briefly, when helium penetrates into the cell at a vacuum, it occupies the entire volume of the cell, so the actual volume of the sample can be determined since the volume

Table 1 Composition of different spray-dried formulations

Formulation number	Drug conc. (%)*	Excipients	Solvent system	Inlet temperature (°C)
1	12.5	cholesterol	Ethanol	80
2	25	cholesterol	Ethanol	80
3	37.5	cholesterol	Ethanol	80
4	37.5	DPPC	Ethanol	80
5	37.5	cholesterol	Water/Ethanol	100
6	37.5	DPPC	Water/Ethanol	100
7	37.5	DPPC + Leucine	Water/Ethanol	100

*Percentage of the total solid content (w/w).

of the cell is known. So, the actual densities of the samples were accurately calculated. Each sample was analyzed thrice.

Aerosol performance of SLmPs

The in vitro pulmonary deposition of the powders was determined by Twin Stage Impinger (TSI) glass apparatus from Copley Scientific (UK). A dry powder formulation device, Novartis Cyclohaler® (Switzerland), was filled with a hard gelatin capsule loaded with 10 mg of each formulation. On the other hand, the mobile phase was introduced to stage 1 (7 mL) and stage 2 (30 mL) of the TSI. Once the assembly had been checked to be tight and vertical, the Cyclohaler® had been inserted to the rubber mouthpiece attached to the throat part of the impinger. The test was operated at 60 L/min for 4 s. The flow rate was achieved using a rotary vein pump from Copley Scientific (UK). After the operation, the impinger components had been washed into separate volumetrics (25 mL for the throat and stage 1, and 50 mL for the device and stage 2) with the same solution. Their contents were assayed for SS, after the lipid had been extracted with certain ratio of chloroform.

Fine particle dose (FPD) was considered as the amount of drug deposited in stage 2 (dae < 6.4 μm). The emitted dose (ED) was determined as a percent of total powder exiting the capsule and the device. The FPF was calculated as the percent of the ratio of FPD to the total amount of drug emitted per capsule.

Determination of drug release from SLmPs

Since the volume of surface liquid in the respiratory tract is relatively low, the conventional European Pharmacopeia methods cannot be used for exact evaluation of dissolution behavior of inhaled drugs due to their large volumes of dissolution media (900–1000 mL) [29]. Hence we used a dispersion method to measure in vitro release of the drug from SLmPs. Briefly, 10 mg of each formulation was suspended individually in 10 mL phosphate buffered saline (PBS, PH = 7.4) in test tubes and incubated in a shaker (Grant instruments, Cambridge, England) at 37°C on 50 rpm. At certain time intervals of 0.25, 0.5, 1, 2, 4, 8, and 12 hours, three tubes were picked and individually assayed for SS after being filtered. The mean value of the tree tubes for each time interval was calculated, and plotted as cumulative amount of SS released over 12 hours.

Statistical analysis

Data for all measurements were considered as the mean ± standard deviation (SD) of at least three separate experiments. One-way analysis of variance (ANOVA) test was used for statistical comparison of the results while $p < 0.05$ was considered significant in all cases.

Results and discussion

Different powder compositions were formulated using the spray drying technique, with the aim of studying the influence of lipid composition and the solvent type on the physiochemical properties and the aerosolization behavior of the powders. Table 1 gives an overview of all the prepared powder formulations. It should be mentioned that the content uniformity test was conducted for both spray-dried formulations and the physical blends, using a conventional invasive sampling method. The active drug content was quantified by HPLC, and ranged between 95 ± 2% and 103 ± 3% for different formulations.

Evaluation of physiochemical properties of aerosol particles

The particle size characteristics of the formulations are summarized in Table 2. The results showed that for the same lipid and solvent composition of the formulations (cholesterol in ethanol), the percentage of SS in the suspensions used for spray drying had no significant effect on the size of resultant SLmPs ($p > 0.05$). Additionally, the D50% of the spray dried formulations obtained from ethanol suspension of the drug were shown to be dependent

Table 2 Particle size measurement obtained by laser diffraction method (mean ± SD)

Formulation number	Drug conc. (%)*	Excipients	Solvent system	Inlet temp. (°C)	D50%	Span
1	12.5	cholesterol	Ethanol	80	3.23 ± 0.48	3.19
2	25	cholesterol	Ethanol	80	5.04 ± 0.66	1.75
3	37.5	cholesterol	Ethanol	80	4.16 ± 0.32	1.66
4	37.5	DPPC	Ethanol	80	1.42 ± 0.15	0.87
5	37.5	cholesterol	Water-Ethanol	100	7.32 ± 0.28	2.26
6	37.5	DPPC	Water-Ethanol	100	4.02 ± 0.18	2.54
7	37.5	DPPC + Leucine	Water-Ethanol	100	4.04 ± 0.25	2.23
C_1	100	-	Ethanol	80	3.70 ± 0.13	2.47
C_2	100	-	Water-Ethanol	100	5.83 ± 0.21	1.82

*Percentage of the total solid content (w/w).

on the type of lipid component, which was much smaller for DPPC-based microparticles than cholesterol ($p < 0.05$). Changing the solvent from ethanol to water-ethanol (30:70 v/v) resulted in an increase in D50% values of both DPPC and cholesterol-based particles ($p < 0.05$). It seems that the enhancement in the inlet temperature of spray drying process has contributed to the particle size enlargement, as it was previously proven that adding in tempe rature will lead to increase in the diameter of particles [30,31]. Furthermore, the laser diffraction particle size analysis showed that co-spray drying of L-leucine with DPPC and SS did not significantly change the particle size distribution with respect to the counterpart sample without L-leucine ($p > 0.05$).

Scanning electron microphotographs of the SLmPs are shown in Figure 1. As shown in Figure 1a-c, changing the solvent in the feed solution did not seriously change the spherical shape of cholesterol-based SLmPs which is typically obtained via spray drying technique [32]. Processing of the drug and DPPC in ethanol produced particles similar to that of cholesterol-based samples (Figure 1d). However, as it is indicated in Figure 1e, applying a mixed solution of water-ethanol (30:70 v/v) in formulations consisted of DPPC resulted in production of wrinkled particles which used to be mostly spherical when pure ethanol was applied as the solvent. It is supposed that the solubility saturation of the formulation components upon former evaporation of the more volatile solvent (ethanol) leads to formation of a primary solid shell which then collapses as the core's water content evaporates [33]. In this case, the surface-active DPPC could have contributed to the formation of this primary solid shell during particle formation stage. Incorporation of L-leucine within this formulation led the spherical shape back to the particles, as it is clearly shown in Figure 1f. It seems that the more tendency of L-leucine to water than ethanol and its subsequent localization in the core of the primary particles inhibited the shell to completely collapse after water evaporation. Figure 2 shows the attachment of SLmPs obtained from water-ethanol (30:70 v/v) solution of DPPC and SS to the large lactose surface. In fact, physical blending of the formulations with lactose monohydrate as the coarse carrier promoted the adhesion of SLmPs onto its surface. This process was expected to aid the deaggregation and dispersion of particles within the respiratory flow [34].

The true density values of the spray dried samples obtained by helium pycnometry are shown in Table 3. SS powders, which were spray dried from both kinds of the solvent systems, were used as controls. The results suggested that utilizing the lipid components along with the drug could result in reduction of the true density of the spray-dried powders. Actually, particle's aerodynamic diameter (d_a) is a function of particle's geometric diameter (d), density (ρ) and morphology (χ, shape factor) according to the following equation:

$$d_a = d\sqrt{(\rho/\chi)}$$

In other words, particles with low density have smaller aerodynamic diameter than their geometric diameter. Thus, it can be of great value to reduce the density and affect the aerodynamic diameter of the particles by changing a DPI formulation composition. In this regard, Scalia et al. had previously reported the true density values of lower than 1 g cm^{-3} for the lipid microparticles obtained by melt emulsification technique [35].

Aerosol performance of the SLmPs

Table 4 shows the ED (%), FPD (μg) and FPF (%) values of the spray dried SLmPs (formulations number 1 to 7) along with the same powders mixed with lactose carrier in the ratio of 1:9 w/w (formulations number 8 to 12). The aerodynamic characteristics were measured using a TSI at the flow rate of 60 L/min after aerosolization by

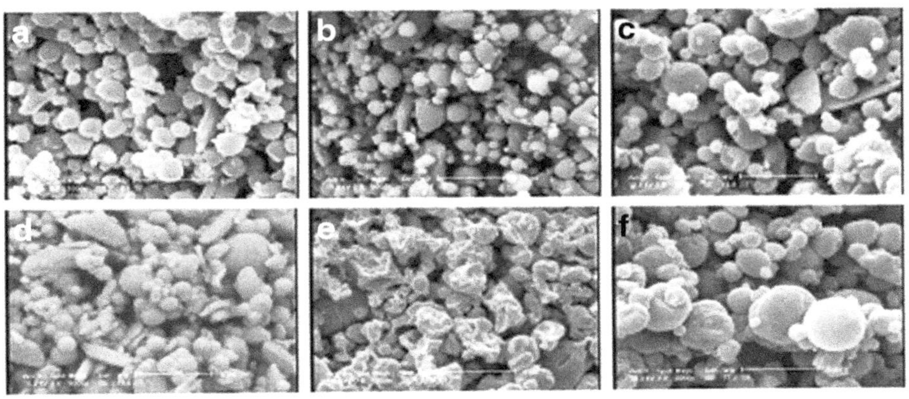

Figure 1 Scanning electron micrographs of SLmPs containing salbutamol sulfate in different formulations: a) F2, b) F3, c) F5, d) F4, e) F6, f) F7.

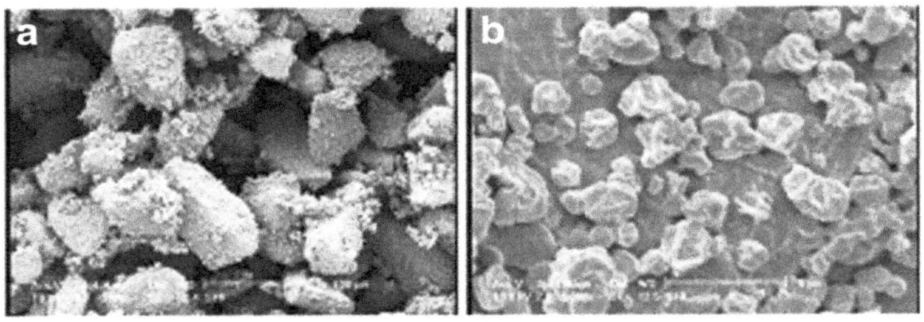

Figure 2 Scanning electron micrographs of SLmPs blended with lactose. a) magnification ×240, **b)** more magnification (×5000) representing SLmPs deposited on the surface of lactose carriers.

Cyclohaler®. It should be noted that SS recoveries from the inhaler and the different parts of the TSI ranged between 90.1-95.2% of the total loaded drug.

It seems that the type of solvent system and lipid excipients had a direct effect on aerosolization properties of the powders. Among the formulations prepared by cholesterol and ethanol, increasing the drug content from 12.5% to 25% did not make a significant change on FPF values ($P > 0.05$), but the initial drug content of 37.5% (Formulation No. 3) appeared to have higher FPF (%) than the others ($P < 0.05$). However, changing the type of cholesterol solvent to 30:70 v/v water-ethanol (Formulation No. 5) resulted in FPF reduction which seems to be due to particle size enlargement of the resultant SLmPs [36,37]. The difference between FPF values associated with the type of solvent was more noticeable when DPPC was used as the lipid excipient. The consequence of changing the solvent from pure ethanol to 30:70 v/v water-ethanol was a noticeable increase in FPF values from 4.1% to 22.5% for DPPC-based formulations ($P < 0.05$). The latter results are not in accordance with the particle size determinations obtained by laser diffraction, since the formulation prepared by the aid of ethanol solution of DPPC had smaller size than that of water-ethanol solution of it. In this case, the particle aggregation of very small particles (D50% =1.42 μm) made up of DPPC as the lipid excipient and ethanol as the solvent, seemed to be the main cause of owning the lowest FPF value. In addition, wrinkled particles usually improve the respirable fraction of a DPI formulation by decreasing the interparticulate cohesion forces as well as enhancing the powder dispersibility [38].

The incorporation of L-leucine to the formulation number 6 which was prepared from 30:70 v/v water-ethanol solution of DPPC and SS resulted in insignificant FPF improvement ($P > 0.05$). As mentioned earlier, both kinds of formulations (F6 and F7) had almost similar particle average diameters, but different shapes. Although L-leucine plays a role of anti-adherent amino acid that can improve the deagglomeration of SLmPs [29], it seems that the corrugated particles made from spray-dried SS and DPPC could compensate the absence of L-leucine and act as favorably as the spherical particles of F7 in the in vitro pulmonary deposition test.

Moreover, simple blending of micron-sized SLmPs with coarse lactose monohydrate terminated in noticeable FPF elevation, compared to the FPF values of uncombined SLmPs. It seems that the absorption of the SLmPs to the surface of lactose, and the subsequent improvement in the dispersibility and deaggregation of them within the airflow resulted in elevated drug deposition in stage 2 of the TSI [24,34]. Finally, we found that co spray-dried DPPC/L-leucine, which had then been blended with coarse lactose (in the ratio of 1:9 w/w), was the most appropriate formulation for SS in term of aerosol performance.

In vitro drug release study

The release profiles of SS from SLmPs are reported in Figure 3. It should be noted that release of pure micronized SS was rapid as nearly all the amount of the drug was

Table 3 True density values obtained by the helium pycnometer

Drug conc. (%)*	Excipients	Solvent system	Inlet temp. (°C)	Density (g/cm^3)
37.5	Cholesterol	Ethanol	80	1.11 ± 0.09
37.5	Cholesterol	Water/Ethanol	100	1.15 ± 0.10
37.5	DPPC	Ethanol	80	1.15 ± 0.08
37.5	DPPC	Water/Ethanol	100	1.18 ± 0.07
100	-	Ethanol	80	1.33 ± 0.11
100	-	Water/Ethanol	100	1.41 ± o.12

*Percentage of the total solid content (w/w).

Table 4 Fine particle dose (FPD), emitted dose (ED) and fine particle fraction (FPF) of salbutamol sulfate after aerosolization from different formulations (mean ± SD)

Formulation number	Lipid excipients	Solvent system**	Inlet temp.(°C)	Blending excipient**	FPF(%)	FPD(μg)	ED(%)
1	Cholesterol	E	80	-	16.7 ± 0.8	165 ± 4.4	79.2 ± 2.1
2	Cholesterol	E	80	-	16.5 ± 1.2	305 ± 5.7	74.1 ± 2.5
3	Cholesterol	E	80	-	21.1 ± 0.9	575 ± 7.3	74.8 ± 1.8
4	DPPC	E	80	-	4.1 ± 0.3	138 ± 3.2	89.3 ± 1.6
5	Cholesterol	W/E	100	-	12.1 ± 0.7	310 ± 4.8	69.1 ± 2.1
6	DPPC	W/E	100	-	22.5 ± 1.3	686 ± 7.5	81.1 ± 2.3
7	DPPC + leucine	W/E	100	-	23.7 ± 1.1	712 ± 6.9	80.2 ± 1.9
8	Cholesterol	E	80	Lac.	24.1 ± 1.4	75 ± 3.1	82.6 ± 2.5
9	Cholesterol	W/E	100	Lac.	20.3 ± 0.8	61 ± 3.5	80.1 ± 2.2
10	DPPC	E	80	Lac.	16.6 ± 0.9	50 ± 2.8	80.1 ± 1.6
11	DPPC	W/E	100	Lac.	33.7 ± 1.5	108 ± 3.7	85.3 ± 2.7
12	DPPC + leucine	W/E	100	Lac.	42.7 ± 1.7	141 ± 4.1	87.9 ± 2.3
C_1^*	-	E	80	Lac.	17.6 ± 1.0	146 ± 2.8	83.4 ± 1.9
C_2^*	-	W/E	100	Lac.	14.4 ± 0.8	116 ± 2.2	81.1 ± 2.1

*C_1 and C_2 are control formulations of 5% (w/v) salbutamol sulfate in spray drying solution.
**E stands for Ethanol, W for Water, and Lac for lactose.

released in less than 30 min, which is in accordance with other studies [35]. In this study, generating inhalable microspheres from SS, cholesterol and ethanol provided a SR profile of the drug. In this regard, several other studies had shown the usefulness of SLmPs in developing SR formulations [7,17,18]. As shown in Figure 3, the release profile of SS from SLmPs produced from cholesterol and ethanol exhibited a burst release of approximately 50%, followed by a sustained SS release pattern over 12 hours, whilst in cholesterol-based SLmPs obtained from water-ethanol solution of SS, no SR profile was observed. This observation can be explained by the fact that the drug has a hydrophilic and ionized nature and does not dissolve in ethanol, so upon application of water and ethanol as the mixed solvent system, the drug mainly partitions into the water phase during the particle formation stage in spray drying chamber, and thus accumulates on the surface of the particle as the water evaporates. However, when the ethanol suspension of the drug is used, it is more likely for SS to be entrapped within the core of SLmPs as it does not dissolve in ethanol and thus does not migrate to lipid surface of the generating microparticles. In contrast, DPPC-based microparticles from ethanol suspension of SS did not show any SR profile, while changing the feed solvent from ethanol to water-ethanol (30:70 v/v) improved the drug entrapment within these DPPC-based SLmPs and exhibited a SR profile over 12 hours with a burst release of nearly 35%. In fact, besides the effect of the solvent, the affinity between the drug and lipid material is another efficient factor, which determines the retention capacity of SLmPs [17]. Herein, DPPC tends to place at the surface of the particles while the drug mostly remains within the aqueous core of the primary particles in the drying chamber before all the water content is subjected to evaporation. Thus, it is possible for DPPC to serve as a SS-retarding carrier in the mentioned inhalable formulation.

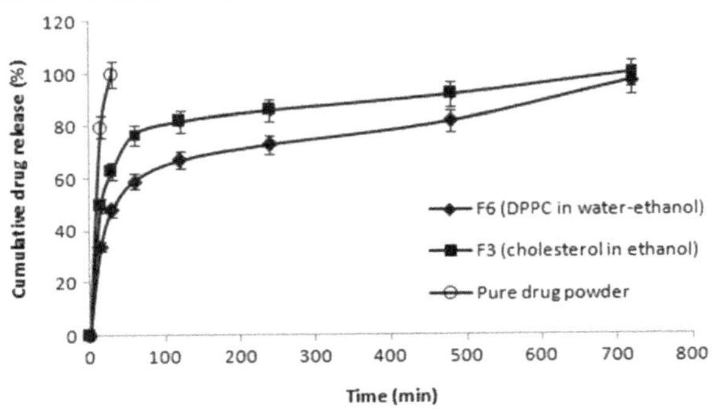

Figure 3 ***In vitro*** **release profile of salbutamol sulfate from different formulations.**

It worth mentioning that, this kind of SR pattern should be justified according to the dissolution rate of the pure drug powder as well as its specific pulmonary delivery rout. In this regard, it can be an acceptable SR pattern for SS DPI formulation since the lung retention time of microparticles is dependent on the generation number of the airway where the inhaled particles are deposited, and our SLmPs showed high FPF indicating that they have the potential to sufficiently penetrate deep into the lungs and avoid mucociliary clearance in the conducting airways. So the prolonged duration of the effect of SS can be expected by the aid of these SLmPs.

Conclusions

The type of lipid, presence of L-leucine in the feed solution, and the solvent system from which the SS-containing SLmPs were spray dried were the factors, which greatly affected the particle morphologies and aerosolization properties. We also observed substantial effects that physical mixing of spray-dried microparticles with coarse carrier can have on the aerosol performance. Among different DPI formulations, powders spray dried from water-ethanol solution of the drug, DPPC and L-leucine which were also physically blended with coarse lactose exhibited the best aerosolization properties. Despite having noticeable burst release during the first hour of the study, some SS-containing SLmPs showed significant release retardation compared the pure drug. The present study suggests that DPPC and L-leucine can be interesting additives for further developments of SS inhalable powder formulations.

Competing interests

The authors declare that they have no competing interests.

Authors' contributions

ZD: Carried out the preparation and characterization of the DPI formulations and drafted the manuscript. KM: Supervisor andparticipated in drafting the manuscript. ARN: Supervisor. HRF: participated in analysis of the drug. MAB: participated in characterization of the powders. All authors read and approved the final manuscript.

Acknowledgements

This study was funded and supported by Tehran University ofMedical Sciences (TUMS); grant no. 87-03-33-7715.

Author details

[1]Aerosol Research Laboratory, Department of Pharmaceutics, School of Pharmacy, Tehran University of Medical Sciences, Tehran, Iran. [2]Medicinal Plants Research Center, Tehran University of Medical Sciences, Tehran, Iran. [3]XRD Research Laboratory, School of Sciences, Tehran University, Tehran, Iran.

References

1. Courrier H, Butz N, Vandamme TF: **Pulmonary drug delivery systems: recent developments and prospects.** *Crit Rev Ther Drug Carrier Syst* 2002, **19:**no. 4–no. 5.
2. Groneberg D, Witt C, Wagner U, Chung K, Fischer A: **Fundamentals of pulmonary drug delivery.** *Resp Med* 2003, **97:**382–387.
3. Labiris N, Dolovich M: **Pulmonary drug delivery. Part I: physiological factors affecting therapeutic effectiveness of aerosolized medications.** *Brit J Clin Pharmacol* 2003, **56:**588–599.
4. Zeng XM, Martin GP, Marriott C: **The controlled delivery of drugs to the lung.** *Int J Pharm* 1995, **124:**149–164.
5. Hardy JG, Chadwick TS: **Sustained release drug delivery to the lungs.** *Clin Pharmacokin* 2000, **39:**1–4.
6. Cook RO, Pannu RK, Kellaway IW: **Novel sustained release microspheres for pulmonary drug delivery.** *J Control Rel* 2005, **104:**79–90.
7. Schreier H, Gonzalez-Rothi RJ, Stecenko AA: **Pulmonary delivery of liposomes.** *J Control Rel* 1993, **24:**209–223.
8. Lu D, Hickey AJ: **Liposomal dry powders as aerosols for pulmonary delivery of proteins.** *AAPS PharmSciTech* 2005, **6:**E641–E648.
9. Abra R, Mihalko PJ, Schreier H: **The effect of lipid composition upon the encapsulation and in vitro leakage of metaproterenol sulfate from 0.2 μm diameter, extruded, multilamellar liposomes.** *J Control Rel* 1990, **14:**71–78.
10. Parthasarathy R, Gilbert B, Mehta K: **Aerosol delivery of liposomal all-trans-retinoic acid to the lungs.** *Cancer Chemother Pharmacol* 1999, **43:**277–283.
11. Pilcer G, Amighi K: **Formulation strategy and use of excipients in pulmonary drug delivery.** *Int J Pharm* 2010, **392:**1–19.
12. Taylor KM, Fan SJ: **Liposomes for drug delivery to the respiratory tract.** *Drug Dev Ind Pharm* 1993, **19:**123–142.
13. Kellaway IW, Farr SJ: **Liposomes as drug delivery systems to the lung.** *Adv Drug Deliv Rev* 1990, **5:**149–161.
14. Niven RW, Schreier H: **Nebulization of liposomes. I. Effects of lipid composition.** *Pharm Res* 1990, **7:**1127–1133.
15. Desai TR, Hancock RE, Finlay WH: **Delivery of liposomes in dry powder form: aerodynamic dispersion properties.** *Eur J Pharm Sci* 2003, **20:**459–467.
16. Jaspart S, Bertholet P, Piel G, Dogné J-M, Delattre L, Evrard B: **Solid lipid microparticles as a sustained release system for pulmonary drug delivery.** *Eur J Pharm Biopharm* 2007, **65:**47–56.
17. Sebti T, Amighi K: **Preparation and in vitro evaluation of lipidic carriers and fillers for inhalation.** *Eur J of Pharm Biopharm* 2006, **63:**51–58.
18. Müller RH, Mäder K, Gohla S: **Solid lipid nanoparticles (SLN) for controlled drug delivery–a review of the state of the art.** *Eur J Pharm Biopharm* 2000, **50:**161–177.
19. Trotta M, Cavalli R, Carlotti M, Battaglia L, Debernardi F: **Solid lipid micro-particles carrying insulin formed by solvent-in-water emulsion–diffusion technique.** *Int J Pharm* 2005, **288:**281–288.
20. Pilcer G, Sebti T, Amighi K: **Formulation and characterization of lipid-coated tobramycin particles for dry powder inhalation.** *Pharm Res* 2006, **23:**931–940.
21. Masters K: *Spray drying handbook.* 5th edition. New York: Longman; 1991.
22. Steckel H, Brandes HG: **A novel spray-drying technique to produce low density particles for pulmonary delivery.** *Int J Pharm* 2004, **278:**187–195.
23. Chow AH, Tong HH, Chattopadhyay P, Shekunov BY: **Particle engineering for pulmonary drug delivery.** *Pharm Res* 2007, **24:**411–437.
24. Son Y-J, McConville JT: **Advancements in dry powder delivery to the lung.** *Drug Dev Ind Pharm* 2008, **34:**948–959.
25. Sanna V, Kirschvink N, Gustin P, Gavini E, Roland I, Delattre L, Evrard B: **Preparation and in vivo toxicity study of solid lipid microparticles as carrier for pulmonary administration.** *AAPS PharmSciTech* 2004, **5:**17–23.
26. Nassimi M, Schleh C, Lauenstein H, Hussein R, Hoymann H, Koch W, Pohlmann G, Krug N, Sewald K, Rittinghausen S: **A toxicological evaluation of inhaled solid lipid nanoparticles used as a potential drug delivery system for the lung.** *Eur J Pharm Biopharm* 2010, **75:**107–116.
27. Smolensky M, D'alonzo G, Kunkel G, Barnes P: **Day-night patterns in bronchial patency and dyspnea: basis for once-daily and unequally divided twice-daily theophylline dosing schedules.** *Chronobiol Int* 1987, **4:**303–317.
28. Chew NY, Shekunov BY, Tong HH, Chow AH, Savage C, Wu J, Chan HK: **Effect of amino acids on the dispersion of disodium cromoglycate powders.** *J Pharm Sci* 2005, **94:**2289–2300.
29. Salama RO, Traini D, Chan H-K, Young PM: **Preparation and characterisation of controlled release co-spray dried drug–polymer microparticles for inhalation 2: Evaluation of in vitro release profiling methodologies for controlled release respiratory aerosols.** *Eur J Pharm Biopharm* 2008, **70:**145–152.
30. Al-Asheh S, Jumah R, Banat F, Hammad S: **The use of experimental factorial design for analysing the effect of spray dryer operating variables on the production of tomato powder.** *Food Bioprod Process* 2003, **81:**81–88.
31. Ståhl K, Claesson M, Lilliehorn P, Lindén H, Bäckström K: **The effect of process variables on the degradation and physical properties of spray dried insulin intended for inhalation.** *Int J Pharm* 2002, **233:**227–237.
32. Vehring R: **Pharmaceutical particle engineering via spray drying.** *Pharm Res* 2008, **25:**999–1022.
33. Lechuga-Ballesteros D, Charan C, Stults CL, Stevenson CL, Miller DP, Vehring R, Tep V, Kuo MC: **Trileucine improves aerosol performance and stability of spray-dried powders for inhalation.** *J Pharm Sci* 2008, **97:**287–302.
34. Srichana T, Brain A, Marriott C, Martin GP: **A study of drug-carrier interactions in dry powder inhaler formulations using the Andersen cascade impactor, X-ray microanalysis and time of flight aerosol beam spectrometry (TOFABS).** *Chem Pharm Bull* 2000, **48:**167–174.
35. Scalia S, Salama R, Young P, Traini D: **Preparation and in vitro evaluation of salbutamol-loaded lipid microparticles for sustained release pulmonary therapy.** *J Microencap* 2012, **29:**225–233.

36. Yu J, Chien YW: **Pulmonary drug delivery: physiologic and mechanistic aspects.** *Crit Rev Ther Drug Carrier Syst* 1997, **14:**395–453.
37. Bosquillon C, Lombry C, Preat V, Vanbever R: **Comparison of particle sizing techniques in the case of inhalation dry powders.** *J Pharm Sci* 2001, **90:**2032–2041.
38. Zeng XM, Martin GP, Marriott C: *Particulate Interactions in Dry Powder Formulation for Inhalation.* London: Taylor & Francis; 2000.

Metabolic effects of newly synthesized phosphodiesterase-3 inhibitor 6-[4-(4-methylpiperidin-1-yl)-4-oxobutoxy]-4-methylquinolin-2(1H)-one on rat adipocytes

Bagher Alinejad[1], Reza Shafiee-Nick[1,2*], Hamid Sadeghian[3] and Ahmad Ghorbani[2]

Abstract

Background: Clinical use of selective PDE3 inhibitors as cardiotonic agents is limited because of their chronotropic and lipolytic side effects. In our previous work, we synthesized a new PDE3 inhibitor named MC2 (6-[4-(4-methylpiperidin-1-yl)-4-oxobutoxy]-4-methylquinolin-2(1H)-one) which produced a high positive inotropic action with a negative chronotropic effect. This work was done to evaluate the effects of MC2 on adipocytes and compare its effects with those of amrinone and cilostamide.

Methods: Preadipocytes were isolated from rat adipose tissue and differentiated to adipocyte in the presence of cilostamide, amrinone or MC2. Lipolysis and adipogenesis was evaluated by measuring glycerol level and Oil Red O staining, respectively. Adipocyte proliferation and apoptosis were determined with MTT assay and Annexin V/PI staining, respectively.

Results: Differentiation to adipocyte was induced by amrinone but not by cilostamide or MC2. Basal and isoproterenol-stimulated lipolysis significantly increased by cilostamide ($p < 0.05$). Similarly, amrinone enhanced the stimulated lipolysis ($p < 0.01$). On the other hand, MC2 significantly decreased both adipogenesis ($p < 0.05$) and stimulated lipolysis ($p < 0.001$). Also, incubation of differentiated adipocytes with MC2 caused the loss of cell viability, which was associated with the elevation in apoptotic rate ($p < 0.05$).

Conclusion: Our data indicate that selective PDE3 inhibitors produce differential effects on adipogenesis and lipolysis. MC2 has proapoptotic and antilipolytic effects on adipocytes and does not stimulate adipogenesis. Therefore, in comparison with the clinically available selective PDE3 inhibitors, MC2 has lowest metabolic side effects and might be a good candidate for treatment of congestive heart failure.

Keywords: Adipogenesis, Amrinone, Cilostamide, Lipolysis, Phosphodiesterases

Introduction

Cyclic nucleotide phosphodiesterases (PDEs) control the level of intracellular cAMP and cGMP, and hence play important roles in cellular signaling pathways. The PDEs are grouped into 11 families which differ in their physiochemical properties, substrate specificities, tissue distributions, and regulatory mechanisms [1]. Among them PDE3 has high expression in heart, airway, liver, pancreas, and adipose tissue and involves in the regulation of cardiovascular functions, insulin secretion, and lipid metabolism [2-5]. Selective PDE3 inhibitors have vasodilatory, antithrombotic, antiproliferative, bronchodilatory, anti-inflammatory, and positive inotropic effects [6-8]. A number of PDE3 inhibitors including cilostamide, cilostazol, milirinone, and amrinone were developed to treat patients with heart failure. However, chronic treatment with these agents was associated with some life-threatening side effects, arrhythmia in particular [7-10]. Therefore, designing new PDE3 inhibitors with

* Correspondence: Shafieer@mums.ac.ir
[1]Department of Pharmacology, School of Medicine, Mashhad University of Medical Sciences, Mashhad, Iran
[2]Pharmacological Research Center of Medicinal Plants, School of Medicine, Mashhad University of Medical Sciences, Mashhad, Iran
Full list of author information is available at the end of the article

desired pharmacological properties and lesser side effects is an attractive subject.

In the previous works we synthesized novel analogs of cilostamide as selective PDE3 inhibitors and evaluated their cardiac and metabolic properties. One of the test compounds, named MC2 (6-[4-(4-methylpiperidin-1-yl)-4-oxobutoxy]-4-methylquinolin-2(1H)-one), produced a potent inotropic action without unwanted effect on basal contraction rate [11-14]. Therefore, it may be a candidate for use as a PDE inhibitor in patients with cardiovascular diseases.

However, in adipose tissue, PDE3 inhibitors increase intracellular cAMP level and thereby increases lipolysis in adipocytes and enhance adipogenesis in preadipocytes [15,16]. Dysregulation of lipid metabolism in adipose tissue may cause deleterious consequences in some pathological conditions such as diabetes mellitus, insulin resistance, fatty liver, and obesity [17-19]. Therefore, as a selective PDE3 inhibitor, MC2 is expected to produce some effects on lipid metabolism which could be a potential risk factor for clinical adverse effect.

Therefore, in the present work, we evaluated the effects of MC2 on adipose tissue functions including adipogenesis and lipolysis, and also on adipocyte viability and apoptosis. Furthermore, the effects of MC2 were compared with the effects of amrinone and cilostamide on adipose tissue.

Materials and method

Chemicals and reagents

Isoproterenol, free glycerol reagent, 4-(2-hydroxyethyl) piperazine-1-ethanesulfonic acid sodium salt (HEPES), 4, 5-Dimethylthiazol-2-yl, 2, 5-diphenyl tetrazolium (MTT), fatty acid-free bovine serum albumin (BSA), and collagenase were purchased from Sigma (USA). Dimethyl sulfoxide (DMSO) and 3-isobutyl-1-methylxanthine (IBMX) were provided from Fluka (Buchs, Switzerland). Dulbecco's modified eagle's medium (DMEM), fetal bovine serum (FBS), penicillin/streptomycin, and Annexin V/PI apoptosis kit were obtained from Invitrogen (USA). Indomethacin, dexamethasone, and insulin were kindly provided by EXIR Company (Iran).

The test compound, MC2, was synthesized based on cilostamide structure by Department of Organic Chemistry, Mashhad University of Medical Sciences (Mashhad, Iran) according to the procedure reported by Sadeghian *et al.* and its PDE3 inhibitory action was assessed by Bioscience Company (BPS Bioscience Inc, San Diego, United States) using PDE assay Kit as described in previous works [14,20]. Figure 1 shows the IC50 of cilostamide, amrinone, and MC2 for PDE3. All the phosphodiesterase inhibitors were dissolved in dimethyl sulfoxide (DMSO) at a final concentration of 0.1% in the medium and equal amounts of carrier were added to control groups of the cells.

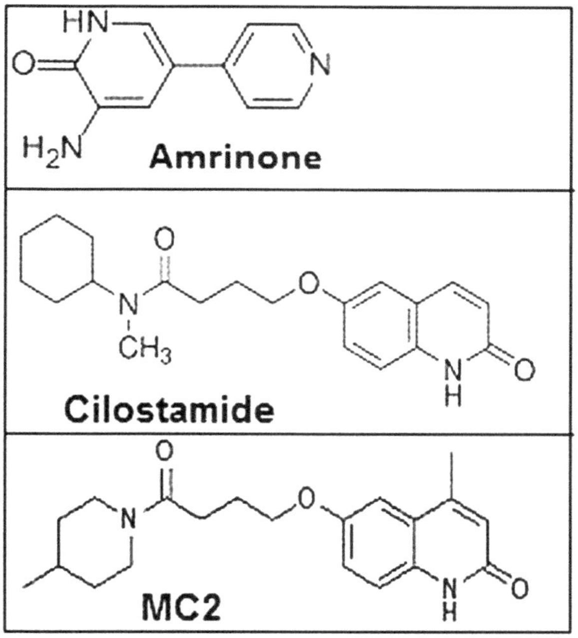

Figure 1 Structure of phosphodiestrase-3 inhibitors amrinone (IC_{50} ~ 50 μM), cilostamide (IC_{50} ~ 0.1 μM) and a new cilostamide derivative MC2 (IC_{50} ~ 1 μM).

Animals

Adult male Wistar rats with weights of 280–300 g were obtained from Laboratory Animal House, Mashhad University of Medical School, Iran. They were housed under a 12/12 h light/dark daily cycle at 22°C and had free access to standard foods and water. All experiments were conducted in accordance with standard ethical guidelines and approved by the local ethics committee of Mashhad University of Medical Sciences.

Preadipocyte preparation and culture

The animals were sacrificed under ether anesthesia and retroperitoneal fat pads were removed immediately and placed in phosphate-buffered saline (PBS) supplemented with 100 U/ml penicillin and 100 μg/ml streptomycin in sterile condition. The tissue was minced into small pieces and incubated for 40 min in PBS containing 2 mg/ml collagenase at 37°C with mild agitation [21,22]. After centrifuging, the floated adipocytes were discarded and the stromal cells were suspended in DMEM medium supplemented with 10% fetal bovine serum, 100 U/ml penicillin and 100 μg/ml streptomycin and cultured in flask. After passage 3, the cells were seeded (at a density of 60000 cells/cm^2) in 12-well plates. On next day, adipogenesis was induced by applying "induction medium" containing DMEM supplemented with 200 nM insulin, 250 μM IBMX, 1 μM dexamethasone, 200 μM indomethacin and 3% FBS. On day 3, the cells were subsequently cultured in "maintenance medium" (induction

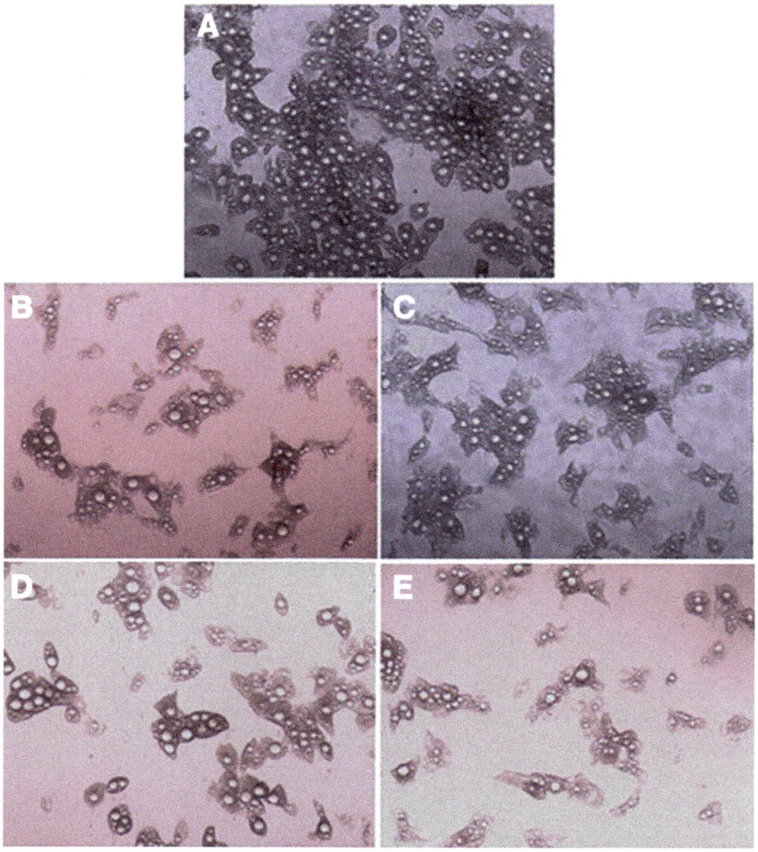

Figure 2 Differentiation of preadipocyte to adipocyte in the presence of (A) IBMX, (B) no PDE inhibitor, (C) amrinone, (D) cilostamide and (E) MC2. Adipogenesis was induced by 3 days incubation in "induction medium"; DMEM supplemented with 3% fetal bovine serum, 200 nM insulin, 250 μM of mentioned PDE inhibitors, 1 μM dexamethasone, 200 μM indomethacin. Then, the cells were subsequently cultured for 6 days in "maintenance medium" (induction medium without phosphodiestrase inhibitors and indomethacin). Magnification: ×100

medium without IBMX and indomethacin) for 9 days and the medium was changed every 3 days.

To investigate the effect of PDE inhibitors on adipogenesis, IBMX was replaced with the same concentration of amrinone, cilostamide, or MC2 in the induction medium during the first three days of incubation. The cellular triglyceride accumulation was measured as an index of the adipocyte differentiation in the presence of PDE3 inhibitors and compared with IBMX.

Oil Red O staining

Oil Red O was used to stain intracellular triglyceride droplets in differentiated adipocytes. Briefly, the cells were washed twice with PBS and fixed with 10% formalin for 30 min. After an additional washing with PBS, the cells were incubated with Oil Red O solution for 20 min [21,23]. Excess stain was removed by washing with distilled water and the stained cells were photographed. Lipid and Oil Red O were extracted using isopropyl alcohol and absorbance was measured using a spectrophotometer at a wavelength of 545 nm. The lipid content for each experimental group is expressed relative to that of IBMX-differentiated cells (adjusted to 100%).

Determination of triglyceride

To support Oil Red O staining, the level of intracellular triglyceride (TG) was evaluated in differentiated adipocytes. Following washing the cells with PBS, intracellular TG was dissolved in 200 μl of 1% Triton X-100/PBS solution. Then, the level of TG was determined by TG assay kit (Pars azma, Co., Ltd., Iran). The protein concentrations were also measured by Bio-Rad protein assay dye reagent (Bio-Rad Laboratories, Inc.). Then the level of TG was normalized to cellular protein content of each treatment group [24]. The TG/protein content (mg/mg) was expressed as percentage compared to IBMX treated group as a control.

Cell proliferation assay

To investigate the effects of the PDE inhibitors on adipocyte proliferation, preadipocytes were seeded (10^4 cell/well) in flat-bottomed 96-well culture plates. After differentiation, adipocytes were incubated with amrinone, cilostamide and

MC2 at the various concentrations (10, 100 and 500 μM) for 6, 12 and 24 h. After completion of the treatment, the cells were incubated with MTT solution for 3 h at 37°C. The supernatants were aspirated, DMSO was added to each well, and the plates were agitated to dissolve the crystal product [25-27]. Absorbance was measured at 545 nm (630 nm as a reference) using a StatFAX303 plate reader.

Annexin V/PI double staining analysis

To detect the apoptosis induced by PDE inhibitors, Annexin V/PI double staining and flow cytometry analysis were used [28]. After adipocyte differentiation in 12-well plates, the cells were exposed to 10, 100 and 500 μM of MC2 for 24 h. After treatment, the cells were washed twice with cold PBS and resuspended in 100 μl binding buffer at a concentration of 1×10^6 cells/ml. Then, 5 μl Annexin V-FITC and 10 μl PI (1 mg/ml) were added to these cells according to manufacturer's instructions. Finally, the cells were analyzed with a FACScalibur flow cytometer (Becton Dickinson) and the distribution of normal, apoptotic and necrotic cells was calculated using WinMDI 2.7 software.

Lipolysis assay

The differentiated adipocytes (cultured in 12-well culture plates) were pre-incubated with serum-free DMEM for 3 h and then bathed with 1 ml Krebs-Ringer bicarbonate buffer containing 5.5 mM glucose, 25 mM HEPES and 2% (w/v) bovine serum albumin. The cells were left untreated (basal lipolysis) or treated with isoproterenol (stimulated lipolysis) and incubated in the absence or presence of PDE inhibitors at 37°C in a humidified chamber under constant shaking for 2 h. Glycerol release in the medium was measured as index of lipolysis using the free glycerol determination kit [29,30].

Statistical analysis

The results are presented as the mean ± standard error. The values were compared using the one-way analysis of variances followed by Dunnett's post hoc test. The results were considered to be statistically significant, if the p-value was less than 0.05.

Results

Effect of PDE inhibitors on adipogenesis

The absence of IBMX in culture medium significantly decreased preadipocyte differentiation to adipocyte comparing to the control medium containing IBMX. Also, the level of adipogenesis in cilostamide and MC2 containing medium was lower than that of control medium. However, the effect of amrinone on preadipocyte differentiation was more than cilostamide and MC2, close to that of IBMX (Figure 2).

Oil Red O staining showed that in the presence of cilostamide and MC2 the level of lipid droplet accumulation was 69 ± 6% and 46 ± 4%, respectively, which was significantly lower than control medium containing IBMX (100 ± 4%, $p < 0.01$-$p < 0.001$) (Figure 3A). These findings were confirmed by measurement of intracellular TG in the differentiated adipocytes. As shown in Figure 3B, the level of intracellular TG in the presence of cilostamide (78 ± 6, $P < 0.05$) and MC2 (43 ± 5, $P < 0.001$) was lower than that of IBMX treated cells (100 ± 10).

Effect of PDE inhibitors on adipocyte proliferation

Incubation of differentiated adipocytes with 10–500 μM of cilostamide, 10–500 μM of amrinoe and 10–100 μM

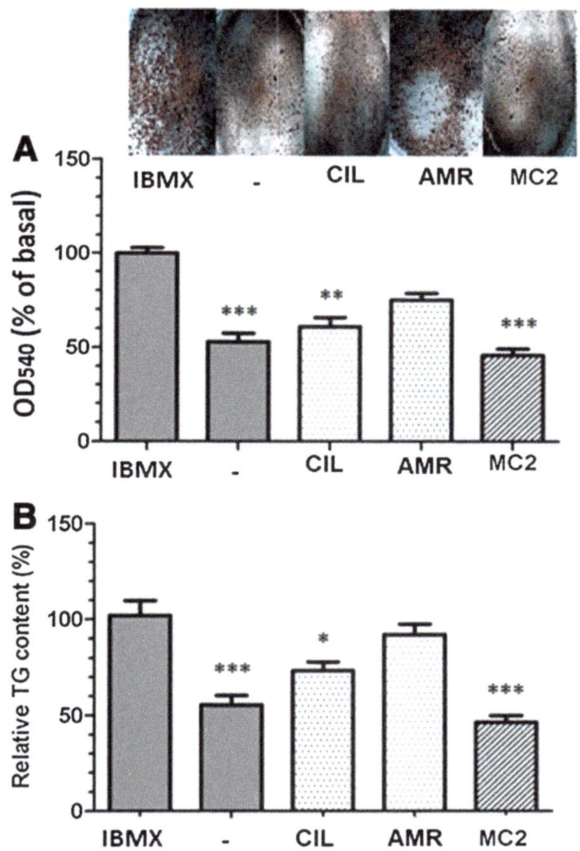

Figure 3 Effects of phosphodiestrase inhibitors on adipogenesis. Differentiation of preadipocytes was induced by 3 days incubation in induction medium; DMEM supplemented with 3% fetal bovine serum, 200 nM insulin, 1 μM dexamethasone, 200 μM indomethacin and 250 μM phosphodiestrase inhibitors (IBMX, amrinone (AMR), cilostamide (CIL), and (MC2). Then, the cells were subsequently cultured for 6 days in "maintenance medium" (induction medium without PDE inhibitors and indomethacin). Lipid accumulation was estimated by measuring the optical density (OD) of Oil Red O stain **(A)** or the level of triglyceride (TG) eluted from adipocytes **(B)**. Data are mean ± SEM of three independent experiments performed in triplicate. *$p < 0.05$,**$p < 0.01$ and ***$p < 0.001$ *vs* control (IBMX).

of MC2 had no effect on their proliferation after 6, 12 and 24 h (Figure 4). MC2 at 500 μM significantly decreased proliferation of differentiated adipocyte to 86 ± 6 ($p < 0.05$), 82 ± 3 ($p < 0.01$) and 79 ± 6 ($p < 0.01$) after 6, 12 and 24 h, respectively.

Effect of MC2 on adipocyte apoptosis

Figure 5A shows the results of bivariate Annexin V/PI flow cytometry of differentiated adipocyte after 24 h incubation with MC2. The lower left quadrant of the histograms shows the viable cells, which exclude PI and are negative for FITC-Annexin V binding. The upper right quadrant represents the early apoptotic cells, which are PI negative and Annexin V positive, indicating integrity of the cytoplasmic membrane. The lower right quadrant represents the non-viable necrotic and late-stage apoptotic cells, which are positive for Annexin V binding and PI uptake. As shown in Figure 5B, incubation of differentiated adipocytes with MC2 caused the loss of cell viability at concentrations of 100 μM ($p < 0.05$) and 500 μM ($p < 0.05$). This effect was associated with the elevation in the number of apoptotic (concentrations of 10 and 100 μM, $p < 0.05$) and necrotic (concentrations of 500 μM, $p < 0.01$) cells.

Effect of PDE inhibitors on lipolysis

The differentiated adipocytes were incubated with different concentrations of PDE inhibitors and glycerol release was measured as index of lipolysis. Amrinone at 100 μM significantly increased isoproterenol-induced (but not basal) lipolysis ($p < 0.05$). Cilostamide at concentration of 100 μM significantly increased basal lipolysis from 100 ± 7% to 334 ± 24% ($p < 0.001$) and also enhanced stimulated lipolysis from 375 ± 48% to 668 ± 34% ($p < 0.01$) (Figure 6A). At the concentration of 10 and 100 μM, basal lipolysis was not changed by MC2. However, it significantly decreased isoproterenol-induced lipolysis from 374 ± 48 to 225 ± 27% ($p < 0.01$) at 100 μM (Figure 6B).

Discussion

The PDEs play an important role in endocrine and cardiovascular functions, cell proliferation, cell differentiation, inflammation, and oxidative stress. Therapeutic application of PDE inhibitors, therefore, ranges from heart failure to pulmonary diseases to erectile dysfunction [31,32]. However, clinical application of these agents is limited because of their side effects, such as arrhythmia, impaired insulin secretion, and alterations in lipid metabolism [4,7]. Therefore, synthesis of new PDE3 inhibitors with desired pharmacological properties and lesser side effects is of great interest. In our previous work, we synthesized MC2 as a new cilostamide derivative and showed that it has inotropic action without unwanted effect on contraction rate [11,13]. In the present work, to assess the effect of synthesized compound on lipid metabolism, we investigated its effects on adipose tissue functions. Our data showed that MC2 unlike

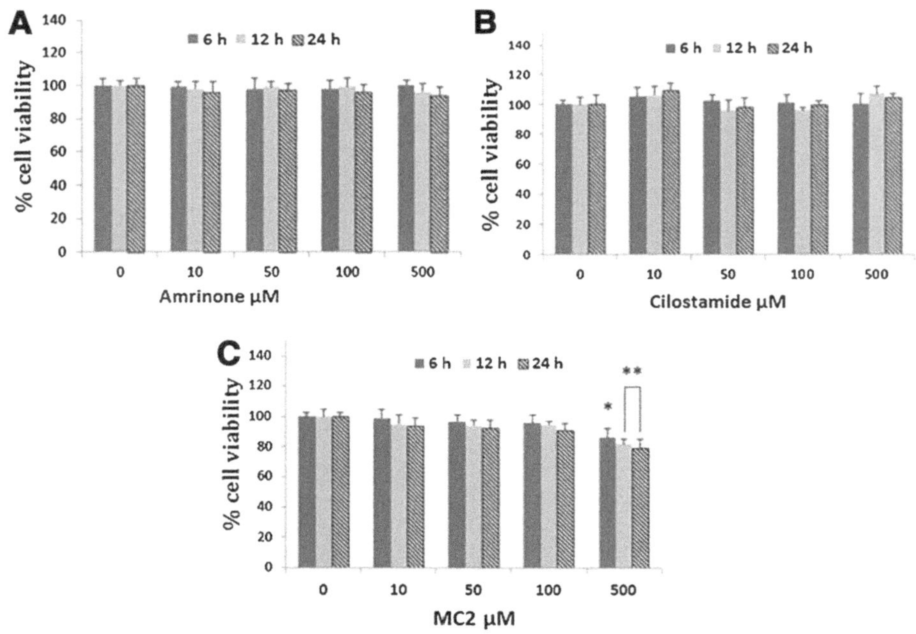

Figure 4 Effects of phosphodiestrase inhibitors on viability of differentiated adipocytes. The cells were incubated with various concentrations of amrinone **(A)**, cilostamide **(B)** and MC2 **(C)** for 6, 12 or 24 h. Cell viability was detected using MTT colorimetric assay. Values are mean ± SEM (n = 9). *$p < 0.05$ and **$p < 0.01$ *vs* control cells (0 μM).

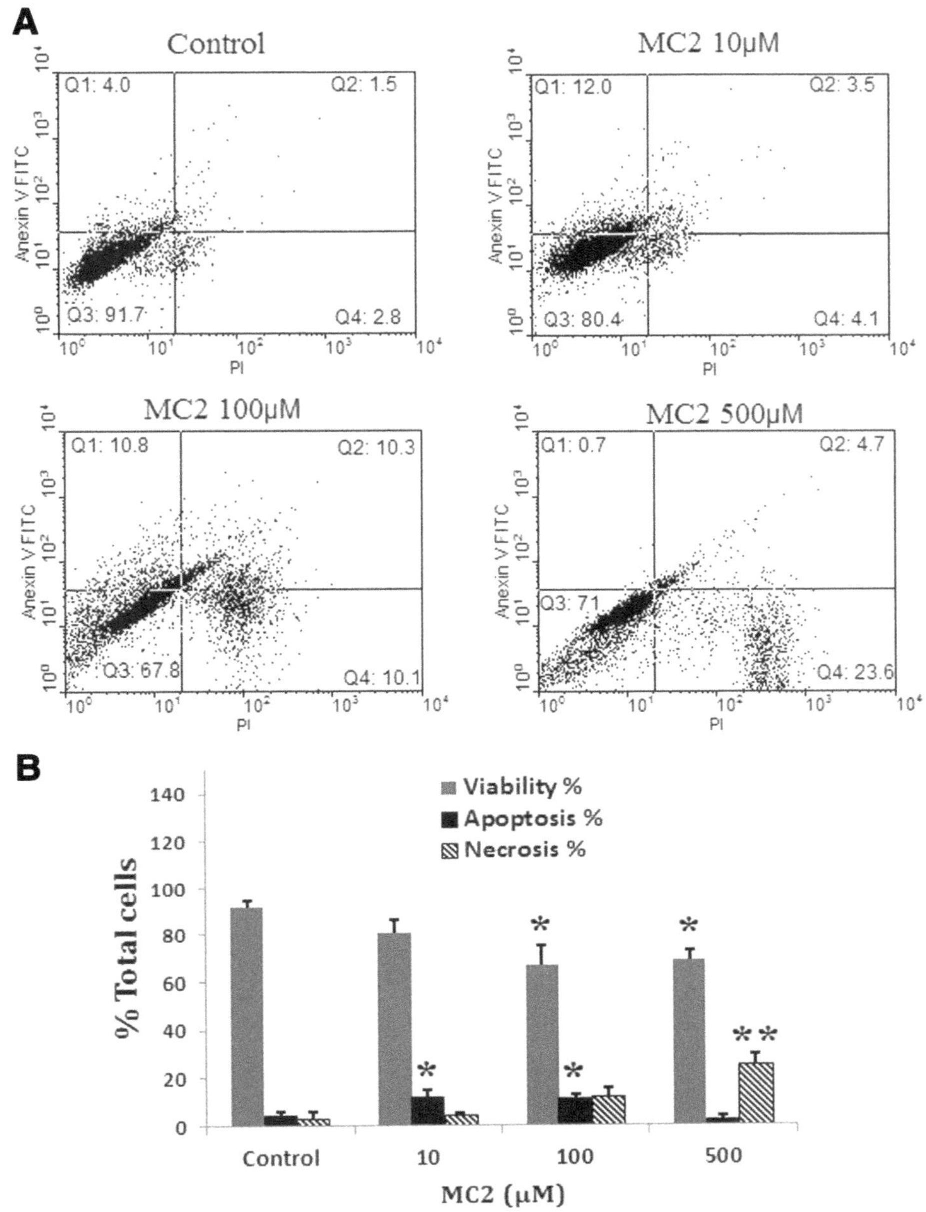

Figure 5 Effect of MC2 on apoptosis of adipocyte. (A) Detection of apoptosis and necrosis assessed with annexin-V-FITC and PI staining. The cells were treated with the indicated concentration of MC2 for 24 h. **(B)** Column bar graph of mean cell florescence for Annexin V-/PI- (Viable cells), Annexin V+/PI- (apoptotic cells), Annexin V+/PI+ (necrotic cells). Data are mean ± SEM of three experiments. *$p < 0.05$ and **$p < 0.01$ *vs* control.

other PDE3 inhibitors does not increase adipogenesis and lipolysis and even has antilipolytic effect.

In agreement with previous reports, in our study the PDE3 inhibitors amrinone and cilostamide potentiated both basal and catecholamine (isoproterenol)-stimulated glycerol release from adipocyte [33]. However, MC2 not only did not increase lipolysis, but inhibited catecholamine-induced glycerol release. Previously, in an *in-vitro* study we showed that MC2 increases liver glycogen storage in rat and mouse which was different from those of other PDE inhibitors [12]. These effects of MC2 cannot be explained with its PDE3 inhibitory action because PDE inhibitors enhance lipolysis via elevation of intracellular cAMP [2].

In our previous studies we found that different PDE3 inhibitors produce differential cardiac and metabolic effects. All of test compounds produced positive inotropic effect but with different efficacies, which were not

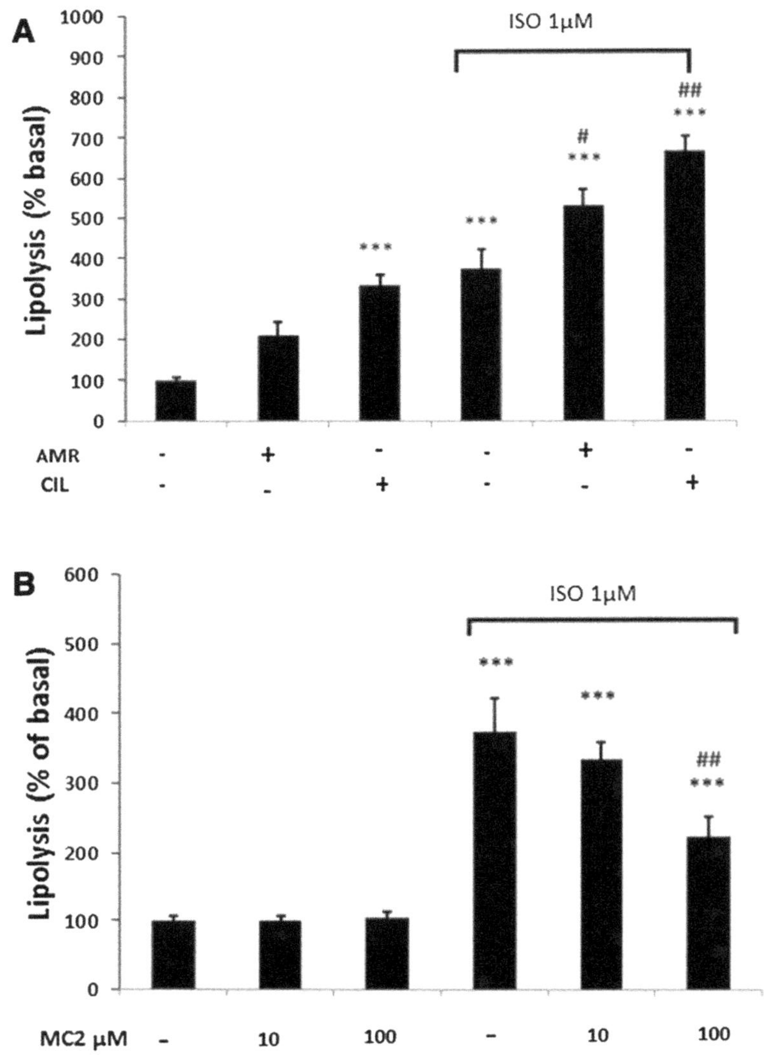

Figure 6 Effects of phosphodiestrase inhibitors on basal and isoproterenol (ISO)-induced lipolysis. Differentiated adipocytes were incubated with 100 μM amrinone (AMR), 100 μM cilostamide (CIL) **(A)** or indicated concentration of MC2 **(B)** for 120 min. Glycerol release in the culture media was assayed as lipolysis indicator. Data are mean ± SEM of three experiments. *P < 0.05 and ***P < 0.001 *vs* Control; #p < 0.05 and ##p < 0.01 vs ISO treated cells.

correlated with their IC_{50} of PDE3 inhibition. Also, they modified atrial contraction rates differently and some of which produced a negative chronotropic effect in spite of having a high positive inotropic effects [11]. Also, in rat hyperglycemic clamp model MC2 increased insulin secretion similar to the other tested PDE inhibitors, but opposite to others it increased the level of glycogen in the liver [12]. These effects implicate that a cAMP-independent signaling pathways may be involved in the biological effects of PDE inhibitors which is manifested by MC2 and may mediate its antilipolytic effect.

In patients with poorly controlled diabetes, deficiency of insulin in conjunction with catecholamine- and glucagon-stimulated lipolysis enhances fatty acid delivery to liver which may lead to ketoacidosis and even death [19]. It is reasonable to conclude that MC2 can decrease the risk of ketoacidosis through inhibition of lipolysis in diabetic patients who are candidate to PDE inhibitor therapy due to cardiovascular diseases.

Consistent with previous reports on the role of PDE inhibitors in adipogenesis [16,34], we found that deprivation of differentiation medium from IBMX attenuated adipogenesis. Neither cilostamide nor MC2 could restore the level of adipocyte differentiation to that of IBMX treated group. It has been revealed that PDEs exist in two forms: soluble (cytosolic) and particulate (membrane-associated) [35]. It is generally accepted that inhibition of soluble but not particulate PDE activity is responsible for IBMX-stimulated differentiation of pre-adipocytes [36]. Therefore, inhibition of PDE3 which predominately exist in the form of particulate cannot mimic the role of IBMX in adipocyte differentiation. On the other hand, similar to what happens in the heart and kidney [37], amrinone, in high concentration may inhibit soluble PDE and therefore could induce adipocyte differentiation approximately to the level induced by IBMX.

The mass of adipose tissue is determined by size and number of adipocytes. The size of adipocytes is reduced by lipolysis and increased by lipogenesis [38,39]. Number of adipocytes is directly related to the rate of adipogenesis and inversely related to the rate of apoptosis. Results of Annexin V/PI and MTT assays showed that MC2 increases adipocyte apoptosis. However, this effect was produced at high concentrations which reduced cell viability and proliferation. Since MC2 cannot increase adipogenesis, its potential proapoptotic effect may reduce total adipocytes number in fat tissue. However, antilipolytic effect of MC2 may prevent severe alteration in the mass of adipose tissue. Future works are needed to address long term effect of MC2 on fat mass.

In conclusion, our data showed that different types of PDE3 inhibitors induce different effects on lipolysis and adipogenesis. Here we introduced MC2 as a new PDE3 inhibitor with potential proapoptotic and antilipolytic effects on adipocytes and without stimulatory action on adipogenesis. These effects of MC2 implicate that, in comparison with amrinone or milrinone, this drug may have lowest metabolic side effect and might be a good candidate for treatment of congestive heart failure.

Competing interests
The authors declare that they have no competing interests.

Authors' contributions
RS-N and AG designed and supervised the study. RSN and HS designed and synthesized the test compounds. BA and AG collected data and wrote the first draft of the manuscript. BA performed the statistical analysis and managed the literature searches. All authors read and approved the final manuscript.

Acknowledgments
This work was a part of the Ph.D. thesis of one of the authors (Bagher Alinejad) and supported by a grant from Research Council of Mashhad University of Medical Sciences, Mashhad, Iran.

Author details
[1]Department of Pharmacology, School of Medicine, Mashhad University of Medical Sciences, Mashhad, Iran. [2]Pharmacological Research Center of Medicinal Plants, School of Medicine, Mashhad University of Medical Sciences, Mashhad, Iran. [3]Department of laboratory Sciences, School of Paramedical Sciences, Mashhad University of Medical Sciences, Mashhad, Iran.

References
1. Francis SH, Turko IV, Corbin JD. Cyclic nucleotide phosphodiesterases: relating structure and function. Prog Nucleic Acid Res Mol Biol. 2001;65:1–52.
2. Snyder BP, Esselstyn JM, Loughney K, Wolda SL, Florio VA. The role of cyclic nucleotide phosphodiesterases in the regulation of adipocyte lipolysis. J Lipid Res. 2005;46:494–503.
3. Palmer D, Maurice DH. Dual expression and differential regulation of phosphodiesterase 3A and phosphodiesterase 3B in human vascular smooth muscle: implications for phosphodiesterase 3 inhibition in human cardiovascular tissues. Mol Pharmacol. 2000;58:247–52.
4. Degerman E, Ahmad F, Chung YW, Guirguis E, Omar B, Stenson L, et al. From PDE3B to the regulation of energy homeostasis. Curr Opin Pharmacol. 2011;11:676–82.
5. Liu H, Maurice DH. Expression of cyclic GMP-inhibited phosphodiesterases 3A and 3B (PDE3A and PDE3B) in rat tissues: Differential subcellular localization and regulated expression by cyclic AMP. Br J Pharmacol. 1998;125:1501–10.
6. Hall IP. Isoenzyme selective phosphodiesterase inhibitors: potential clinical uses. Br J Clin Pharmacol. 1993;35:1–7.
7. Movsesian M, Wever-Pinzon O, Vandeput F. PDE3 inhibition in dilated cardiomyopathy. Curr Opin Pharmacol. 2011;11:707–13.
8. Boswell-Smith V, Spina D, Page CP. Phosphodiesterase inhibitors. Br J Pharmacol. 2006;147:S252–7.
9. Curfman GD. Inotropic therapy for heart failure-an unfulfilled promise. New Engl J Med. 1991;325:1509–60.
10. Smith AH, Owen J, Borgman KY, Fish FA, Kannankeril PJ. Relation of milrinone after surgery for congenital heart disease to significant postoperative tachyarrhythmias. Am J Cardiol. 2011;108:1620–4.
11. Hosseini A, Shafiee-Nick R, Parsaee H, Sadeghian H. Inotropic and chronotropic effects of new cilostamide derivatives on isolated rat atria. Iran J Physiol Pharmacol. 2011;15:341–50.
12. Hosseini A, Shafiee-Nick R, Pour Ali Behzad N, Sadeghian H. Differential metabolic effects of novel cilostamide analogs, methyl carbostiryl derivatives, in mouse and hyperglycemic rat. Iran J Basic Med Sci. 2012;15:916–25.
13. Mansouri SM, Shafiee-Nick R, Parsaee H, Seyedi SM, Saberi MR, Sadeghian H. Inotropic and chronotropic effects of 6-hydroxy-4-methylquinolin-2(1H)-one derivatives in isolated rat atria. Iran Biomed J. 2008;12:77–84.
14. Sadeghian H, Seyedi SM, Saberi MR, Nick RS, Hosseini A, Bakavoli M, et al. Design, synthesis and pharmacological evaluation of 6-hydroxy-4-methylquinolin-2 (1H)-one derivatives as inotropic agents. J Enzyme Inhib Med Chem. 2008;24:918–29.
15. Chaves VE, Frasson D, Kawashita NH. Several agents and pathways regulate lipolysis in adipocytes. Biochimie. 2011;93:1631–40.
16. Jia B, Madsen L, Petersen RK, Techer N, Kopperud R. Activation of Protein kinase A and exchange protein directly activated by cAMP promotes adipocyte differentiation of human mesenchymal stem cells. PLoS One. 2012;7:e34114.
17. Arner P, Langin D. Lipolysis in lipid turnover, cancer cachexia, and obesity-induced insulin resistance. Trends Endocrinol Metab. 2014;25:255–62.
18. Fabbrini E, Mohammed BS, Magkos F, Korenblat KM, Patterson BW, Klein S. Alterations in adipose tissue and hepatic lipid kinetics in obese men and women with nonalcoholic fatty liver disease. Gastroenterology. 2008;134:424–31.
19. Perilli G, Saraceni C, Daniels MN, Ahmad A. Diabetic ketoacidosis: a review and update. Curr Emerg Hosp Med Rep. 2013;1:10–7.
20. Degerman E, Belfrage P, Newman AH, Rice KC, Manganiello VC. Purification of the putative hormone-sensitive cyclic AMP phosphodiesterase from rat adipose tissue using a derivative of cilostamide as a novel affinity ligand. J Biol Chem. 1987;262:5797–807.
21. Ghorbani A, Hadjzadeh MR, Rajaei Z, Zendehbad SB. Effects of fenugreek seeds on adipogenesis and lipolysis in normal and diabetic rat. Pakistan J Biol Sci. 2014;17:523–8.
22. Ghorbani A, Feizpour A, Hashemzahi M, Gholami L, Hosseini M, Soukhtanloo M, et al. The effect of adipose derived stromal cells on oxidative stress level, lung emphysema and white blood cells of guinea pigs model of chronic obstructive pulmonary disease. DARU J Pharm Sci. 2014;22:26.

23. Ghorbani A, Jalali SA, Varedi M. Isolation of adipose tissue mesenchymal stem cells without tissue destruction: a non-enzymatic method. Tissue Cell. 2014;46:54–8.
24. Okazaki H, Igarashi M, Nishi M, Tajima M, Sekiya M, Okazaki S, et al. Identification of a novel member of the carboxylesterase family that hydrolyzes triacylglycerol: a potential role in adipocyte lipolysis. Diabetes. 2006;55:2091–7.
25. Mortazavian SM, Ghorbani A. Antiproliferative effect of viola tricolor on neuroblastoma cells in vitro. Aust J Herbal Med. 2012;24:93–6.
26. Mortazavian SM, Ghorbani A, Hesari TG. Effect of hydro-alcoholic extract of *Viola tricolor* and its fractions on proliferation of uterine cervix carcinoma cells. Iranian J Obstet Gynecol Infertility. 2012;15:9–16.
27. Forouzanfar F, Goli AA, Assadpour E, Ghorbani A, Sadeghnia HR. Protective effect of *Punica granatum* L. against serum/glucose deprivation-induced PC12 cells injury. Evid Based Complement Alternat Med. 2013;2013:716730.
28. Vermes I, Haanen C, Steffens-Nakken H, Reutelingsperger C. A novel assay for apoptosis flow cytometric detection of phosphatidylserine expression on early apoptotic cells using fluorescein labelled annexin V. J Immunol Methods. 1995;184:39–51.
29. Ghorbani A, Abedinzade M. Comparison of *in vitro* and *in situ* methods for studying lipolysis. ISRN Endocrinol. 2013;2013:205385.
30. Ghorbani A, Omrani GH, Hadjzadeh MR, Varedi M. Proinsulin C-peptide inhibits lipolysis in diabetic rat adipose tissue through phosphodiestrase-3B enzyme. Horm Metab Res. 2013;45:221–5.
31. Lugnier C. PDE inhibitors: a new approach to treat metabolic syndrome? Curr Opin Pharmacol. 2011;11:698–706.
32. Rajiv M, Vinod K. Phosphodiesterase inhibitors and their role in therapeutics. J Res Med Educ Ethics. 2013;3:115–23.
33. Ghorbani A, Omrani GH, Hadjzadeh MR, Varedi M. Effects of rat C-peptide-II on lipolysis and glucose consumption in cultured rat adipose tissue. Exp Clin Endocrinol Diabetes. 2011;119:343–7.
34. Jeon YH, Heo YS, Kim CM, Hyun YL, Lee TG. Phosphodiesterase: overview of protein structures, potential therapeutic applications and recent progress in drug development. Cell Mol Life Sci. 2005;62:1198–220.
35. Elks ML, Manganiello VC. A role for soluble cAMP phosphodiesterases in differentiation of 3 T3-L1 adipocytes. J Cell Physiol. 1985;124:191–8.
36. Sun L, Nicholson AC, Hajjar DP, Gotto Jr AM, Han J. Adipogenic differentiating agents regulate expression of fatty acid binding protein and CD36 in the J744 macrophage cell line. J Lipid Res. 2003;44:1877–86.
37. Ghosh R, Sawant O, Ganpathy P, Pitre S, Kadam V. Phosphodiesterase inhibitors: their role and implications. 2009;1:1148-1160
38. Rayalam S, Della-Fera MA, Baile CA. Phytochemicals and regulation of the adipocyte life cycle. J Nutr Biochem. 2008;19:717–26.
39. Ghorbani A, Varedi M, Hadjzadeh MR, Omrani GH. Type-1 diabetes induces depot-specific alterations in adipocyte diameter and mass of adipose tissues in the rat. Exp Clin Endocrinol Diabetes. 2010;118:442–8.

Design, synthesis, docking study and cytotoxic activity evaluation of some novel letrozole analogs

Mohsen Vosooghi[1], Loghman Firoozpour[2], Abolfazl Rodaki[2], Mahboobeh Pordeli[3], Maliheh Safavi[4], Sussan K Ardestani[3], Armin Dadgar[1], Ali Asadipour[5], Mohammad Hassan Moshafi[5] and Alireza Foroumadi[5,6*]

Background: Breast cancer is the most common type of female cancer. One class of hormonal therapy for breast cancer drugs -non steroidal aromatase inhibitors- are triazole analogues. In this work, some derivatives of these drugs was designed and synthesized. All synthesized compounds were evaluated for their cytotoxic activities on breast cancer cell lines (MDA-MB-231, T47D and MCF-7).

Methods: Our synthetic route for designed compounds started from 4-bromotolunitrile which was reacted with 1*H*-1,2,4-triazole to afford 4-(4-cyanobenzyl)-1,2,4-triazole. The reaction of later compound with aromatic aldehydes led to formation of the designed compounds. Eleven novel derivatives 1a-k were tested for their cytotoxic activities on three human breast cancer cell lines.

Results: Among the synthesized compound, 4-[2-(3-chlorophenyl)-1-(1*H*-1,2,4-triazol-1-yl)ethenyl]benzonitrile (**1c**) showed the highest activity against MCF-7 and MDA-MB-231 cell lines and 4-[2-(4-methoxyphenyl)-1-(1*H*-1,2,4-triazol-1-yl)ethenyl]benzonitrile (**1 h**) exhibited highest activity against T47D cell line. According to cytotoxic activities results, compound 4-[2-(4-dimethylamino)-1-(1*H*-1,2,4-triazol-1-yl)ethenyl]benzonitrile (**1 k**) showed comparative activity against T47D and MDA-MB-231 cell lines with compound (**1 h**) and our reference drug Etoposide.

Conclusion: In the process of anti-cancer drug discovery, to find new potential anti-breast cancer agents, we designed and synthesized a novel series of letrozole analogs. Cytotoxicity evaluation revealed that compounds (**1c**) and (**1 k**) were the most potent compounds with comparative activity with Etoposide. The results revealed that π-π interactions are responsible for the enzyme inhibitions of compounds (**1 c**) and (**1 k**).

Keyword: Breast cancer, Non-steroidal aromatase inhibitor, Cytotoxic activity

Background

Breast cancer is the most common female cancer. According to the American cancer society's report about 12% of women in the U.S. will develop some invasive breast cancer during their lifetime. However breast cancer treatment has a complicated process and problems, chemotherapy resistance, surgery and available anti-tumor drugs side effects make it more difficult to gain the appropriate treatment regimen; consequently, there is great demand to introduce new active compounds with more anticancer activity and less unwanted reaction [1,2].

* Correspondence: aforoumadi@yahoo.com
[5]Neuroscience Research Center, Institute of Neuropharmacology, Kerman University of Medicinal Sciences, Kerman, Iran
[6]Pharmaceutical Sciences Research Center, Tehran University of Medical Sciences, Tehran, Iran
Full list of author information is available at the end of the article

There is some different type of systemic therapy for breast cancer, one kind is hormonal therapy. Hormonal therapy can be given to women whose breast cancers test positive for estrogen to lower estrogen levels. Letrozole is a third generation of non-steroidal aromatase inhibitor – one class of hormonal therapy drugs- that was first introduces by Novartis to the market as Femara® for the treatment of local or metastatic breast cancer [3-5].

Non-steroidal aromatase inhibitors (as shown in Figure 1) are triazole or imidazole analogues that bind to the active site of enzyme by coordinating the heme iron atom of active site through a heterocyclic nitrogen lone pair [5,6].

As it shown in Figure 1, 1-benzyl-1*H*-1,2,4-triazole scaffold is a conservative section of aromatase inhibitors which contains various moieties attached to the aliphatic carbon part of this scaffold. In continuation of our research program to find a novel anticancer agent [7-11], and considering the above mentioned data, in the current study, we

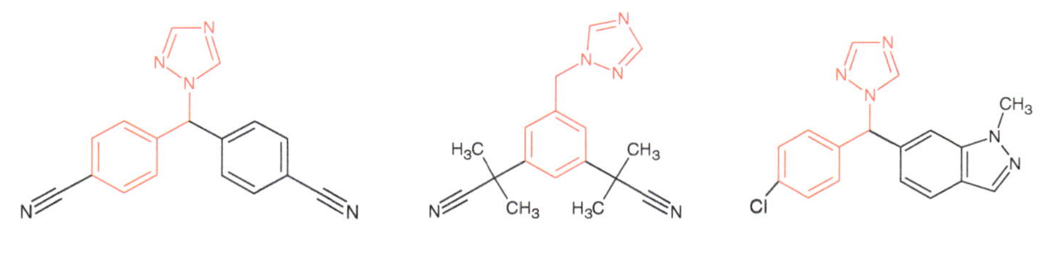

Figure 1 Structure of non-steroidal aromatase inhibitors.

report the synthesis of a novel series of substituted ethenylbenzene derivatives which linked tol-benzyl-1*H*-1,2,4-triazole (**1a-k**) and evaluated against three human breast cancer cell lines (Scheme 1).

Methods

Chemistry

All raw-materials, solvents and reagents were provided from Aldrich Chemicals and Merck AG. A Kofler hot stage apparatus was used for determination of melting points. The IR and ^{1}HNMR Spectra were determined on a Shimadzu 470 (potassium bromide disks) and a Bruker 500 spectrophotometer respectively. Tetramethylsilane (TMS) was used as internal standard and chemical shifts are reported in ppm relative to it. The elemental analysis for C, H and N were taken by a Perkin-Elmer 843 spectrometer with using KBr as diluent. Electrospray ionization mass spectra (ESI-MS) were recorded by using Agilent 6410 Triple Quad. LC/MS.

Key intermediate 4-(4-cyanobenzyl)-1,2,4-triazole was prepared according to Doiron J. and his collogues report [12].

General procedure for preparing of 4[2-aryl-1-(1H-1, 2, 4-triazol-1-yl)ethenyl]benzonitrile (1a-k)

4-(4-Cyanobenzyl)-1,2,4-triazole (1Gr) and 1,4-Dioxane (10 mL) were added to the reaction vessel and stirred. Sodium hydride (0.27 Gr 60%) was added to the reaction mixture in 0–5°C and stirred for 30 minutes. Corresponding aldehyde (0.5 mmol) was added to the mixture and stirred at room temperature for 30 minutes. Ethanol (3 mL) was added to the reaction mixture at 60°C and stirred for an hour. Reaction mixture cooled to room temperature and mixture of ice-water (25 Gr) was added. Precipitate was filtered and recrystallized in ethanol to yield corresponding compound (**1a-k**).

4-[2-Phenyl-1-(1H-1, 2, 4-triazol-1-yl)ethenyl]benzonitrile (1a)

Yield: 73%, mp 141–146°C. IR (KBr, cm^{-1}) ν_{max}: 2245 (nitrile), 1630 (C = C). ^{1}H NMR (500 MHz, $CDCl_3$): δ 8.25(s, 1H, triazole), 8.05 (s, 1H, triazole), 7.70-7.68 (d, *J* = 8.55 Hz,2H, benzonitrile), 7.35-7.33 (d, *J* = 8.55 Hz, 2H, benzonitrile), 7.30-7.26 (m, phenyl and ethenyl), 6.88-6.87 (d, *J* = 7.3 Hz, 1H, phenyl), ESI-Mass *m/z*: 272 $[M]^+$.

4-[2-(2-Chlorophenyl)-1-(1H-1,2,4-triazol-1-yl)ethenyl] benzonitrile (1b)

Yield: 70%, mp 141–144°C. IR (KBr, cm^{-1}) ν_{max}: 2240 (nitrile), 1622 (C = C). ^{1}H NMR (500 MHz, $CDCl_3$): δ 8.16(s, 1H, triazole), 7.96 (s, 1H, triazole), 7.72-7.71 (d , *J* = 8.45 Hz, 2H, benzonitrile), 7.43 (s, 1H, ethenyl), 7.45 (d, *J* = 7.75 Hz, 1H, phenyl), 7.40-7.39 (d, *J* = 8.45 Hz, 2H, benzonitrile), 7.27-7.23 (t, *J* = 7.9 Hz, 1H, phenyl), 7.08-7.05 (t, J = *J* = 7.15 Hz, 1H, phenyl), 6.61-6.59 (d, *J* = 7.75 Hz, 1H, phenyl), ESI-Mass *m/z*: 306 $[M]^+$.

4-[2-(3-Chlorophenyl)-1-(1H-1,2,4-triazol-1-yl)ethenyl] benzonitrile (1c)

Yield: 74%, mp 137–140°C. IR (KBr, cm^{-1}) ν_{max}: 2242 (nitrile), 1631 (C = C).^{1}H NMR (500 MHz, $CDCl_3$): δ 8.25(s, 1H, triazole), 8.04 (s, 1H, triazole), 7.70-7.69 (d, *J* = 8.5 Hz, 2H, benzonitrile), 7.35-7.33 (d, *J* = 8.5 Hz, 2H, benzonitrile), 7.29-7.26 (m, 1H, phenyl), 7.22 (s, 1H, phenyl), 7.20-7.18 (d, *J* = 7.95 Hz, 1H, phenyl), 6.93 (s, 1H,

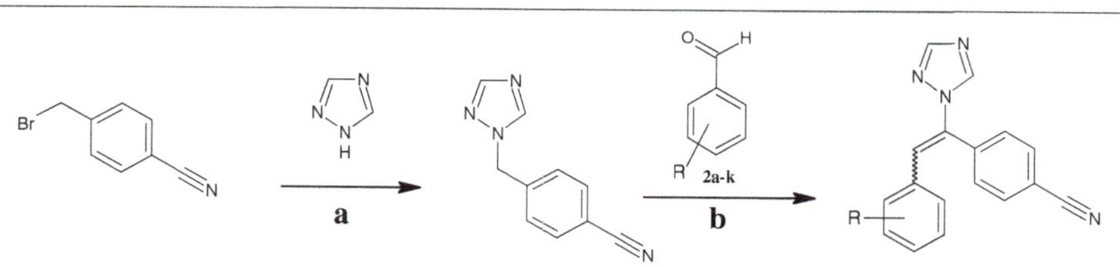

Scheme 1 The Synthesis rout of 4-[2-aryl-1-(1*H*-1,2,4-triazol-1-yl)ethenyl] benzonitriles 1a-k. (a) MeOH, KOH, DMF, **(b)** 1,4-Dioxane, recrystallized in EtOH.

ethenyl), 6.69-6.68 (d, $J = 8.2$ Hz, 1H, phenyl), ESI-Mass m/z: 306 $[M]^+$.

4-[2-(4-Chlorophenyl)-1-(1H-1,2,4-triazol-1-yl)ethenyl] benzonitrile (1d)

Yield: 71%, mp 139–146°C. IR (KBr, cm^{-1}) ν_{max}: 2237 (nitrile), 1630 (C = C).^{1}H NMR (500 MHz, $CDCl_3$) δ 8.25(s, 1H, triazole), 8.04 (s, 1H, triazole), 7.70-7.69 (d, $J =$ 8.86 Hz,2H, benzonitrile), 7.34-7.33 (d, $J = 8.6$ Hz, 2H, benzonitrile), 7.27-7.25 (d, $J = 8.5$ Hz, 2H, phenyl),7.24 (s, 1H, ethenyl), 6.80-6.79(d, $J = 8.5$ Hz, 2H, phenyl), ESI-Mass m/z: 306 $[M]^+$.

4-[2-(2,4-Dichlorophenyl)-1-(1H-1,2,4-triazol-1-yl)ethenyl] benzonitrile (1e)

Yield: 74%, mp 150–153°C. IR (KBr, cm^{-1}) ν_{max}: 2248 (nitrile), 1629 (C = C).^{1}H NMR (500 MHz, $CDCl_3$): δ 8.16 (s, 1H, triazole), 7.96 (s, 1H, triazole), 7.74-7.72 (d, $J =$ 8.35 Hz, 2H, benzonitrile) , 7.42-7.40 (m, 4H, benzonitrile and ethenyl), 7.04-7.01 (m, 1H, phenyl), 6.56-6.55 (m, 1H, phenyl), ESI-Mass m/z: 340 $[M]^+$.

4-[2-(3-Fluorophenyl)-1-(1H-1,2,4-triazol-1-yl)ethenyl] benzonitrile (1f)

Yield: 74%, mp 145–150°C. IR (KBr, cm^{-1}) ν_{max}: 2244 (nitrile), 1634 (C = C).^{1}H NMR (500 MHz, $CDCl_3$): δ 8.25 (s, 1H, triazole), 8.05 (s, 1H, triazole), 7.71-7.69 (d, $J =$ 8.5 Hz,2H, benzonitrile), 7.35-7.33 (d, $J = 8.5$ Hz, 2H, benzonitrile), 7.30-7.26 (m, 1H, phenyl), 7.25 (s, 1H, ethenyl), 7.03-6.99 (m, 1H, phenyl), 6.68-6.66 (d, $J = 7.75$ Hz, 1H, phenyl), 6.58-6.56 (d, $J = 7.8$ Hz, 1H, phenyl), ESI-Mass m/z: 290 $[M]^+$.

4-[2-(3-Methoxyphenyl)-1-(1H-1,2,4-triazol-1-yl)ethenyl] benzonitrile (1 g)

Yield: 74%, mp 128–132°C. IR (KBr, cm^{-1}) ν_{max}: 2242 (nitrile), 1631 (C = C).^{1}H NMR (500 MHz, $CDCl_3$): δ 8.24 (s, 1H, triazole), 8.05 (s,1H, triazole), 7.69-7.67 (d, $J =$ 8.1 Hz, 2H, benzonitrile), 7.34-7.33 (d, $J = 8.1$ Hz, 2H, benzonitrile), 7.27 (s, 1H, ethenyl), 7.21-7.18 (t, $J = 7.9$ Hz, 1H, phenyl), 6.86-6.84 (d, $J = 7.6$ Hz, phenyl), 6.54-6.53 (d, $J = 7.43$ Hz, phenyl), 6.31 (s, 1H, phenyl), 3.66 (s,3H,OMe), ESI-Mass m/z: 302 $[M]^+$.

4-[2-(4-Methoxyphenyl)-1-(1H-1,2,4-triazol-1-yl)ethenyl] benzonitrile (1 h)

Yield: 74%, mp 140–143°C. IR (KBr, cm^{-1}) ν_{max}: 2244 (nitrile), 1632 (C = C).^{1}H NMR (500 MHz, $CDCl_3$) δ 8.27 (s, 1H, triazole), 8.08 (s,1H, triazole), 7.67-7.65 (d, $J =$ 8.7 Hz,2H, benzonitrile) , 7.30-7.29 (d , $J = 8.7$ Hz, 2H, benzonitrile), 7.25 (s, 1H, ethenyl), 6.80-6.78 (d, $J = 9.2$ Hz, 2H, phenyl), 6.77-6.76 (d, $J = 9.2$ Hz, 2H, phenyl), 3.80 (s,3H, OMe), ESI-Mass m/z: 302 $[M]^+$.

4-[2-(2,4-Dimethoxyphenyl)-1-(1H-1,2,4-triazol-1-yl)ethenyl] benzonitrile (1i)

Yield: 74%, mp 158–161°C. IR (KBr, cm^{-1}) ν_{max}: 2239 (nitrile), 1632 (C = C). ^{1}H NMR (500 MHz, $CDCl_3$): δ 8.22 (s, 1H, triazole), 8.06 (s,1H, triazole), 7.66-7.65 (d, $J =$ 8.3 Hz,2H, benzonitrile), 7.50 (s, 1H, ethenyl), 7.31-7.30 (d, $J = 8.3$ Hz, 2H, benzonitrile), 6.44-6.27 (m, 3H, phenyl), 3.84 (s,3H, OMe), 3.79 (s,3H, OMe), ESI-Mass m/z: 332 $[M]^+$.

4-[2-(2,3,4-Trimethoxy)-1-(1H-1,2,4-triazol-1-yl)ethenyl] benzonitrile (1j)

Yield: 75%, mp 188–191°C. IR (KBr, cm^{-1}) ν_{max}: 2246 (nitrile), 1634 (C = C).^{1}H NMR (500 MHz, $CDCl_3$): δ 8.20 (s, 1H, triazole), 8.09 (s,1H, triazole), 7.67-7.65 (d, $J =$ 8.3 Hz,2H, benzonitrile), 7.51 (s, 1H, ethenyl), 7.33-7.30 (d, $J = 8.3$ Hz, 2H, benzonitrile), 6.46-6.25 (m, 2H, phenyl), 3.86 (s,3H, OMe), 3.81 (s,3H, OMe), 3.76 (s,3H, OMe), ESI-Mass m/z: 3362 $[M]^+$.

4-[2-(4-Dimethylamino)-1-(1H-1,2,4-triazol-1-yl)ethenyl] benzonitrile (1 k)

Yield: 72%, mp 158–161°C. IR (KBr, cm^{-1}) ν_{max}: 2241 (nitrile), 1633 (C = C).^{1}H NMR (500 MHz, $CDCl_3$) δ 8.26 (s, 1H, triazole), 8.05 (s,1H, triazole), 7.66-7.65 (d, $J =$ 8.5 Hz,2H, benzonitrile), 7.32-7.27 (d, $J = 8.5$ Hz, 2H, benzonitrile), 7.25 (s, 1H, ethenyl), 6.79-6.75 (d, $J = 9.1$ Hz, 2H, phenyl), 6.74-6.72 (d, $J = 9.1$ Hz, 2H, phenyl), 3.79-3.75 (m,6H, Me), ESI-Mass m/z: 315 $[M]^+$.

Physicochemical prediction

Marvin was used for chemical drawing, displaying and characterizing chemical structures, calculator plugins were used for structure property prediction and calculation, (version: Marvin 6.0.3, 2013, ChemAxon scientific package, http://www.chemaxon.com).

Molecular modeling study

Docking studies for selected compounds were performed using Autodock Vina (ver. 1.1.1) [13]. The crystal structure of human placental aromatase cytochrome P450 in complex with androstenedione (code ID: 3EQM, resolution [Å]: 2.90) was retrieved from protein data bank [14-17]. Crystal structure was cleaned from Co-crystallized ligand and water molecules and the protein was converted to pdbqt format using Autodock Tools (1.5.4) [18]. 2Dstructures of ligands converted to 3D in pdbqt format by Openbabel (ver. 2.3.1) [18]. The docking parameters were set on vina docking parameter as follow: center_x = 85.027; center_y = 54.737; center_z = 46.428; size_x =50; size_y =50; size_z =50;. The other parameters were left as default for the program. Finally, the conformation for the best free energy of binding was selected for analyzing the interactions between the macromolecule and selected inhibitors. 3D

Table 1 Target structures and physicochemical properties

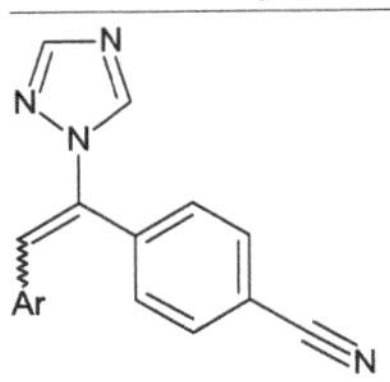

No.	Comp. Code	Ar	MW	Formula	Vander Waals Surface	Polar Surface	Log P
1.	1a	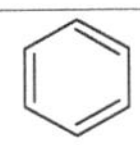	272	$C_{17}H_{12}N_4$	363.21	54.50	3.12
2.	1b	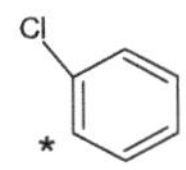	306.75	$C_{17}H_{11}ClN_4$	376.65	54.50	3.72
3.	1c	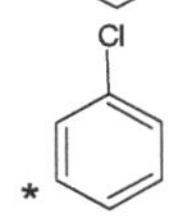	306.75	$C_{17}H_{11}ClN_4$	378.12	54.50	3.72
4.	1d	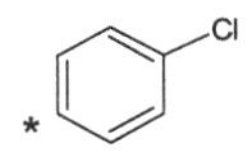	306.75	$C_{17}H_{11}ClN_4$	378.12	54.50	3.72
5.	1e	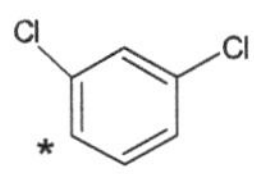	341.19	$C_{17}H_{10}Cl_2N_4$	393.15	54.50	4.33
6.	1f	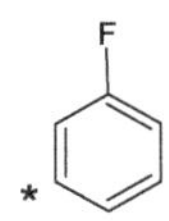	290.29	$C_{17}H_{11}FN_4$	369.04	54.50	3.22
7.	1g	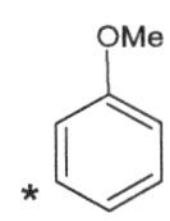	302.33	$C_{18}H_{14}ON_4$	410.22	63.73	2.96
8.	1h	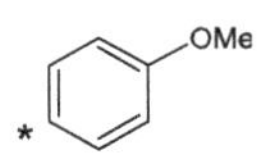	302.33	$C_{18}H_{14}ON_4$	409.36	63.73	2.96
9.	1i	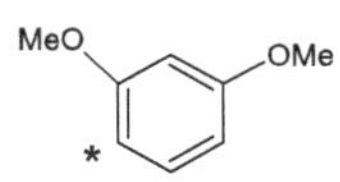	332.36	$C_{19}H_{16}O_2N_4$	457.69	72.96	2.80
10.	1j	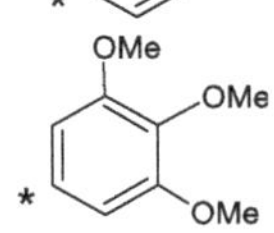	362.38	$C_{20}H_{18}O_3N_4$	504.76	82.19	2.65
11.	1k	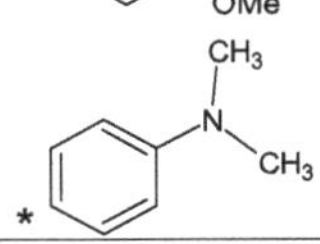	315.37	$C_{19}H_{17}N_5$	448.10	57.74	3.23

models of ligand-receptor interactions are generated by using the Autodock Tools (1.5.4) [19].

Biological assay

Cell lines and cell culture

Three human breast cancer cell lines including MDA-MB-231, MCF-7 and T-47D were obtained from National Cell Bank of Iran (NCBI, Iran). The cells were grown in RPMI-1640 medium supplemented with 10% heat-inactivated fetal calf serum (GibcoeBRL, UK), 100 mg/ml streptomycin and 100 U/ml penicillin at 37°C/95% rh/5% CO_2.

In vitro cytotoxicity assay

The in-vitro cytotoxic activity of all synthesized compounds **1a-k** was achieved against three human breast cancer cell lines using MTT colorimetric assay according

Table 2 *In vitro* cytotoxic activity (IC_{50}, μg/ml) of compounds 1a-k against breast cancer cell lines[a]

No.	Comp. Code	Cell lines		
		MCF-7	MDA-MB-231	T-47D
1.	1a	57.1 ± 2.1	87.5 ± 2.5	64.3 ± 1.9
2.	1b	63.2 ± 2.6	97.3 ± 3.1	77.1 ± 2.8
3.	1c	27.1 ± 1.2	14.5 ± 2.1	76.25 ± 7.0
4.	1d	52.3 ± 2.2	43.3 ± 3.4	83.3 ± 5.2
5.	1e	78.3 ± 5.7	83.3 ± 7.2	92.3 ± 6.2
6.	1f	72.3 ± 5.5	85.3 ± 7.4	87.3 ± 7.5
7.	1 g	40.3 ± 2.8	77.4 ± 6.5	69.4 ± 5.7
8.	1 h	74.6 ± 6.5	82.3 ± 7.4	14.3 ± 1.1
9.	1i	75.3 ± 4.4	89.4 ± 6.1	79.1 ± 7.7
10.	1j	69.3 ± 5.3	45.05 ± 6.2	63.3 ± 6.6
11.	1 k	55.3 ± 5.1	19.7 ± 1.8	16.8 ± 2.1
12.	Etoposide	7.9 ± 0.5	11.1 ± 1.1	8 ± 0.8

[a]The IC_{50} values represent an average of three independent experiments (mean ± SD).

to the method of Mosman [20]. Cells were seeded in 96-well plates (Nunc, Denmark) and incubated overnight in a humidified air atmosphere at 37°C with 5% CO_2 to allow cell attachment. The cells were then incubated for another 48 h with various concentrations of compounds **1a-k**. The final concentration of DMSO in the highest concentration of the applied compounds was 1%. In each plate, there were three control wells (cells without test compounds) and three blank wells (the medium with 1% DMSO) for cell viability. Etoposide were used as positive controls for cytotoxicity. After 48 h, the culture medium was removed and 200 μl phenol red-free medium containing MTT (final concentration 0.5 mg/mL) was added to wells, followed by 4 h incubation.

After incubation, the culture medium was then replaced with 100 μl of DMSO and the absorbance of each well was measured by using a microplate reader at 492 nm. For each compound, the concentration causing 50% cell growth inhibition (IC_{50}) compared with the control containing 1% DMSO was calculated from concentration response curves by regression analysis.

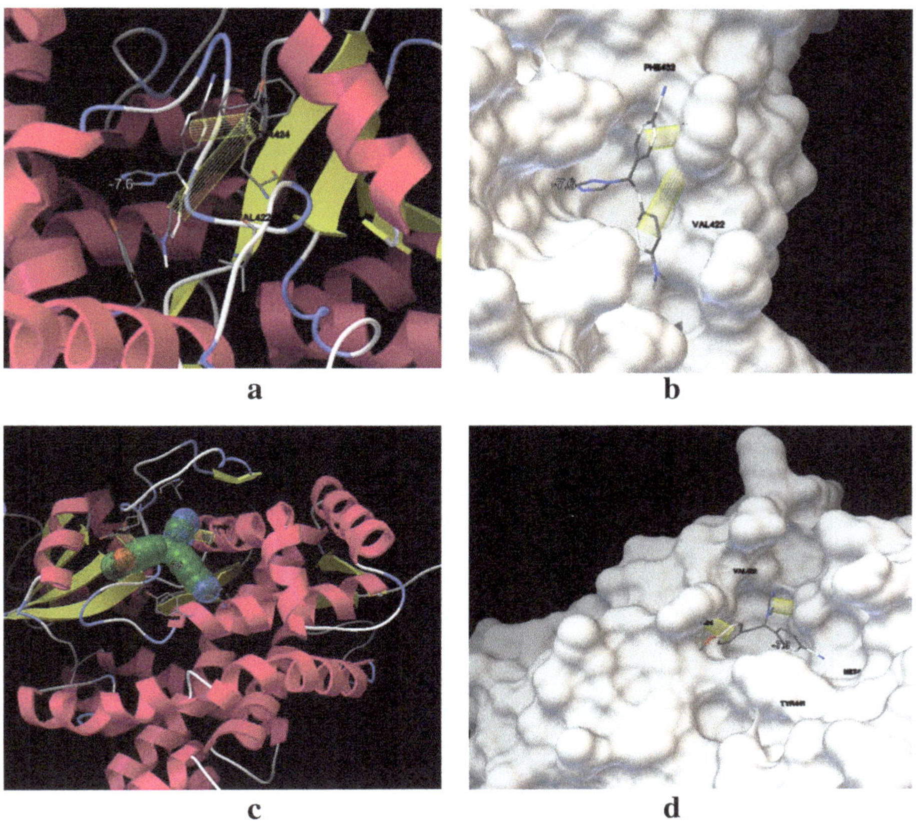

Figure 2 Presentation of compounds (1c) and (1 k) with aromatase enzyme, π-π interactions showed in yellow cylindrical shape. **(a, b)** visualization of compound **(1c)** in enzyme with ribbon and molecular surface views; **(c, d)** binding mode of **(1 k)** in enzyme with ribbon and molecular surface views.

Results and discussions

Chemistry

4-Bromotolunitrile was converted to 4-(4-cyanobenzyl)-1,2,4-triazole and subsequently to corresponding product, 4-[2-aryl-1-(*1H*-1,2,4-triazol-1-yl)ethenyl]benzonitrile (**1a-k**) according to the procedure presented in Scheme 1. Chemical structures, molecular formula and molecular weight of compounds (**1a-k**) are illustrated in Table 1. Reaction yields are presented in chemistry section of methods in this report.

Physicochemical prediction

In order to investigate the physicochemical properties of products, Vander Waals surface, polar surface and partition-coefficient (Log P) of compounds (**1a-k**) were predicted by Marvin program and are reported in Table 1. As it shown primary physicochemical criteria were passed by all designed compounds (**1a-k**).

Cytotoxic activity

The *in vitro* cytotoxic activity of 4[2-aryl-1-(*1H*-1,2,4-triazol-1-yl)ethenyl]benzonitrile (**1a-k**), were tested against three human breast cancer lines including MDA-MB-231, T47D and MCF-7. The various concentrations of the synthetic compounds (final concentration 5, 10, 20, 40, 80 and 100 μg/ml) were applied to calculate IC_{50}. The 50% growth inhibitory concentration (IC_{50}) for products were calculated and depicted in Table 2.

According to MTT assay results in Table 2, 4-[2-(3-chlorophenyl)-1-(*1H*-1,2,4-triazol-1-yl)ethenyl]benzonitrile (**1c**) showed the highest activity against MCF-7 and MDA-MB-231 cell lines with IC_{50} values of 27.1 ± 1.2 and 14.5 ± 2.1 μg/ml, respectively and 4-[2-(4-methoxyphenyl)-1-(*1H*-1,2,4-triazol-1-yl)ethenyl]benzonitrile (**1 h**) exhibited highest activity against T47D cell line with IC_{50} value of 14.3 ± 1.1 μg/ml. As can be seen in Table 2, compound 4-[2-(4-dimethylamino)-1-(*1H*-1,2,4-triazol-1-yl)ethenyl]benzonitrile (**1 k**), showed comparative activity against T47D and MDA-MB-231 cell lines with compound **1 h** and Etoposide withIC_{50} values of 16.8 ± 2.1 and 19.7 ± 1.8 μg/ml, respectively. As it shown in MTT assay results all other synthesized compound did not show good activity against tested cell lines.

Docking study

In order to understand the binding mode of active compounds in the active site pocket of aromatase, docking study was performed using Autodock Vina. To attain this aim, the potent compounds, **1c** and **1 k** were docked into target enzyme. Docking strongly suggested that the π-π interaction between adjacent phenyl rings and hydrophobic moieties in enzyme residues –Tyrosine 424 and Tyrosine 361- are effective in activity of biologically active synthesized compounds. According to Figure 2, selected compounds fit in the pocket of aromatase enzyme completely, however missing the potentially hydrogen bond between ligands and macromolecule is responsible for moderate activities of compounds (**1c**) and (**1 k**).

Conclusion

In the process of anti-cancer drug discovery, to find new potential anti-breast cancer agents, we designed and synthesized a novel series of letrozole analogs. Cytotoxicity evaluation revealed that compounds (**1c**) and (**1 k**) were the most potent compounds with comparative activity with Etoposide. Physicochemical properties of products predicted and the binding mode of (**1c**) and (**1 k**) were predicted by docking simulation; the results revealed that π-π interactions are responsible for the enzyme inhibitions of compounds (**1c**) and (**1 k**).

Competing interests

The authors declare that they have no competing interests.

Authors' contributions

MV: design and synthesis of the title compound, manuscript preparations. LF: computational design for prediction of physicochemical properties. AR: collaboration in the synthesis of the target compounds. MP: collaboration in cytotoxic assay. MS: collaboration in cytotoxic assays and IC_{50} calculations. SKA: supervision of the pharmacological part. AD: reporting the spectra and writing experimental section. AA: collaboration in the synthesis of intermediates. KD: collaboration in cytotoxic assays. AF: design of target compounds and the synthetic rout. All authors read and approved the final manuscript.

Acknowledgments

This work was supported by a grant from Iran National Science Foundation (INSF).

Author details

[1]Department of Medicinal Chemistry, Faculty of Pharmacy, Tehran University of Medical Sciences, Tehran, Iran. [2]Drug Design and Development Research Center, Tehran University of Medical Sciences, Tehran, Iran. [3]Institute of Biochemistry and Biophysics, University of Tehran, PO Box 13145-1384, Tehran, Iran. [4]Department of Biotechnology, Iranian Research Organization for Science and Technology, Tehran, Iran. [5]Neuroscience Research Center, Institute of Neuropharmacology, Kerman University of Medicinal Sciences, Kerman, Iran. [6]Pharmaceutical Sciences Research Center, Tehran University of Medical Sciences, Tehran, Iran.

References

1. Dutta U, Pant K: **Aromatase inhibitors: past, present and future in breast cancer therapy.** *Med Oncol* 2008, **25**:113–124.
2. Vicini F, Beitsch P, Quiet C, Gittleman M, Zannis V, Fine R, Whitworth P, Kuerer H, Haffty B, Keisch M, Lyden M: **Five-year analysis of treatment efficacy and cosmesis by the American society of breast surgeons mammo site breast brachytherapy registry trial in patients treated with accelerated partial breast irradiation.** *Int J Radiant Oncol Biol Phys* 2011, **79**:808–817.
3. Smith GL, Xu Y, Buchholz TA, Giordano SH, Jiang J, Shih YC, Smith BD: **Association between treatment with brachytherapy vs. whole-breast irradiation and subsequent mastectomy, complications , and survival among older women with invasive breast cancer.** *JAMA* 2012, **307**:1827–1837.
4. Cox JA, Swanson TA: **Current modalities of accelerated partial breast irradiation.** *Nat Rev Clin Oncol* 2013, **10**:344–356.
5. Caporuscio F, Rastelli G, Imbriano C, Delrio A: **Structure-based design of potent aromatase inhibitors by high-throughput docking.** *J Med Chem* 2011, **54**:4006–4017.

6. Dowsett M, Cuzick J, Ingle J, Coates A, Forbes J, Bliss J, Buyse M, Baum M, Buzdar A, Colleoni M, Coombes C, Snowdon C, Gnant M, Jakesz R, Kaufmann M, Boccardo F, Godwin J, Davies C, Peto R: **Meta-analysis of breast cancer outcomes in adjuvant trials of aromatase inhibitors versus tamoxifen.** *J Clin Oncol* 2010, **28:**509–518.
7. Zonouzi A, Mirzazadeh R, Safavi M, Kabudanian Ardestani S, Emami S, Foroumadi A: **2-Amino-4-(nitroalkyl)-4H-chromene-3-carbonitriles as New Cytotoxic Agents.** *Iran J Pharm Res* 2013, **12:**679–685.
8. Vosooghi M, Yahyavi H, Divsalar K, Shamsa H, Kheirollahi A, Safavi M, Ardestani SK, Sadeghi-Neshat S, Mohammadhosseini N, Edraki N, Khoshneviszadeh M, Shafiee A, Foroumadi A: **Synthesis and In vitro cytotoxic activity evaluation of (*E*)-16-(substituted benzylidene) derivatives of dehydroepiandrosterone.** *Daru J Pharm Sci* 2013, **21:**34.
9. Ketabforoosh S H M E, Kheirollahi A, Safavi M, Esmati N, Ardestani S K, Emami S, Firoozpour L, Shafiee A, A Foroumadi A: **Synthesis and anti-cancer activity evaluation of new dimethoxylated chalcone and flavanone analogs.** *Arch. Pharm. (Weinheim)* 2014, in press: doi:10.1002/ardp.201400215.
10. Noushini S, Alipour E, Emami S, Safavi M, Ardestani SK, Gohari AR, Shafiee A, Foroumadi A: **Synthesis and cytotoxic properties of novel (*E*)-3-benzylidene-7-methoxychroman-4-one derivatives.** *Daru J Pharm Sci* 2013, **2:**31.
11. Alipour E, Mousavi Z, Safaei Z, Pordeli M, Safavi M, Firoozpour L, Mohammadhosseini N, Saeedi M, Ardestani SK, Shafiee A, Foroumadi A: **Synthesis and cytotoxic evaluation of some new[1,3]dioxolo[4,5-g] chromen-8-one derivatives.** *Daru J Pharm Sci* 2014, **22:**41.
12. Doiron J, Soultan AH, Richard R, Touré MM, Picot N, Richard R, Cuperlović-Culf M, Robichaud GA, Touaibia M: **Synthesis and structure-activity relationship of 1- and 2-substituted-1,2,3-triazole letrozole-based analogues as aromatase inhibitors.** *Eur J Med Chem* 2011, **46:**4010–4024.
13. Trott O, Olson AG: **Software news and update AutoDockVina: improving the speed and accuracy of docking with a new scoring function, efficient optimization, and multithreading.** *J Comput Chem* 2010, **31:**455–461.
14. Ghosh D, Griswold J, Erman M, Pangborn W: **Structural basis for androgen specificity and oestrogen synthesis in human aromatase.** *Nature* 2009, **457:**219–223.
15. Suvannang N, Nantasenamat C, Isarankura-Na-Ayudhya C, Prachayasittikul V: **Molecular docking of aromatase inhibitors.** *Molecules* 2011, **16:**3597–3617.
16. Thakur A, Timiri AK: **Designing of potential new aromatase inhibitor for estrogen dependent disease: a computational approach.** *World J Pharm Sci* 2014, **2:**13–24.
17. Mirzaie S, Chupani L, Barzegari Asadabadi E, Shahverdi AR, Jamalan M: **Novel inhibitor discovery against aromatase through virtual screening and molecular dynamic simulation: a computational approach in drug design.** *EXCLI J* 2013, **12:**168–183.
18. Sanner MF: **Python: a programming language for software integration and development.** *J Mol Graph Mod* 1999, **17:**57–61.
19. O'Boyle NM, Banck M, James CA, Morley C, Vandermeersch T, Hutchison GR: **Open babel: an open chemical toolbox.** *J Cheminform* 2011, **3:**33.
20. Mosmann T: **Rapid colorimetric assay for cellular growth and survival: application to proliferation and cytotoxicity assays.** *J Immunol Methods* 1983, **65:**55–63.

Beneficial effects of pioglitazone and metformin in murine model of polycystic ovaries via improvement of chemerin gene up-regulation

Nahid Kabiri[1], Mohammad Reza Tabandeh[2*] and Seyed Reza Fatemi Tabatabaie[1]

Abstract

Background: Polycystic ovary syndrome (PCO) is recognized as the most common endocrinopathy in female. Chemerin is a novel adipocytokine that is expressed in ovary and upregulated in adipose tissue of obese, PCO patients. To date there is no report about the regulation of ovarian chemerin gene expression after PCO induction and treatment by insulin sensitizing drugs including pioglitazone and metformin.
Thirty female rats were divided into six experimental groups with five rats in each group including control group, PCO group (i.m injection of 4 mg estradiol benzoate for 40 days), metformin treated (200 mg/kg/day for 21 days), pioglitazone treated (20 mg/kg/day, for 21 days), PCO + metformin and PCO + pioglitazone. PCO was detected by microscopic observation of vaginal smear and treatment by metformin and pioglitazone was initiated one week after that. Ovarian chemerin expression was analyzed by real time PCR and western blotting.

Results: Our results demonstrated that PCO induction resulted in elevation of chemerin mRNA and protein levels in ovary in concomitant with incidence of insulin resistance and increasing androgen and progesterone production. We observed that metformin and pioglitazone attenuated ovarian chemerin expression and improved insulin resistance and abnormal steroid production in PCO rats.

Conclusion: Based on data presented here we concluded that alteration of ovarian chemerin expression may has important role in PCO development and manipulation of chemerin expression or signaling by pioglitazone or metformin can be a novel therapeutic mechanism in the treatment of PCO patients by these drugs.

Keywords: PCO, Chemerin, Gene expression, Ovary, Pioglitazone, Metformin

Background

Polycystic ovary syndrome (PCO) is recognized as the most common endocrinopathy in female during the reproductive age. PCO is characterized by reproductive dysfunction symptoms such as hyperandrogenic chronic anovulation due to excess androgen production, menstrual disturbances, infertility or subfertility and the presence of enlarged, sclerocystic ovaries. Obesity, insulin resistance, pancreatic-cell dysfunction and impaired glucose tolerance occur at least in 50% of women with PCO [1,2]. Previous reports have shown that hyperinsulinemia in these patients dysregulates LH secretion and promotes ovarian androgen secretion resulting in elevation of free androgen level [3].

Over the past decade it has been shown that adipocytes are secretory cells that produce a variety of proteins with hormonal actions, which collectively have been called adipocytokines. These cytokines have important roles in male and female reproductive physiology by regulation of carbohydrate and lipid metabolism in adipose or reproductive tissues such as hypothalamus-pituitary axis, ovary, uterus and embryo [4,5]. Among them, adiponectin, leptin, resistin and visfatin are the major adipocytokines which their changes in serum or adipose tissue have been identified in patients with obesity, insulin resistance and PCO [6,7]. Various secretion or gene expression patterns of adipocytokines or their receptors have been detected in adipose tissue or ovary of PCO patients [8,9].

* Correspondence: m.tabandeh@scu.ac.ir
[2]Department of Biochemistry and Molecular Biology, Faculty of Veterinary Medicine, Shahid Chamran University of Ahvaz, Ahvaz, Iran
Full list of author information is available at the end of the article

Chemerin is a novel adipocytokine which is predominantly expressed by adipocytes and its gene expression elevates in the adipose tissue of obese animals and human [7]. High correlations have been found between plasma chemerin level and different features of metabolic syndrome including body mass index, plasma triglycerides and blood pressure in human [10]. Chemerin knockdown animals demonstrate impaired adipocyte gene expression and unregulated glucose and carbohydrate metabolism [11]. Recent data demonstrate that recombinant chemerin promotes angiogenesis; a mechanism which is essential for adipose tissue expansion in obese patients [11,12]. Recently, inhibitory action of chemerin on FSH or IGF-1 induced steroidogenesis have been reported in granulosa cells [13-15]. Serum chemerin increases in women with PCO [16].

Insulin-sensitizing drugs (ISDs) such as metformin or thiazolidinediones (TZDs) ameliorate reproductive abnormalities, restore ovulation and regular estrous cycle, increase pregnancy rates and reduce androgenic symptoms in women with PCO [17,18]. The positive actions of these insulin-sensitizing agents on adipocytokine secretion or expression in adipose tissue or ovaries of PCO patients have been described. However the full mechanism of action of these two drugs in ovaries of PCO patient is still unraveled and further investigations remain to elucidate the precise mechanism of actions of these drugs at molecular levels.

To our knowledge, no study is available that identify the changes of chemerin gene expression in ovaries of animals or human with PCO and that compare the effects of pioglitazone and metformin on its gene expression in experimental model of PCO. Here for the first time we showed that ovarian chemerin gene expression changed after PCO induction and pioglitazone or metformin treatment.

Methods

Rat treatment regimes

Thirty Female Sprague-Dawley rats (3 month of age) weighing 150-180 g were housed in a temperature-controlled room (23 ± 1°C) with a 12 h light/dark cycle and were provided rat chow (Pars, Tehran, Iran) and water at libitum.

All animals used were cared for according to the Guide for the Care and Use of Laboratory Animals by the National Academy of Sciences (National Institutes of Health publication No. 86-23). The rats were allowed to acclimatize for 10 days before the beginning of the experiment. The estrous cyclicity was monitored by vaginal smears obtained between 08:00 and 12:00 hours and the rats with abnormal cyclicity were dismissed from the experiment.

The rats were divided into six experimental groups with five rats in each group: 1) healthy control (vehicle control), 2) PCO, 3) metformin treated 4) pioglitazone treated, 5) PCO and metformin treated and 6) PCO and pioglitazone treated. PCO was induced by a single i.m injection of 4 mg estradiol valerate (Loghman Pharmaceutical & Hygienic Co, Karaj, Iran) in 0.2 ml sesame oil (Barij Essense, Kashan, Iran) for 40 days [19] and detected by microscopic observation of vaginal smear. The presence of prolonged cornified cells for at least two consecutive estrous cycles was used as successful PCO induction. Treatment with metformin and pioglitazone was initiated one week after PCO induction.

Animals in metformin treated groups (groups 3 and 5) were received 200 mg/kg/day metformin (Loghman Pharmaceutical & Hygienic Co, Karaj, Iran) by gavage method for 21 days. Pioglitazone (Dorsa Pharmaceutical Co. Tehran, Iran) was daily used for the 21 days duration as the same method as metformin groups with dose of 20 mg/kg/day. Dosages of pioglitazone and metformin were chosen based on dosages that were clinically used in human patients (25-30 mg/kg/day for pioglitazone and 200-300 mg/kg/day for metformin).

Tissue and serum sampling

Animals were anesthetized by chloroform and serum samples were obtained by cardiac puncture, separated by centrifuging at 5,000 rpm for 5 minutes and stored at -20°C for the subsequent assays. Both ovaries were carefully trimmed of adhering fat and connective tissue, pooled and immediately frozen in liquid nitrogen at -80°C. The body weight and length (nose to anus lenght) of all rats were determined at the end of study and body mass index (BMI) was calculated by using following formula as described previously; body weight (g)/Length^2 (cm^2) [20]. Control ovaries were collected from rats at estrous or proestrous stages of cycle.

Ovarian morphology

Some ovary was removed, cleaned of adherent connective fat tissue, and fixed in 4% formaldehyde buffer for at least 24 hours. Thereafter the samples were dehydrated and imbedded in paraffin. The ovaries were partially longitudinally sectioned (4 μm, every tenth section mounted on the glass slide), stained with hematoxylin and eosin and the presence of healthy and atretic follicles, follicular cysts and corpora lutea was assayed. Antral follicles with pyknotic granulosa and theca layers, unhealthy, degenerative oocyte and filled in antral cavity with numerous apoptotic derbies were characterized as atretic follicles. Preantral follicles with degenerative oocyte and pyknotic granulosa layer were assigned as atretic follicles.

Hormone and glucose assays

Serum insulin levels were measured by using the Rat ELISA kits (Mercodia, Sweden) according to the manufacturer's recommendation. Insulin concentration was expressed as μg/L. The limit of detection of insulin was 0.01 μg/L and the intra-assay and interassay coefficients of variation were less than 4% and 8.13%, respectively. The calibrator ranges were between 0-10 μg/L (first calibrator at 0.01 μg/L).

The progesterone (P4) and testosterone (T) concentrations were determined by using a commercial radioimmunoassay kit (Immunotech, Radiová, Czech Republic). The limit of detection of P4 was 0.1 ng/ml, and the intra-assay and interassay coefficients of variation were less than 10% and 11%, respectively. The calibrator ranges were between 0 - 100 ng/mL (first calibrator at 0.1 ng/mL). The limit of detection of T was 0.1 ng/ml, and the intra-assay and interassay coefficients of variation were less than 12.1% and 11.2%, respectively. The calibrator ranges were between 0 – 25 ng/mL (first calibrator at 0.1 ng/mL). Blood glucose was determined by glucose oxidase method (Pars Azmoon, Tehran, Iran) as described by manufacturer.

HOMA-IR estimation

HOMA-IR was estimated through previously described formula (fasting glucose × fasting insulin/22.5) and represented by unit of mmol/L × μU/ml [21].

RNA preparation

Total RNA was extracted from ovaries using TriPure total RNA isolation kit according to the manufacturer's procedure (Roche Molecular System, USA), dissolved in dimethyl pyrocarbonate treated water and quantified at a wavelength of 260 nm by nanodrop spectrophotometry (Eppendorf, Hamburg, Germany). The RNA with optical density absorption ratio OD260 nm/OD280 nm between 1.8 and 2.0 was used for reverse transcription (RT) reaction. Genomic DNA was removed by treating 1 μg of isolated RNA with 2 units of DNase I (Fermentas Inc, Vilnius, Lithuania).

Reverse transcription – polymerase chain reaction

Reverse transcription was done in a total volume of 20-μl by using an AmpliSence cDNA synthesis kit (AmpliSens Enterovirus-Eph, Russia) as recommended by the manufacturer. The PCR reactions was performed in a 25-μl reaction using Taq DNA polymerase (Cinagen Co, Iran) and a thermal cycler (Eppendorf Mastercycler, Hamburg, Germany). Specific sets of primers (BIONEER, Seoul, South Korea) that used for amplification of rat chemerin were as follows; forward: 5′-ATG GCGGGCAACGGCGCCAT-3′ and reverse: 5′-CCAT CAACGTCGTCAACTAA-3′. Thermal conditions for amplification of chemerin were 35 cycles consisting of denaturing at 94°C for 1 min, annealing at 58°C for 1 min, extension at 72°C for 1 min, with an initial denaturing step at 95°C for 10 min and a final extension step at 72°C for 10 min. cDNA from adipose tissue was used as positive control. Expression of chemerin in rat ovaries was confirmed by visualization of PCR product on agarose gel electrophoresis (1%).

Real time PCR

To evaluate the levels of chemerin gene expression in ovaries of different animals quantitative real-time PCR (qRT-PCR) was performed using the ABI Step One plus real-time PCR detection system (ABI plus; Applied Biosystems, USA), and qPCR™ Green master kit for SYBR Green I® (Applied Biosystems, USA). Relative expression level of chemerin transcript was compared to GAPDH as housekeeping gene. Specific sets of primers (Macrogen, Seoul, South Korea) that were used for amplification of rat GAPDH [GenBank: NM_017008.4] and chemerin [GenBank: NM_001013427] genes were designed using Beacon Designer 7.1. Sequences of primers for amplification of rat GAPDH and chemerin (BIONEER, Seoul, South Korea) were as follows; rat chemerin: 5′-TGTGGACAGTGCTGATGACCTGTT-3′ and 5′-CAGT TTGATGCAGGCCAGGCATTT-3′ and rat GAPDH: 5′-CTCATCTACCTCTCCATCGTCTG-3′ and 5′-CCTGC TCTTGTCTGCCGGTGCTTG-3′ Real time PCR reactions were performed with the following settings: 5 minutes of pre-incubation at 95°C followed by 40 cycles for 15 seconds at 95°C and 45 second at 60°C. Reactions were performed in triplicate. A reaction without cDNA was performed in parallel as negative control.

Relative quantification was performed according to the comparative $2^{-\Delta\Delta Ct}$. For analysis of qRT-PCR results based on ΔΔCt method StepOne™ software was used. The result for the gene expression was given by a unitless value through the formula $2^{-\Delta\Delta Ct}$. Validation of assay to check that the primer for the GAPDH and chemerin had similar amplification efficiencies was performed as described previously [22].

Western blotting

Total protein from isolated ovaries was precipitated after RNA and DNA isolation using TriPure total RNA isolation kit according to the manufacturer's procedure (Roche Molecular System, USA) and its concentration was measured using Bradford method as described previously [23]. Twenty five μl of each protein sample (1 μg/μl) were mixed with 25 μl Laemmli sample buffer supplemented with 2-mercaptoethanol at a final concentration of 7.5% (vol/vol). The samples were heated for 15 min at 65°C, separated by 10% SDS-PAGE and electrophoretically transferred to a nitrocellulose membrane (Schleicher & Schuell, Inc., Keene, NH). The filters were blocked by incubation for 1 h in PBS with 5% nonfat milk. Blots were then washed in PBS-Tween and immunoblotted with primary antibody against mouse chemerin (Abcam,

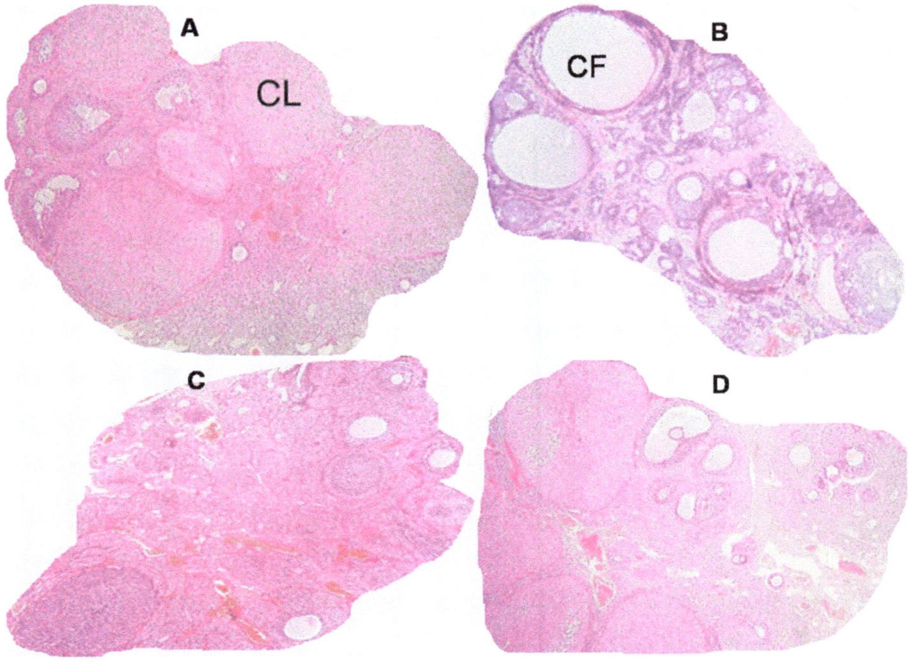

Figure 1 Ovarian features in normal rats (A), estradiol induced PCO rats, (B) PCO rats treated with pioglitazone (C) and PCO rats treated with metformin (D). Normal rats displayed follicles at different stages and the presence of corpora lutea (CL) **(A)**, while estradiol treatment resulted in formation of higher numbers of atretic and cystic follicles (CF) and the absence of CL **(B)**. Metformin and pioglitazone treated rats **(C and D)** exhibited lower numbers of CF, higher numbers of antral follicles and growing young CL. H & E staining (magnification × 40).

Cambridge, UK, Art No: ab112450) at 1:500 ratio. Detection of primary antibody was done using goat anti rabbit HRP-conjugated antibody (Abcam, Cambridge, UK, Art No; ab98467) at 1:1000 ratio and DAB reagent (Sigma Aldrich, Germany). Densitometric quantification of chemerin proteins in relation to GAPDH as calibrator was performed using Image J software (National Institutes of Health). Western blot was done in three independent experiments for each sample.

Statistical analyses

Data analyses were done using the SPSS 16.0 software package (SPSS Inc., Chicago, IL, USA). Two-way analysis of variance (ANOVA) and general linear model was fit to evaluate the effect of PCO status (PCO vs. control) and treatments (treatment with metformin or pioglitazon vs. no treatment) on each variable. The two-way ANOVA model is given by $Yijk = \mu + \alpha_i + \beta_j + (\alpha\beta)_{ij}$, where α_i and β_j represent the effects of PCO induction and treatment, and $(\alpha\beta)_{ij}$ represents the interaction of two factors. The Spearman rank correlation coefficient was used to estimate the correlation between chemerin gene expression and different parameters. All experimental data were presented as the mean ± SD. The level of significance for all tests was set at $P < 0.05$.

Result

The ovaries in the control group exhibited a typically normal appearance with small and medium sized antral follicles and corpora lutea (Figure 1A). The ovaries in the PCO group displayed typical PCO-like changes including presence of higher numbers of atretic and cystic follicles compared with the control group (Figure 1B). Metformin and pioglitazone treated rats exhibited lower numbers of atretic and cystic follicles, higher numbers of antral follicles and growing young corpora lutea compared with PCO group (Figure 1C-D). Restoration of normal follicular appearance was more pronounced in metformin treated rats compared with pioglitazon treated animals (Figure 1C-D).

The real time-PCR and western blot results demonstrated that chemerin mRNA and protein levels were elevated in ovaries of PCO rats when compared to that in healthy animals ($P < 0.05$) (Figure 2). The chemerin gene expression levels were decreased in ovaries of PCO rats in response to treatment with metformin and pioglitazone compared to untreated PCO rats ($p < 0.05$) (Figure 2). Metformin and pioglitazone had no effects on the levels of chemerin mRNA and protein in healthy treated rats in relation to healthy untreated animals regardless of PCO status (Figure 2) ($p > 0.05$).

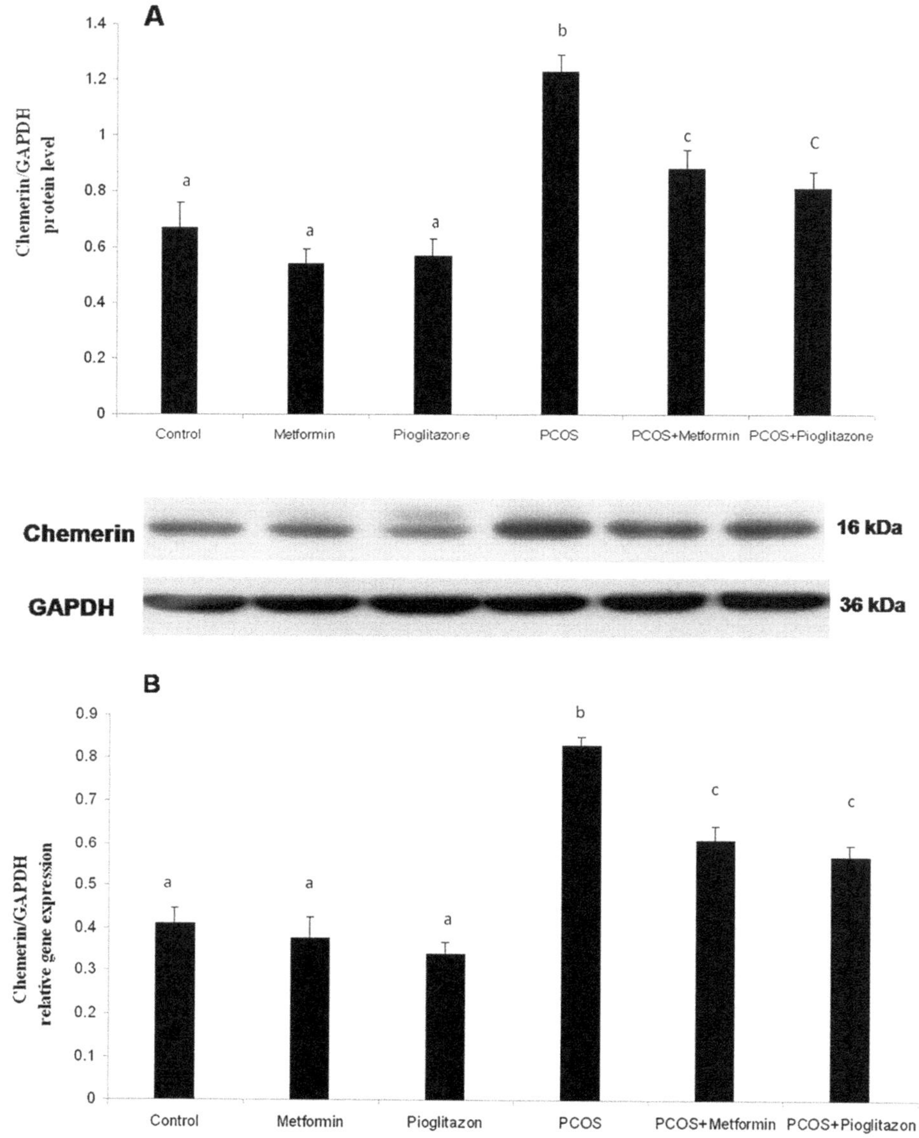

Figure 2 Chemerin protein (A) and mRNA levels (B) in rat ovaries after PCO induction and treatment with pioglitazone and metformin (n = 5 in each group). Chemerin was up-regulated in ovary of PCO rats compared with control animals, whereas its level decreased after treatment with metformin and pioglitazone. Data were presented as the mean ± SD. Different letters denote differences among groups at $P < 0.05$.

As shown in Figures 3 and 4 plasma glucose and insulin levels were higher in the PCO induced rats (1.92 ± 0.38 fold) when compared with normal untreated group ($p < 0.05$) after controlling for the effect of treatment. Treatment of PCO rats with metformin and pioglitazone resulted in reduction of glucose (1.36 ± 0.27) and insulin (1.82 ± 0.36) levels in relation to PCO untreated rats ($p < 0.05$) (Figures 3 and 4). In healthy treated groups plasma insulin and glucose levels had no differences with healthy untreated animals (Figures 3 and 4), ($p > 0.05$) after controlling for PCO status.

The HOMA-IR index, which reflects whole body insulin resistance, was increased in PCO animals (3.63 ± 0.41 fold) ($p < 0.05$) (Figure 5) regardless of treatments. Metformin and pioglitazone induced reduction of HOMA-IR in PCO rats about 2.8 fold compared with untreated PCO animals ($p < 0.05$) (Figure 5). Healthy treated rats did not show clear changes in HOMA-IR level in relation to healthy untreated rats after controlling PCO status.

The plasma concentrations of T and P4 are shown in Figures 6 and 7 respectively. We found a 1.8 ± 0.3 fold increase of plasma T and a 6.9 ± 0.8 fold increase of P4

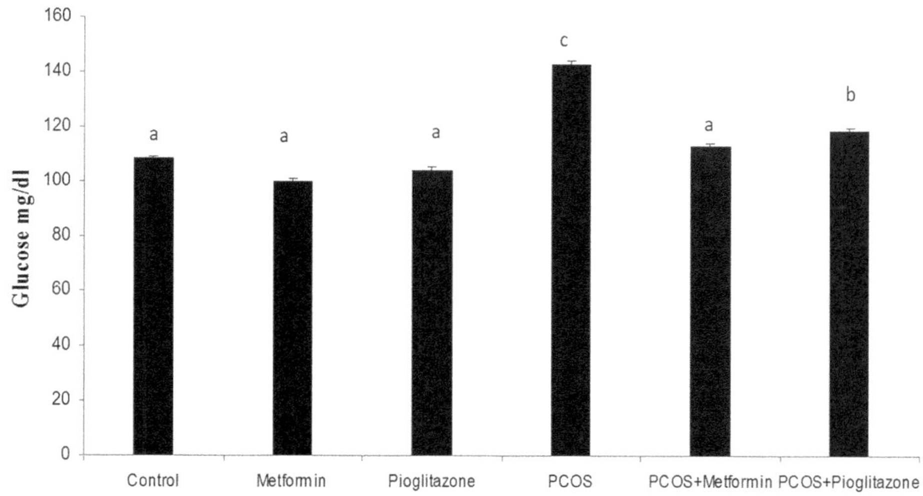

Figure 3 Serum glucose levels (mg/dl) in normal rats (n = 5), PCO induced rats (n = 5) and treated rats with metformin and pioglitazone (n = 5). Serum glucose was elevated in PCO rats compared with control animals. Treatment of PCO rats with metformin and pioglitazone resulted in reduction of glucose level in relation to PCO untreated rats. Data were presented as the mean ± SD. Different letters denote differences among groups at P < 0.05.

rats after induction of PCO ($p < 0.05$) (Figures 6 and 7) regardless of treatments. We found that in treated PCO rats, T concentrations were decreased by 1.2 ± 0.3 fold and 1.9 ± 0.5 fold after metformin and pioglitazone treatment respectively ($p < 0.05$) (Figure 6). The reduction of T level was more pronounced in PCO rats in the presence of pioglitazone compared with metformin ($p < 0.05$) (Figure 6), while metformin was more effective in reducing P4 concentration in this group ($p < 0.05$) (Figure 7).

Spearman Rank correlation analyses demonstrated that ovarian chemerin gene expression was positively associated with P4 ($p < 0.01$), HOMA-IR, BMI, insulin and glucose levels ($p < 0.05$) (Table 1). Δ chemerin gene expression in treated PCO animals had positive correlation with Δ insulin, Δ HOMA-IR and Δ P4 ($p < 0.05$) (Table 1).

Discussion

PCO is a heterogeneous syndrome characterized by hyperandrogenism, insulin resistance and obesity [24]. The mechanism that is responsible for insulin resistance is unclear and several hypotheses have been suggested. Because obesity is linked to insulin resistance and many women with PCO are obese, it is possible that, at least in a subgroup of patients, insulin resistance is worsened by excessive adipose mass or abnormal secretion or action of adipocytokines [25]. Chemerin is a newly identified

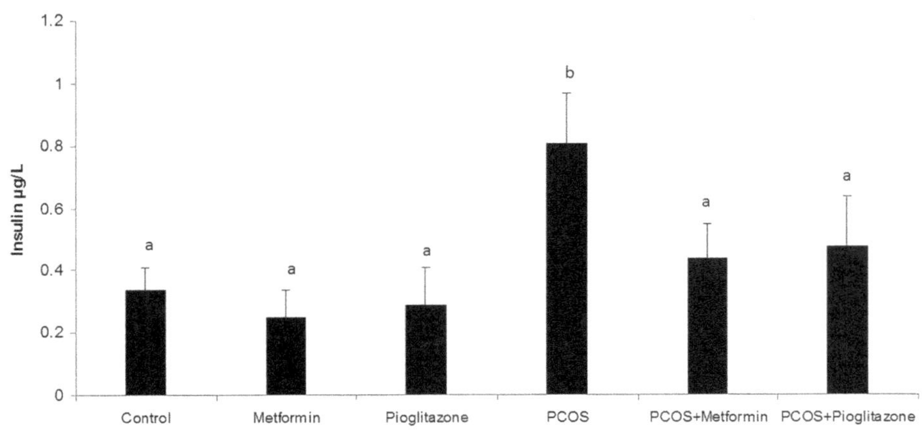

Figure 4 Serum insulin levels (ug/L) in normal rats (n = 5), PCO induced rats (n = 5) and treated rats with metformin and pioglitazone (n = 5). Serum insulin level was considerably higher in PCO rats compared with that in normal animals. Treatment of PCO rats with metformin and pioglitazone decreased the over-secretion of insulin in relation to PCO untreated rats. Data were presented as the mean ± SD. Different letters denote differences among groups at P < 0.05.

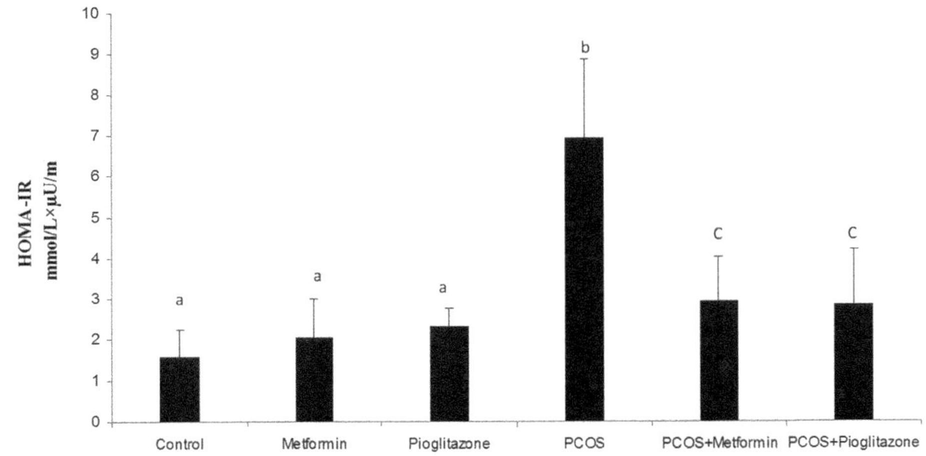

Figure 5 HOMA-IR index (mmol/L × uU/ml) in normal rats (n = 5), PCO induced rats (n = 5) and treated rats with metformin and pioglitazone (n = 5). Rats with PCO showed insulin resistance compared with normal rats, while treatment of those with metformin and pioglitazone attenuate insulin resistance in relation to PCO untreated rats. Data were presented as the mean ± SD. Different letters denote differences among groups at P < 0.05.

adipokine whose systemic levels are elevated in obesity and positively correlate with markers of the metabolic syndrome such as body mass index, triglycerides, high-sensitivity C-reactive protein [15,26]. Recently Tan et al demonstrated an increase of serum and subcutaneous and omental adipose tissue chemerin expression in women with PCO [10]. Chemerin is also expressed in ovary of animal and human, but few data exists on regulation of chemerin gene expression in polycystic ovaries [14,27]. Here we present novel data showing an increase of chemerin gene expression in rat ovary after induction of PCO. The animals in PCO group gained more weight, had higher plasma insulin and glucose levels and showed an elevation of HOMA-IR; an index of insulin resistance. Our findings was in agreement with results of Wang et al which has shown the higher level of chemein expression in the ovary of dihydrotestosterone (DHT) induced PCO rats [15]. Several experiments have demonstrated that chemerin may play a role in pathophysiology of PCO in animal or human by direct action on ovary [10,13,14]. We know that formation of polycystic ovaries is critically associated with abnormal steroidogenesis. It has been found that chemerin decreases estradiol secretion and suppressed FSH-induced progesterone and estradiol secretion in preantral follicles and granulosa cells by inhibition of aromatase and p450scc expression [13].

It is also well recognized that development of polycystic ovaries is associated with new blood vessel formation

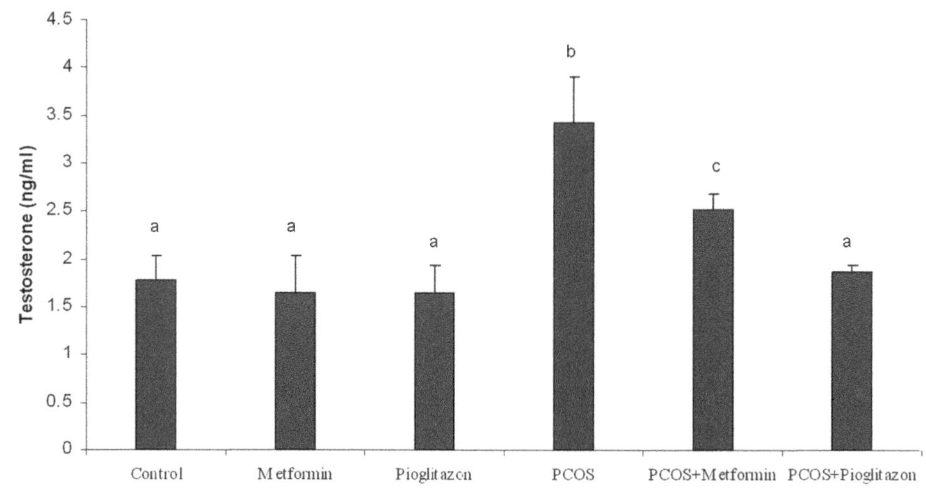

Figure 6 Serum testosterone (T) levels (ug/L) in normal rats (n = 5), PCO induced rats (n = 5) and treated rats with metformin and pioglitazone (n = 5). Induction of PCO caused an increasing the T level, while metformin and pioglitazone attenuated over secretion of T. Data were presented as the mean ± SD. Different letters denote differences among groups at P < 0.05.

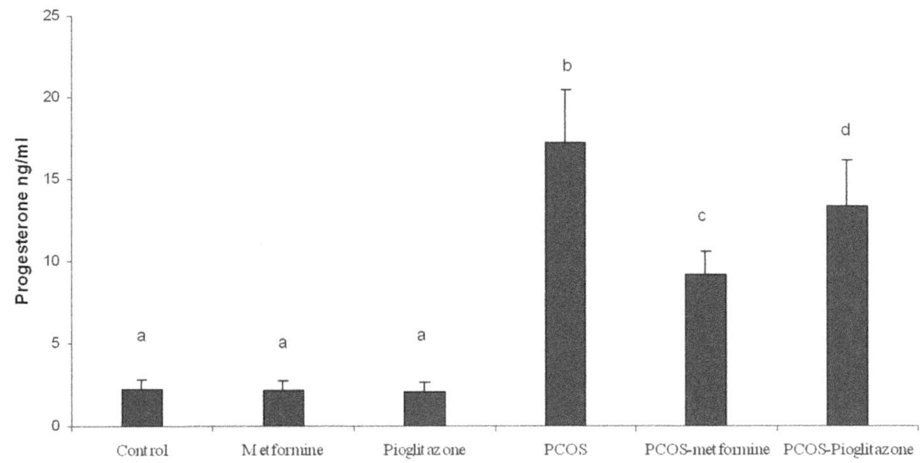

Figure 7 Serum progesterone (P) levels (ug/L) in normal rats (n = 5), PCO induced rats (n = 5) and treated rats with metformin and pioglitazone (n = 5). Induction of PCO caused an increasing the P level, while metformin and pioglitazone attenuated over secretion of T. Data were presented as the mean ± SD. Different letters denote differences among groups at P < 0.05.

[28]. Although there is no data about the effect of chemerin on ovarian angiogenesis, however it is plausible that chemerin may act as angiogenic factor. Recently Bozauglo et al using an *in vitro* angiogenesis assay has shown that chemerin induced the formation of capillary-like structures, a process which occur in obese patient and result in adipose tissue expansion [12]. These observations lead to the hypothesis that increasing the chemerin gene expression in ovary of PCO rats may alter ovarian steroidogenesis or angiogenesis and may play a role in the development and progression of this reproductive disorder.

It has been demonstrated that alteration of metabolic and endocrine function of adipocytes result in a higher secretion of proinflammatory substances including tumor necrosis factor alpha (TNF-α) and interleukin-6 (IL-6)

Table 1 Correlation between chemerin gene expression in ovaries of PCO rats with insulin, glucose, HOMA-IR index, testosterone, progesterone and body mass index (BMI) after PCO induction and treatment of PCO rats with pioglitazone and metformin

ΔChemerin mRNA (after treatment)		Chemerin mRNA (PCOS)		Variables
p	r	p	r	
0.0847	0.361	0.0327	0.661*	Glucose (mg/dl)
0.0432	0.578*	0.0087	0.754**	Insulin (μg/l)
0.0916	0.291	0.0414	0.523*	Testosterone (ng/ml)
0.0382	0.619*	0.0091	0.827**	Progesterone (ng/ml)
0.0478	0.564*	0.0276	0.678*	HOMA-IR
0.0739	0.378	0.0312	0.654*	BMI

*Correlation is significant at the 0.05 level.
**Correlation is significant at the 0.01 level.
Correlation coefficient (r) and statistical significance (P) are indicated.
(Δ) change in chemerin gene expression level after treatment.

[29]. Many reports have demonstrated that these potent inflammatory compounds alter normal physiology of ovary such as steroidogenesis and enhance the risk of PCO development [17,30]. Presence a positive association between increasing body weight and ovarian chemerin gene expression in this study raises the possibility that alteration of chemerin gene expression in ovary of PCO animals may be, in some part, due to increasing fat mass and releasing higher inflammatory mediators such as IL-6 and TNF-α. This hypothesis is supported by the fact that TNF-α increases adipocyte chemerin and elevation of serum TNF-α leads to higher systemic chemerin in mice [31].

We also found the higher plasma insulin level in animals with PCO compared with healthy rats and its positive association with ovarian chemerin gene expression. Interestingly, insulin elevates chemerin in human adipose tissue explants *in vitro*, and systemic chemerin increases after prolonged hyperinsulinemia in healthy individuals. This finding suggests that hyperinsulinemia which occur in our experiment may enhance the chemerin gene expression in polycystic ovaries and it may have role in progression of impaired steroid production [32].

Consistent with previous results, our study showed that chemerin has role in PCO development and manipulation of chemerin gene expression or its signaling may be a novel therapeutic approaches in the treatment of PCO patients. To clarify this hypothesis we test the effect of pioglitazone and metformin on the ovarian chemerin gene expression in normal and PCO animals. To our knowledge, this is the first report demonstrating that treatment of PCO rat with pioglitazone and metformin alter chemerin gene expression in the ovary. Here we reported for the first time that 21 days treatment of PCO rats with metformin and pioglitazone reduced ovarian chemerin mRNA and protein abundance with a concomitant decrease in insulin resistance in PCO animals. Reduction of chemerin gene expression was more pronounced in PCO rats in the presence of pioglitazone compared with metformin, while these drugs had no effects on the basal levels of ovarian chemerin mRNA and protein in healthy animals. We also found improvement of insulin resistance in animals treated with pioglitazone or metformin. Animals in these groups showed lower plasma insulin and glucose level and HOMA-IR compared with PCO animals.

Pioglitazone and metformin are the most important insulin-sensitizing agents currently used most often in clinical practice to improve insulin resistance of PCO patients via different mechanisms which are not thoroughly understood [33,34]. A diverse beneficial effect of pioglitazone and metformin on the treatment of PCO has been described in recent years [35]. Alteration of numerous genes involved in different ovarian functions such as cell proliferation, steroid production and new blood formation by these drugs have been detected and it demonstrate that their positive effects on ovarian function in PCO patients may be multifactorial [35,36]. Recently it has been found that troglitazone or metformin reduce the secretion of chemerin from adipoe tissue and metformin can also reduces chemerin blood levels in concomitant with improving insulin sensivity and decreasing BMI in women with PCO [10]. It has also been demonstrated that both drugs have anti-angiogenic actions, suppresses ovarian androgen production and reduce the secretion of proinflammatory factors including IL-6 and TNF-α [37-39]. Given our findings and those from other groups we hypothesized that these drugs may improve functional and endocrine disturbances of polycystic ovaries, in some part, by suppression of ovarian chemerin gene expression and attenuation of its adverse effect on normal functions of polycystic ovaries.

Conclusion

In conclusion, using a murine model of PCO, we provided novel evidence that chemerin is an important adipocytokine which may contribute to the dysregulation of ovarian function in PCO. Our study indicated that ovarian chemerin gene expression is associated with several key parameters of the metabolic syndrome in PCO status. Oral administration of pioglitazone and metformin to PCO rats altered the ovarian expression of chemerin genes. These results suggest that some therapeutic effects of metformin and pioglitazone in PCO may be due to their direct actions on ovarian chemerin gene expression.

Competing interests

The authors declare that they have no competing interests.

Authors' contributions

SRFT and MRT were the supervisors and designed the study. MRT carried out the molecular studies. SRFT carried out the hormone assays. All authors read and approved the final manuscript.

Acknowledgements

This work was funded by a Grant from Shahid Chamran University of Ahvaz research Council (Grant No: 636410, 1391.4.6).

Author details

[1]Department of Physiology, Faculty of Veterinary Medicine, Shahid Chamran University of Ahvaz, Ahvaz, Iran. [2]Department of Biochemistry and Molecular Biology, Faculty of Veterinary Medicine, Shahid Chamran University of Ahvaz, Ahvaz, Iran.

References

1. Kumar A, Woods KS, Bartolucci AA, Azziz R: **Prevalence of adrenal androgen excess in patients with the polycystic ovary syndrome (PCO).** *Clin Endocrin* 2005, **62**:644–649.
2. David A, Ehrmann DM: **Polycystic ovary syndrome.** *New Engl J Med* 2005, **352**:1223–1236.
3. Barnes RB, Rosenfield RL, Ehrmann DA, Cara JF, Cuttler L, Levitsky LL, Rosenthal IM: **Ovarian hyperandrogenism as a result of congenital adrenal virilizing disorders: evidence for perinatal masculinization of neuroendocrine function in women.** *J Clin Endocrin Metabol* 1994, **79**:1328–1333.
4. Galic S, Oakhill JS, Steinberg GR: **Adipose tissue as an endocrine organ.** *Mol Cell Endocrinol* 2010, **316**:129–139.
5. Mitchell M, Armstrong DT, Robker RL, Norman RJ: **Adipokines: implications for female fertility and obesity.** *Reproduction* 2005, **130**(5):583–597.
6. Gnacińska M, Małgorzewicz S, Stojek M, Łysiak-Szydłowska W, Sworczak K: **Role of adipokines in complications related to obesity.** *Adv Med Sci* 2009, **54**(2):150–157.
7. Goralski KB, McCarthy TC, Hanniman EA, Zabel BA, Butcher EC, Parlee SD, Muruganandan S, Sinal CJ: **Chemerin, a novel adipokine that regulates adipogenesis and adipocyte metabolism.** *J Biol Chem* 2007, **282**:28175–28188.
8. Bideci A, Camurdan MO, Yeşilkaya E, Demirel F, Cinaz P: **Serum ghrelin, leptin and resistin levels in adolescent girls with polycystic ovary syndrome.** *J Obstet Gynaecol Res* 2008, **34**:578–584.
9. Carmina E, Orio F, Palomba S, Cascella T, Longo RA, Colao AM, Lombardi G, Lobo RA: **Evidence for altered adipocyte function in polycystic ovary syndrome.** *Eur J Endocrin* 2005, **152**:389–394.
10. Tang T, Lord JM, Norman RJ, Yasmin E, Balen AH: **Insulin-sensitising drugs (metformin, rosiglitazone, pioglitazone, D-chiro-inositol) for women with polycystic ovary syndrome, oligo amenorrhoea and subfertility.** *Cochrane Database Syst Rev* 2012, **16**:5. CD003053.
11. Kaur J, Adya R, Tan BK, Chen J, Randeva HS: **Identification of chemerin receptor (ChemR23) in human endothelial cells: Chemerin-induced endothelial angiogenesis.** *Biochem Biophys Res Commun* 2010, **391**:1762–1768.
12. Bozaoglu K, Joanne E, Curran Claire J, Mohamed S, Zaibi S, Segal D, Konstantopoulos N, Morrison S, Carless M, Dyer TD, Shelley A, Cole Harald HH, Eric G, Moses K: **Chemerin, a Novel Adipokine in the Regulation of Angiogenesis.** *J Clin Endocrinol Metab* 2010, **95**:2476–2485.
13. Kim JY, Xue K, Cao M, Wang Q, Liu JY, Leader A, Han JY, Tsang BK: **Chemerin Suppresses Ovarian Follicular Development and Its Potential Involvement in Follicular Arrest in Rats Treated Chronically with Dihydrotestosterone.** *Endocrinilogy* 2013. doi:10.1210/en. 1001.
14. Tan BK, Chen J, Farhatullah S, Adya R, Kaur J, Heutling D, Lewandowski CK, Ohare PJ, Lehnert H, Randeva SH: **Insulin and metformin regulate circulating and adipose tissue chemerin.** *Diabetes* 2009, **58**:1971–1978.
15. Wittamer V, Franssen JD, Vulcano M, Mirjolet JF, Le Poul E, Migeotte I, Brézillon S, Tyldesley R, Blanpain C, Detheux M, Mantovani A, Sozzani S, Vassart G, Parmentier M, Communi D: **Specific recruitment of antigen-presenting cells by chemerin, a novel processed ligand from human inflammatory fluids.** *J Exp Med* 2003, **198**:977–985.
16. Haghighi N, Yaghmaei S, Hashemi P, Saadati F, Tehrani N, Ramezani F, Hedayati M: **The association between serum chemerin concentration and polycystic ovarian syndrome.** *Tehran Univ Med J* 2012, **70**(5):320–324.
17. Checa MA, Requena A, Salvador C, Tur R, Callejo J, Espino JJ, Bregues FF, Herrero J: **Insulin-sensitizing agenets: use in pregnancy as therapy in polycystic ovary syndrome.** *Hum Reprod Update* 2005, **11**(4):375–390.
18. Rezvanfar MA, Rezvanfar MA, Ahmadi A, Saadi HA, Baeeri M, Abdollahi M: **Mechanistic links between oxidative/nitrosative stress and tumor necrosis**

factor alpha in letrozole-induced murine polycystic ovary: biochemical and pathological evidences for beneficial effect of pioglitazone. *Hum Exp Toxicol* 2012, **31**:887–897.

19. Brawer JR, Munoz M, Farookhi R: Development of the polycystic ovarian condition (PCO) in the estradiol valerate-treated rat. *Biol Reprod* 1986, **35**:647–655.
20. Mani F, Fernandes AAH, Cicogna AC, Novelli Filho JLVB: Anthropometrical parameters and markers of obesity in rats. *Lab Anim* 2007, **41**:111–119.
21. Katsuki A, Sumida Y, Gabazza EC, Murashima S, Furuta M, Araki- Sasaki R, Hori Y, Yano Y, Adachi Y: Homeostasis model assessment is a reliable indicator of insulin resistance during follow-up of patients with type 2 diabetes. *Diabetes Care* 2001, **24**(2):362–365.
22. Livak K: *ABI Prism 7700 Sequence Detection System*. Foster City, CA: User Bulletin 2. PE. Applied Biosystems; 1997.
23. Bradford MM: A rapid and sensitive for the quantitation of microgram quantitites of protein utilizing the principle of protein-dye binding. *Anal Biochem* 1976, **72**:248–254.
24. Barber TM, McCarthy MI, Wass JAH, Franks S: Obesity and polycystic ovary syndrome. *Clin Endocrin* 2006, **65**:137–145.
25. Bozaoglu K, Segal D, Shields KA, Cummings N, Curran JE, Comuzzie AG, Mahaney MC, Rainwater DL, Vandeberg JL, MacCluer JW, Collier G, Blangero J, Walder K, Jowett JBM: Chemerin is associated with metabolic syndrome phenotypes in a Mexican-American population. *J Clin Endocrinol Metab* 2009, **95**:2476–2485.
26. Ernst MC, Sinal CJ: Chemerin: at the crossroads of inflammation and obesity. *Endocrin Metabol* 2010, **21**:660–667.
27. Bozaoglu K, Bolton K, McMillan J, Zimmet P, Jowett J, Collier G, Walder K, Segal L: Chemerin is a novel adipokine associated with obesity and metabolic syndrome. *Endocrinology* 2007, **148**(10):4687–4694.
28. Douglas NC, Nakhuda GS, Sauer MV, Zimmermann RC: Angiogenesis and Ovarian Function. *J Fertil Reprod* 2005, **13**(4):7–15.
29. González F, Rote NS, Minium J, Kirwan JP: Evidence of proatherogenic inflammation in polycystic ovary syndrome. *Metabolism* 2009, **58**(7):954–962.
30. González F: Inflammation in Polycystic Ovary Syndrome: underpinning of insulin resistance and ovarian dysfunction. *Steroids* 2010, **77**(4):300–305. 10.
31. Parlee SD, Ernst MC, Sinal CJ, Goralski KB: TNFα enhances the expression and secretion of chemerin from adipocytes. *FASEB J* 2009, **755**:5.
32. Rezvanfar MA, Saadi HAS, Gooshe M, Abdolghaffari AH, Baeeri MB, Abdollahi M: Ovarian aging-like phenotype in the hyperandrogenism-induced murine model of polycystic ovary. *Oxid Med Cell Long* 2014, **2014**:1–10.
33. Iuorno MJ, Nestler JE: Insulin-lowering drugs in polycystic ovary syndrome. *Obst Gynecol Clin North Am* 2001, **28**(1):153–164.
34. De Leo V, La Marca A, Petraglia F: Insulin-lowering agents in the management of polycystic ovary syndrome. *Endoc Rev* 2003, **24**(5):633–667.
35. Glueck CJ, Moreira A, Goldenberg N, Sieve L, Wang P: Pioglitazone and metformin in obese women with polycystic ovary syndrome not optimally responsive to metformin. *Human Reprod* 2003, **18**(8):1618–1625.
36. Wang Q, Leader A, Tsang BK: Inhibitory Roles of Prohibitin and Chemerin in FSH-Induced Rat Granulosa Cell Steroidogenesis. *Endocrinol* 2013. doi:10.1210/en.1836.
37. Angelidis G, Dafopoulos K, Messini KI, Valotassiou V, Tsikouras P, Vrachnis N, Psimadas D, Georgoulias P, Messinis IE: The Emerging Roles of Adiponectin in Female Reproductive System-Associated Disorders and Pregnancy. *Reprod Sci* 2013, **20**:872–881.
38. Libby P, Plutzky J: Inflammation in diabetes mellitus: role of peroxisome-proliferator-activated receptor-alpha and peroxisome-proliferator-activated receptor-gamma agonists. *Am J Cardiol* 2007, **99**:27–40.
39. Nestler JE, Jakubowicz DJ, Evans WS, Pasquali R: Effects of metformin on spontaneous and clomiphene-induced ovulation in the polycystic ovary syndrome. *N Engl J Med* 1998, **338**:1876–1880.

Anti-hyperlipidemic and anti-atherosclerotic effects of *Pinus eldarica* Medw. nut in hypercholesterolemic rabbits

Hasan Fallah Huseini[1], Maryam Sotoudeh Anvari[2], Yaser Tajallizadeh khoob[3], Shahram Rabbani[4], Farshad Sharifi[5], Seyed Masoud Arzaghi[5] and Hossein Fakhrzadeh[5*]

Abstract

Background: Previous studies suggest that chemical constituents present in *Pinus eldarica* Medw (*P. eldarica*) nut possess antioxidant properties that may positively influence lipid profile.
The present study was conducted to evaluate the efficacy of *P. eldarica* nut on the experimental atherosclerosis development in hypercholesterolemic rabbits.

Methods: Forty male 6 months old white New Zealand rabbits (1.8–2 kg) were randomly assigned into five equal groups. One group was kept as control (normal) group, fed on standard rabbit diet and other 4 groups were fed on high cholesterol diet (HCD). Out of four HCD groups one group was kept as control (HCD) and other three groups were treated with different doses (50, 100 and 200 mg/kg/day) of *P. eldarica* nut for 8 weeks. Percentage of aortic wall area changes as indication of atherosclerosis development and fasting blood cholesterol, LDL, HDL and triglyceride levels were determined in all groups.

Results: The results indicate that fasting blood cholesterol and aortic atherosclerotic involvements in 200 mg/kg/day and 100 mg/kg/day *P. eldarica* nut extract treated groups significantly decreased as compared to the high cholesterol-diet control group.

Conclusion: *P. eldarica* nut lowers blood cholesterol level and aortic atherosclerotic involvement in hypercholesterolemic rabbits.

Keywords: *Pinus eldarica* nut, Rabbits, Atherosclerosis, Hypercholesterolemia

Introduction

Atherosclerotic vascular disease is a major cause of morbidity and mortality worldwide [1]. Dyslipidemia is a crucial risk factor for atherosclerosis and oxidative stress following free radical-mediated oxidation of low-density lipoproteins is associated with progression of atherogenesis and its vascular complications [2–4]. In the search for plant foods that provide cardiovascular benefits, nuts have recently enticed attention. Among nuts, the Iranian pine, *Pinus eldarica* Medw (*P. eldarica*) nuts are used as food. *P. eldarica* belongs to the botanical family pinaceae and naturally grows in the Transcaucasian region between Europe and Asia, and it is also spread in Iran, Afghanistan and Pakistan [5, 6].

In Russia and the Central Asian countries the *P. eldarica* needles, buds, resin and nuts have been widely used in traditional medicine for the treatment of bronchial asthma, and various skin diseases [7, 8]. Several components such as β-caryophyllene, α-pinene, longifolene, α-humulene, δ-3-carene and β-pinene with antioxidant properties have been reported in the *P. eldarica* nut oil [9].

In our previous study high concentrations of total polyphenols and fatty acids have been detected in *P. eldarica* nut as indication of its antioxidant properties [10]. Experimental studies strongly support the efficacy of polyphenols and unsaturated fatty acids in the treatment of chronic diseases including cardiovascular disorders

* Correspondence: Fakhrzad@tums.ac.ir
[5]Elderly Health Research Center, Endocrinology and Metabolism Population Sciences Institute, Tehran University of Medical Sciences, 4th floor, No 4, Ostad Nejatollahi Street, Engelab Avenue, Tehran, Iran
Full list of author information is available at the end of the article

[11–14]. The present study was conducted to evaluate the possible anti-hypercholesterolemic and anti-atherosclerotic effects of *P. eldarica* nut in hypercholesterolemic rabbits.

Methods

Chemicals

Methanol, phosphoric acid, chloroform, acetonitril and sodium chloride were purchased from Merck Company (India) nn. Ethyl acetate was purchased from Sinopharm Chemical Reagent Company (China). Polyphenol standards: (+) - catechin, (–) - epicatechin, Gallic acid, vanillic acid, *para* coumaric acid, ferullic acid, *ortho* coumaric acid and tyrosol were purchased from Sigma-Aldrich Corporation (Germany). Cholesterol powder was purchased from Solvay Duphar Co., Belgium.

Plant material

P. eldarica cones were collected from Chitgar Forest Park (West of Tehran). The cones were collected between June and July of 2010. The plant was identified by M. Ahvazi and herbarium specimen was preserved in the herbarium of Medicinal Plants Institute (ACECR) with Herbarium code of 689. *P. eldarica* cones were dried in a dark place at room temperature. The nuts were removed from cones and grounded to powder by grinder.

Plant extract

The hydroalcholic extract of *P. eldarica* nut powder was prepared using 70 % ethanol in water, using percolation method at room temperature. The powdered plant material was soaked initially in a solvent in a percolator and then sufficient amount of the solvent was added to cover material and kept for 24 h with occasional stirring. Then the outlet of the percolator was opened and the liquid contained therein was allowed to drip slowly. The procedure was repeated twice and the combined extractions were clarified by filtration and concentrated to dryness on rotary evaporator at a maximum of 40 °C temperature and under reduced pressure.

Polyphenol determination

The polyphenol content of *P. eldarica* nut was determined by the High-performance liquid chromatography (HPLC) method developed by Dogan et al. [15]. In brief a standard solution was prepared by dissolving 10 mg of (+) catechin (sigma), epicatechin (sigma), and other phenolic compounds in 10 ml methanol and diluting this solution with methanol HPLC grade. The range of concentration was between 50 and 1000 μg/ml and standard curve was linear ($R^2 \geq 0.998$). Then 20 μL of sample solution was injected to the HPLC and the chromatogram was recorded at 280 nm. First, 20 μl of standard solution was injected and the chromatogram was recorded at 280 nm. Next, we compared the area of the peaks in standard and sample chromatograms and calculated the amount of polyphenols in *P. eldarica*. Total phenol was computed from measurement of individually detected phenols [16].

Animals and diet

Forty male 6-month-old white New Zealand rabbits (1.8–2 kg) were purchased from Razi Research Institute, Karaj, Iran. High cholesterol diet (HCD) was prepared by adding of 1 g cholesterol powder and 3 g corn oil to 96 g of standard laboratory food.

General procedures

Rabbits were housed individually in cages in temperature-controlled room (24 °C) under a 12-h light/dark cycle with free access to food and water in the Animal Research Center of Institute of Medicinal Plants. The experimental protocol was approved by the Iranian Institutional Animal Ethics Committee and was conducted according to the Iranian Institutional Animal Care Guidelines for the use and care of experimental animal, drug, dose, and treatment schedule.

After a 2-week adaptation period, rabbits were randomly assigned to five equal groups: control (normal) group fed on standard a diet, HCD control group fed on HCD (1 % cholesterol), and three groups fed on HCD and treated with *P. eldarica* nut in three different doses (50, 100 and 200 mg/kg/day). The extract in the dosages of 50, 100, 200 mg was mixed with little amount of rabbit pellets and fed orally one hour before feeding. The whole experiment lasted 8 weeks. Upon termination of the study biochemical analysis of serum lipids and pathological evaluation of aortas were performed.

Biochemical analysis

At the end of the study, the overnight fasting blood sample was taken from marginal ear veins for lipid analysis. Fasting blood cholesterol (Cho) LDL, HDL and triglyceride (TG) levels in sera were measured using enzyme assay kits (Pars Azmun Co., Iran).

Pathological analysis

At the end of the study, rabbits were killed by chloroform (overdose) and their aortas were separated up to diaphragm. The aortas were then divided into the proximal, middle, and distal segments. The aortic specimens were dehydrated in a graded series of alcohol xylene and embedded in paraffin for light microscopic examination. From each paraffin block, four sections of 4 mm^2 were cut and stained with hematoxylin and eosin. All sections were evaluated microscopically for fatty streak, foam cells, extracellular lipid core, as atheromatous plaque elements. The degree of vascular injury and atherosclerosis was

Table 1 Percent of polyphenols in *P. eldarica* nut mean ± SD [16]

Polyphenols	Percent
Catechin	10.1 ± 0.18
Epicatechin	10.3 ± 0.18
Gallic acid	1.6 ± 0.09
P. coumaric acid	1.4 ± 0.12
Ferullic acid	1.7 ± 0.21
O. coumaric acid	0.12 ± 0.02
Tyrosol	29.1 ± 0.08
Dimers of catechin and epicatechin	7.5 ± 1.06
Unknown	38.18 ± 0.28
Total phenols (ppm)	483 ± 27

quantitatively measured based on lesion area (on scale of mm^2) with use of a color image analyzer (E200; Nikon, Tokyo, Japan) [17]. Both the surgeon and the pathologist were blinded to the control and experiment groups.

Statistical analysis

All values are expressed as means ± SE. Data were analyzed by one way ANOVA, and all differences were inspected by Duncan's multiple test. Differences were considered to be significant at $p < 0.05$.

Results

The polyphenol content of the *P. eldarica* nut is presented in Table 1. Considering this method more than 8 polyphenols were identified in *P. eldarica* nut in which catechin, epicatechin and tyrosol were highest in concentration.

Results show that feeding the rabbits for 8 weeks with HCD leads to a significant increase in their blood serum total cholesterol, LDL-C and to a lesser extent in TG levels. Results indicate that serum total cholesterol and LDL-C levels significantly decrease in the groups treated with 200 mg/kg/day and 100 mg/kg/day of *P. eldarica* compared to the control group; although it is of note that all of the aortic samples from HCD-fed rabbits showed some degree of atherogenesis and none of them were normal. There were no significant changes in fasting blood TG and HDL-C levels in *P. eldarica* treated groups compared to control group (Table 2) (Fig. 1).

Morphological changes of the aortic wall atherosclerotic involvement are shown in Fig. 1. The aortic wall area percent in groups treated with 200 mg/kg/day and 100 mg/kg/day *P. eldarica* nut decreased significantly compared to the control group (Table 2).

Discussion

The results suggest that *P. eldarica* nut extract reduced total cholesterol, LDL-C and extent of aortic atherosclerotic involvement in hypercholesterolemic rabbits. The mechanism underlying inhibition of aortic atherosclerotic progression by *P. eldarica* nut extract may not be solely due to its lipid lowering effect, as the levels of serum total cholesterol and LDL-C were remarkably higher in cholesterol-fed rabbits than in normal ones. Other mechanisms may also play a role for such effect. Increases in serum cholesterol and LDL-C and consequent oxidation of LDL-C are essential steps for development of atherosclerotic plaques [2]. In fact formation of oxidatively-modified LDL-C is the first step of atherogenesis in so-called "oxidation hypothesis" [17].

Table 2 The fasting blood parameters and aortic wall area percent (mm^2) after 8 weeks of high cholesterol diet (HCD) fed rabbits treated with *P. eldarica* nut extract at dosages of 50, 100, 200 mg/kg compared with high control HCD fed rabbits (mean ± SD)

Groups	Triglyceride (mg/dl)	Cholesterol (mg/dl)	LDL (mg/cl)	HDL (mg/dl)	Aortic wall area percent (mm^2)	Percent of aortic wall area changes
Control (normal)	60.4 ± 15.8	31.4 ± 4.5	9.2 ± 4.7	13.2 ± 3.2	0.247 ± 0.032	
Control (HCD)	91.2 ± 48.9	1545.6 ± 510.6	1060.6 ± 360.5	113.4 ± 55.8	0.296 ± 0.049	16.55↑ Compared with control (normal)
	P = 0.218*	P = 0.003*	P = 0.016*	P = 0.003*	P = 0.005*	
P. eldarica nut extract 50 mg/kg	93.6 ± 31.2	1253.0 ± 578.0	834.4 ± 201.2	87.6 ± 17.7	0.276 ± 0.048	6.76↓ compared with control (HCD)
	P = 0.929**	P = 0.421**	P = 0.544**	P = 0.351**	P = 0.350**	
P. eldarica nut extract 100 mg/kg	102.2 ± 37.7	834.4 ± 201.2	552.4 ± 158.2	90.2 ± 15.9	0.261 ± 0.038	11.83↓ compared with control (HCD)
	P = 0.700**	P = 0.020**	P = 0.034**	P = 0.410**	P = 0.048**	
P. eldarica nut extract 200 mg/kg	108.8 ± 28.0	710.4 ± 448.0	438.4 ± 292.2	99.4 ± 11.8	0.259 ± 0.042	12.50↓compared with control (HCD)
	P = 0.505**	P = 0.025**	P = 0.020**	P = 0.47**0	P = 0.032**	

$P < 0.05$ was considered as statistically significant
*compared with control (normal) group
**compared with control (HCD) group

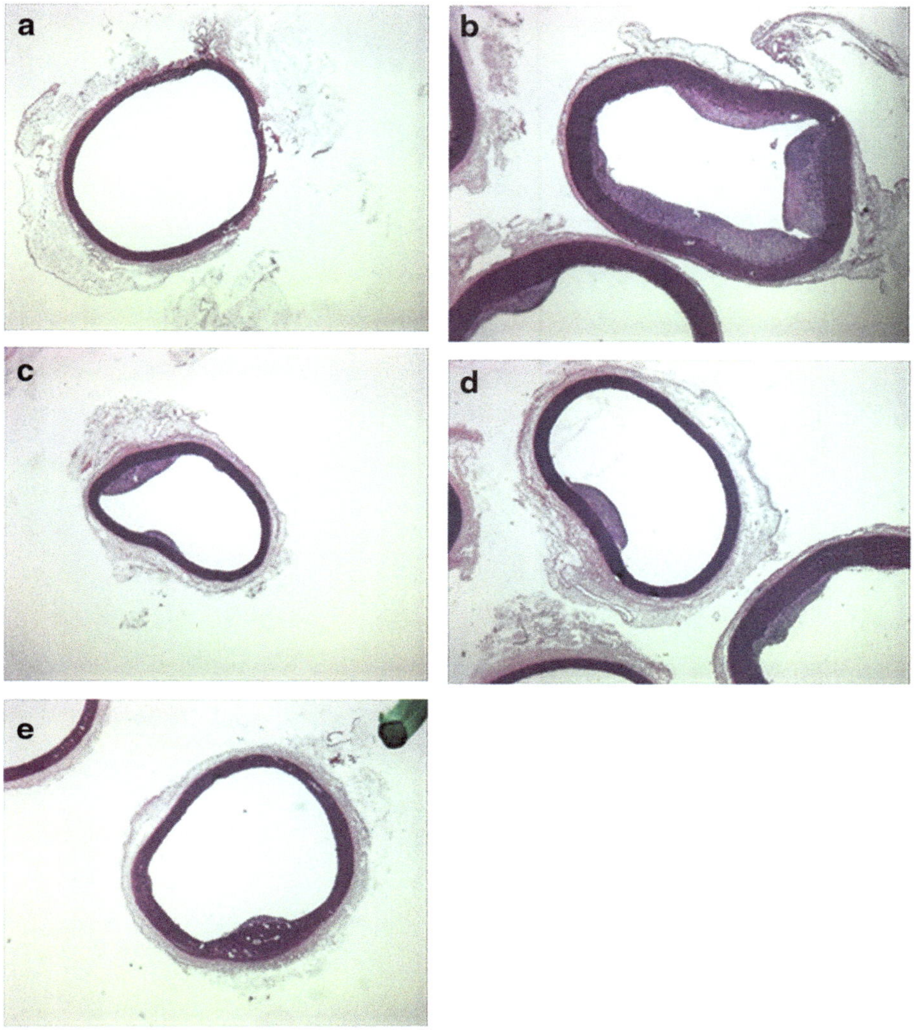

Fig. 1 Morphological changes of the aortic wall atherosclerotic involvement. **a** Normal rabbits fed on standard laboratory diet, **b** Rabbits fed on HCD; **c** Rabbits fed on HCD and treated with 50 mg/kg of *P. eldarica*; **d** Rabbits fed on HCD and treated with 100 mg/kg of *P. eldarica*; **e** Rabbits fed on HCD and treated with 200 mg/kg of *P. eldarica*

Moreover it has been shown that susceptibility of LDL-C to oxidation independently correlates with the extent of atherosclerosis [18]. It is now established that inhibition of oxidative stress and lipid oxidation could have beneficial effects on regression of atherogenesis [19]. *P. eldarica* nuts contain high concentrations of polyphenols and flavonoids (Table 1) [10]. Several data suggested that, flavonoids improve dyslipidemia, inhibit low-density lipoprotein cholesterol oxidation and protect vascular endothelium against oxidative damage [20–22]. Furthermore, catechin and epicatechin which are found in high concentrations in *P. eldarica* nuts are also main chemical constituent of other Pinus species barks such as French matitime pine bark extract (pycnogenol) [23]. Several studies have shown the beneficial effects of pycnogenol for health to be mainly due to its antioxidant properties and consequent excellent free radical scavenging function [24–26]. In addition other components such as tyrosol with antioxidant properties which are present in high concentrations in *P. eldarica* nuts may directly or indirectly influence lipoprotein and cellular metabolism against atherogenesis [10, 27].

On the other hand, the observed anti-atherogenic effects of *P. eldarica* nut in the rabbits may also be in part due to appreciable amounts of essential oils such as α-pinene, β-pinene and β-caryophyllene present in this nut [9]. The antioxidant properties of α-pinene, β-pinene and β-caryophyllene are reported in other studies [28]. Of note the limitations of this study were lack of determination of the essential oil components and antioxidant properties of *P. eldarica* nut extract. To our knowledge this is the first trial on the anti-atherosclerotic and hypolipidemic effects of *P. eldarica* extracts on hypercholesterolemic rabbits. In a similar study we also have recently shown the beneficial effects of *Pinus eldarica* nut extract on blood glucose and cholesterol levels in hypercholesterolemic alloxan-induced diabetic rats [29]. As *P. eldarica* nuts are usually safe and used as food, further investigation of their clinical efficacy in the treatment of hypercholesterolemia is suggested.

Competing interests

The authors declare that they have no competing interests.

Authors' contributions

HFH performed the field trial and preparation of the manuscript, MSA performed the pathological analysis, YTk contributed in preparing the research proposal, SR prepared aortic specimens for pathological analysis, FS performed the statistical analysis, SMA contributed in the field trial and laboratory analysis, HF was the principle investigator who conceived the idea and prepared the research proposal and helped in the preparation of the manuscript. All authors read and approved the final manuscript.

Acknowledgements

This research was supported by a grant from the Endocrinology and Metabolism Research Institute, Tehran University of Medical Sciences Tehran, Iran and the Institute of Medicinal Plants (ACECR), Karaj.

Author details

[1]Medicinal Plants Research Center, Institute of Medicinal Plants, ACECR, Karaj, Iran. [2]Clinical and Surgical Pathology Department Tehran Heart Center, Tehran University of Medical Sciences, Tehran, Iran. [3]Endocrinology and Metabolism Research Center, Endocrinology and Metabolism Clinical Sciences Institute, Tehran University of Medical Sciences, Tehran, Iran. [4]Experimental Research Center, Tehran Heart Center, Tehran University of Medical Sciences, Tehran, Iran. [5]Elderly Health Research Center, Endocrinology and Metabolism Population Sciences Institute, Tehran University of Medical Sciences, 4th floor, No 4, Ostad Nejatollahi Street, Engelab Avenue, Tehran, Iran.

References

1. Finegold JA, Asaria P, Francis DP. Mortality from ischaemic heart disease by country, region, and age: statistics from World Health Organisation and United Nations. Int J Cardiol. 2012;168(2):934–45.
2. Badimon L, Vilahur G. LDL-cholesterol versus HDL-cholesterol in the atherosclerotic plaque: inflammatory resolution versus thrombotic chaos. Ann N Y Acad Sci. 2012;1254:18–32.
3. Stocker R, Keaney Jr JF. Role of oxidative modifications in atherosclerosis. Physiol Rev. 2004;84(4):1381–478.
4. Chen K, Keaney Jr JF. Evolving concepts of oxidative stress and reactive oxygen species in cardiovascular disease. Curr Atheroscler Rep. 2012;14(5):476–83.
5. Zargary A. Medicinal plants. 5th ed. Tehran: Tehran University Press; 1996. p. 9–12.
6. Mozaffarian W. Tree and shrubs of Iran. 1st ed. Tehran Iran: Farhang Moaser Press; 1983. p. 563–5.
7. Mamedov N, Craker LE. Medicinal plants used for the treatment of bronchial asthma in Russia and Central Asia. J Herbs Spices Med Plants. 2001;8:91–117.
8. Mamedov N, Gardner Z, Craker LE. Medicinal plants used in Russia and Central Asia for the treatment of selected skin conditions. J Herbs Spices Med Plants. 2005;11:191–222.
9. Afsharypour S, Sanaty F. Essential oil constituents of leaves and fruits of Pinus eldarica Medw. J Essent Oil Res. 2005;17:327–8.
10. Sadeghi Afjeh M, Fallah Huseini H, Tajalizadekhoob Y, Mirarefin M, Sharifi F, Taheri E, et al. Determination of phenolic compounds in Pinus eldarica by HPLC. J Med Plant Res. 2014;49:23–33.
11. Pandey KB, Rizvi SI. Plant polyphenols as dietary antioxidants in human health and disease. Oxid Med Cell Longev. 2009;2(5):270–8.
12. Pandey KB, Rizvi SI. Current understanding of dietary polyphenols and their role in health and disease. Curr Nutr Food Sci. 2009;5(4):249–63.
13. Tavakoli R, Mohadjerani M, Hosseinzadeh R, Tajbakhsh M, Naqinezhad A. Essential-oil and fatty-acid composition, and antioxidant activity of extracts of Ficaria kochii. Chem Biodivers. 2012;9(12):2732–41.
14. Causey JL. Korean pine nut fatty acids induce satiety-producing hormone release in overweight human volunteers, American Chemical Society National Meeting & Exposition. 2006. p. 26–30.
15. Dogan S, Diken ME, Dogan M. Antioxidant, phenolic and protein contents of some medicinal plants. J Med Plant Res. 2010;4:2566–73.
16. Sadeghi Afjeh M, Fallah Huseini H, Tajallizadekhoob Y, Mirarefin M, Taheri E, Saeednia S, et al. Determination of phenolic compounds in Pinus Eldarica by HPLC. J Med Plant Res. 2014;13(49):22–33.
17. Kumar V, Abbas AK, Fausto N. Pathologic basis of disease. 7th ed. Philadelphia: Saunders; 2005. p. 25–6.
18. Regnström J, Nilsson J, Tornvall P, Landou C, Hamsten A. Susceptibility to low- density-lipoprotein oxidation and coronary atherosclerosis in man. Lancet. 1992;339:1183–6.
19. Heinecke JW. Oxidants and antioxidants in the pathogenesis of atherosclerosis: implications for the oxidised low density lipoprotein hypothesis. Atheroscler. 1998;141:1–15.
20. Loke WM, Proudfoot JM, Hodgson JM, McKinley AJ, Hime N, Magat M, et al. Specific dietary polyphenols attenuate atherosclerosis in apolipoprotein E-knockout mice by alleviating inflammation and endothelial dysfunction. Arterioscler Thromb Vasc Biol. 2010;30(4):749–57.
21. Martin S, Andriantsitohaina R. Cellular mechanism of vasculo-protection induced by polyphenols on the endothelium. Ann Cardiol Angeiol (Paris). 2002;51(6):304–15.
22. Mulvihill EE, Huff MW. Antiatherogenic properties of flavonoids: implications for cardiovascular health. Can J Cardiol. 2010;26:17A–21.
23. Yesli-Celiktas O, Ganzera M, Akgun I, Sevimli C, Korkmaz KS, Bedir E. Determination of polyphenolic constituents and biological activities of bark extracts from different Pinus species. J Sci Food Agric. 2009;89(8):1339–45.
24. Rohdewald P. A review of the French matitime pine bark extract (Pycnogenol), a herbal medication with a diverse pharmacology. Int J Clin Pharmacol Ther. 2002;40:158–68.
25. Sato M, Yamada Y, Matsuoka H, Nakashima S, Kamiya T, Ikeguchi M, et al. Dietary pine bark extract inhibit atherosclerotic lesion development in male Apo-E-deficient mice by lowering the serum cholesterol level. Biosci Biotechnol Biochem. 2009;73:1314–7.
26. Maritim A, Dene BA, Sanders RA, Watkins JB. Effects of Pycnogenol treatment on oxidative stress in streptozotocin-induced diabetic rats. J Biochem Mol Toxicol. 2003;17:193–9.
27. Giovannini C, Straface E, Modesti D, Coni E, Cantafora A, De Vincenzi M, et al. Tyrosol, the major olive oil biophenol, protects against oxidized-LDL-induced injury in Caco-2 cells. J Nutr. 1999;129(7):1269–77.
28. Miguel MG. Antioxidant and anti-inflammatory activities of essential oils: a short review. Molecules. 2010;15(12):9252–87.
29. Fallah Huseini H, Mehrzadi S, Ghaznavi H, Tajallizadehkhoob Y, Fakhrzadeh H. Effects of pinus eldarica medw: nut extract on blood glucose and cholesterol levels in hypercholesterolemic alloxan-induced diabetic rats. J Med Plant Res. 2013;1(45):68–74.

Phthalimide analogs as probable 15-lipoxygenase-1 inhibitors: synthesis, biological evaluation and docking studies

Alireza Aliabadi[1,2*], Ahmad Mohammadi-Farani[1,3], Zeinab Hosseinzadeh[2,4], Hamid Nadri[5], Alireza Moradi[5] and Farahnaz Ahmadi[1,3]

Abstract

Background: Recent studies have been explained the role of lipoxygenases (LOX) in the origin of cancer. Among the lipoxygenases, the 5-LOX, 12-LOX and 15-LOX are more important in the cause of neoplastic disorders. In the present investigation, a new series of anticancer agents with 1,3,4-thiadiazole and phthalimide substructures were synthesized and their *in vitro* cytotoxicity was evaluated by MTT assay. Moreover, enzyme inhibitory potency was also assessed by enzymatic protocol towards 15-LOX-1. Molecular docking was performed to explore *in silico* binding mode of the target compounds.

Results: Tested compounds showed a better cytotoxic activity against HT29 cell line (colorectal cancer) in comparison with other cell lines (PC3: prostate carcinoma; SKNMC: neuroblastoma). Unfortunately, all of the tested derivatives rendered lower inhibitory potency than quercetin towards 15-LOX-1. Four hydrogen bonds were detected in docking studies for compound **4d** as the most potent derivative in enzymatic assay.

Conclusions: The biological results of reported compounds in this research were not so satisfactory. But, further structural modifications are necessary to improve the bioactivity of these derivatives.

Keywords: Synthesis, Phthalimide, 1,3,4-Thiadiazole, Lipoxygenase, Anticancer

Background

Arachidonic acid is a fatty acid released from membrane phospholipids during cell stimulation. Arachidonic acid is metabolized mainly by two groups of enzymes consist of lipoxygenases (LOX, which includes 5-LOX, 12-LOX, and 15-LOX) and cyclooxygenase (COX). Inhibition of cyclooxygenases delays tumorigenesis in animals and humans [1, 2]. Various epidemiological and animal studies have confirmed that there is a close relationship between high fat consumption with an increased incidence and growth of tumors at several specific organ sites like breast. More recent studies also presented that patients with consumption of diets with a high proportion of polyunsaturated ω-6 fatty acid (n-6 PUFA), such as arachidonic acid and linoleic acid are associated with a more advanced disease stage at the time of diagnosis of breast cancer [2]. The LOXs convert polyunsaturated fatty acids like arachidonic and linoleic acids into biologically active metabolites that affects various cellular events such as signaling, structure and metabolism. According to the later tumorigenesis studies, it is likely that polyunsaturated fatty acids may enhance tumorigenesis via oxidative metabolism. Eicosanoids derived from the arachidonic acid cascade have been implicated in the pathogenesis of a variety of human diseases, including cancer, and are now believed to play important roles in tumor promotion, progression, and metastatic disease [3–5]. Vigorous expression of the enzymes (LOXs & COXs) that synthesize bioactive lipid metabolites from unsaturated fatty acids (arachidonic acid and linoleic acid) appears to be related to the development of prostate carcinoma remarkably. Other research have also reported that 15-LO-2 is expressed in normal prostate tissue, but poorly expressed in prostate tumors. Thus, 15-LO-1 is highly expressed in prostate tumors while 15-LO-2 is highly expressed in normal tissue. 15-LO-1 in prostate cancer tumors

* Correspondence: aliabadi.alireza@gmail.com
[1]Pharmaceutical Sciences Research Center, School of Pharmacy, Kermanshah University of Medical Sciences, Kermanshah, Iran
[2]Department of Medicinal Chemistry, Faculty of Pharmacy, Kermanshah University of Medical Sciences, Kermanshah, Iran
Full list of author information is available at the end of the article

converts linoleic acid, its preferred substrate to 13-*S*-hydroxy-octadecadienoic acid (13-(*S*)-HODE) and other metabolites. These metabolites appear to alter cellular signaling pathways, and thus the inappropriate expression might alter biological events and contribute to tumor development [6–8]. On the basis of this information, the drugs with capability of interaction with pathways related to the production of lipoxygenases metabolites or signaling functions of lipoxygenases products may be effective pharmaceutical agents in prevention or treatment of cancer.

Literature reviews declare that 1,3,4-thiadiazole ring as 5-membered heterocycle have diverse biological effects such as anti-inflammatory, anticonvulsant, antibacterial, antileshmanial, antioxidant and anticancer [9–20]. On the other hands, phthalimide moiety is another heterocyclic residue derived from the isoindole ring. This moiety has also exhibited several pharmacological activities like anticonvulsant, antitubercular, anti-inflammatory, anti-acetylcholinesterase as well as anticancer effects [21–31]. In the current investigation, we encouraged to synthesize a new series of chemical entities bearing 1,3,4-thiadiazole and phthalimide (isoindoline-1,3-dione) residues as potential anticancer agents.

Methods

Chemistry

The corresponding chemical reagents and starting materials were purchased from the commercial companies such as Merck and Sigma-Aldrich. The purification of the prepared compounds was carried out by column chromatography using ethyl acetate/petroleum ether. Spectroscopic methods were applied for characterization of the synthesized compounds. ^{1}H NMR spectra were acquired by Bruker 250 MHz in deutrated chloroform ($CDCl_3$) and the obtained data were expressed as δ (ppm) compared to tetramethylsilane (TMS) as internal standard. Infrared (IR) spectra of the prepared compounds were obtained by Shimadzu 470 with preparing potassium bromide (KBr) disk. The mass spectra were run on a Finigan TSQ-70 spectrometer (Finigan, USA) at 70 eV. Melting points were determined using electrothermal 9001 melting point analyzer apparatus and are uncorrected.

Synthesis of 2-(1,3-Dioxoisoindolin-2-yl)acetic acid (2)

5 g (33.8 mmol) of phthalic anhydride, 2.53 g (33.8 mmol) glycine and 4.67 ml (33.8 mmol) triethylamine (Et_3N) were mixed in toluene (100 ml) and the reaction mixture was refluxed overnight (Scheme 1). The reaction was monitored by thin layer chromatography (TLC). Toluene was evaporated by rotary evaporator apparatus under reduced pressure. The obtained residue was washed by diethyl ether (Et_2O) and *n*-hexane. The obtained white powder was used for the next step without any extra purification [32].

^{1}HNMR ($CDCl_3$, 250 MHz) δ (ppm): 4.3 (s, 2H, $-CH_2-$), 7.70 (dd, 2H, $J = 8.4$ Hz, $J = 2.4$ Hz, $H_{5,6}$-Phthalimide), 7.85

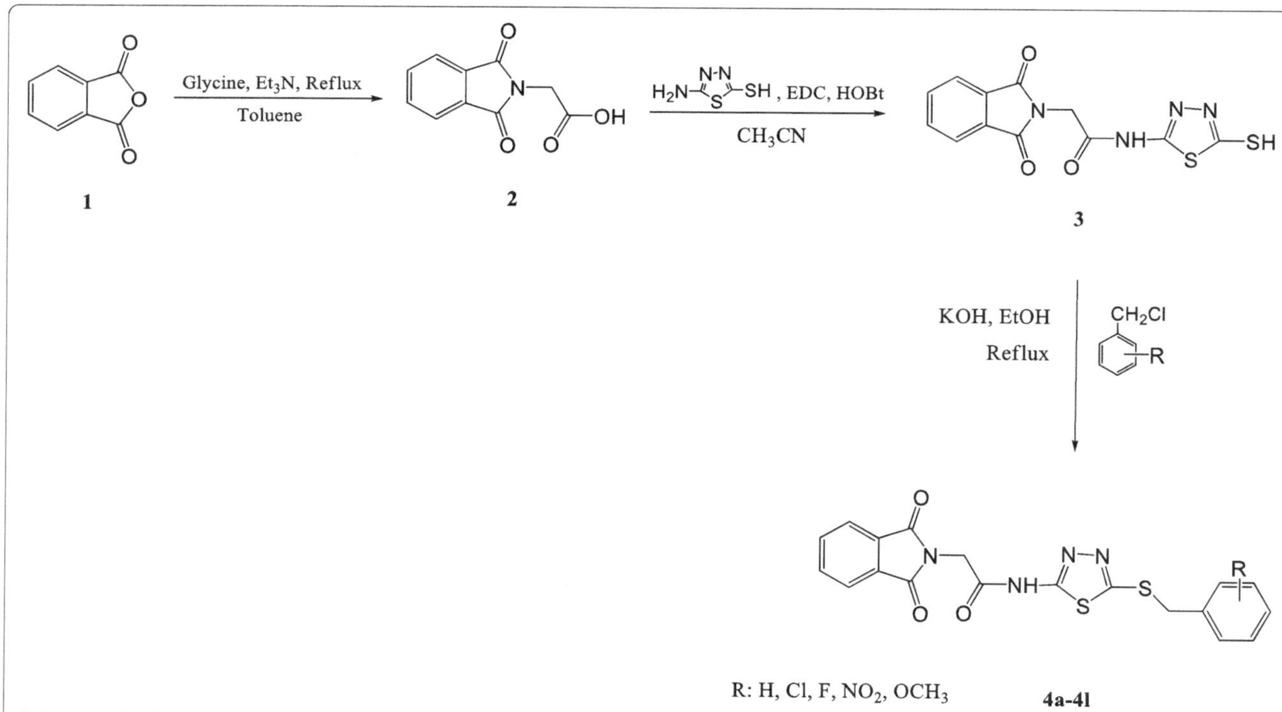

Scheme 1 Synthetic pathway for preparation of compounds 4a-4 l

(dd, 2H, $J = 8.4$ Hz, $J = 2.4$ Hz, $H_{4,7}$-Phthalimide), 11.97 (brs, –COOH). IR (KBr, cm^{-1}) ῡ: 3468 (OH, acid), 3155, 2989, 2939, 1705 (C=O, acid). MS (*m/z*, %): 205 (M^+, weak), 160 (100), 133 (20), 104 (40), 76 (35), 50 (20).

Synthesis of 2-(1,3-Dioxoisoindolin-2-yl)-N-(5-mercapto-1,3,4-thiadiazol-2-yl)acetamide (3)

3 g (14.63 mmol) of 2-(1,3-dioxoisoindolin-2-yl)acetic acid (compound **2**), 2.80 g (14.63 mmol) *N*-ethyl-*N*-dimethylaminopropyl carbodiimide (EDC) and 1.98 g (14.63 mmol) hydroxybenzotriazole (HOBt) were mixed in 70 ml acetonitrile (CH_3CN) and the obtained mixture was stirred for 30 min. Then, 1.95 g (14.63 mmol) of 5-amino-1,3,4-thiadiazole-2-thiol was added to the reaction mixture and the stirring was continued for 24 h. The reaction end was proved by thin layer chromatography (TLC). Then, acetonitrile was evaporated using rotary evaporator and the residue was washed by diethyl ether and *n*-hexane. More purification was done by column chromatogaraphy (petroleum ether/ethyl acetate 70/30) to afford a yellowish powder [33–35].

^{1}HNMR ($CDCl_3$, 250 MHz) δ (ppm): 4.81 (s, 2H, –CH_2-CO-), 3.82 (s, 1H, SH), 7.89 (dd, 2H, $J = 8.4$ Hz, $J = 2.4$ Hz, $H_{5,6}$-Phthalimide), 7.94 (dd, 2H, $J = 8.4$ Hz, $J = 2.4$ Hz, $H_{5,6}$-Phthalimide), 13.81 (brs, NH). IR (KBr, cm^{-1}) ῡ: 3201, 3070, 2924, 1739, 1608, 1554, 1465, 1377, 1307, 1053, 717. MS (*m/z*, %): 320 (10), 287 (80), 263 (60), 231 (100), 160 (80), 159 (60), 121 (40), 104 (40), 76 (45).

General procedure for synthesis of compounds 4a-4 l

In a flat bottom flask, 0.2 g (0.625 mmol) of 2-(1,3-dioxoisoindolin-2-yl)-*N*-(5-mercapto-1,3,4-thiadiazol-2-yl)acetamide (compound **3**) was treated with 0.035 g (0.625 mmol) potassium hydroxide in absolute ethanol and heated for 5 min, then equimolar (0.625 mmol) quantity of appropriate benzyl chloride derivative was added to the reaction medium and reflux condition was performed for 24 h. Thin layer chromatography (TLC) was carried out to determine the reaction end. Then, crushed ice was added to the reaction flask and the formed precipitate was filtered and collected. Crystallization was performed using ethanol [35].

2-(1,3-Dioxoisoindolin-2-yl)-N-(5-(2-nitrobenzylthio)-1,3,4-thiadiazol-2-yl)acetamide (4a)

^{1}HNMR ($CDCl_3$, 250 MHz) δ (ppm): 4.79 (s, 2H, –S-CH_2-), 4.89 (s, 2H, –CH_2-CO-), 7.45 (t, 1H, H_4-2-Nitrophenyl), 7.57 (m, 2H, $H_{5,6}$-2-Nitrophenyl), 7.81 (dd, 2H, $J = 8.4$ Hz, $J = 2.4$ Hz, $H_{5,6}$-Phthalimide), 7.95 (dd, 2H, $J = 8.4$ Hz, $J = 2.4$ Hz, $H_{5,6}$-Phthalimide), 8.06 (d, 1H, $J = 10$ Hz, H_3-2-Nitrophenyl). IR (KBr, cm^{-1}) ῡ: 3414, 3325, 3170, 3035, 2927, 2854, 2742, 1774, 1720, 1573, 1523, 1415, 1346, 1303, 1195, 952, 713.

2-(1,3-Dioxoisoindolin-2-yl)-N-(5-(3-nitrobenzylthio)-1,3,4-thiadiazol-2-yl)acetamide (4b)

^{1}HNMR ($CDCl_3$, 250 MHz) δ (ppm): 4.45 (s, 2H, –S-CH_2-), 4.77 (s, 2H, –CH_2-CO-), 7.48-7.59 (m, 2H, 3-Nitrophenyl), 7.73 (dd, 2H, $J = 8.4$ Hz, $J = 2.4$ Hz, $H_{5,6}$-Phthalimide), 7.92 (d, 1H, $J = 7.5$ Hz, H_4-3-Nitrophenyl), 8.24 (dd, 2H, $J = 8.4$ Hz, $J = 2.4$ Hz, $H_{4,7}$-Phthalimide), 8.36 (s, 1H, H_2-3-Nitrophenyl). IR (KBr, cm^{-1}) ῡ: 3429, 3209, 3066, 2924, 2854, 1774, 1708, 1527, 1411, 1350, 1296, 1195, 1053, 952, 717. MS (*m/z*, %): 455 (M^+, Weak), 398 (15), 268 (100), 235 (35), 193 (45), 136 (55), 109 (15), 89 (30), 60 (35).

2-(1,3-Dioxoisoindolin-2-yl)-N-(5-(4-nitrobenzylthio)-1,3,4-thiadiazol-2-yl)acetamide (4c)

^{1}HNMR ($CDCl_3$, 250 MHz) δ (ppm): 4.42 (s, 2H, –S-CH_2-), 4.79 (s, 2H, –CH_2-CO-), 7.52 (d, 2H, $J = 10$ Hz, $H_{2,6}$-4-Nitrophenyl), 7.79 (dd, 2H, $J = 8.4$ Hz, $J = 2.4$ Hz, $H_{5,6}$-Phthalimide), 7.91 (dd, 2H, $J = 8.4$ Hz, $J = 2.4$ Hz, $H_{4,7}$-Phthalimide), 8.2 (d, 2H, $J = 10$ Hz, $H_{2,6}$-4-Nitrophenyl). IR (KBr, cm^{-1}) ῡ: 3421, 3352, 3113, 2927, 2850, 1774, 1720, 1519, 1415, 1346, 1303, 1107, 952, 713. MS (*m/z*, %): 455 (M^+, Weak), 398 (12), 268 (100), 235 (20), 193 (90), 136 (30), 109 (25), 89 (60), 60 (40).

2-(1,3-Dioxoisoindolin-2-yl)-N-(5-(3-methoxybenzylthio)-1,3,4-thiadiazol-2-yl)acetamide (4d)

^{1}HNMR ($CDCl_3$, 250 MHz) δ (ppm): 3.74 (s, 3H, –OCH_3), 4.38 (s, 2H, –S-CH_2-), 4.86 (s, 2H, –CH_2-CO-), 6.77 (d, 1H, $J = 10$ Hz, H_4-3-Methoxyphenyl), 6.92 (m, 2H, H_2, H_6 -3-Methoxyphenyl), 7.20 (t, 1H, $J = 7.5$ Hz, H_5-3-Methoxyphenyl), 7.77 (dd, 2H, $J = 8.4$ Hz, $J = 2.4$ Hz, $H_{5,6}$-Phthalimide), 7.92 (dd, 2H, $J = 8.4$ Hz, $J = 2.4$ Hz, $H_{4,7}$-Phthalimide). IR (KBr, cm^{-1}) ῡ: 3425, 3329, 3170, 3035, 2927, 2850, 1720, 1624, 1577, 1415, 1303, 1269, 1159, 1049, 952, 713. MS (*m/z*, %): 440 (M^+, 10), 160 (40), 121 (100), 104 (45), 92 (20), 76 (35), 65 (60), 52 (55).

2-(1,3-Dioxoisoindolin-2-yl)-N-(5-(4-methoxybenzylthio)-1,3,4-thiadiazol-2-yl)acetamide (4e)

^{1}HNMR ($CDCl_3$, 250 MHz) δ (ppm): 3.76 (s, 3H, –OCH_3), 4.35 (s, 2H, –S-CH_2-), 4.85 (s, 2H, –CH_2-CO-), 6.82 (d, 2H, $J = 7.5$ Hz, $H_{3,5}$-4-Mehoxyphenyl), 7.28 (d, 2H, $J = 7.5$ Hz, $H_{2,6}$-4-Mehoxyphenyl), 7.77 (dd, $J = 8.4$ Hz, $J = 2.4$ Hz, 2H, $H_{5,6}$-Phthalimide), 7.92 (dd, 2H, $J = 8.4$ Hz, $J = 2.4$ Hz, $H_{5,6}$-Phthalimide). IR (KBr, cm^{-1}) ῡ: 3325, 3248, 3132, 3035, 2927, 2850, 1774, 1705, 1627, 1577, 1419, 1307, 1246, 1195, 1180, 1064, 952. MS (*m/z*, %): 440 (M^+, Weak), 249 (10), 193 (10), 160 (60), 121 (100), 104 (30), 92 (40), 76 (75), 65 (70), 52 (45).

***2-(1,3-Dioxoisoindolin-2-yl)-N-(5-(2-fluorobenzylthio)-1,3,4-thiadiazol-2-yl)acetamide* (4f)**

^{1}HNMR ($CDCl_3$, 250 MHz) δ (ppm): 4.47 (s, 2H, S-CH_2-), 4.83 (s, –CH_2-CO-), 7.04-7.09 (m, 4H, 2-Fluorophenyl), 7.79 (dd, 2H, $J = 8.4$ Hz, $J = 2.4$ Hz, $H_{5,6}$-Phthalimide), 7.91 (dd, 2H, $J = 8.4$ Hz, $J = 2.4$ Hz, $H_{4,7}$-Phthalimide). IR (KBr, cm^{-1}) ῡ: 3429, 3329, 3170, 2924, 2854, 2738, 1774, 1720, 1624, 1573, 1492, 1415, 1303, 1195, 952, 759. MS (*m/z*, %): 428 (M^{+}, 12), 371 (25), 241 (20), 166 (30), 109 (100), 83 (10).

***2-(1,3-Dioxoisoindolin-2-yl)-N-(5-(3-fluorobenzylthio)-1,3,4-thiadiazol-2-yl)acetamide* (4 g)**

^{1}HNMR ($CDCl_3$, 250 MHz) δ (ppm): 4.39 (s, 2H, –S-CH_2-), 4.85 (s, 2H, –CH_2-CO-), 6.92 (t, 1H, $J = 7.5$ Hz, H_5-3-Fluorophenyl), 7.11 (m, 2H, H_4, H_6 -3-Fluorophenyl), 7.24 (m, 1H, H_2-3-Fluorophenyl), 7.77 (dd, 2H, $J = 8.4$ Hz, $J = 2.4$ Hz, $H_{5,6}$-Phthalimide), 7.92 (dd, 2H, $J = 8.4$ Hz, $J = 2.4$ Hz, $H_{5,6}$-Phthalimide), 13.70 (brs, NH). IR (KBr, cm^{-1}) ῡ: 3444, 3170, 3035, 2924, 2854, 1774, 1720, 1566, 1415, 1300, 952, 713. MS (*m/z*, %): 428 (M^{+}, 15), 371 (30), 241 (40), 166 (25), 109 (100), 83 (10).

***2-(1,3-Dioxoisoindolin-2-yl)-N-(5-(4-fluorobenzylthio)-1,3,4-thiadiazol-2-yl)acetamide* (4 h)**

^{1}HNMR ($CDCl_3$, 250 MHz) δ (ppm): 4.36 (s, 2H, –S-CH_2-), 4.86 (s, 2H, –CH_2-CO-), 6.99 (t, 2H, $H_{2,6}$-4-Fluorophenyl), 7.32 (t, 2H, $H_{3,5}$-4-Fluorophenyl), 7.77 (dd, 2H, $J = 8.4$ Hz, $J = 2.4$ Hz, $H_{5,6}$-Phthalimide), 7.92 (dd, 2H, $J = 8.4$ Hz, $J = 2.4$ Hz, $H_{4,7}$-Phthalimide). IR (KBr, cm^{-1}) ῡ: 3433, 3329, 3159, 3039, 2927, 2850, 1774, 1720, 1624, 1573, 1508, 1415, 1303, 1226, 1087, 952, 831, 713. MS (*m/z*, %): 428 (10), 371 (20), 241 (10), 166 (40), 109 (100), 83 (12).

***N-(5-(2-Chlorobenzylthio)-1,3,4-thiadiazol-2-yl)-2-(1,3-dioxoisoindolin-2-yl)acetamide* (4i)**

^{1}HNMR ($CDCl_3$, 250 MHz) δ (ppm): 4.54 (s, 2H, –S-CH_2-), 4.87 (s, 2H, –CH_2-CO-), 7.20 (m, 2H, $H_{3,6}$-2-Chlorophenyl), 7.35 (t, 1H, H_4-2-Chlorophenyl), 7.43 (t, 1H, H_5-2-Chlorophenyl), 7.77 (dd, 2H, $J = 8.4$ Hz, $J = 2.4$ Hz, $H_{5,6}$-Phthalimide), 7.92 (dd, 2H, $J = 8.4$ Hz, $J = 2.4$ Hz, $H_{4,7}$-Phthalimide). IR (KBr, cm^{-1}) ῡ: 3475, 3429, 3170, 3051, 2927, 2858, 2738, 1774, 1720, 1566, 1469, 1415, 1300, 1195, 952, 713. MS (*m/z*, %): 446 (M^{+}+2, 4), 444 (M^{+}, 10), 284 (12), 162 (10), 160 (85), 125 (100), 104 (10), 76 (15).

***N-(5-(3-Chlorobenzylthio)-1,3,4-thiadiazol-2-yl)-2-(1,3-dioxoisoindolin-2-yl)acetamide* (4j)**

^{1}HNMR ($CDCl_3$, 250 MHz) δ (ppm): 4.37 (s, 2H, –S-CH_2-), 4.85 (s, 2H, –CH_2-CO-), 7.24 (m, 3H, 3-Chlorophenyl), 7.41 (s, 1H, H_2-3-Chlorophenyl), 7.77 (dd, 2H, $J = 8.4$ Hz, $J = 2.4$ Hz, $H_{5,6}$-Phthalimide), 7.92 (dd, 2H, $J = 8.4$ Hz, $J = 2.4$ Hz, $H_{4,7}$-Phthalimide). IR (KBr, cm^{-1}) ῡ: 3325, 3170, 3055, 2927, 2850, 1720, 1627, 1573, 1400, 1300, 1203, 1111, 1083, 1049, 956, 713, 648. MS (*m/z*, %): 446 (M^{+}+2, 5), 444 (M^{+}, 15), 162 (25), 160 (50), 125 (100), 104 (30), 76 (35).

***N-(5-(4-Chlorobenzylthio)-1,3,4-thiadiazol-2-yl)-2-(1,3-dioxoisoindolin-2-yl)acetamide* (4 k)**

^{1}HNMR ($CDCl_3$, 250 MHz) δ (ppm): 4.35 (s, 2H, –S-CH_2-), 4.85 (s, 2H, –CH_2-CO-), 7.28 (dd, 4H, 4-Chlorophenyl), 7.77 (dd, 2H, $J = 8.4$ Hz, $J = 2.4$ Hz, $H_{5,6}$-Phthalimide), 7.91 (dd, 2H, $J = 8.4$ Hz, $J = 2.4$ Hz, $H_{5,6}$-Phthalimide). IR (KBr, cm^{-1}) ῡ: 3325, 3155, 3059, 3035, 2927, 2850, 1774, 1720, 1627, 1573, 1492, 1303, 1091. MS (*m/z*, %): 446 (M^{+}+2, 5), 444 (M^{+}, 12), 284 (5), 162 (15), 160 (90), 125 (100), 104 (20), 76 (25).

***N-(5-(Benzylthio)-1,3,4-thiadiazol-2-yl)-2-(1,3-dioxoisoindolin-2-yl)acetamide* (4 l)**

^{1}HNMR ($CDCl_3$, 250 MHz) δ (ppm): 4.39 (s, 2H, –S-CH_2-), 4.86 (s, 2H, –CH_2-CO-), 7.23-7.37 (m, 5H, Phenyl), 7.77 (dd, 2H, $J = 8.4$ Hz, $J = 2.4$ Hz, $H_{5,6}$-Phthalimide), 7.92 (dd, 2H, $J = 8.4$ Hz, $J = 2.4$ Hz, $H_{4,7}$-Phthalimde). IR (KBr, cm^{-1}) ῡ: 3425, 3329, 3170, 3032, 2927, 2850, 1720, 1627, 1573, 1546, 1415, 1396, 1303, 1195, 1111, 952, 709. MS (410, M^{+}), 160 (75), 91 (100), 77 (10).

MTT assay

Synthesized derivatives (compounds **4a-4 l**) were tested for cytotoxic activity at 0.1-100 μM concentration in three human cancer cell lines of PC3 (Prostate carcinoma), HT29 (Colorectal cancer) and SKNMC (Neuroblastoma). Cells were purchased from the Pasteur Institute of Iran. Cells from different cell lines were seeded in 96-well plates at the density of 8000–10,000 viable cells per well and incubated for 24 h to allow cell attachment. The cells were then incubated for another 24 h with various concentrations of compounds **4a-4 l**. Cells were then washed in PBS, and 20 μL of MTT (3–(4,5-dimethylthiazol-2-yl)-2,5-diphenyl tetrazolium bromide solution (5 mg/mL) were added to each well. An additional 4 h of incubation at 37 °C were done, and then the medium was discarded. Dimethyl sulfoxide (60 μL) was added to each well, and the solution was vigorously mixed to dissolve the purple tetrazolium crystals. The absorbance of each well was measured by plate reader (Anthous 2020; Austria) at a test wavelength of 550 nm against a standard reference solution at 690 nm. The amount of produced purple formazan is proportional to the percentage of cell viability [33–35].

15-Lipoxygenase-1 assay

The basis of this method is oxidative coupling of 3-methyl-2-benzothiazolinone hydrazone (MBTH) with 3 (dimethylamino) benzoic acid (DMAB) in a hemoglobin catalyzed reaction. This reaction is initiated in the presence of lipoxygenase reaction product, linoleic acid hydroperoxide and results in a blue color formation which has a peak absorbtion at 590 nm [36]. Quercetin was used as the reference compound. Linoleic acid and two stock solutions (A and B) were prepared first. Solution A contained 50 mM DMAB and l00 mM phosphate buffer (pH = 7.0). Solution B was prepared by mixing 10 mM MBTH (3 mL) and hemoglobin (5 mg/mL, 3 mL) in 50 mM phosphate buffer at pH 5.0 (25 mL). A linoleic acid solution (1 mg/ml) was prepared by diluting 5 mg linoleic acid (solubilised in 0.5 ml ethanol) with KOH 100 mM.

For each compound the samples were solved in ethanol (25 μl) and mixed in a test tube with SLO (4000 units/mL, prepared in 50 mM phosphate buffer pH = 7.0, 25 μL) and phosphate buffer (50 mM, pH = 7, 900 μL). After a 5 min delay at room temperature, 50 μL linoleic acid was added to the mixture to start the hydroperoxidation reaction. After 8 min, solution A (270 μL) and solution B (130 μL) were added to the above mixture. 5 min later, 200 μL of SDS solution (2 %) was added to stop the reaction. The absorbance at 590 nm was compared with control (ethanol without sample).

Docking

The related protein structure was downloaded from brookhaven protein data bank (http://RCSB.org). Namely, 15-Lipoxygenase-1 in complex with dihydroxybenzoic acid (pdb code: 1N8Q) was utilized. ArgusLab software 4.0 was used for drawing the chemical structures and then energy minimization was carried out using AM1 as semiemperical method [37]. The related ligand groups as well as binding site groups were defined. The binding location of dihydroxybenzoic aicd was defined as binding site for searching the best pose and conformation for all ligands. The geometry optimization of the protein structure was done by universal force field (UFF) as molecular mechanic method. Binding mode and related interactions of ligands with lipoxygense enzyme were explored in ArgusLab software.

Results and discussion

Chemistry

According to the Table 1 all intermediate and final compounds were prepared with an average yield. Compound **4a** with *ortho* nitro moiety obtained with a low yield (39 %) and compound **4c** with *para* nitro moiety prepared with an acceptable yield (74 %). For affording compound **2**, phthalic anhydride was reacted with glycine in the presence of triethylamine in toluene under reflux conditions to perform a Gabriel reaction. The white powder of compound **2** was treated with *N*-ethyl-*N*-dimethylaminopropyl carbodiimide (EDC) and hydroxybenzotriazole (HOBt) in acetonitrile and after 30 min, 5-amino-1,3,4-thiadiazole-2-thiol was added to form an amidic bond. The obtained thiol derivative was used for synthesis of the final products **4a–4 l** in alkaline medium that generated by potassium hydroxide in refluxing ethanol.

Synthesized compounds were characterized by spectroscopic methods such as ^{1}H NMR, IR and MS and corresponding melting points were also measured. Compound **4a** with *ortho* nitro moiety rendered the lowest melting point (179 °C) among the final products and compounds **4e** with *para* methoxy group demonstrated the highest melting point (259 °C) in these series. ^{1}H NMR spectra were acquired in deutrated chloroform ($CDCl_3$). In the most cases the acidic property of the proton of the amidic bond (NH group) was caused to not be appeared in the NMR spectra. Phthalimide group as well as 1,3,4-thiadiazole ring function as electron withdrawing groups and these have an important role in

Table 1 Properties of synthesized compounds

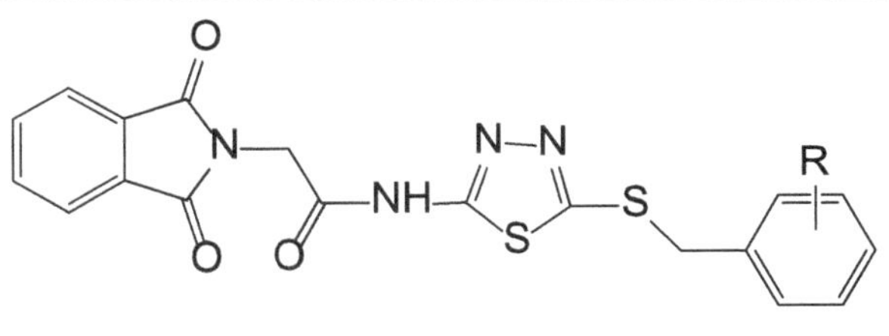

Compound	(R)	Closed formula	MW (g/mol)	m.p (°C)	Yield (%)
2	-	$C_{10}H_7NO_4$	205.4	115	70
3	-	$C_{12}H_8N_4O_3S_2$	320.3	220	48
4a	*o*-NO_2	$C_{19}H_{13}N_5O_5S_2$	455.4	179	39
4b	*m*-NO_2	$C_{19}H_{13}N_5O_5S_2$	455.4	243	46
4c	*p*-NO_2	$C_{19}H_{13}N_5O_5S_2$	455.4	204	74
4d	*m*-OCH_3	$C_{20}H_{16}N_4O_4S_2$	440.5	186	43
4e	*p*-OCH_3	$C_{20}H_{16}N_4O_4S_2$	440.5	259	41
4f	*o*-F	$C_{19}H_{13}FN_4O_3S_2$	428.4	190	48
4 g	*m*-F	$C_{19}H_{13}FN_4O_3S_2$	428.4	173	40
4 h	*p*-F	$C_{19}H_{13}FN_4O_3S_2$	428.4	154	57
4i	*o*-Cl	$C_{19}H_{13}ClN_4O_3S_2$	444.9	205	47
4j	*m*-Cl	$C_{19}H_{13}ClN_4O_3S_2$	444.9	188	57
4 k	*p*-Cl	$C_{19}H_{13}ClN_4O_3S_2$	444.9	155	45
4 l	H	$C_{19}H_{14}N_4O_3S_2$	410.4	187	53

enhancing the acidic property of the hydrogen of NH group.

Cytotoxicity evaluation

Three cancerous cell lines were used to test the anticancer activity of the final compounds **4a-4 l**. PC3 (Prostate carcinoma), HT29 (colorectal cancer) and SKNMC (neuroblastoma) was cultured and intended derivatives were assessed at concentration 0.1-100 μM and the obtained results were compared to doxorubicin as reference drug. None of the tested compounds showed superior cytotoxic effect than doxorubicin at tested concentrations towards the utilized cell lines. Generally tested derivatives exerted a better cytotoxic activity against HT29 cell line compared to other cell lines. PC3 and SKNMC cell lines were the most resistant cell lines to the tested compounds. None of the introduced moieties containing electron withdrawing groups and electron donating groups on the phenyl residue were efficacious to produce a remarkable anticancer activity.

Enzymatic assay

An enzyme inhibitory assay was performed towards 15-lipoxygenase-1 and obtained results were presented as percent of inhibition and provided in Table 2. Unfortunately, none of the tested derivatives demonstrated superior inhibitory effect than quercetin as reference compound and natural product inhibitor of the enzyme. Compound **4d** with *meta* positioning of the methoxy moiety was the most potent inhibitor in this series (38 % inhibition). Moving the position of the methoxy to the *para* decreased the inhibitory effect of the compound significantly as observed in compound **4e**. Nitro containing derivatives (**4a, 4b, 4c**) and compound **4 k** with *para* positioning of the chlorine substituent did not show any inhibitory activity against 15-lipoxygenase-1.

Molecular modeling

All prepared derivatives were docked by ArgusLab software into the active site of 15-lipoxygenase-1. Compound **4d** (m-OCH_3) as representative of synthesized compounds in this series that showed a superior enzyme inhibitory activity in enzymatic assay has been shown in Fig. 1. Four hydrogen bonds were detected with Ser 582, Ser 586 and Ala 587. One of the nitrogen atom of the 1,3,4-thiadiazole ring has participated in hydrogen bonding interaction with Ser 582. Amino acid Ser 586 has also formed two hydrogen bonding interactions with oxygen of the methoxy group. The first one is with oxygen atom of the hydroxyl group in the side chain of this amino acid and the second one is with related NH_2 group of the Ser 586. Finally, Ala 587 is responsible for the fourth hydrogen bond interaction. The NH of the amidic bond between Ala 587 and Ser 586 has the role of hydrogen bond donor to the oxygen of the methoxy group. This potential and probable hydrogen bonds maybe a logical reason for higher enzyme inhibitory potency of compound **4d** compared to others.

Structure activity relationship

Enzyme inhibitory effect of the final prepared compounds was investigated towards 15-lipoxygense-1 and obtained results were listed in Table 2. None of the tested derivatives exerted favorable inhibitory potency towards 15-LOX-1 at 200 μM concentration compared to quercetin as reference compound. Quercetin as

Table 2 Biological data of synthesized compounds. Results of the cytotoxicity assay were reported as $IC_{50} \pm SD$ (μM)

Compound	R	15-Lipoxygenase-1 (% of inhibition)[a]	PC3	HT29	SKNMC
4a	*o*-NO_2	NA[b]	100<	100<	100<
4b	*m*-NO_2	NA	>100	100<	100<
4c	*p*-NO_2	NA	100<	100<	100<
4d	*m*-OCH_3	38	100<	100<	100<
4e	*p*-OCH_3	11	100<	100<	100<
4f	*o*-F	31	100<	10.91 ± 4.1	100<
4 g	*m*-F	26	100<	100<	50.2 ± 5.4
4 h	*p*-F	35	88.83 ± 4.3	100<	100<
4i	*o*-Cl	17	81.92 ± 4.7	100<	100<
4j	*m*-Cl	18.5	89.21 ± 5.7	100<	100<
4 k	*p*-Cl	NA[a]	>100	24.06 ± 3.1	69.7 ± 3.6
4 l	H	19	>100	100<	100<
Doxorubicin	-	-	3.8 ± 0.75	2.1 ± 0.26	1.3 ± 0.4
Quercetin	-	100	-	-	-

a:The percent of inhibition was determined at 200 μM concentration
b:No activity

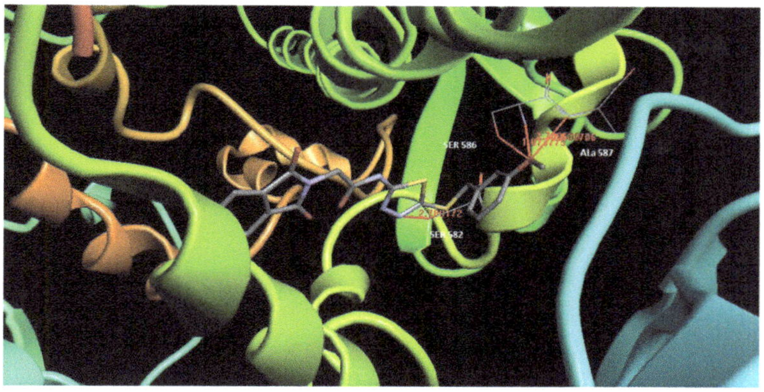

Fig. 1 Structure of docked compound 4d (m-OCH_3) into the active site of 15-lipoxygenase. Four hydrogen bonds were detected with Ser 582 (one), Ser 586 (two) and Ala 587 (one)

naturally occurring compound showed 100 % inhibition at 200 μM concentration. Among the tested derivatives, compound **4d** with *meta* positioning of the methoxy group afforded the highest inhibitory effect (38 %). Movement of the methoxy to the *para* position caused a detrimental effect and decreased the inhibitory activity. Nitro containing compounds (**4a, 4b, 4c**) as well as *para* chlorine containing compound (**4 k**) did not demonstrated any inhibitory activity at tested concentration. Fluorine containing derivatives also exhibited a high inhibitory activity compared to others. This inhibitory activity was more observable while the fluorine substituted at position *ortho* and *para*. It is probable that electron withdrawing effect of this moiety is a critical factor to increase the enzyme inhibitory effect. Replacement of the fluorine substituent with chlorine caused a decrease in activity. Chlorine atom has a greater size and lipophilicity than fluorine and it is likely that these parameters induce a negative effect on interaction of the ligands to the corresponding receptor.

Three cancerous cell lines were used to evaluate the *in vitro* cytotoxicity potency of synthesized derivatives. Unfortunately, tested compounds did not display a remarkable activity against utilized cell lines (Table 2). Only compounds **4f** (*ortho* fluorine) and **4 k** (*para* chlorine) rendered an acceptable cytotoxic potency against HT29 cell line. None of the nitro and methoxy substituted derivatives exerted an inhibitory potency (IC_{50}) up to 100 μM concentration. Substitution of the fluorine at *meta* position of the phenyl residue caused an enhancement in cytotoxic activity towards SKNMC cell line. *Para* positioning of the fluorine was also caused a brief increase in anticancer activity in PC3 cell line. A descending trend in IC_{50} was seen from compound **4i** (*o*-Cl) to **4 k** (*p*-Cl) against PC3 cell line. But, a reverse trend was demonstrated for chlorinated derivatives against HT29 and SKNMC cell lines. Steric factor and lipophilicity effects produced by chlorine atom maybe a probable reason for this observation.

Based on the above mentioned information, there is not any direct correlation between the cytotoxic activity and inhibition of lipoxygenase. According to the previously reported literature [34, 35], it could be hypothesized that inhibition of tyrosine kinases is the probable of cytotoxicity of these compounds.

Conclusions

A new series of compounds with combination of 1,3,4-thiadiazole and phthalimide substructures were synthesized and their cytotoxicity was evaluated *in vitro* using MTT protocol. Furthermore, synthesized derivatives were tested in an enzymatic assay for exploration of the inhibitory activity towards 15-lipoxygenase-1. According to the obtained results in MTT assay as well as enzymatic experiment, the investigated compounds did not show a favorable anticancer activity. Amongst them, only compounds **4f** (*ortho* fluorine) and **4 k** (*para* chlorine) exhibited an acceptable cytotoxic potency towards HT29 cell line. Hence, further structural modifications are needed to achieve derivatives with superior activity.

Competing interests

The authors declared that they have no competing interest.

Authors' contributions

AA: Synthesis Molecular Modelling. AM-F: Cytotoxicity assay. ZH: Contributor in all parts. HN: Enzymatic assay. AM: Enzymatic assay. FA: Cytotoxicity assay.

Acknowledgements

The authors are acknowledged from the research council of Kermanshah University of Medical Sciences due to financial support of the current research. This work was performed in partial fulfillment of the requirement for PharmD of Mrs Zeinab Hossseinzadeh.

Author details

[1]Pharmaceutical Sciences Research Center, School of Pharmacy, Kermanshah University of Medical Sciences, Kermanshah, Iran. [2]Department of Medicinal Chemistry, Faculty of Pharmacy, Kermanshah University of Medical Sciences, Kermanshah, Iran. [3]Department of Pharmacology, Toxicology and Medical Services, Faculty of Pharmacy, Kermanshah University of Medical Sciences, Kermanshah, Iran. [4]Students Research Committee, Kermanshah University of Medical Sciences, Kermanshah, Iran. [5]Neurobiomedical Research Center, Yazd Shahid Sadoughi University of Medical Sciences, Yazd, Iran.

References

1. Rioux N, Castonguay A. Inhibitors of lipoxygenase: a new class of cancer chemopreventive agents. Carcinogenesis. 1998;8:1393–400.
2. Tong WG, Ding XZ, Adrian TE. The mechanisms of lipoxygenase inhibitor-induced apoptosis in human breast cancer cells. Biochem Biophys Res Commun. 2002;296:942–8.
3. Steele VE, Holmes CV, Hawk ET, Kopelovich L, Lubet RA, Crowell JA. Lipoxygenase inhibitors as potential cancer chemopreventives. Cancer Epidemiol Biomarkers Prev. 1999;8:467–83.
4. Shureiqi I, Chen D, Jack Lee J, Yang P, Newman RA, Brenner DE, et al. 15-LOX-1: a novel molecular target of nonsteroidal anti-inflammatory drug-Induced apoptosis in colorectal cancer cells. J Natl Cancer Inst. 2000;14:1136–42.
5. Shureiqi I, Lippman SM. Lipoxygenase modulation to reverse carcinogenesis. Cancer Res. 2001;61:6307–12.
6. Kelavkar UP, Nixon JB, Cohen C, Dillehay D, Eling TE, Badr KF. Overexpression of 15-lipoxygenase-1 in PC-3 human prostate cancer cells increases tumorigenesis. Carcinogenesis. 2001;11:1765–73.
7. Shureiqi I, Xu X, Chen D, Lotan R, Morris JS, Fischer SM. Nonsteroidal anti-Inflammatory drugs induce apoptosis in esophageal cancer cells by restoring 15-Lipoxygenase-1 expression. Cancer Res. 2001;61:4879–84.
8. Mahdavi M, Shirazi MS, Taherkhani R, Saeedi M, Alipour E, Moghadam FH, et al. Synthesis, biological evaluation and docking study of 3-aroyl-1-(4-sulfamoylphenyl)thiourea derivatives as 15-lipoxygenase inhibitors. Eur J Med Chem. 2014;82:308–13.
9. Asadipour A, Edraki N, Nakhjiri M, Yahya-Meymandi A, Alipour E, Saniee P, et al. Anti-Helicobacter pylori activity and structure-activity relationship study of 2-Alkylthio-5-(nitroaryl)-1,3,4-thiadiazole derivatives. Iran J Pharm Res. 2013;3:281–7.
10. Mohammadhosseini N, Saniee P, Ghamaripour A, Aryapour H, Afshar F, Edraki N, et al. Synthesis and biological evaluation of novel benzyl piperazine derivatives of 5-(5-nitroaryl)-1,3,4-thiadiazoles as Anti-Helicobacter pylori agents. Daru: J Pharm Sci. 2013;1:66.
11. Moshafi MH, Sorkhi M, Emami S, Nakhjiri M, Yahya-Meymandi A, Negahbani AS, et al. 5-Nitroimidazole-based 1,3,4-thiadiazoles: heterocyclic analogs of metronidazole as anti-Helicobacter pylori agents. Arch Pharm Chem Life Sci. 2011;344(3):178–83.
12. Rajak H, Deshmukh R, Aggarwal N, Kashaw S, Kharya MD, Mishra P. Synthesis of novel 2,5-disubstituted 1,3,4-thiadiazoles for their potential anticonvulsant activity: pharmacophoric model studies. Arch Pharm Chem Life Sci. 2009;342:453–61.
13. Abdel-Aziz M, Aly OM, Khan SS, Mukherjee K, Bane S. Synthesis, Cytotoxic properties and tubulin polymerization inhibitory activity of novel 2-pyrazoline derivatives. Arch Pharm Chem Life Sci. 2012;345:535–48.
14. Mishra G, Singh AK, Jyoti K. Review article on 1,3,4-Thiadiazole derivatives and its pharmacological activities. Int J Chem Tech Res. 2011;3:1380–93.
15. Singh AK, Mishra G, Jyoti K. Review on Biological Activities of 1,3,4-Thiadiazole derivatives. J App Pharm Sci. 2011;5:44–9.
16. Kalidhar U, Kaur A. 1,3,4-Thiadiazole derivatives and their biological activities: A Review. Res J Pharm Biol Chem. 2011;4:1091–106.
17. Siddiqui N, Ahuja P, Ahsan W, Pandeya SN, Alam MS. Thiadiazoles: progress report on biological activities. J Chem Pharm Res. 2009;1:19–30.
18. Behrouzi-Fardmoghadam M, Poorrajab F, Kaboudanian Ardestani S, Emami S, Shafiee A, Foroumadi A. Synthesis and in vitro anti-leishmanial activity of 1-[5-(5-nitrofuran-2-yl)-1,3,4-thiadiazol-2-yl]- and 1-[5-(5-nitrothiophen-2-yl)-1,3,4-thiadiazol-2-yl]-4-aroylpiperazines. Bioorg Med Chem. 2008;16:4509–15.
19. Poorrajab F, Kaboudanian Ardestani S, Emami S, Behrouzi-Fardmoghadam M, Shafiee A, Foroumadi A. Nitroimidazolyl-1,3,4-thiadiazole-based anti-leishmanial agents: Synthesis and in vitro biological evaluation. Eur J Med Chem. 2009;4:1758–62.
20. Mirzaei J, Siavoshi F, Emami S, Safari F, Khoshayand MR, Shafiee A, et al. Synthesis and in vitro anti-Helicobacter pylori activity of *N*-[5-(5-nitro-2-heteroaryl)-1,3,4-thiadiazol-2-yl]thiomorpholines and related compounds. Eur J Med Chem. 2008;8:1575–80.
21. Kok SHL, Gambari R, Chui CH, Yuen MCW, Lin E, Wong RSM, et al. Synthesis and anti-cancer activity of benzothiazole containing phthalimide on human carcinoma cell lines. Bioorg Med Chem. 2008;16:3626–31.
22. Yang YJ, Yang YN, Jiang JS, Feng ZM, Liu HY, Pan XD, et al. Synthesis and cytotoxic activity of heterocycle-substituted phthalimide derivatives. Chin Chem Lett. 2010;21:902–4.
23. Machado AL, Lima LM, Araújo-Jr JX, Fraga CAM, Koatzc VLG, Barreiroa EJ. Design, synthesis and antiinflammatory activity of novel phthalimide derivatives, structurally related to thalidomide. Bioorg Med Chem Lett. 2005;15:1169–72.
24. Malgorzata W, Katarzyna K. Synthesis and anticonvulsant evaluation of some *N*-substituted phthalimides. Acta Pol Pharm. 2009;3:249–57.
25. Lee N-J, Jeong I-C, Cho M-Y, Jeon C-W, Yun B-C, Kim Y-O, et al. Synthesis and *in vitro* antitumor activity of phthalimide polymers containing podophyllotoxin. Eur Polym J. 2006;42:3352–9.
26. Lima LM, Brito FCF, Souza SD, Miranda ALP, Rodrigues CR, Fragaa CAM, et al. Novel phthalimide derivatives, designed as leukotriene D_4 receptor antagonists. Bioorg Med Chem Lett. 2002;12:1533–5.
27. Santos JL, Yamasaki PR, Chin CM, Takashi CH, Pavan FR, Leite CQF. Synthesis and in vitro anti mycobacterium tuberculosis activity of a series of phthalimide derivatives. Bioorg Med Chem. 2009;17:3795–9.
28. Mohammadi-Farani A, Ahmadi A, Nadri H, Aliabadi A. Synthesis, docking and acetylcholinesterase inhibitory assessment of 2-(2-(4-Benzylpiperazin-1-yl)ethyl)isoindoline-1,3-dione with potential anti-alzheimer effects. Daru J Pharm Sci. 2013;21:47–55.
29. Foroumadi A, Mohammadi-Farani A, Garmsiri Mahvar M, Aliabadi A. Synthesis and evaluation of anti-acetylcholinesterase activity of 2-(2-(4-(2-Oxo-2-phenylethyl)piperazin-1-yl)ethyl)isoindoline-1,3-dione derivatives with potential anti-Alzheimer effects. Iran J Basic Med Sci. 2013;10(16):1049–54.
30. Aliabadi A, Gholamine B, Karimi T. Synthesis and antiseizure evaluation of isoindoline-1,3-dione derivatives in mice. Med Chem Res. 2014;23:2736–43.
31. Aliabadi A, Foroumadi A, Safavi M, Kaboudian Ardestani S. Synthesis, molecular docking and cytotoxicity evaluation of 2-(4-substituted-benzyl)isoindoline-1,3-dione derivatives as anticancer agents. J Rep Pharm Sci. 2012;1:19–22.
32. Ragavendran JV, Sriram D, Patel SK, Reddy IV, Bharathwajan N, Stables J. Design and synthesis of anticonvulsants from a combined phthalimide-GABA-anilide and hydrazone pharmacophore. Eur J Med Chem. 2007;42:146–51.
33. Mohammadi-Farani A, Foroumadi A, Rezvani Kashani M, Aliabadi A. *N*-Phenyl-2-*p*-tolylthiazole-4-carboxamide derivatives: Synthesis and cytotoxicity evaluation as anticancer agents. Iran J Basic Med Sci. 2014;17:502–8.
34. Aliabadi A, Eghbalian E, Kiani A. Synthesis and cytotoxicity evaluation of a series of 1,3,4-thiadiazole based compounds as anticancer agents. Iran J Basic Med Sci. 2013;11:1133–8.
35. Aliabadi A, Hasanvand Z, Kiani A, Mirabdali SS. Synthesis and *in vitro* cytotoxicity assessment of *N*-(5-(Benzylthio)-1,3,4-thiadiazol-2-yl)-2-(4-(trifluoromethyl)phenyl)acetamide with potential anticancer activity. Iran J Pharm Res. 2013;4:687–93.
36. Anthon GE, Barrett DM. Colorimetric method for the determination of lipoxygenase activity. J Agric Food Chem. 2001;49:32–7.
37. ArgusLab 4.0 Mark A. Thompson Planaria Software LLC, Seattle, WA http://www.arguslab.com.

Chitosan and chitosan chlorhydrate based various approaches for enhancement of dissolution rate of carvedilol

Amol S Shete[1*], Adhikrao V Yadav[2] and Srinivasa M Murthy[3]

Abstract

Background and the purpose of the study: Carvedilol nonselective β-adrenoreceptor blocker, chemically (±)-1-(Carbazol-4-yloxy)-3-[[2-(o-methoxypHenoxy) ethyl] amino]-2-propanol, slightly soluble in ethyl ether; and practically insoluble in water, gastric fluid (simulated, TS, pH 1.1), and intestinal fluid (simulated, TS without pancreatin, pH 7.5) Compounds with aqueous solubility less than 1% W/V often represents dissolution rate limited absorption. There is need to enhance the dissolution rate of carvedilol. The objective of our present investigation was to compare chitosan and chitosan chlorhydrate based various approaches for enhancement of dissolution rate of carvedilol.

Methods: The different formulations were prepared by different methods like solvent change approach to prepare hydrosols, solvent evaporation technique to form solid dispersions and cogrind mixtures. The prepared formulations were characterized in terms of saturation solubility, drug content, infrared spectroscopy (FTIR), differential scanning calorimetry (DSC), powder X-ray diffraction (PXRD), electron microscopy, *in vitro* dissolution studies and stability studies.

Results: The practical yield in case of hydrosols was ranged from 59.76 to 92.32%. The drug content was found to uniform among the different batches of hydrosols, cogrind mixture and solid dispersions ranged from 98.24 to 99.89%. There was significant improvement in dissolution rate of carvedilol with chitosan chlorhdyrate as compare to chitosan and explanation to this behavior was found in the differences in the wetting, solubilities and swelling capacity of the chitosan and chitosan salts, chitosan chlorhydrate rapidly wet and dissolve upon its incorporation into the dissolution medium, whereas the chitosan base, less water soluble, would take more time to dissolve.

Conclusion: This technique is scalable and valuable in manufacturing process in future for enhancement of dissolution of poorly water soluble drugs.

Keywords: Solubility, Dissolution, Carvedilol, Hydrosols, Chitosan and chitosan chlorhydrate

Background

The rate of absorption and bioavailability of poorly water soluble drugs is often controlled by the rate of dissolution of the drug in gastrointestinal tract. Many technological methods of enhancing the dissolution characteristics of slightly water soluble drugs have been reported in literature. These include reducing particle size to increase the surface area [1], solublization in surfactant system [2], formation of water soluble complexes [3], use of prodrug, drug derivatization and manipulation of solid state of drug substance to improve drug dissolution i.e. by decreasing drug crystallinity [4] or crystal engineering [5-7]. Chitosan is a linear polycationic copolymer of b [1-4] linked 2-acetamido-2-deoxy-b-D-glucopyranose and 2- amino-2-deoxy-b-D-glucopyranose obtained from deacetylation of chitin, a structural polysaccharide which is very abundantly distributed in nature [8]. In recent year's chitosan and chitosan derivatives has gained increasing interest in the pharmaceutical field due to its favorable biological properties such as biocompatibility, biodegradability, and

* Correspondence: amol.shete@rediffmail.com
[1]Department of Pharmaceutics, Shree Santkrupa College of Pharmacy, Ghogaon, Tal. Karad Dist, Satara, MS, India
Full list of author information is available at the end of the article

Table 1 Composition of carvedilol- chitosan and chitosan chlorhydrtate hydrosol formulations

Batch code	Carvedilol (mg)	Chitosan (%)	Chitosan chlorhydrate (%)	Glacial acetic acid (ml)	Sodium citrate (2% w/v) (ml)
C1	500	0.05	-	20	100
C2	500	0.2	-	20	100
C3	500	0.4	-	20	100
C4	500	0.6	-	20	100
C5	500	1	-	20	100
C6	500	-	0.05	20	100
C7	500	-	0.2	20	100
C8	500	-	0.4	20	100
C9	500	-	0.6	20	100
C10	500	-	0.8	20	100
C11	500	-	1	20	100
C12	500	-	-	20	100

lack of toxicity, together with its wide availability, low cost and high versatility of use [9,10] Previously chitosan was largely used as an excipient for oral drug solid dosage forms, due to its binder, anti-adherent and disintegrant properties [11-13].

Chitosan, being cationic polysaccharide in neutral or basic pH conditions, contains free amino group and hence insoluble in water. In acidic pH, amino group can undergo protonation thus making it soluble in water. It breaks down slowly to harmless products amino sugars, which are completely absorbed by the human body [14]. Chitin, a structural Moreover, its ability in improving the dissolution properties and bioavailability of poorly-soluble drugs has been proved [14-17]. Carvedilol nonselective β-adrenoreceptor blocker, chemically (±)-1-(Carbazol-4-yloxy)-3-[[2-(o-methoxyphenoxy) ethyl] amino]-2-propanol, slightly soluble in ethyl ether; and practically insoluble in water, gastric fluid (simulated, TS, pH 1.1), and intestinal fluid (simulated, TS without pancreatin, pH 7.5)

Compounds with aqueous solubility less than 1% w/v often represents dissolution rate limited absorption [18,19]. The solid systems for several drugs using chitosan have been reported with solid dispersions, co-ground mixtures and solid complexes, physical mixture and co- ground products and spray dried products at different ratios. There are reports on the improvement of dissolution rate and bioavailability of poorly water soluble drugs by precipitation of chitosan using solvent change method [20-22]. Hence objectives of present investigation were (i) To assess the feasibility of chitosan and chitosan chlorhydrate in enhancing dissolution rate of carvedilol by preparing hydrosols using solvent change method. (ii) To compare efficacy low molecular weight chitosan (chitosan chlorhydrate) and chitosan in enhancement of dissolution of carvedilol. (iii) To compare effect of different methods like solvent change approach, co- ground mixture and solid dispersions on dissolution rate of carvedilol.

Methods

Materials

Carvedilol was obtained as gift sample from Lupin Pharma. Ltd. Pune. India. Chitosan (85% deactylated), chitosan chlorhydrate obtained from mehtani chitosan India. Hydrochloric acid (35-38%), glacial acetic acid (99.5%), sodium citrate (99.5%) was purchased from Loba chemicals. Mumbai, India. All other chemicals were analytical grade.

Methods

Preparation of hydrosols

The composition of different batchhes is given in Table 1. Chitosan solution was prepared by soaking chitosan and

Table 2 Composition of carvedilol - chitosan and chitosan chlorhydrtate cogrind mixture

Batch code	Carvedilol (mg)	Chitosan (mg)	Chitosan chlorhydrate (mg)
C13	500	5	-
C14	500	20	-
C15	500	40	-
C16	500	60	-
C17	500	100	-
C18	500	-	5
C19	500	-	20
C20	500	-	40
C21	500	-	60
C22	500	-	80
C23	500	-	100
C24	500	-	-

chitosan chlorhydrate in 1% glacial acetic acid for 3 hrs. a weighed amount of drug was dispersed in chitosan solution by stirring at 4000 rpm for 25 min. then dispersion was added to sodium citrate solution to precipitate chitosan on drug to form hydrosols. The precipitate obtained was filtered through Whatmann No. 1 filter paper using vacuum filtration unit and dried at 45°C for 24 h. the dried product then passed through sieve No. 60 to obtain uniform size distribution. A control hydrosol formulation without chitosan was also prepared (C12) (Table 1). The practical yield of prepared hydrosols was calculated.

Preparation of co-grind mixture

The composition of different batches is given in Table 2. Listed amount of carvedilol was accurately weighed and co grinded with chitosan and chitosan chlorhydrate in mortar for 30 min. Product then passed through sieve No. 60 to obtain uniform size distribution. A control formulation without chitosan was also prepared (C24) (Table 2).

Preparation of solid dispersions

The composition of different batches is given in Table 3. Chitosan solution was prepared by soaking chitosan and chitosan chlorhydrate in 1% glacial acetic acid for 3 hrs. A weighed amount of drug was dispersed in chitosan solution by stirring at 4000 rpm for 25 min, and then dispersion was dried at 45°C for 24 hrs. The dried product then passed through sieve No. 60 to obtain uniform size distribution. A control dispersion formulation without chitosan was also prepared (C36) (Table 3).

Table 3 Composition of carvedilol- chitosan and chitosan chlorhydrtate solid dispersions

Batch code	Carvedilol (mg)	Chitosan (%)	Chitosan chlorhydrate (%)	Glacial acetic acid (ml)
C25	500	0.05	-	20
C26	500	0.2	-	20
C27	500	0.4	-	20
C28	500	0.6	-	20
C29	500	1	-	20
C30	500	-	0.05	20
C31	500	-	0.2	20
C32	500	-	0.4	20
C33	500	-	0.6	20
C34	500	-	0.8	20
C35	500	-	1	20
C36	500	-	-	20

Table 4 Practical yield, drug content and solubility data in water and SGF for the pure drug and prepared hydrosols, cogrind mixture and solid dispersions

Formulation code	% Yield	Drug content	Water (mg/ml)	SGF (mg/ml)
Carvedilol	-	-	0.13 ± 0.002	0.43 ± 0.001
C1	85.62	99.23 ±0.58	0.21 ± 0.001	0.41 ± 0.004
C2	80.32	99.12 ± 0.76	0.37 ± 0.002	0.39 ± 0.004
C3	75.86	99.45 ± 0.68	0.39 ± 0.004	1.2 ± 0.002
C4	64.83	99.78 ± 0.98	0.36 ± 0.004	1.03 ± 0.002
C5	59.76	98.24 ± 1.23	0.35 ± 0.001	1.04 ± 0.004
C6	86.86	98.45 ± 0.98	0.31 ± 0.005	1.00 ± 0.004
C7	82.23	99.14 ± 1.45	0.72 ± 0.001	0.86 ± 0.001
C8	73.32	99.56 ± 1.02	0.74 ± 0.005	0.41 ± 0.001
C9	69.46	99.89 ± 1.13	0.60 ± 0.005	0.42 ± 0.006
C10	63.23	99.25 ± 0.87	0.54 ± 0.005	0.41 ± 0.001
C11	59.21	98.78 ± 0.96	0.68 ± 0.004	0.42 ± 0.002
C12	93.32	99.63 ± 1.96	0.14 ± 0.001	0.41 ± 0.004
C13	100	98.32 ± 1.06	0.43 ± 0.002	0.42 ± 0.007
C14	100	99.32 ± 1.23	0.78 ± 0.001	0.45 ± 0.004
C15	100	98.65 ± 0.98	2.36 ± 0.004	0.46 ± 0.003
C16	100	99.12 ± 1.24	1.2 ± 0.001	0.55 ± 0.004
C17	100	98.56 ± 0.91	1.40 ± 0.001	0.46 ± 0.002
C18	100	99.12 ± 0.85	0.45 ± 0.002	0.41 ± 0.003
C19	100	98.95 ± 0.89	1.23 ± 0.004	0.42 ± 0.002
C20	100	99.12 ± 0.92	2.01 ± 0.004	0.50 ± 0.004
C21	100	99.17 ± 1.44	3.21 ± 0.001	0.33 ± 0.008
C22	100	98.32 ± 1.56	2.14 ± 0.006	0.40 ± 0.002
C23	100	99.32 ± 0.97	3.45 ± 0.003	0.33 ± 0.001
C24	100	99.10 ± 1.12	0.23 ± 0.002	0.43 ± 0.002
C25	98.35	98.56 ± 0.97	0.42 ± 0.003	0.46 ± 0.004
C26	99.56	99.45 ± 1.35	0.78 ± 0.004	0.47 ± 0.001
C27	99.00	99.78 ± 1.65	1.38 ± 0.004	0.36 ± 0.002
C28	99.23	99.87 ± 0.94	1.53 ± 0.001	0.45 ± 0.002
C29	99.65	98.92 ± 0.96	0.97 ± 0.004	0.47 ± 0.004
C30	98.32	98.23 ± 0.98	0.26 ± 0.002	0.48 ± 0.005
C31	99.32	99.15 ± 0.0.91	0.54 ± 0.003	0.45 ± 0.007
C32	99.23	99.25 ± 1.25	0.65 ± 0.001	0.40 ± 0.003
C33	99.78	99.42 ± 1.32	0.68 ± 0.002	0.47 ± 0.002
C34	99.65	99.89 ± 1.20	0.89 ± 0.004	0.48 ± 0.004
C35	99.21	99.47 ± 1.02	1.62 ± 0.002	0.42 ± 0.003
C36	98.96	99.56 ± 1.05	0.13 ± 0.006	0.42 ± 0.004

Solubility, drug content determination

An excess amount of carvedilol or prepared formulations was placed in the vials containing 10 ml of different solvents (water and simulated gastric fluid (SGF) without enzymes pH 1.2) the vials were agitated in a

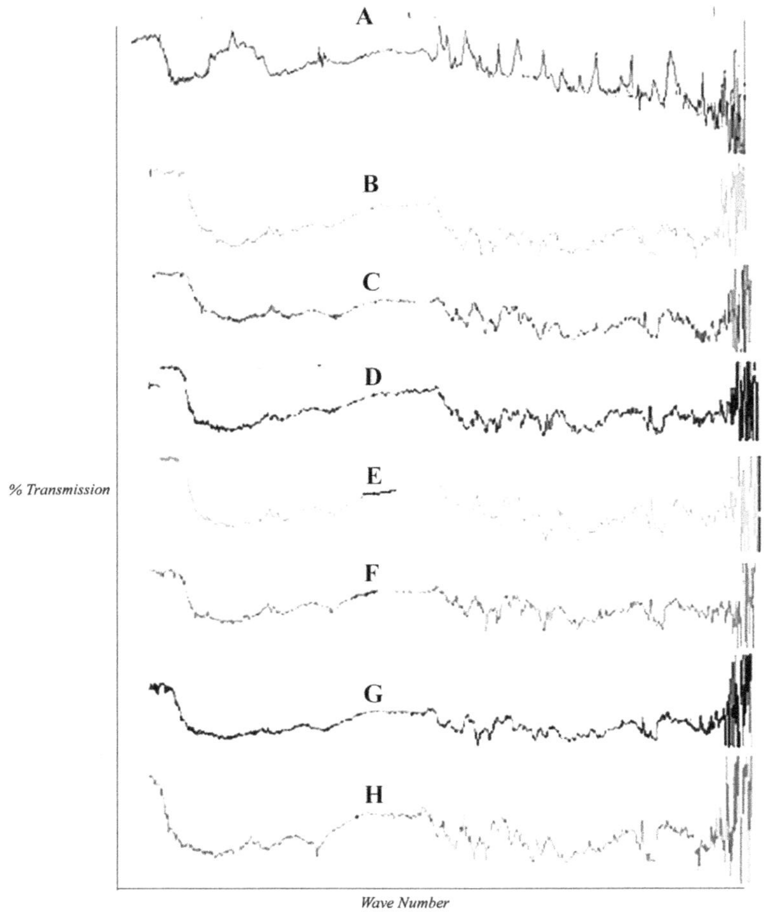

Figure 1 Comparative FTIR pattern of carvedilol and Chitosan based hydrosols, solid dispersions and co grinding mixture. **A**. chitosan, **B**. Carvedilol, **C**.0.2% chitosan hydrosols, **D**. 0.4% Ch-chlorhydrate hydrosols, **E**. SD 0.4% chitosan, **F**. SD 0.8% Ch-chlorhydrate, **G**. 0.4% chitosan cogrind mixture, **H**. 0.4% ch-chlorhydrate cogrind mixture.

incubator shaker (100 rpm/min) for 24 hrs. The solution was filtered through a membrane filter (0.45 μm) the amount of drug solublized was analyzed spectrophotometrically (JASCO, V-530, Japan) at 241.5 nm. This study was carried out to determine the saturation solubility of carvedilol in water and SGF.

For determination of drug content, prepared hydrosols, solid dispersions and co-ground mixture (10 mg) were triturated with SGF and finally volume was made up to 100 ml with the same. The solution was filtered through a membrane filter (0.45 μm) the amount of drug solublized was analyzed spectrophotometrically (JASCO, V-530, Japan) at 241.5 nm after sufficient dilutions with SGF.

Infrared (IR) spectroscopy

IR spectroscopy was conducted using a Shimadzu FTIR 8300S Spectrophotometer (Shimadzu, Tokyo, Japan) and the spectrum was recorded in the wavelength region of 4000–400 cm^{-1}. The procedure consisted of dispersing a sample (drug, mixture of drug and polymer and prepared hydrosols) in KBr and compressing into discs by applying a pressure of 5 t for 5 min in a hydraulic press. The pellet was placed in the light path and the spectrum was recorded. All spectra were collected as an average of three scans at a resolution of 2 cm^{-1}.

Differential scanning colorimetry (DSC)

DSC was performed using DSC-60A (Shimadzu, Tokyo, Japan) calorimeter to study the thermal behavior of drug alone and prepared co-hydrosols. The samples were heated in hermetically sealed aluminum pans under nitrogen flow (30 ml/min) at a scanning rate of 10°C/min from 50°C to 300°C. Empty aluminum pan was used as a reference. The physical mixture of drug with excipients for compatibility studies was prepared by triturating the drug with excipients in a dried mortar for 5 min.

Powder X- Ray diffraction (PXRD)

The X-ray diffraction patterns of pure drug and the optimized hydrosols formulation were recorded using PHilips analytical X-ray diffractometer (Model: PW 3710) (PHilips, Almelo, The Netherlands) with a copper target over the interval of 5–70° $2\theta^{-1}$. The conditions were: voltage 40 kV; current 30 mA; scanning speed 2°/min; temperature of acquisition: room temperature; detector: scintillation counter detector; sample holder: non-rotating holder.

Electron microscopy (EM)

The surface characteristics of the pure drug and prepared hydrosols were studied by binocular EM (NIKON, Tokyo, Japan) at 100 × .

In vitro dissolution study

The dissolution rate of Carvedilol alone and prepared formulations were measured in triplicate in a dissolution apparatus (Lab India, Model Disso 2000 Tablet dissolution test apparatus, Mumbai, India) using apparatus USP Type II. Dissolution studies were carried out using 900 mL SGF (Simulated gastric fluid pH 1.2) at 37° ± 0.5°C at 50 rpm. 30 mg carvedilol or its equivalent amount formulations were placed in 900 mL of SGF. 5 mL samples were withdrawn after 15, 30, 45 min. Replaced each time with 5 mL fresh SGF to maintain a proper sink condition. The solutions were immediately filtered through 0.45 μm membrane filter, diluted and the concentration of carvedilol was determined spectro-photometrically at 241.5 nm.

Stability study

After determining the drug content, the optimized formulations were charged for accelerated stability studies as per ICH guidelines. The samples (each 100 mg, n = 3) were kept for stability studies at 40 ± 2°C and 75 ± 5% RH for a period of 6 months in environmental test chamber (HMG INDIA, Mumbai). The samples were kept in glass vials sealed with rubber plugs. 10 mg of stored hydrosols were taken out at 15, 30, 60, 90 and 180 days, they were analyzed for drug content and physical change.

Results and discussion

The solubility, dissolution behavior and permeability of a drug are the key determinants of its oral bioavailability. The solubility data of Carvedilol reveals that it is poorly soluble in water. Therefore, the improvement of carvedilol dissolution from its oral solid dosage forms is of great concern. The practical yield in case of hydrosols was ranged from 59.76 to 92.32% (Table 4).

The practical yield was found to be decreased with the increase in polymer concentration due to the formation of a thick viscous chitosan solution from which separation of the drug hydrosols was difficult. The drug content was found to be good and uniform among the different batches of hydrosols, cogrind mixture and solid dispersions ranged from 98.24 to 99.89% (Table 4). The solubility studies of the chitosan cogrind mixture, C-15 showed highest solubility of drug in both water (2.36 mg/ml) in comparison with pure drug (0.13 mg/ml). If we compare solubility data of chitosan and chitosan chlorhydrtae batch C21 showed better aqueous solubility (3.21 mg/ml). No difference was observed in case of solubility in simulated gastric fluid. The difference in aqueous solubility of chitosan and chitosan chlorhydrate may be due to better enhanced wetting property due to salting out, low molecular weight of chitosan chlorhydrate. In addition, as the concentration of chitosan or chitosan

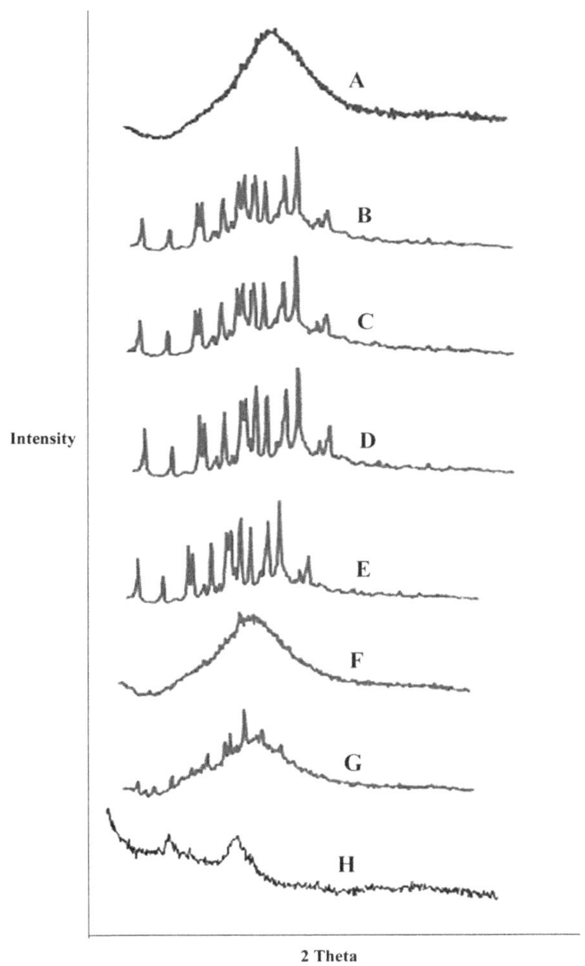

Figure 2 Comparative P-XRD pattern of carvedilol and Chitosan based hydrosols, solid dispersions and co grinding mixture. A. Carvedilol, **B**. 0.2% chitosan hydrosols, **C**. 0.4% Ch-chlorhydrate hydrosols, **D**. SD 0.4% chitosan, **E**. SD 0.8% Ch-chlorhydrate, **F**. 0.4% chitosan cogrind mixture, **G**. 0.4% ch-chlorhydrate cogrind mixture, H. chitosan.

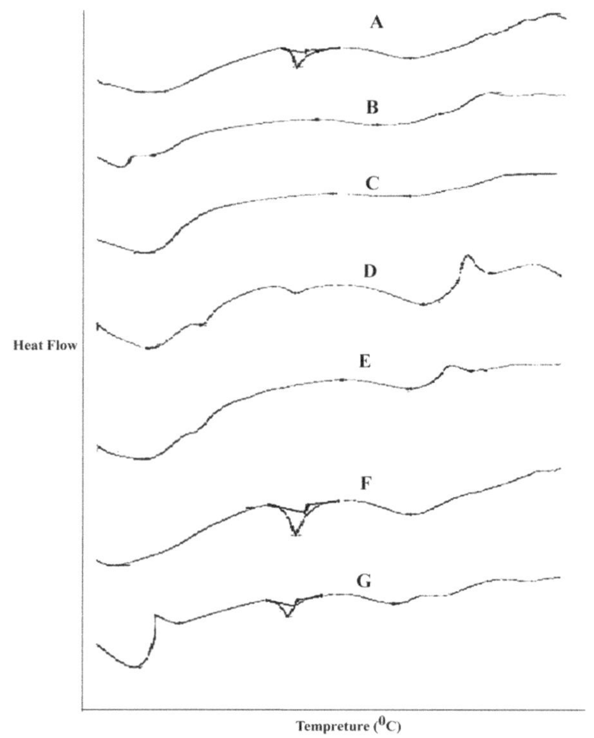

Figure 3 Comparative DSC of carvedilol and formulations A. Carvedilol, **B.** 0.2% Chitosan hydrosols, **C.** 0.4% Chitosan chlorhydrate hydrosols, **D.** 0.2% Chitosan solid dispersions, **E.** 0.8% Chitosan chlorhydrate solid dispersions, **F.** 0.4% Chitosan Co-grinding, **G.** 0.4% Chitosan chlorhydrate Co-grinding.

chlorhydrtae increased in the formulation, the solubility gradually increased up to a certain concentration followed by decrease in the solubility. If we compare the methods of formulation co-grind mixture showed higher solubility data than solid dispersions and hydrosols, this might due to micronization or sustained supersaturation of material in media for cogrind mixture.

The possible interaction between drug and chitosan as hydrosol formers were studied by IR spectroscopy (Figure 1). The pure carvedilol showed peaks at 3300–3500 cm^{-1}, onset around 1600 cm^{-1}, other around 1500 cm¯1, 1000–1300 cm^{-1} due to presence of N-H stretch, O-H stretch, consistent with aromatic compounds and C-OH stretch respectively. It was observed that all important peaks due to functional group of drug are present in the hydrosols along with some new intense peaks indicating the presence of hydrogen bonding. Also there are peaks observed in the range of 400–800 cm^{-1} in hydrosols prepared from chitosan chlorhydrate indicative of halogen hydrogen interaction.

The PXRD patterns of the pure drug and the hydrosols are shown in Figure 2. The XRD scan of carvedilol showed intense peak of cystallanity at 22.7° (2θ) with peak intensity of 1832 indicating its crystalline nature. The relative degree of crystllanity values of carvedilol hydrosols at specific angle are 1.22, 1.08, 1.18, 0.833, 1.04, 1.00 for prepared chitosan and chitosan chlorhydrate hydrosols as shown in Figure 2 respectively. It indicates crystalline nature of carvedilol in prepared hydrosols.

The results of DSC studies are given in Figure 3 and Table 5. Pure carvedilol showed a sharp endotherm at 155.94°C corresponding to its melting point. There was no appreciable change in the melting endotherms of the cogrind mixture as compare pure drug. However there is disappearance of melting endothermic peaks of carvedilol when formulated into hydrosols and solid dispersions meaning is that drug has been converted into amorphous form and chitosan and chitosan chlorhydtare in crystalline form. The endothermic peaks for chitosan and chitosan chlorhydrate were observed in the range of 200–225°C.

The photomicrographs of pure carvedilol and the selected crystal formulations are given in Figure 4. The pure carvedilol was characterized by hydrosols of bigger size and regular shape with an apparently smooth surface. In contrast hydrosols were present in the form of fine powder. Additionally, solid dispersions were porous and with rough surface which might have resulted in the enhanced dissolution rate as compared to pure drug. The size of hydrosols was comparatively less than carvedilol.

The increase in the carvedilol solubility, although little, and dramatically increase in its dissolution rate from prepared hydrosols, cogrind mixture and solid dispersions can be explained as follow (as shown in Figures 5 & 6):

Chitosan has been proposed as a useful excipient for enhancing the bioavailability of poorly water-soluble compounds [23]. Chitosan and its derivatives have been reported as a good vehicle for enhancing the solubility and dissolution of poorly water-soluble drugs [24-26]. Chitosan dissolves readily in most of the acid solutions and upon dissolution, amine groups of the polymer become protonated, resulting in a positively charged

Table 5 Melting endotherms of carvedilol and prepared formulations

Formulations	Melting endotherm at (°C)
Carvedilol	**155.94**
0.2% Chitosan hydrosols	**Nil**
0.4% Chitosan chlorhydrate hydrosols	**Nil**
0.2% Chitosan solid dispersions	**Nil**
0.8% Chitosan chlorhydrate solid dispersions	**Nil**
0.4% Chitosan Co-grinding	**153.78**
0.4% Chitosan chlorhydrate Co-grinding	**152.97**

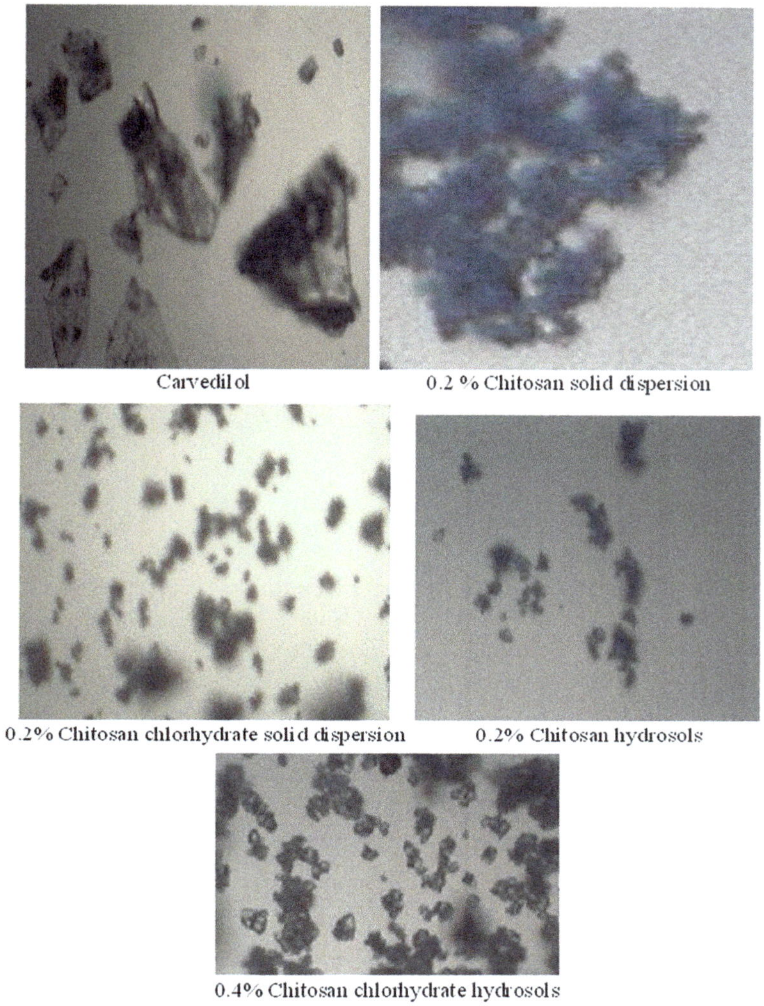

Figure 4 **Electronic microphotographs of optimized formulations.**

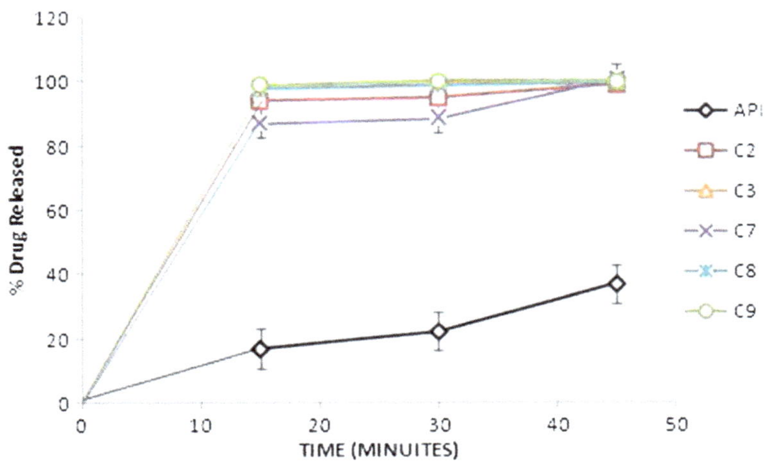

Figure 5 ***In vitro*** **release of carvedilol from the prepared hydrosol formulations in SGF.** The points represent mean values, n = 3.

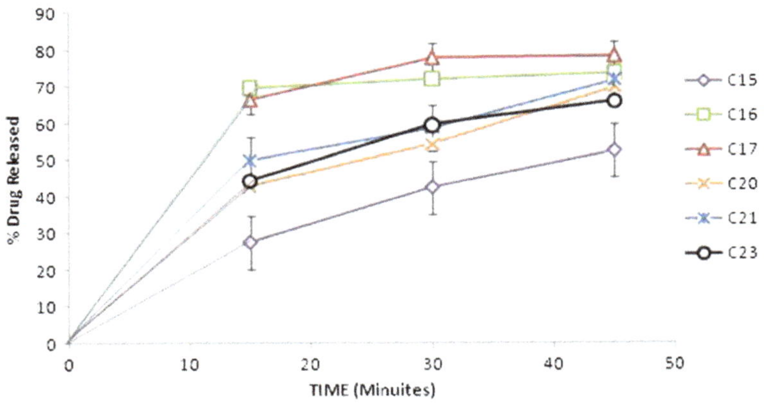

Figure 6 In vitro release of carvedilol from the prepared cogrind formulations in SGF. The points represent mean values, n = 3.

polysaccharide (RNH3+) and chitosan salts (chloride, glutamate, etc.) that are soluble in water [27].

The earlier literature reveals that dissolution rate not only depends on the surface area and particle size of the processed powder, but is greatly affected by crystal morphhology and wettability [27] So increased wettability of the drug by the adsorption of chitosan and chitosan chlorhydrate onto the hydrophobic surface of the drug is the first reason. In a previous study also, chitosan showed increased solubility and dissolution rate of naproxen due to adsorption on its surface [26]. One interesting case was observed all solid dispersions showed 100% drug release within 15 minutes. Carvedilol exhibited pH dependent solubility. Its solubility decreases with increasing pH then starts decreasing after pH 4. At lower pH values protonated form of carvedilol and its salts generated *in situ* will determine its solubility. Hydrochloride salt generated *in situ* in an acidic medium might be less soluble in this medium than the protonated carvedilol itself. At basic pH as the pH increases from 9.2 to 11 its solubility remains more or less constant [28]. In formulation of solid dispersions glacial acetic acid was used so acetic acid incorporates acidity to the formulation that's why there might be possibility of enhancement of dissolution rate of carvediol [28].

The difference in dissolution rate enhancement by chitosan and chitosan chlorhydrate can be explained as, the trend found was that for the two types of chitosan (base and salt), the lower the *M*w, the faster was the drug dissolution. This behavior was predictable taking into account the relationship between *M*w and viscosity of polymer solution [29].

Upon contact with the acidic medium; chitosan swells and forms a gel. The diffusion of the drug through the gel into the release medium would be retarded by increasing the viscosity of the polymer, and hence of the gel [30]. On the other hand, the chitosan chlorhydrate led to faster drug dissolution than chitosan. The explanation to this behavior was found in the differences in the wetting rate, solubilities and swelling capacity of the chitosan and chitosan salts, chitosan chlorhydrate rapidly wet and dissolve upon its incorporation into the dissolution medium, whereas the CS base, less water soluble, would take more time to dissolve. In order to clarify the causes of significant difference in the dissolution rate, the surface morphology of the hydrosols was examined by electronic microscope (EM). Thus the fine and fluffy physical state of C-3 hydrosols along with their porous and rough surface as supported by EM might also have contributed to the enhanced solubility and dissolution rate of carvedilol from these hydrosols.

The physical stability of optimized formulations was compared with the drug. The formulations were found

Table 6 Drug content of formulations after stability studies

Storage condition 30 ± 2°C /65 ± 5% RH	Drug Content (%) of formulations						
	Carvedilol	0.2% Chitosan hydrosols	0.4% Chitosan chlorhydrate hydrosols	0.2% chitosan solid dispersions	0.8% chitosan chlorhydrate solid dispersions	0.4% Chitosan Co-grinding	0.4% Chitosan chlorhydrate Co-grinding
Time 0 days	99.56 ± 1.16	98.77 ± 1.31	98.19 ± 2.13	99.66 ± 1.24	98.17 ± 1.14	99.46 ± 1.11	98.86 ± 1.15
Time 90 days	99.46 ± 1.38	98.67 ± 1.44	98.09 ± 2.34	99.76 ± 1.32	98.67 ± 1.43	99.27 ± 1.12	98.66 ± 1.34
Time 180 days	99.26 ± 1.10	98.47 ± 1.22	97.69 ± 2.01	99.16 ± 1.16	98.97 ± 1.25	99.29 ± 1.14	99.10 ± 1.17

to be stable during the study periods there was no any change in color was found. The drug content in all the formulations was found to be within the limit. The drug content within the formulations is shown in the Table 6.

Conclusions

The present study investigated successful and simple methods to enhance the dissolution rate of carvedilol by using chitosan and chitosan chlorhydrate. If this process can be scaled-up to manufacturing level, this technique has the potential to develop into an invaluable technology in future.

Competing interests

The authors report no competing interests. The authors alone are responsible for the content and writing of the paper.

Authors' contributions

SAS: carried out the formulation studies, characterized the samples for evaluation parameters participated in the sequence alignment and drafted the manuscript. YAV participated in sequence alignment. MSM participated in its design and coordination and helped to draft the manuscript and interpretation of spectral analysis. All authors read and approved the final manuscript.

Acknowledgement

The authors are thankful to Lupin Research Park, Pune,Maharashtra, India, for providing gift sample of Carvedilol. The authors are also thankful to Prof. Dr. R.C. Doijad, Principal, Shree Santkrupa College of Pharmacy, Ghogaon, Karad, Dist. Satara, and Maharashtra, India for providing research facilities.

Author details

[1]Department of Pharmaceutics, Shree Santkrupa College of Pharmacy, Ghogaon, Tal. Karad Dist, Satara, MS, India. [2]Gourishankar Institute of Pharmaceutical Education and Research, Limb, Satara 415002, India. [3]Vignan Institute of Pharmaceutical sciences, Deshmukhi, 508284, Nalgonda Dist, India.

References

1. Xi H, Chinmay G, Daniel T, Yuhua C, Dave R: **Simultaneous micronization and surface modification for improvement of flow and dissolution of drug particles.** *Int J Pharm* 2011, **415:**185–195.
2. Nokhodchi A: **The effect of type and concentration of vehicle on dissolution rate of poorly water soluble drug (indomethacin) from liquid solid compacts.** *J Pharm Pharmaceut Sci* 2005, **8:**18–25.
3. Kakran M, Sahoo NG, Li L: **Dissolution enhancement of quercetin through nanofabrication, complexation, and solid dispersion.** *Colloids Surf B: Biointerfaces* 2011, **88:**121–130.
4. Andre FA, Bruno GG, Chris V, Jean Paul R: **Gelucire 44/14 based immediate release formulations for poorly water-soluble drugs.** *Drug Dev Ind Pharm* 2012, doi:10.3109/03639045.2012.709251. Posted online on August 8.
5. Blagden N, de Matas M, Gavan P, York P: **Crystal engineering of active pharmaceutical ingredients to improve solubility and dissolution rates.** *Adv Drug Deli Rev* 2007, **59:**617–630.
6. Jagadeesh Babu N, Nangia A: **Solubility advantage of amorphous drugs and pharmaceutical cocrystals.** *Crystal Growth & Design* 2011, **11:**2662.
7. Chadha R, Saini A, Arora P, Bhandari S: **Pharmaceutical cocrystals: A novel approach for oral bioavailability enhancement of drugs.** *Crit Rev Ther Drug Carrier Syst* 2012, **29:**183–218.
8. Felt O, Buri P, Gurny R: **Chitosan: a unique polysaccharide for drug delivery.** *Drug Dev Ind Pharm* 1998, **24:**979–993.
9. Nicolas D, Julien R, Raphael R, Pierre G, Jean-Marc S, Christine J, Jean-François G, Véronique P: **Tocol modified glycol chitosan for the oral delivery of poorly soluble drugs.** *Int J Pharm* 2012, **423:**452–460.
10. Mukhopadhyay P, Mishra R, Rana D, Kundu P: **Strategies for effective oral insulin delivery with modified chitosan nanoparticles: A review.** *Prog Polym Sci.* Available online 16 May 2012 In Press, Corrected Proof.
11. Nagai T, Sawayanagi Y, Nambu N: **Applications of chitin and chitosan to pHarmaceutical preparations.** In *Chitin, Chitosan and Related Enzymes.* Edited by Zizakis JP. Orlando, FL: Academic Press; 1984:21–39.
12. Ritthidej GC, Chomto P, Pummangura S, Menasveta P: **Chitin and chitosan as disintegrants in paracetamol tablets.** *Drug Dev Ind Pharm* 1994, **20:**2109–2134.
13. Upadrashta SM, Katikaneni PR, Nuessle NO: **Chitosan as a tablet binder.** *Drug Dev Ind PHarm* 1992, **18:**1701–1708.
14. Sawayanagi Y, Nambu N, Nagai T: **Dissolution properties and bioavailability of pHenytoin from ground mixtures with chitin or chitosan.** *Chem Pharm Bull* 1983, **31:**2062–2068.
15. Shiraishi S, Arahira M, Imai T, Otagiri M: **Enhancement of dissolution rates of several drugs by low molecular chitosan and alginate.** *Chem Pharm Bull* 1990, **38:**185–187.
16. Acarturk F, Sencan A, Celebi N: **Evaluation of the effect of low molecular weight chitosan on the solubility and dissolution characteristics of spironolactone.** *Pharmazie* 1993, **48:**605–607.
17. Portero A, Remunãn-Lopez C, Vila-Jato JL: **Effect of chitosan and chitosan glutamate enhancing the dissolution properties of the poorly water soluble drug nifedipine.** *Int J Pharm* 1998, **175:**75–84.
18. Horter D, Dressman JB: **Influence of physicochemical properties on dissolution of drugs in the gastrointestinal tract.** *Adv Drug Deli Rev* 2001, **46:**75–87.
19. Anal AK, Stevens WF: **Chitosan–alginate multilayer beads for controlled release of ampicillin.** *Int J Pharm* 2005, **290:**45–54.
20. Mutalik S, Prambil A, Krishnan M, Achuta NU: **Enhancement of dissolution rate and bioavailability of aceclofenac: a chitosan based solvent change approach.** *Int J Pharm* 2008, **350:**279–90.
21. Talari R, Varshosaz J, Abolfazl Mostafavi S, Nokhodchi A: **Gliclazide microcrystals prepared by two methods of *in situ* micronization: pharmacokinetic studies in diabetic and normal rats.** *AAPS PharmTech* 2010, **11:**786–792.
22. Ahmed NA, Viviane FN, Safaa S: **Formulation and physicochemical characterization of chitosan/Acyclovir co-crystals.** *Pharm Dev Technol* 2011.
23. Mura P, Zerrouk N, Mennini N, Maestrelli F, Chemtob C: **Development and characterization of naproxen-chitosan solid systems with improved drug dissolution properties.** *Eur J Pharm Sci* 2003, **19:**67–75.
24. Maestrelli F, Zerrouk N, Chemtob C, Mura P: **Influence of chitosan and its glutamate and hydrochloride salts on naproxen dissolution rate and permeation across Caco-2 cells.** *Int J Pharm* 2004, **271:**257–267.
25. Kumar VSG, Mishra DN: **Preparation characterization and *in vitro* dissolution studies of solid systems of valdecoxib with chitosan.** *Chem Pharm Bull* 2006, **54:**2–12.
26. Rowe RC, Sheskey PJ, Owen SC: *Handbook of PHarmaceutical excipients.* London, United Kingdom: PHarmaceutical Press; 2006.
27. Perrut M, Jung J, Leboeuf F: **Enhancement of dissolution rate of poorly-soluble active ingredients by supercritical fluid processes. Part I. Micronization of neat particles.** *Int J Pharm* 2005, **288:**3–10.
28. Shewale BD, Sapkal NA, Raut NJ, Gaikwad RA: **Effect of hydroxy propyl B- Cyclodextrin on solubility of carvedilol.** *Indian J PHarm Sci* 2008, **70:**255–257.
29. Adusumilli PS, Bolton SM: **Evaluation of chitosan citrate complexes as matrices for controlled release formulations using a 3^2 full factorial design.** *Drug Dev Ind PHarm* 1991, **17:**1931–1945.
30. Imai T, Shiraishi S, Saito H, Otagiri M: **Interaction of indomethacin with low-molecular weight chitosan and improvement of some pHarmaceutical properties of indomethacin by low-molecular weight chitosans.** *Int J Pharm* 1991, **67:**11–20.

Derivative spectrophotometric method for simultaneous determination of clindamycin phosphate and tretinoin in pharmaceutical dosage forms

Maliheh Barazandeh Tehrani[1*], Melika Namadchian[1], Sedigheh Fadaye Vatan[2] and Effat Souri[1]

Abstract

A derivative spectrophotometric method was proposed for the simultaneous determination of clindamycin and tretinoin in pharmaceutical dosage forms. The measurement was achieved using the first and second derivative signals of clindamycin at (^{1}D) 251 nm and (^{2}D) 239 nm and tretinoin at (^{1}D) 364 nm and (^{2}D) 387 nm. The proposed method showed excellent linearity at both first and second derivative order in the range of 60–1200 and 1.25–25 μg/ml for clindamycin phosphate and tretinoin respectively. The within-day and between-day precision and accuracy was in acceptable range (CV<3.81%, error<3.20%). Good agreement between the found and added concentrations indicates successful application of the proposed method for simultaneous determination of clindamycin and tretinoin in synthetic mixtures and pharmaceutical dosage form.

Keywords: Clindamycin, Tretinoin, Derivative spectrophotometry, Pharmaceutical dosage form

Background

Clindamycin, (methyl-7-chloro-6,7,8-trideoxy-6-{[(4*R*)-1-methyl-4-propyl-L-prolyl]amino}-1-thio-L-threo-α-D-galacto-octopyranoside), (Figure 1) is a semi-synthetic derivative of lincomycin. Clindamycin reveals potent activity against many gram-positive and gram-negative bacterial infections. Topical clindamycin is used for the treatment of acne vulgaris which typically leads to suppression of cutaneous propionibacterium acnes [1].

Tretinoin, (3,7-dimethyl-9-(2,6,6-trimethyl-1-cyclohexenyl)-nona-2,4,6,8-tetraenoic acid) (Figure 1) is a derivative of vitamin A. Tretinoin could reduce the hyperkeratinization in the sebaceous follicle and accordingly decrease the sebum secretion and inflammation [1].

Acne vulgaris is a common dermatologic problem which could be treated with systemic or topical drugs. More importantly the combination therapy of topical clindamycin and tretinoin is more beneficial for the treatment of mild to moderate stages of acne vulgaris [2].

There are some reported articles in the literature for the determination of clindamycin [3-8] or tretinoin [9,10] alone or via the combination of the two drugs [11] by HPLC and gas chromatography in bulk or in pharmaceutical dosage form. HPLC method has been used in the USP35- NF30 for determination of clindamycin phosphate and tretinoin in separate gel dosage form but no simultaneous method is reported [12]. The literature survey revealed that although there were some spectrophotometric methods for the determination of clindamycin [13,14] or tretinoin [15,16] alone, no validated spectrophotometric method for simultaneous determination of clindamycin and tretinoin was reported. The spectrophotometric technique is a highly preferable method for routine analysis due to its simplicity and economical advantages. Since the spectrophotometric quantitative analysis of two or more compounds with overlapping spectra will likely prove difficult, thus the derivative spectrophotometry is a fairly useful method for analysis of a multi-compound mixture.

* Correspondence: barazand@sina.tums.ac.ir
[1]Department of Medicinal Chemistry, Faculty of Pharmacy and Pharmaceutical Sciences Research Center, Tehran University of Medical Sciences, Tehran, Iran
Full list of author information is available at the end of the article

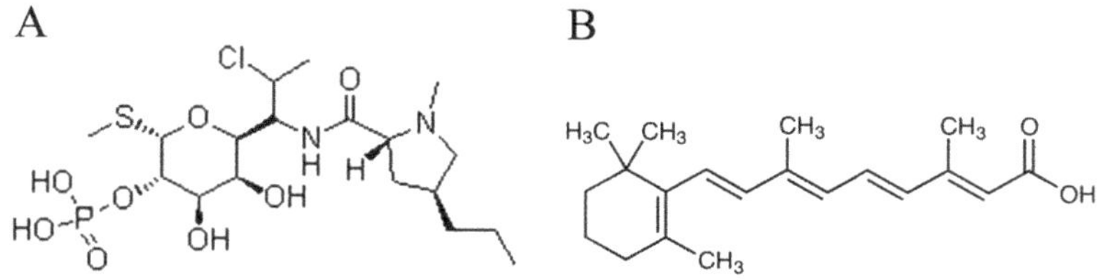

Figure 1 **Chemical structure of A) Clindamycin phosphate and B) Tretinoin.**

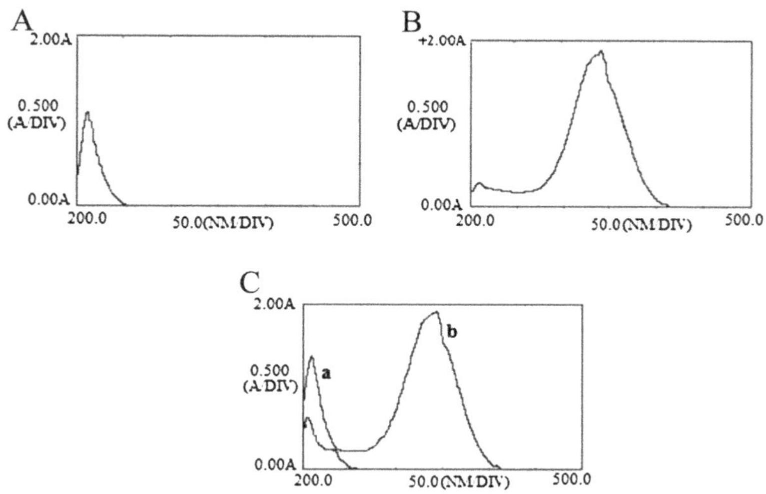

Figure 2 **Zero-order spectra of clindamycin phosphate (A), tretinoin (B) and overlapped spectra (C).**

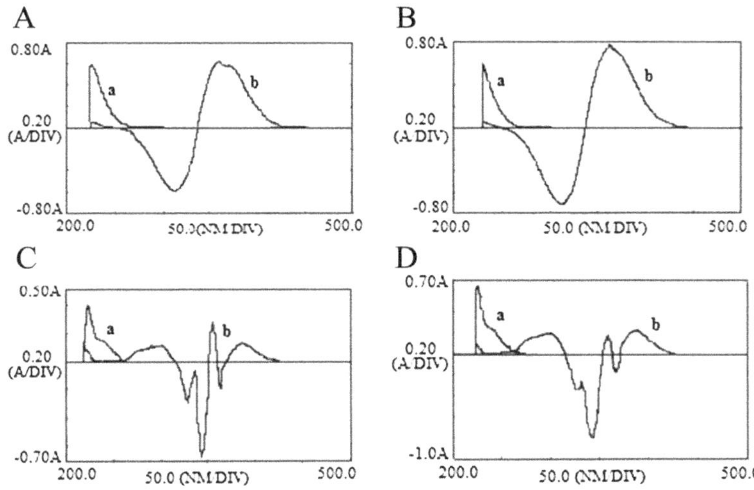

Figure 3 **Derivative spectra of clindamycin phosphate (a) and tretinoin (b); (A) First order spectra (Δλ=16); (B) First order spectra (Δλ=20); (C) Second order spectra (Δλ=10.5); (D) second order spectra (Δλ=14).**

Table 1 Statistical data of calibration curves of clindamycin in the presence of tretinoin (12.5 μg/ml)

Parameters	$^{1}D^{*}$ (Δλ=16) (λ=252 nm)	^{1}D (Δλ=20) (λ=251 nm)	$^{2}D^{**}$ (Δλ=10.5) (λ=234 nm)	^{2}D (Δλ=14) (λ=239 nm)
Linearity range	60–1200 μg/ml	60–1200 μg/ml	60–1200 μg/ml	60–1200 μg/ml
Regression equation	$Y= 0.000120X-9.761\times10^{-5}$	$Y= 0.000185X-0.00098$	$Y= 0.00024X-3.912\times10^{-5}$	$Y= 0.0004282X- 0.038$
SD of slope	1.41×10^{-6}	1.63×10^{-7}	1.60×10^{-6}	7.80×10^{-6}
RSD of slope (%)	0.170	0.088	0.65	1.82
SD of intercept	0.000839	0.000210	0.003403	0.005001
Correlation coefficient	0.999	0.999	0.998	0.998

* First derivative order.
**Second derivative order.

In this study a derivative spectrophotometric method based on zero-crossing is used for simultaneous determination of clindamycin and tretinoin.

Experimental

Chemicals

Both drugs were favorably provided by Kish Medipharm Pharmaceutical Co., Kish, Iran. The purity of clindamycin and tretinoin which were used in the proposed method was 97.43 and 101.1% respectively based on the standard USP 32, NF 27 assay method.

The excipients used in the formulation of Acnomis® gel and a blank gel without active ingredients were also provided by Kish Medipharm Pharmaceutical Co. NaOH, methanol and acetonitrile were of analytical grade and purchased from Merck (Darmstadt, Germany).

The Acnomis® gel containing clindamycin phosphate (1.2 g/100 g) and tretinoin (25 mg/100 g) was also prepared by Kish Medipharm Pharmaceutical Co.

Instruments

A double beam UV-Visible spectrophotometer (160A, Shimadzu, Japan) with a fixed 2 nm band width and 1 cm quartz cell were utilized for spectrophotometric measurement. A Waters (Milford,USA)HPLC system (A Model 510 pump, a model 717 plus auto-sampler and a model 418 UV-Visible detector) was used for HPLC determination.

Standard solutions

Stock solutions of clindamycin phosphate and tretinoin were prepared separately in a mixture of methanol and 0.1 M NaOH (50:50) to reach a concentration of 1.2 and 250 μg/ml respectively. Synthetic mixtures of varying concentration of clindamycin phosphate (60, 120, 240, 360, 480, 720, 960 and 1200 μg/ml) in the presence of tretinoin (12.5 μg/ml) and also varying concentration of tretinoin (1.25, 2.5, 5, 7.5, 10, 15, 20 and 25 μg/ml) in the presence of clindamycin phosphate (600 μg/ml) were prepared for construction of calibration curves. The standard solutions of clindamycin and tretinoin in the synthetic mixtures for determination of relative recovery were constructed with respect to their ratio in the pharmaceutical dosage form.

Accuracy and precision

The within-day and between-day precision and accuracy of the proposed method were calculated by analyzing three sets of synthetic mixtures of clindamycin phosphate and tretinoin in one day and three consecutive days.

Application of the method in dosage form

A 0.5 g sample of gel formulation containing propylene glycol, butylated hydroxytoluene, simethicon, clindamycin phosphate (1.2 g/100) and tretinoin (25 mg/100) was weighed and transmitted to a 50 ml volumetric flask. The

Table 2 Statistical data of calibration curves of tretinoin in the presence of clindamycin (600 μg/ml)

Parameters	$^{1}D^{*}$ (Δλ=16) (λ=364 nm)	^{1}D (Δλ=20) (λ=364 nm)	$^{2}D^{**}$ (Δλ=10.5) (λ=386 nm)	^{2}D (Δλ=14) (λ=387 nm)
Linearity range	1.25–25 μg/ml	1.25–25 μg/ml	1.25–25 μg/ml	1.25–25 μg/ml
Regression equation	$Y= 0.05086X-0.00035$	$Y= 0.06260X-0.0024$	$Y= 0.010585X+ 0.00035$	$Y= 0.018587X+ 0.00437$
SD of slope	3.44×10^{-5}	7.12×10^{-5}	1.38×10^{-4}	1.38×10^{-4}
RSD of slope (%)	0.067	0.113	1.300	0.740
SD of intercept	0.000774	0.000736	0.00146	0.00259
Correlation coefficient	0.999	0.999	0.999	0.998

* First derivative order.
**Second derivative order.

Table 3 Accuracy and precision data for determination of clindamycin in the presence of tretinoin (12.5 μg/ml) by different order derivative spectrophotometry

Added (μg/ml)	Within-day (n = 3)			Between-day (n = 9)		
	Found (μg/ml)	CV (%)	Error (%)	Found (μg/ml)	CV (%)	Error (%)
$^{1}D^{*}$ (Δλ=16)						
60.00	60.50±1.58	2.62	0.83	59.96±1.76	2.94	−0.07
480.00	474.31±9.72	2.05	−1.18	479.44±7.89	1.64	−0.11
1200.00	1205.56±1.73	0.14	0.46	1201.55±4.13	0.34	0.13
^{1}D (Δλ=20)						
60.00	60.20±0.64	1.07	0.33	59.10±1.09	1.85	−1.49
480.00	482.20±1.30	0.26	0.46	480.99±2.40	0.50	0.20
1200.00	1203.68±2.12	0.18	0.30	1205.51±2.18	0.18	0.46
$^{2}D^{**}$ (Δλ=10.5)						
60.00	60.81±2.20	3.61	1.35	59.91±1.72	2.88	−0.14
480.00	480.06±16.34	3.40	0.01	471.36±18.00	3.81	−1.80
1200.00	1201.46±6.50	0.54	0.12	1201.87±9.63	0.80	0.15
^{2}D (Δλ=14)						
60.00	60.23±1.40	2.32	0.38	61.36±1.80	2.93	2.26
480.00	467.14±3.70	0.80	−2.67	465.89±4.06	0.87	−2.94
1200.00	1215.98±18.00	1.48	1.33	1224.42±11.96	0.97	2.03

* First derivative order.
**Second derivative order.

Table 4 Accuracy and precision data for determination of tretinoin in the presence of clindamycin (600 μg/ml) by different order derivative spectrophotometry

Added (μg/ml)	Within-day (n = 3)			Between-day (n = 9)		
	Found (μg/ml)	CV (%)	Error (%)	Found (μg/ml)	CV (%)	Error (%)
$^{1}D^{*}$ (Δλ=16)						
1.25	1.22±0.02	1.64	−2.37	1.21±0.02	1.63	−3.2
5.00	4.88±0.004	0.09	−2.38	4.88±0.01	0.21	−2.38
15.00	14.98±0.081	0.54	−0.13	14.95±0.05	0.34	−0.33
^{1}D (Δλ=20)						
1.25	1.27±0.008	0.64	1.60	1.26±0.01	1.02	0.80
5.00	4.85±0.018	0.37	−2.94	4.84±0.02	0.41	−3.20
15.00	15.02±0.036	0.24	0.13	15.00±0.03	0.21	0.00
$^{2}D^{**}$ (Δλ=10.5)						
1.25	1.23±0.02	1.61	−1.60	1.23±0.03	2.44	−1.60
5.00	4.86±0.062	1.28	−2.8	4.89±0.08	1.64	−2.23
15.00	15.35±0.11	0.72	2.33	15.39±0.16	1.07	2.64
^{2}D (Δλ=14)						
1.25	1.22±0.002	0.16	−2.40	1.21±0.02	1.65	−3.20
5.00	4.97±0.005	0.11	−0.60	4.88±0.08	1.67	−2.37
15.00	15.29±0.40	2.62	1.93	15.39±0.49	3.18	2.63

* First derivative order.
**Second derivative order.

Table 5 Relative recovery of clindamycin (1.2 g) and tretinoin (25 mg)

Derivative order	Recovery (%) (n=4)	
	Tretinoin	Clindamycin
$^{1}D^{*}$ ($\Delta\lambda$ =16)	99.3 ± 1.6	98.3 ± 1.3
^{1}D ($\Delta\lambda$ =20)	98.5 ± 2.6	97.3 ± 2.6
$^{2}D^{**}$ ($\Delta\lambda$ =10.5)	98.6 ± 1.4	95.6 ± 1.9
^{2}D ($\Delta\lambda$ =14)	95.2 ± 4.9	94.3 ± 0.5

* First derivative order.
**Second derivative order.

sample was dissolved in a mixture of methanol and 0.1 M NaOH (50:50) by sonicating for 10 min. The mixture was made up to required volume with the same solvent and centrifuged for 10 min at 4000 rpm. The clear solution was used for determination of clindamycin and tretinoin by the proposed method and also pharmacopoeial method reported for determination of clindamycin or tretinoin alone. A solution of blank gel treated by the same procedure was used as blank in spectrophotometric method.

Results and discussion

Selection of solvent

Tretinoin was not soluble in water. Both clindamycin and tretinoin were soluble in alcohol and chloroform but their solubility in non-aqueous solvents was lower than in methanol [17]. Their solubility was improved by adding NaOH to the methanol and consequently, a mixture of methanol and 0.1 M NaOH (50:50) was selected as a proper solvent to prepare the standard solutions.

Absorption spectra

The zero-order spectra of clindamycin (600 μg/ml) and tretinoin (12.5 μg/ml) solutions were separately measured at 200–500 nm using the solvent (methanol: 0.1 M NaOH 50:50) as a blank.

To give a clear picture, the absorption spectra of clindamycin phosphate and tretinoin are shown in Figure 2 where the zero-order spectra demonstrated a marked overlapping. As a result, simultaneous determination of two drugs will not be possible by direct measurement of absorbance signals. The first to fourth order derivative spectra of those solutions were obtained in the same range at different $\Delta\lambda$ values.

Zero-crossing points were assigned from the first to fourth order derivative spectra of clindamycin and tretinoin. The suitable zero-crossing points were selected based on the best linear response to the clindamycin concentration in the presence of tretinoin or the tretinoin concentration in the presence of clindamycin.

Selection of suitable wavelengths

As it is shown in Figure 3, the first and second order spectra of clindamycin and tretinoin revealed zero-crossing points for their simultaneous determination. The zero-crossing points of clindamycin and tretinoin in the first order derivative were found to be 252 ($\Delta\lambda$=16), 251 ($\Delta\lambda$=20) and 364 nm ($\Delta\lambda$=16) and in the second order derivative were 234($\Delta\lambda$=10.5), 239 nm ($\Delta\lambda$=14) and 386 ($\Delta\lambda$=10.5), 387 nm ($\Delta\lambda$=14) respectively.

Method validation

The validation was done according to ICH recommendations for linearity, range, accuracy and precision, limit of detection (LOD), limit of quantification (LOQ) robustness and relative recovery [18].

Linearity

To verify the validation of Beer's law, six series of calibration curves were plotted using the first and second order spectra in the range of 60–1200 μg/ml and 1.25–25 μg/ml for clindamycin and tretinoin respectively.

The results of calibration curves in four different $\Delta\lambda$ and wavelengths are given in Table 1 and 2. These data illustrate that the first and second derivative spectra measurements with $\Delta\lambda$ = 16, 20, 10.5 and 14 can be meaningfully usable. The correlation coefficient of the calibration curves (n=6) for both drugs in all wavelengths was greater than 0.998%.

Table 6 Assay results of containing Clindamycin (1.2 g) and Tretinoin (25 mg) using derivative spectrophotometry and HPLC method

Derivative order		Clindamycin (g/100)		Tretinoin (mg/100)	
		Mean± SD	(%) Recovery	Mean± SD	(%) Recovery
UV/VIS	$^{1}D^{*}$ ($\Delta\lambda$=16)	1.16± 0.03	96.66	24.54± 0.03	98.16
	^{1}D ($\Delta\lambda$=20)	1.15± 0.06	95.83	24.85± 0.03	99.40
	$^{2}D^{**}$ ($\Delta\lambda$=10.5)	1.14±0.03	95.00	24.11± 0.02	96.44
	^{2}D ($\Delta\lambda$=14)	1.16± 0.02	96.67	23.95± 0.06	95.80
HPLC		1.15±0.07	95.83	24.62±0.97	98.49

* First derivative order.
**Second derivative order.

The high values of correlation coefficient and the values of y-intercepts close to zero indicate the good linearity of the calibrations.

Accuracy and precision

In order to study the accuracy and precision, the proposed method was applied for simultaneous determination of varying concentrations of clindamycin (60, 480 and 1200 μg/ml) in the presence of tretinoin (12.5 μg/ml) and varying concentrations of tretinoin (1.25, 5 and 15 μg/ml) in the presence of clindamycin (600 μg/ml). The within-day and between-day precision and accuracy were calculated (Tables 3 and 4).

The percentage of coefficients of variations obtained was in the range of 0.09–3.81 and the percent of error was lower than 3.2% for both drugs in all the three selected concentrations which indicate good accuracy and precision of the method.

Limit of detection & limit of quantification

The limit of detection measured based on the standard deviation of the response and slope, was in the range of 3.4-42.5 μg/ml and 0.05–0.42 μg/ml in the first and second derivative order for clindamycin phosphate and tretinoin respectively. The quantitation limit was 60 μg/ml for clindamycin phosphate and 1.25 μg/ml for tretinoin.

Robustness

The robustness of the proposed method was assessed by changes in the ratio of methanol and NaOH and also the molarity of NaOH up to 10 percent. There was no significant difference between the results.

Relative recovery

The recovery was determined using standard addition method. The recoveries in different derivative conditions ranged from 94.3 to 98.3% for clindamycin and 95.2–99.3% for tretinoin (Table 5).

Application

The proposed method was applied successfully for the analysis of clindamycin and tretinoin in pharmaceutical dosage form (Acnomis® gel) containing 1.2 g clindamycin and 25 mg tretinoin (Table 6). The results obtained from the first and second derivative order indicate the percentage of recovery to be between 94.3-99.3 in all evaluations. This technique of analysis was compared with a HPLC method [11]. Using the two-tailed t-test method it was revealed that there was no significant difference between the results obtained from these two methods (p-value>0.05).

Conclusion

It was concluded that the first and second order derivative UV spectrophotometric method at $\Delta\lambda$= 16, 20, 10.5 and 14 could be used for simultaneous determination of clindamycin phosphate and tretinoin in their combined pharmaceutical products. This method could be used for rapid analysis of active ingredients in process and for quality control samples.

Competing interest

The authors declare that they have no competing interest.

Authors' contributions

MBT has guided the project and prepared the manuscript. MN carried out the analysis and method development. SFV prepared sample and standard solutions and collaborate in analysis. ES made substantial contributions for study design, data interpretation and involved in drafting the manuscript. All authors read and approved the final manuscript.

Acknowledgment

This study was part of a M.D. thesis supported by Tehran University of Medical Sciences (grant No: 17724).

Author details

[1]Department of Medicinal Chemistry, Faculty of Pharmacy and Pharmaceutical Sciences Research Center, Tehran University of Medical Sciences, Tehran, Iran. [2]R & D Department, Kish Medipharm Company, No. 64, Kish free zone island, Iran.

References

1. Brunton L, Parker KL: *Goodman and Gilman's Manual of Pharmacology and Therapeutics*. Twelfth edition. USA: The McGraw-Hill Companies; 2008:1078–1083.
2. Fu LW, Vender RB: **Newer Approaches in topical combination therapy for acne.** *Skin Therapy Lett* 2011, **16**(9):4–6.
3. Hornedo-Nunez A, Getek TA, Korfmacher WA, Simenthal F: **High-performance liquid chromatography of clindamycin and clindamycin phosphate with electrochemical detection.** *J Chromatogr* 1990, **503**:217–225.
4. Vladimirov S, Markovic L, Agbaba D, Zivanov-Stakic D, Brboric J: **High performance liquid chromatographic determination of clindamycin in pharmaceutical formulations.** *J Serbian Chem Soc* 1997, **62**:177–181.
5. Fieger- Buschges H, Schubler G, Larsimont V, Blume H: **Determination of clindamycin in human plasma by high-performance liquid chromatography using coupled columns.** *J Chromatogr B: Biomedical Sciences and Applications* 1999, **724**:281–286.
6. Batzias GC, Delis GA, Koutsoviti-Papadopoulou M: **A new HPLC/UV method for determination of clindamycin in dog blood serum.** *J Pharm Biomed Anal* 2004, **35**:545–554.
7. Platzer DJ, White BA: **Development and validation of a gradient HPLC method for the determination of clindamycin and related compounds in a novel tablet formulation.** *J Pharm Biomed Anal* 2006, **41**:84–88.
8. Bharathi C, Jayaram P, Raj JS, Saravana Kumar M, Bhargavi V, Handa VK, Dandala R, Naidu A: **Indentification, isolation and characterization of impurities of clindamycin palmitate hydrochloride.** *J Pharm Biomed Anal* 2008, **48**:1211–1218.
9. Tashtoush BM, Jacobson EL, Jacobson MK: **A rapid HPLC method for simultaneous determination of tretinoin and isotretinoin in dermatological formulations.** *J Pharm Biomed Anal* 2007, **43**:859–864.
10. Tashtoush BM, Jacobson EL, Jacobson MK: **UVA is the major contributor to the photo degradation of tretinoin and isotretinoion: Implications for development of improved pharmaceutical formulations.** *Int J Pharm* 2008, **352**:123–128.
11. Ye YR, Bektic E, Buchta R, Houlden R, Hunt B: **Simultaneous determination of tretinoin and clindamycin phosphate and their degradation products in topical formulations by reverse phase HPLC.** *J Sep Sci* 2004, **27**:71–77.
12. Shefter E: **The United States Pharmacopeia 35-The National Formulary. 30.** 2012, **3**:2707–4921.
13. Amin AS: **Spectrophotometric and conductometric determination of clindamycin hydrochloride in pure form and in pharmaceutical preparations.** *Analusis* 1995, **23**:415–417.

14. El-Yazbi FA, Blaih SM: **Spectrophotometric and titrimetric determination of clindamycin hydrochloride in pharmaceutical preparations.** *Analyst* 1993, **118**:577–579.
15. Gupta A, Gulati M, Pandey NK: **A validated UV spectrophotometric method for simultaneous estimation of tretinoin and benzoyl peroxide in bulk and semisolid dosage form.** *Rasayan J Chem* 2009, **2**(3):649–654.
16. Patel P, Kabra P, Kimbahune R, Urmila GH: **Quantitative estimation of isotretinoin in bulk and formulation by UV-visible spectrophotometry.** *Res J Pharm Biol Chem Sci* 2011, **2**(1):167–172.
17. O'Neil MJ: *The Merck Index.* 13th edition. USA, NJ: Merck Research Laboratories; 2001:2377–8251.
18. ICH: *Validation of Analytical Procedures: Methodology, International Conference on Harmonization.* Geneva: IFPMA; 1996.

A New extractive spectrophotometric method for determination of rizatriptan dosage forms using bromocresol green

Effat Souri[1*], Abbas Kaboodari[1], Noushin Adib[2] and Massoud Amanlou[1]

Abstract

Background and the purpose of the study: Rizatriptan is used effectively for the treatment of migraine headache. In this study, a simple, rapid and low cost spectrophotometric method based on the ion-pair complexation is proposed for the determination of rizatriptan in raw material and dosage forms.

Methods: The ion-pair complexation using bromocresol green as reagent was performed in a buffer solution and the absorbance was measured by a spectrophotometer. The ion-pair formation conditions were optimized and the accuracy and precision of the method were calculated.

Results and major conclusion: Best results were achieved by using 6 ml of the bromocresol green reagent in the presence of phosphate buffer (pH 3.0). The stoichiometry of the resulted complex was 1:1. The within-day and between-day precision values were lower than 2.9 and 1.8 percent for the calibration range of 0.5–50 and 10–100 µg/ml, respectively. The proposed method was successfully used for the determination of rizatriptan in dosage forms without any interference.

Keywords: Rizatriptan, Bromocresol green, Lon-pair complexation, Spectrophotometry

Introduction

Rizatriptan benzoate (Figure 1), N, N-dimethyl-5-(1H, 1, 2, 4-triazol-1-ylmethyl)-1H-indole-3-ethanamine benzoate, binds selectively with high affinity to human 5-hydroxytryptamine 1B/1D receptor. Clinical trials have demonstrated the effectiveness of oral rizatriptan for the treatment of migraine headache [1-3].

Several analytical methods based on liquid chromatography/ tandem mass spectrometry [4,5] or high performance liquid chromatography with fluorescence detection [6] has been reported for determination of rizatriptan in biological fluids. HPLC [7-9] and HPTLC [10] methods have also been used for quantitative determination of rizatriptan in bulk drug or pharmaceutical dosage forms. Furtheremore, few spectrophotometric methods were reported in the literature for the determination of rizatriptan in dosage forms [11-16]. Some of these methods are based on ion-pair complexation, redox-complexation reaction in the presence of iron ion and also oxidative coupling reactions. In most previously reported spectrophotometric methods a relatively narrow linear range or high limit of quantification has been obtained.

As rizatriptan is not official in USP or BP, there is still a demand for new simple, sensitive and rapid methods in order to determine the drug in pharmaceutical dosage forms. The present study deals with the development and validation of a sensitive extractive spectrophotometric method using bromocresol green (BCG) as ion-pair complexation reagent. The BCG reagent is relatively cheap and has been used before in our laboratory for determination of some other drugs [17-19]. Spectrophotometric methods are rapid, cost effective, simple and acceptable which use very routine and available instruments in every quality control laboratory. The validated method could be successfully used for routine quality control analysis without any special sample preparation before determination.

* Correspondence: souri@sina.tums.ac.ir
[1]Department of Medicinal Chemistry, Faculty of Pharmacy and Drug Design and Development Research Center, Tehran University of Medical Sciences, Tehran 14155-6451, Iran
Full list of author information is available at the end of the article

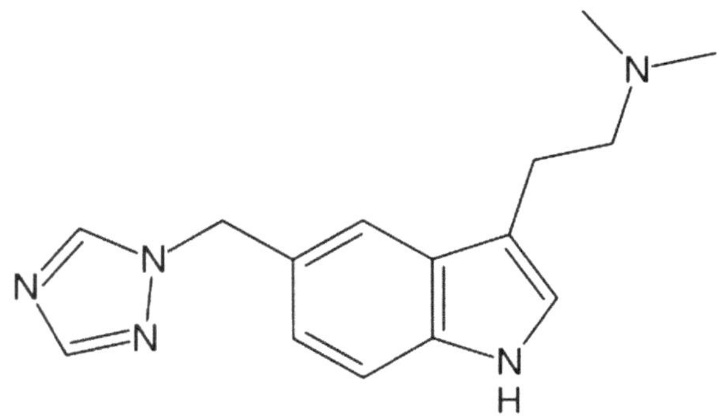

Figure 1 Chemical structure of rizatriptan.

Materials and methods

Apparatus

A double beam UV-visible spectrophotometer (UV-160, Shimadzu, Japan) in the wavelength range of 200–800 was used for spectrophotometric measurements.

A Waters HPLC system consisting of a Model 515 pump, a Model 717 plus Autosampler and a Model 486 UV-visible detector (All from Waters, Milford, USA) were used. Multi-channel Chrom&Spec software for chromatography (version 1.5×) was used for data processing.

Chemicals

Rizatriptan benzoate (purity 99.8%) was from Merck (Batch No: 000705126 0048038) and was kindly provided by Food and Drug Laboratory Research Center, Ministry of Health, Tehran, Iran. Bromocresol green (BCG) and the other analytical grade chemicals were purchased from Merck (Darmstadt, Germany).

Standard solutions

A standard solution of rizatriptan benzoate (5×10^{-4} M) was prepared by dissolving 13.5 mg of the drug in 100 ml of distilled water.

A 5×10^{-4} M solution of BCG was prepared by dissolving 349 mg of BCG in 1000 ml of distilled water by adding 2 ml of 0.1 M NaOH for better solubility.

The phosphate buffer (0.1 M) was prepared by dissolving 1.78 g of NaH_2PO_4 in 1000 ml of distilled water. The pH value was adjusted to 3.0.

The Britton- Robinson buffers in the pH range of 2–7 were prepared from an equal mixture of 0.1 M acetic acid, 0.1 M boric acid and 0.1 M phosphoric acid. The pH value was adjusted using a 1 M NaOH solution.

General procedure for sample preparation

An aliquot of 2 ml of rizatriptan solution (5×10^{-4} M), 1 ml of buffer solution (pH 3), 6 ml of BCG reagent (5×10^{-4} M), and 1 ml of distilled water were transferred to a 100 ml separating funnel. The mixture was extracted three times using 5, 3 and 2 ml portions of chloroform. The separating funnel was vigorously shacked for 30 seconds for extraction. The organic phase was separated and dehydrated by passing over anhydrous sodium sulfate and was transferred to a 10 ml volumetric flask. The volume was completed with chloroform and the absorbance was measured at 416 nm against a reagent blank.

Optimization of the reaction conditions

Selection of the optimum pH

The effect of pH on ion-pair complex formation was studied by using the general procedure and Britton-Robinson buffers in the range of 2–7. Also, different kinds of buffers (phthalate, acetate, phosphate) at the same pH value were studied to find out the effect of buffer type.

Selection of the reagent amount

Using 2 ml of rizatriptan solution (5×10^{-4} M) and 1 ml of phosphate buffer (pH 3.0), different amounts of BCG reagent (0.5–7 ml) were added and after extraction, the

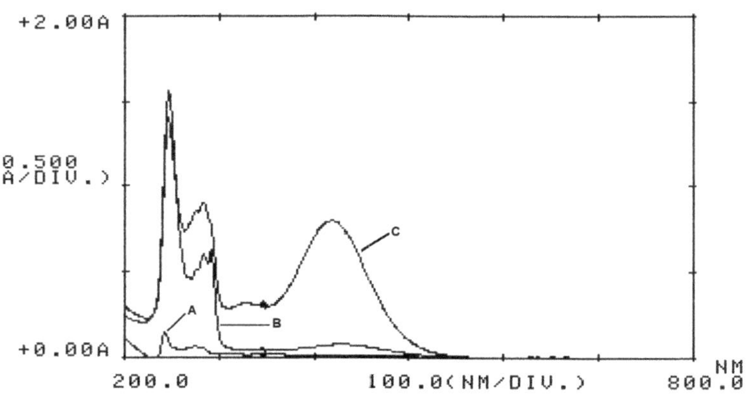

Figure 2 (A) Absorption spectra of rizatriptan, (B) BCG, and (C) the ion-pair complex of rizatriptan and BCG using 2 ml of rizatriptan (5×10^{-4} M) and 6 ml of BCG (5×10^{-4} M).

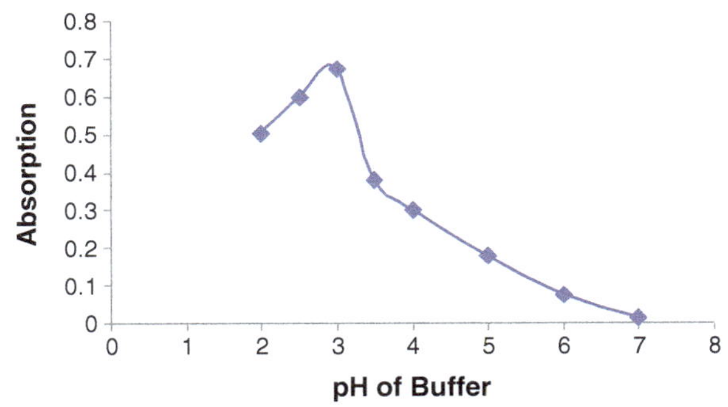

Figure 3 The effect of pH of the buffer (Britton-Rabinson) on the ion-pair complex formation using 2 ml of rizatriptan (5×10^{-4} M) and 4 ml of BCG (5×10^{-4} M).

absorbance of the resulting solution was measured at 416 nm.

Selection of the extracting solvent

To find out the best extracting solvent, chloroform; dichloromethane; ethyl acetate; and diethyl ether were used as extracting solvents and the absorbance of the resulting ion-pair complexes were compared.

The effect of the reaction time

The effect of time on the ion-pair complex formation was studied at various time intervals in the range of 0–60 min.

Stoichiometric relationship

The Job's method of continuous variations was applied to find out the stoichiometric ratio of the ion-pair complexation. Different volumes of rizatriptan and BCG, at equal molar concentrations (4×10^{-4} M), were mixed with a fixed total volume and the absorbance of the resulting ion-pair complex was measured according to the general procedure. The resulting absorbance was plotted over the mole ratio of rizatriptan.

Determination of rizatriptan in dosage forms

Twenty Rizatriptan tablets (5 mg) (Farabi Pharmaceutical Co, Iran) were finely powdered using a mortar and pestle. Next, an amount of the resulted power equivalent to one tablet (5 mg of rizatriptan) was accurately weighed and transferred to a 100 ml volumetric flask and about 70 ml of distilled water was added. The mixture was sonicated for 15 min and made up to volume by the same solvent. After filtration through a 0.45 μm syringe filter, the concentration of rizatriptan was measured according to the general procedure. The amount of rizatriptan was calculated by comparing the obtained absorbance with a standard solution at the same concentration. The same procedure was also performed for determination of rizatriptan by HPLC using a previously published method [20].

Relative recovery

The relative recovery of rizatriptan from dosage form was evaluated by standard addition method. Rizatriptan standard solution at concentration level of 40 μg/ml was added to a solution obtained from tablet powder equal to one tablet. After ion-pair complexation and according to the general procedure, the absorbance of this solution was compared with a standard solution at 40 μg/ml after subtraction of the absorbance of a tablet powder. The relative recovery was then calculated.

Linearity

Six series of rizatriptan solutions in the range of 0.5–50 μg/ml and also 10–100 μg/ml were prepared and the absorbance was measured according to the general procedure. The calibration curves were constructed and the statistical data were calculated. For calibration curves in the range of 0.5–50 μg/ml, 5 ml (instead of 2 ml) of rizatriptan solution were used.

Precision and accuracy

To find out the precision and accuracy, three sets of different solutions of rizatriptan at three different concentration levels for each calibration range were prepared in triplicate and measured for 3 days. The within-day and between-day precision and accuracy were calculated.

Results and discussion

Absorption spectra

The absorption spectra of the yellow ion-pair complex between rizatriptan and BCG extracted with chloroform measured in the range of 200–800 nm against the blank solution showed a maximum absorbance at 416 nm (Figure 2). This wavelength was used for spectrophotomertic measurements. No absorption was observed in the visible region for rizatriptan or BCG solutions alone. As the maximum absorbance of the formed ion-pair complex between rizatriptan and BCG was observed in

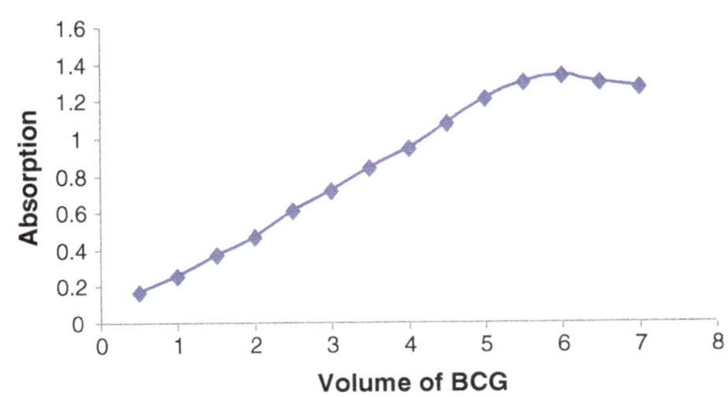

Figure 4 The effect of BCG (5×10^{-4} M) amount on the absorbance of the ion-pair complex at 416 nm using 2 ml of rizatriptan (5×10^{-4} M).

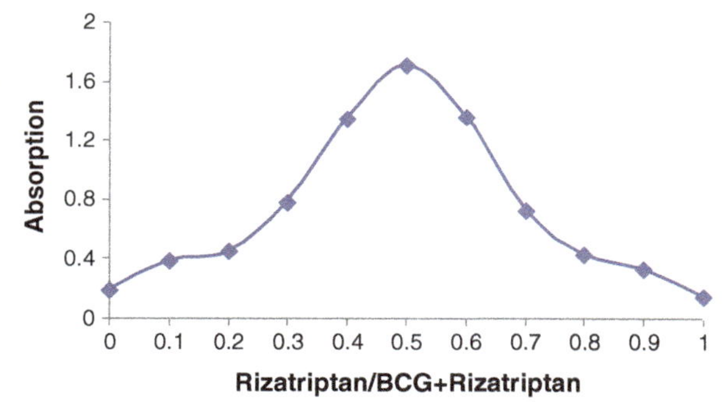

Figure 5 **Stoichiometry of the ion-pair complex of rizatriptan (4×10^{-4} M) and BCG (4×10^{-4} M) by Job's continuous variation method.**

Table 1 Statistical data of calibration curves of rizatriptan in standard solutions (n = 6)

Parameters	Low range	High range
Linearity range	0.50–50 μg/ml	10–100 μg/ml
Regression equation	y = 0.025x + 0.004	y = 0.0107x + 0.0036
Standard deviation of slope	0.00033	0.00016
Relative standard deviation of slope (%)	1.32	1.53
Standard deviation of intercept	0.0015	0.0097
Correlation coefficient (r^2)	0.9997	0.9998
Limit of Quantification (LOQ)	0.50	10.00
Limit of Detection (LOD)	0.17	3.33
Extinction coefficient (ε)	2.1×10^4	2.1×10^4

the visible region, the interference of the excipients was within the minimum range.

Selection of the suitable pH

The ion-pair complexation was performed according to the general procedure using Britton-Robinson buffer in the range of 2–7. The results are demonstrated in Figure 3. The maximum absorbance value was obtained at pH 3.0. Using different kinds of buffers (phthalate, Britton-Robinson or phosphate) at the same pH value, the best results were observed in the presence of 1 ml of phosphate buffer. It was also observed that higher absorption intensity was achieved when the buffer solution was added after rizatriptan and BCG solution.

Selection of the reagent amount

To achieve complete reaction and maximum absorbance, solutions of fixed concentrations of rizatriptan and varied volumes (0.5–7 ml) of the BCG reagent were tested. The results showed that maximum response was achieved by using 6 ml of BCG reagent (Figure 4). Higher amounts had no effect on the complex formation.

Selection of the extracting solvent

Different extracting solvents (chloroform, dichloromethane, diethyl ether and ethyl acetate) were used. Maximum absorbance and higher selective extraction of the ion-pair complex were achieved using chloroform as the extracting solvent. It was also found that three times extraction with 5, 3 and 2 ml of solvent produced better results in comparison to one time extraction with 10 ml of chloroform.

The effect of reaction time

Performing the ion-pair complexation in different time intervals (0, 5, 10, 20, 30 and 60 min), showed that the maximum absorbance was achieved immediately after mixing the rizatriptan solution and BCG reagent in the presence of buffer solution.

Stability of the ion-pair complex

The stability of the rizatriptan-BCG ion-pair complex was evaluated for 24 h at room temperature. The results showed that the formed complex was relatively stable for at least 8 h (recovery > 95%).

Composition of the ion-pair complex

The Job's method of continuous variations by using varied volumes of equimolar solutions of rizatriptan (4×10^{-4} M) and BCG (4×10^{-4} M) was employed to find out the stoichiometry of the ion-pair complex.

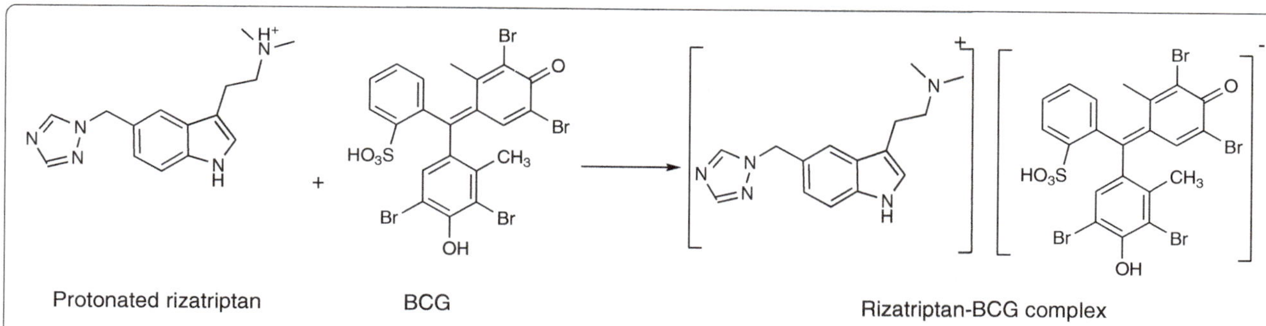

Figure 6 **Structure of the formed ion-pair complex of rizatriptan and BCG.**

Table 2 Precision and accuracy of the method for determination of rizatriptan in standard solutions (n=9; 3 sets for 3 days)

Concentration added (μg/ml)	Within-day (n=3)			Between-day (n=9)		
	Found (μg/ml)	CV (%)	Error (%)	Found (μg/ml)	CV (%)	Error (%)
0.50	0.49 ± 0.11	2.24	−2.00	0.49 ± 0.01	2.85	−2.00
5.00	5.01 ± 0.08	1.59	0.20	5.08 ± 0.10	1.96	1.60
50.00	50.32 ± 0.65	1.30	0.64	50.37 ± 0.88	1.75	0.74
10.00	9.86 ± 0.09	0.91	−1.40	9.94 ± 0.18	1.81	−0.60
50.00	49.83 ± 0.89	1.79	−0.34	50.33 ± 0.78	1.55	0.66
100.00	99.13 ± 1.52	1.53	−0.87	99.54 ± 1.79	1.80	−0.46

The absorbance was plotted over the mole ratio of rizatriptan (Figure 5). The plot reached a maximum value at a mole fraction of 0.5 which indicated an equimolar (1:1) basis of the ion-pair complexation. The proposed structure of the ion-pair complex is displayed in Figure 6.

Method validation

Linearity

The calibration curves in the range of 0.5–50 μg/ml and 10–100 μg/ml were linear according to the statistical parameters shown in Table 1. High values of correlation coefficient and small values of the intercept were achieved.

Precision and accuracy

The within-day and between-day precision and accuracy were evaluated for selected concentrations of rizatriptan in one day and three consecutive days. The results are summarized in Table 2. Low values of CV and error indicated the acceptable precision and accuracy of the proposed method.

Relative recovery

The relative recovery of rizatriptan from tablet samples was about 98 percent which showed no interferences from the excipients.

Application of the method

The proposed method was used for determination of rizatriptan in tablet dosage forms. The proposed spectrophotometric procedure was compared with a previously published HPLC method [20]. No significant differences ($p<0.05$) were observed using both methods.

Conclusion

The proposed spectrophotomertic method is relatively simple, rapid, and cost effective and it is also accurate and sensitive for determination of rizatriptan in bulk powder and tablet dosage forms. No special sample preparation is needed and no interferences from tablet excipients were observed. The limit of determination of this method is lower than other previously reported spectrophotometric methods. Therefore, the validated method could be useful for routine quality control assay of rizatriptan in pharmaceutical raw material and dosage forms.

Competing interests

There are no other conflicts of interest related to this publication.

Authors' contribution

All authors contributed to the concept and design, making and analysis of data, drafting, revising and final approval. ES is responsible for the study registration. AK has done the experiments. NA provides test samples, reference material and data analysis. ES and MA are responsible for interpretation and manuscript writing and administrative support. All authors read and approved the final manuscript.

Acknowledgement

This work was supported by grant from the Research Council of Tehran University of Medical Sciences.

Author details

[1]Department of Medicinal Chemistry, Faculty of Pharmacy and Drug Design and Development Research Center, Tehran University of Medical Sciences, Tehran 14155-6451, Iran. [2]Department of Pharmaceutics, Food and Drug Laboratory Research Center, Ministry of Health, Tehran, Iran.

References

1. Brunton L, Parler K, Blumenthal D, Buxton I: *Goodman and Gillman's Manual of Pharmacology and Therapeutics*. USA: McGraw-Hill Medical Publishing Division; 2008.
2. Barbanti P, Fofi L, Dall'Armi V, Aurilia C, Egeo G, Vanacore N, Bonassi S: **Rizatriptan in migraineurs with unilateral cranial autonomic symptoms: a double-blind trial.** *J Headache Pain* 2012, **13**:407–414.
3. Seeburger JL, Taylor FR, Friedman D, Newman L, Ge Y, Zhang Y, Hustad CM, Lasorda J, Fan X, Hewitt D, Ho T, Connor KM: **Efficacy and tolerability of rizatriptan for the treatment of acute migraine in sumatriptan non-responders.** *Cephalalgia* 2011, **31**:786–796.
4. Guo JF, Zhang AJ, Zhao L, Sun XH, Zhao YM, Gao HZ, Liu ZY, Qiao SY: **Determination of rizatriptan in human plasma by liquid chromatographic-electrospray tandem mass spectrometry: application to a pharmacokinetic study.** *Biomed Chromatogr* 2006, **20**:61–66.
5. Chen Y, Miao H, Lin M, Fan G, Hong Z, Wu H, Wu Y: **Development and validation of a selective and robust LC-MS/MS method for high-throughput quantifying rizatriptan in small plasma samples: Apllication to a clinical pharmacokinetic study.** *J Chromatogr B* 2006, **844**:268–277.
6. Chen J, Jiang X, Jiang W, Mei N, Gao X, Zhang Q: **Liquid chromatographic method for the determination of rizatriptan in human plasma.** *J Chromatogr B* 2004, **805**:169–173.

7. Mallikarjuna Rao B, Sangaraju S, Srinivasu MK, Madhavan P, Lalitha Devi M, Rajendra Kumar P, Chandrasekhar KB, Arpitha C, Satya Balaji J: **Development and validation of a specific stability indicating high performance liquid chromatographic method for rizatriptan benzoate.** *J Pharm Biomed Anal* 2006, **41**:1146–1151.
8. Joseph Sunder Raj T, Bharathi C, Saravana Kumar M, Prabahar J, Naveen Kumar P, Kumar Sharma H, Parikh K: **Identification, isolation and characterization of process-related impurities in rizatriptan benzoate.** *J Pharm Biomed Anal* 2009, **49**:156–162.
9. Ramzia IE-B, Nashwah GM, Heba AN: **Two chromatographic methods for the determination of some antimigraine drugs.** *Anal Chem Insights* 2012, **7**:13–20.
10. Syama Sundar B, Suneetha A: **Development and validation of HPLC method for the estimation of rizatriptan benzoate in bulk and tablets.** *Ind J Pharm Sci* 2010, **72**:798–801.
11. Khedkar A, Rajendra V, Kulkarni A, Dehghan MH, Saifee M, Lahoti S: **Spectrophotomertic method for analysis of rizatriptan benzoate.** *Int J Ph Sci* 2009, **1**:307–309.
12. Kumari AS, Subhasish S, Kaushik DK, Annapurna MM: **UV-spectroscopic methods for estimation of rizatriptan benzoate in pharmaceutical preparations.** *Int J ChemTech Res* 2010, **2**:653–659.
13. Shanmukha Kumar JV, Ramachandran D, Settaluri VS, Lakshmi Lavanya A, Shechinah Felice C: **Validation of analytical procedures for determination of rizatriptan benzoate.** *The Pharma Res* 2010, **4**:28–37.
14. Ramzia IE-B, Nashwah GM, Heba AN: **Fluorimetric and colorimetric methods for the determination of some antimigraine drugs.** *J Chem Pharm Res* 2011, **3**:304–314.
15. Shanmukha Kumar JV, Prasad KRS, Ramachandran D, Settaluri VS: **Development and validation of spectrophotometric methods for determination of maxalt (rizatriptan benzoate) in pure and pharmaceutical formulation.** *IJPI's Anal Chem* 2011, **1**:1–5.
16. Prashanth KN, Basavaiah K, Vinay KB: **Sensitive and selective spectrophotometric assay of rizatriptan benzoate in pharmaceuticals using three sulphonphthalein dyes.** *Arabian J Chem* 2011, in press.
17. Amanlou M, Khosraian P, Souri E, Ghorban Dadrass O, Dinarvand R, Alimord MM, Akbari H: **Determination of buprenorphine in raw material and pharmaceutical products using ion-pair formation.** *Bull Korean Chem Soc* 2007, **28**:183–187.
18. Amanlou M, Hoseinzadeh N, Azizan H, Souri E, Farsam H: **Determination of ketotifen fumarate in raw material and pharmaceutical products using ion-pair formation.** *Anal Letters* 2007, **40**:3267–3279.
19. Amanlou M, Souri E, Izady S, Farsam H: **Spectrophotometric determination of tropicamide in bulk and pharmaceutical formulations.** *IJPR* 2007, **3**:43–50.
20. Jagtap SS, Gopu CL, Mahadik KR, Mahadik MV: **Stability indication reversed-phase high-performance liquid chromatographic method for the determination of rizatriptan benzoate in bulk powder and in pharmaceutical formulations.** *Res J Pharm Biol Chem Sci* 2010, **1**:385–395.

Surface modification of PLGA nanoparticles via human serum albumin conjugation for controlled delivery of docetaxel

Saeed Manoochehri[1], Behrad Darvishi[1], Golnaz Kamalinia[2], Mohsen Amini[3], Mahdieh Fallah[4], Seyed Naser Ostad[5], Fatemeh Atyabi[1,2] and Rassoul Dinarvand[1,2*]

Abstract

Background: Poly lactic-co-glycolic acid (PLGA) based nanoparticles are considered to be a promising drug carrier in tumor targeting but suffer from the high level of opsonization by reticuloendothelial system due to their hydrophobic structure. As a result surface modification of these nanoparticles has been widely studied as an essential step in their development. Among various surface modifications, human serum albumin (HSA) possesses advantages including small size, hydrophilic surface and accumulation in leaky vasculature of tumors through passive targeting and a probable active transport into tumor tissues.

Methods: PLGA nanoparticles of docetaxel were prepared by emulsification evaporation method and were surface conjugated with human serum albumin. Fourier transform infrared spectrum was used to confirm the conjugation reaction where nuclear magnetic resonance was utilized for conjugation ratio determination. In addition, transmission electron microscopy showed two different contrast media in conjugated nanoparticles. Furthermore, cytotoxicity of free docetaxel, unconjugated and conjugated PLGA nanoparticles was studied in HepG2 cells.

Results: Size, zeta potential and drug loading of PLGA nanoparticles were about 199 nm, −11.07 mV, and 4%, respectively where size, zeta potential and drug loading of conjugated nanoparticles were found to be 204 nm, −5.6 mV and 3.6% respectively. Conjugated nanoparticles represented a three-phasic release pattern with a 20% burst effect for docetaxel on the first day. Cytotoxicity experiment showed that the IC50 of HSA conjugated PLGA nanoparticles (5.4 μg) was significantly lower than both free docetaxel (20.2 μg) and unconjugated PLGA nanoparticles (6.2 μg).

Conclusion: In conclusion surface modification of PLGA nanoparticles through HSA conjugation results in more cytotoxicity against tumor cell lines compared with free docetaxel and unconjugated PLGA nanoparticles. Albumin conjugated PLGA nanoparticles may represent a promising drug delivery system in cancer therapy.

Keywords: PLGA nanoparticles, Surface modification, Human serum albumin, Emulsion evaporation, Tumor targeting, Docetaxel

* Correspondence: dinarvand@tums.ac.ir
[1]Department of Pharmaceutics, Faculty of Pharmacy, Tehran University of Medical Sciences, Tehran 1417614411, Iran
[2]Nanotechnology Research Centre, Tehran University of Medical Sciences, Tehran, Iran
Full list of author information is available at the end of the article

Background

Polymeric nanoparticles are considered as one of the most promising carrier systems for cytotoxic drug delivery and have received a great deal of attention during the recent years. Poly lactic-co-glycolic acid (PLGA) based nanoparticulate system is one of the most successful and interesting colloidal systems. PLGA nanoparticles (NPs) protect the therapeutic agents and increase their stability and can be used for controlled delivery of therapeutics with improved pharmacokinetic and pharmacodynamic profile. Furthermore, PLGA is approved by United States Food and Drug Administration (FDA) and European Medicine Agency (EMA) for various drug delivery formulations. However, PLGA NPs, suffer from a significant limitation due to their high level of opsonization by reticuloendothelial system (RES) [1]. To address this negative aspect, several methods and procedures have been utilized for surface modification of PLGA NPs in order to produce PLGA based nanoparticulate systems which are not readily recognized by RES. This goal has been achieved by PLGA NPs surface coating with more hydrophilic agents to cover their hydrophobic surface and provide stealth nanoparticles. Various agents have been used for this purpose including polyethylene glycol (PEG), poloxamers and chitosan molecules to neutralize or reduce the negative zeta potential of PLGA NPs and reduce their phagocytosis by RES [2]. However, surface modified PLGA NPs have been found to highly localize in liver tissue due to the rigidity of the PLGA core which has triggered many research studies to improve surface modification methods for achieving better outcomes [3,4].

Among various available agents, human serum albumin (HSA) seems to be a promising molecule for surface modification of PLGA NPs. HSA is known to be the most abundant native protein in human body which has various advantages including ready availability, biodegradability, and low toxicity and immunogenicity [5]. HSA has received special interest in drug delivery studies due to its ability for passive targeting through enhanced permeation and retention (EPR) effect which is related to both "enhanced permeation" of macromolecules through the fenestrated structure of tumor vasculature in addition to an "enhanced retention" which is considered to be related to the lack of effective lymphatic drainage in tumor tissues [6]. Furthermore it has been postulated that active targeting of HSA coated nanoparticles occurs through special albumin receptors on tumor cell membranes [7].

Surface modification of PLGA NPs by grafting protein molecules has been previously reported and various proteins including transferrin and wheat germ agglutinin have been coated on the surface of PLGA NPs through covalent conjugation. The created stealth NPs have successfully increased the cellular uptake of PLGA NPs and have resulted in a greater antiproliferative activity and better cytotoxicity in vitro. In addition in vivo experiments have confirmed a higher tumor accumulation for the above surface coated NPs [8-10]. HSA coating by non-covalent interactions have also been studied where protein molecules only saturate the nanoparticles surface and no covalent linking occurs [11].

Herein, docetaxel (DTX), a cytostatic agent with very low water solubility was encapsulated in PLGA NPs produced by a modified emulsification evaporation method and was subjected to surface modification by HSA molecules through a carbodiimide conjugation reaction. Surface modification created a stealth core shell structure and was used to reduce the negative charge on PLGA NPs along with an increase in drug efficiency through passive targeting. These newly developed fully biodegradable HSA coated PLGA NPs can increase DTX water solubility and will eliminate the need for Tween 80 utilization in DTX formulations which has been taken responsible for many of DTX injections side effects including hypersensitivity reactions [12]. The nanoparticles were further evaluated for their cytotoxic effect in HepG2 cell line. The present evidences suggest that HSA stealth PLGA NPs may represent a promising nanoparticulate drug delivery system for DTX and other anticancer agents.

Methods

Materials

PLGA (50:50, 504H, MW = 48 kDa) was purchased from Boehringer-Ingelheim (Ingelheim, Germany). HSA, 1-ethy1-3-(3-dimethylaminopropyl) carbodiimide (EDC), N–hydroxysuccinimide (NHS) and 3-(4,5-dimethyathiazol-2-yl)-2,5-diphenyltetrazoliumbromide (MTT) were purchased from Sigma-Aldrich (St. Louis, MO, USA). Dulbecco's modified eagle's medium (DMEM), fetal bovine serum (FBS) and penicillin and streptomycin antibiotic mixture were obtained from Life technologies (grand Island, NY, USA).Polyvinyl alcohol (PVA) was obtained from Acros (Geel, Belgium). 2-(N-morpholinoethansulfonicacid) (MES) was purchased from Fluka (St. Louis, MO, USA). DTX was from Cipla (Mumbai, India). All other solvents and reagents unless otherwise stated were from Merck (Darmstadt, Germany).

Preparation of PLGA nanoparticles

PLGA NPs were fabricated using a modified emulsification/ evaporation method [12]. Briefly, PVA (0.5% w/w) was dissolved in deionized water providing the aqueous phase where MES buffer (50 mmol) was used for pH adjustment (pH = 5). In organic phase, PLGA and docetaxel were dissolved in mixtures with various ratios of acetone and dichloromethane and the resulting organic phase was slowly added to the aqueous phase using an ultrasonic probe (Misonix, USA) equipped with a microtip (power: 11 watt, time: 5 min). During sonication, the whole system was placed in an ice bath to prevent any loss of the oil phase due to evaporation and the mixture was magnetically stirred overnight. The experiment was conducted with 10% and 20% organic phase to water phase ratio to evaluate the effect of oil: water ratio on the formed nanoparticles characteristics. Purification of nanoparticles was achieved by three times centrifugation with a high speed centrifuge (21,000 g for 30 minutes) at 10°C (Sigma 3 K30, Ostrode, Germany) to remove any extra PVA from the NPs surface. The isolated NPs were then lyophilized into a fine cake.

Surface modification of PLGA NPs by HSA conjugation

PLGA NPs were conjugated with HSA through a carbodiimide coupling reaction. For this purpose, PLGA carboxylic functional groups were first activated through exposure with 15 mg EDC and 12 mg NHS for 5 h right after their preparation in a medium consisting of MES buffer (pH = 5, 50 mmol). The activated NPs were then purified by three times centrifugation (21,000 g for 30 minutes) at 10°C to remove any remnants of PVA, EDC and NHS.

The activated PLGA nanoparticles were then exposed to HSA solution in 40 ml phosphate buffered saline (PBS, pH = 7.4) with an equimolar concentration in a dropwise manner and under constant stirring. The conjugated NPs were then isolated by a centrifugation step (15,000 g for 30 minutes) at 10°C and the supernatant was removed. Conjugated NPs were then subjected to the lyophilization process for long term storage.

Determination of HSA conjugated PLGA NPs molecular structure

For determining the number of free carboxylic moieties in activated PLGA NPs and further calculation of the activation ratio a Bruker 500 MHz ^{1}H-NMR system (Bruker, Germany) was used and the resulting nuclear magnetic resonance (NMR) spectrum was utilized to characterize the substitution degree of activated PLGA.

Fourier transform infrared (FT-IR) spectroscopy was used to characterize the molecular structure of PLGA NPs conjugated with HSA and to confirm the structural changes occurred after HSA conjugation. Lyophilized samples were placed on KBr disks and their FT-IR spectra were recorded by a Nicolet (Magna IR-550, USA) spectrophotometer.

NPs characterization and morphology evaluation

PLGA and PLGA NPs conjugated with HSA were fully characterized and their size, poly dispersity index (PDI) and zeta potential were determined by dynamic light scattering (DLS) (Malvern Zetasizer, ZS, Malvern, UK).

To evaluate the particles morphology, PLGA NPs were coated with gold under vacuum conditions and their morphology was evaluated by scanning electron microscopy (SEM) (FE-SEM, S4160, Hitachi, Japan).

Furthermore, transmission electron microscope (TEM) (Zeiss EM10C, Carl Zeiss AG, Oberkochen, Germany) was used to evaluate the surface morphology of PLGA NPs conjugated with HSA.

Differential scanning calorimetry (DSC) was performed for PLGA NPs conjugated with HSA in addition to a physical mixture of PLGA, HSA and DTX with a Mettler DSC 823 unit (Mettler Toledo, Switzerland) and a Julabo thermocryostate model FT100Y (Julabo labortechnik, Germany) where Indium was utilized for instrument calibration. The scanning took place between 20 to 200°C with a thermal scan rate of 10°C per minute.

Determination of DTX concentration, drug loading and entrapment efficiency in nanoparticles

The extent of DTX loading in PLGA and PLGA NPs conjugated with HSA was investigated by a previously published method [13]. Briefly, a small amount of PLGA NPs (2 mg) was dispersed in 2 ml acetonitrile resulting in PLGA and DTX dissolution in acetonitrile medium. In the next step methanol was added to the above mixture and resulted in PLGA precipitation. This solution only contained DTX and was injected to high pressure liquid chromatography (HPLC) (Knauer apparatus model K-1001 Wellchrome (Berlin, Germany) equipped with a PDA K-2700 ultraviolet Detector (Knauer, Berlin, Germany). A C18 column (internal diameter: 0.46 cm, length: 25 cm, pore size: 5 μm, ODS 3-MZ, Germany) was used as stationary phase and acetonitrile: water mixture (65: 35) was used as the mobile phase. The analysis was performed in 230 nm wavelength at 25°C and DTX concentration was evaluated accordingly. Furthermore, "drug loading" which is calculated as the ratio between DTX (expressed as μg) and the PLGA NPs (expressed as mg) in addition to "entrapment efficiency" or the percent of drug loaded in PLGA nanoparticles to the initial amount of DTX were determined.

DTX release from PLGA nanoparticles

Dialysis technique was used to evaluate drug release from PLGA NPs [14]. A dialysis tube (molecular weight cut-off: 8 kDa) containing 2 mg of nanoparticles suspended in 5 ml PBS (pH = 7.4) was dipped in a medium consisting of 20 ml PBS (pH =7.4) containing 0.1% Tween 80 and was continuously stirred on a shaker incubator for over 14 days at 37°C. At selected time intervals, 15 mL of the medium was removed and the medium was replenished with freshly prepared PBS. The aliquots were then exposed to dichloromethane for liquid-liquid extraction of DTX. The extraction procedure was repeated three times and the extracted organic phase was evaporated and the remnants were dissolved in 200 μl acetonitrile and were subjected to

HPLC analysis. Drug release data were expressed as the percentage of the cumulative amount of drug release.

In vitro cytotoxicity of DTX encapsulated NPs

HepG2 (Human hepatocellular carcinoma) cells were obtained from Pasteur Institute of Iran (Tehran, Iran) and were cultivated and maintained in DMEM growth media supplemented with 10% FBS and 1% penicillin streptomycin antibiotic mixture. The cells were incubated at 37°C in a humidified atmosphere with 5% CO_2 and the culture media was exchanged every other day. Cells were seeded in 96 wells with a density of 1×10^4 cells per well and were incubated for 24 h to allow cellular attachment. Cells were then treated with different concentrations of free DTX, PLGA NPs and PLGA NPs conjugated with HSA for 96 hand were then exposed to 20 μL of MTT reagent (5 mg/mL per well) for an additional 4 h. The culture media was then discarded and 200 μL dimethylsulfoxide was added to each well to dissolve the formed formazan crystals. Optical density was then measured at 570 nm with a 660 nm background using a microplate reader (Anthos 2020; Anthos Labtec Instruments, Wals, Austria). Each experiment was performed in triplicate and cellular viability was expressed as the percentage of viable cells to control. IC50 was calculated from the cell viability data as the drug concentration in which cell growth was inhibited by 50%. Furthermore similar MTT assays were performed with drug free PLGA NPs and conjugated PLGA NPs with HSA to assess any intrinsic carrier toxicity.

Results and Discussion

PLGA nanoparticles preparation and characterization

PLGA nanoparticles were prepared by a modified emulsification evaporation method (Figure 1). In this method the organic phase solution containing DTX and PLGA provides the oil phase (O) and PVA aqueous solution serves as the water phase (W) in an O/W emulsion. Physical sonication induction reduces the size of nano droplets in this emulsion. The particulate characteristics of prepared PLGA NPs in addition to their drug loading and entrapment efficiency are shown in Table 1. As it is observed PLGA NPs had an average size of 180 to 221 nm and were monodispersed as confirmed by their PDI amounts which was less than or equal to 0.23. Nanoparticles drug loading was achieved by drug incorporation into PLGA NPs during the production process and a maximum 5.35% drug loading with about 48% entrapment efficiency was achieved. The formed NPs carried a negatively charged zeta potential of about -11mv.

Size is the most important and effective parameter in determining the cellular uptake and biological functions of colloidal systems where a reduced size will usually result in significantly better uptake of nanoparticles by tumor cells [15]. It has been demonstrated that emulsion fabrication is the most critical step during the preparation of nanoparticles where the size of emulsion droplets is directly relevant to the final nanoparticles size [16,17]. Various factors may affect the size of PLGA NPs including the stabilizer type and the oil phase solvent mixture composition.

The oil phase solvent mixture here was composed of various ratios of dichloromethane and acetone. As shown in Figure 2A, nanoparticles size decreased as a result of reducing the acetone to dichloromethane ratio in the oil phase mixture where the smallest size was achieved by a 40:60 (acetone: dichloromethane) ratio. This may be due to a decrease in the interfacial tension between the oil phase and aqueous phase with increasing the portion of acetone in the oil phase mixture. It has been reported that

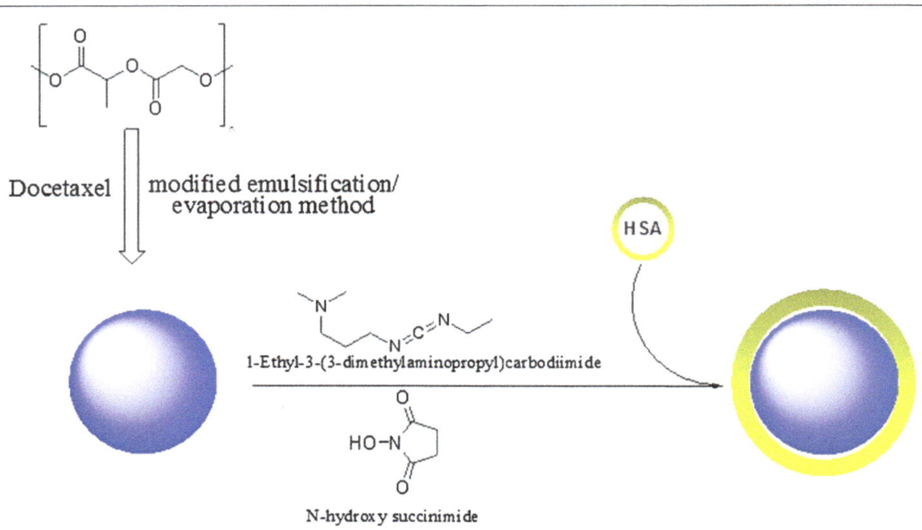

Figure 1 PLGA and conjugated PLGA nanoparticles with HSA formation process.

Table 1 PLGA nanoparticles and PLGA nanoparticles conjugated with HSA characteristics (DCM: dichloromethane, O: oil phase, W: water phase, HSA: human serum albumin, PLGA: Poly (lactic-co-glycolic acid), PDI: polydispersity index and EE: entrapment efficiency)

Sample	Acetone: DCM	O:W ratio (%)	HSA:PLGA	Size (nm)	PDI	Zeta potential (mv)	E.E (%)	Loading (μg/mg)
1	2.5:97.5	20	-	221 ± 25	0.23 ± 0.02	−13.48 ± 1.8	18.5 ± 2.1	2.06 ± 0.18
2	10:90	20	-	195 ± 19	0.15 ± 0.01	−11.71 ± 2.1	25.2 ± 1.8	2.8 ± 0.41
3	20:80	20	-	188 ± 28	0.14 ± 0.01	−15.32 ± 2.3	9.3 ± 1.6	1.0 ± 0.2
4	40:60	20	-	180 ± 29	0.20 ± 0.02	−11.13 ± 1.9	6.2 ± 1.1	0.7 ± 0.05
5	5:95	10	-	204 ± 20	0.15 ± 0.02	−11.52 ± 1.5	13.5 ± 1.1	1.5 ± 0.1
6	10:90	10	-	199 ± 22	0.17 ± 0.01	−11.07 ± 1.8	48.2 ± 2.3	5.35 ± 0.33
7	20:80	10	-	189 ± 19	0.18 ± 0.02	−9.83 ± 1.3	9.46 ± 1.4	1.05 ± 0.07
8	30:70	10	-	186 ± 22	0.16 ± 0.01	−11.08 ± 1.4	2.8 ± 0.7	0.3 ± 0.03
9	40:60	10	-	180 ± 21	0.20 ± 0.02	−11.02 ± 1.7	7.6 ± 1.5	0.85 ± 0.1
10	10:90	10	50:50	204 ± 15	0.14 ± 0.01	−5.6 ± 0.21	33.7 ± 2.6	3.62 ± 0.42
11	10:90	10	75:25	221 ± 24	0.17 ± 0.01	−5.45 ± 0.24	34.2 ± 2.1	3.53 ± 0.37

during the emulsification process the two organic and aqueous phases are not in equilibrium and the acetone concentration is not homogenous at the interface of oil and water phases. Acetone diffuses through the higher viscosity oil phase resulting in an acetone concentration gradient which creates some perturbation and turbulence in the interface of the two phases. This perturbation further results in a larger interface area between the oil droplets and aqueous medium and creates extremely fine nano droplets which result in the formation of small sized nanoparticles. The interfacial tension decrease between the oil and water phases due to the presence of acetone in the organic solvent mixture in addition to acetone passive diffusion from nano droplets and the subsequent spontaneous mixing will result in PLGA NPs formation with a much smaller size [17].

Besides the size of NPs, loading and entrapment efficiency are also affected by acetone to dichloromethane ratio. As it is observed in Figure 2B, loading is decreased with increasing the acetone: dichloromethane ratio from 10:90 to 40:60. In addition entrapment efficiency shows the same trend and a decrease in this parameter is observed with increasing acetone to dichloromethane ratio. DTX has poor water solubility and favors the organic phase during oil in water emulsion preparation. This higher drug affinity to the oil core results in a higher drug loading and better entrapment efficiency [18]. However when acetone to dichloromethane ratio is very low, both loading and entrapment efficiency are significantly decreased which may be related to the high DTX solubility in acetone solutions [19]. On the other hand when acetone to dichloromethane ratio is increased, some of the drug molecules dissolved in the oil core may disperse out along with acetone. This results in some sort of drug leak and will decrease the drug loading [17].

In addition to the oil phase composition, the ratio of oil to water is another factor which may impact the evaporation phase and nanoparticles formation process. Decreasing the

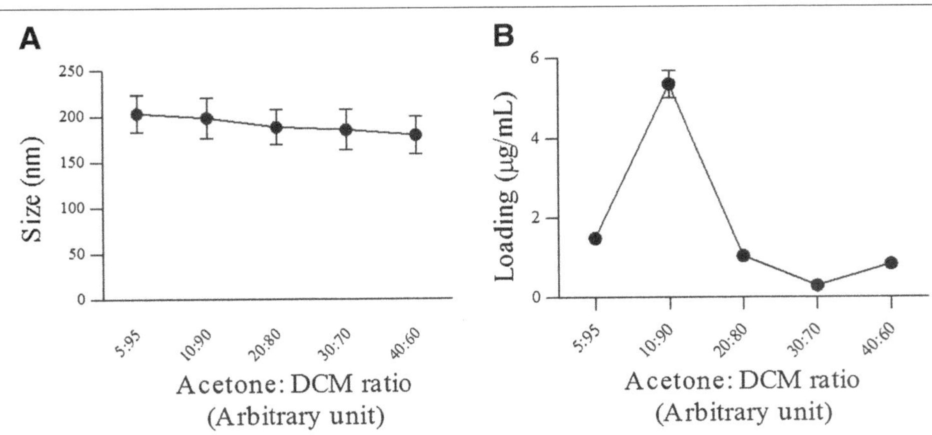

Figure 2 The effect of acetone to dichloromethane ratio on PLGA nanoparticles size (A) and drug loading (B).

oil to water ratio from 20% to 10% has mildly increased the nanoparticles size along with a slight increase in their entrapment efficiency and drug loading (Table 1). It has been postulated that when the aqueous phase volume is increased in relation to oil phase, the droplets external energy which is the cause of droplets breakage is distributed in a higher volume and a lower droplet breakage and an elevated particle size will be achieved [20,21].

Nanoparticles stabilization and protection of the droplets is another important step in the emulsification process which is achieved by addition of surfactant molecules. These surfactants prevent drops coalescence and result in a better size. In this study 0.5% PVA was used as a stabilizer to create a cover between organic and aqueous phases interface and provide effective stabilization [22,23].

PLGA NPs size and morphology was further evaluated by SEM microscopy which showed roughly spherical particles (Figure 3). It is noteworthy that NPs showed a larger size when evaluated by DLS compared to SEM images which may be due to the swelling of particles when dispersed in the aqueous medium [16].

Characterization of PLGA nanoparticles conjugated with HSA

HSA was conjugated to carboxylic functional groups on PLGA structure through a carbodiimide meditated coupling reaction Figure 1). FT-IR spectra of PLGA, HSA, their physical mixture and PLGA NPs conjugated with HSA are shown in Figure 4. As it can be seen, free PLGA ester and acid bonds absorption peaks can be observed in 1760 (cm^{-1}) and 1713 (cm^{-1}). In free HSA the amide bond stretch region was observed in 1650 (cm^{-1}). When HSA conjugated PLGA nanoparticles spectrum was evaluated, 1760 (cm^{-1}), 1713 (cm^{-1}) and 1650 (cm^{-1}) absorption peaks were observed which confirms the presence of both PLGA and HSA structures in the conjugated NPs.

Activated PLGA NPs structure was further evaluated by its ^1H NMR spectra to predict the ratio of covalently conjugated carboxylic functional groups on PLGA NPs. For this purpose area under the curve of NHS peak at 2.0 ppm was compared with area under the curve of PLGA peaks at 5.4, 4.9 and 1.5 ppm in activated PLGA NMR spectra. It was found that about 30% of PLGA carboxylic acid moieties were involved in PLGA activation reaction where about 70% of carboxylic functional groups remained free. This suggests a 30% conjugation ratio between PLGA and HSA.

To further evaluate HSA conjugated PLGA nanoparticles, size and zeta potential of these particles were evaluated and were compared with unconjugated PLGA NPs (Table 1). As it is observed, the size of PLGA NPs conjugated with HSA was slightly increased in comparison to PLGA NPs.

Zeta potential which is another important nanoparticle characteristic and can influence particle stability and cell adhesion was also measured in PLGA NPs conjugated with HSA [24]. As shown in Table 1, the zeta potential of PLGA NPs conjugated with HSA showed a negative zeta potential, which was smaller than that of PLGA NPs (-11.07 ± 1.8 mV vs. -5.6 ± 0.21 mV). This decrease in negative zeta potential is probably due to the involvement of carboxylic functional groups on PLGA NPs in amide bond formation with amino moieties on lysine amino acids in HSA primary structure [25].

Entrapment efficiency and loading of PLGA NPs and PLGA NPs conjugated with HSA are shown in Table 1. As it is shown, the entrapment efficiency and drug loading in PLGA NPs conjugated with HSA were slightly less than PLGA NPs.

PLGA NPs morphology was evaluated by TEM imaging (Figure 5). As it is observed PLGA NPs were almost spherical with a size of about 200 nm where HSA conjugated NPs showed a slightly larger size. PLGA NPs were uniform but a notable outer layer was observed in

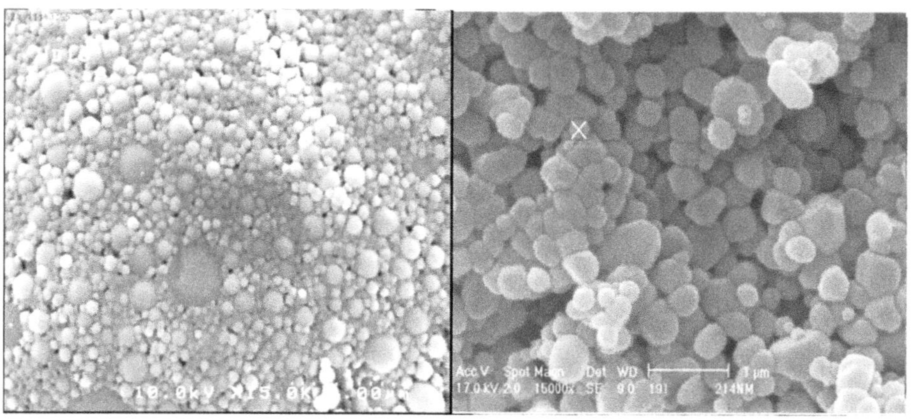

Figure 3 Poly (lactic-co-glycolic acid) (PLGA) nanoparticles morphology acquired by scanning electron microscopy with 15,000 times magnification.

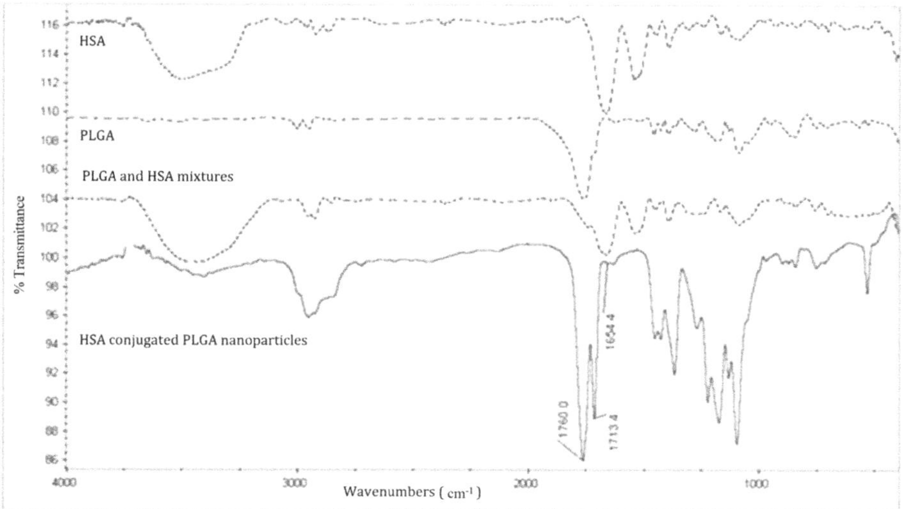

Figure 4 **FT-IR spectrum of HSA, PLGA, their physical mixture and PLGA NPs conjugated with HSA (PLGA major absorption peaks are observed in 1760 (cm^{-1}) and 1713 (cm^{-1}) where HSA major absorption peak comes in 1650 (cm^{-1})).**

conjugated NPs. It seems that HSA, have formed a mushroom structure on NPs surface which is in accordance with the predicted core-shell structure and may be able to prevent PLGA NPs opsonization more effectively [26].

Drug polymer mixtures may exist in various forms and structures for example amorphous or crystalline drug in combination with an amorphous or crystalline polymer [27]. DSC was utilized here to examine the thermal transitions in PLGA NPs and PLGA NPs conjugated with HSA.

Figure 6 shows DSC thermograms of PLGA, DTX, HSA, PLGA NPs and PLGA NPs conjugated with HSA in addition to a physical mixture of PLGA, DTX and HSA. As it can be seen, PLGA has an endothermic glassy transition temperature around 50°C. Glassy transition endothermic process for HSA conjugated NPs was observed at about 60°C. In the physical mixture thermogram a peak is observed in 160°C which stands for DTX melting point peak in its crystalline form. This peak is not observed in PLGA NPs and PLGA NPs conjugated with HSA which suggests an absence of crystallinity and an amorphous structure for DTX molecules in these NPs [28,29].

DTX release pattern from PLGA and HSA conjugated PLGA NPs

Various factors may affect drug release behavior from PLGA NPs including the polymer type and composition and drug-polymer interactions. In vitro drug release pattern from PLGA and PLGA NPs conjugated with HSA is shown as the cumulative percentage of release in Figure 7. DTX release from PLGA NPs followed a bi-phasic pattern. As shown in Figure 7, a burst release occurs within 10 h when roughly 40% of the drug was released from the

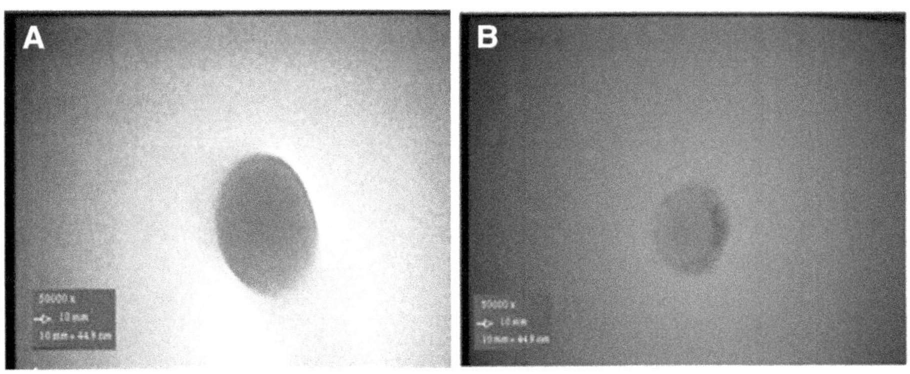

Figure 5 **Appearance of A) PLGA nanoparticle and B) PLGA nanoparticle conjugated with HSA acquired by transmission electron microscopy with 50,000 times magnification (Conjugation has occurred in the surface of PLGA nanoparticles where phase contrast is clearly observe).**

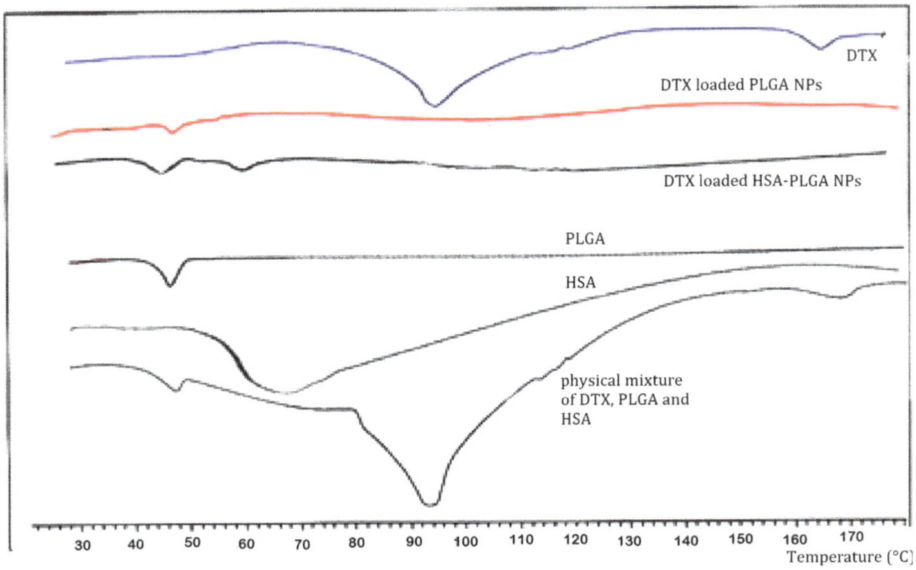

Figure 6 DSC thermograms of PLGA, HSA, DTX and DTX loaded in PLGA NP conjugated with HSA (Peaks of PLGA, HSA, and DTX was observed at 48°C, 60°C and 160°C. In DTX encapsulated HSA-PLGA nanoparticles, PLGA peak was observed at 48°C, HSA peak was observed at 60°C and no peak was observed at 160°C indicating the amorphous structure of DTX in this nanoparticulate formulation).

nanoparticles. The rest of DTX was released with a slower rate within 12 days. This initial burst release may be related to the portion of DTX molecules which are adsorbed on nanoparticle's surface and the diffusion controlled drug dissolution of drug molecules at nanoparticles and medium interface [30]. In addition the release of DTX molecules which are encapsulated near the surface of PLGA NPs may also contribute in this initial burst release. The slower second phase is related to the entrapped DTX inside the polymeric NPs.

The release profile of DTX from PLGA NPs conjugated with HSA exhibited a three-phasic pattern (Figure 7). 20% initial burst release occurred at the first day and in the next 8 days 75% of DTX was released. The rest of the drug was eventually released within 4 days. Comparing the release pattern of these two nanoparticles demonstrated that the release rate of DTX from conjugated NPs was slower and followed a three phasic pattern including an initial burst phase, a second release phase and a much slower final drug release phase.

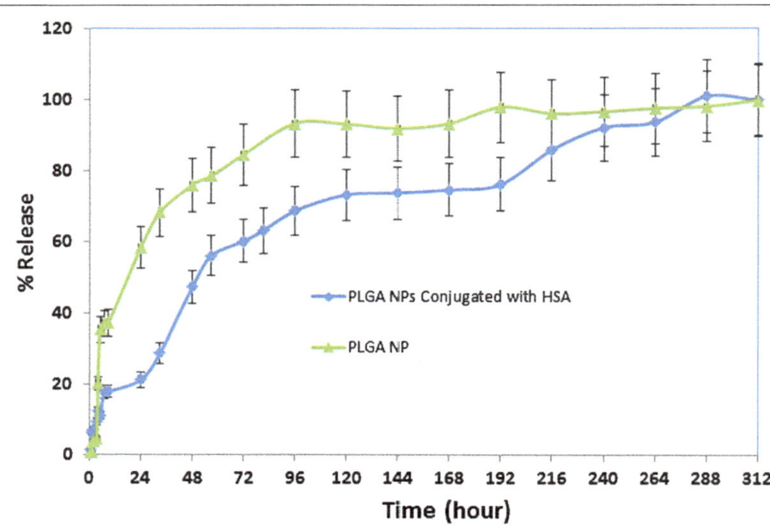

Figure 7 DTX release pattern from PLGA NPs and PLGA NPs conjugated with HSA in PBS medium (pH = 7.4). In PLGA NPs, 40% burst release of DTX occurred in the first 10 hours. The drug was then released slowly within 12 days (green line); In PLGA NPs conjugated with HSA, 20% burst release of DTX occurred within 24 hours and the overall release rate was much slower compared to PLGA NPs (blue line).

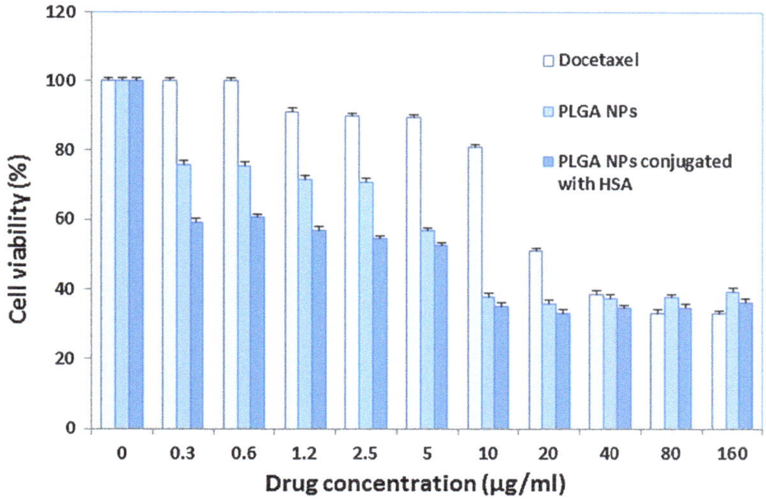

Figure 8 Cell viability in HepG2 cell line in exposure to free DTX, DTX encapsulated PLGA NPs and DTX encapsulated HSA-PLG NPs with various concentrations against Hep-G2 assessed by MTT assay (n = 3).

The graph shows that surface treatment with HSA molecules has resulted in a reduced initial burst where only 20% of drug is released during the first 24 h from HSA conjugated NPs in comparison to around 60% in unconjugated NPs. This lower burst effect is probably due to a decrease in the amount of drug which is adsorbed on the surface of conjugated NPs [9].

In vitro cytotoxicity assay

To assess the cellular cytotoxicity of PLGA NPs and PLGA NPs conjugated with HSA, HepG2 cell line was used. HepG2 cell line has been recognized as a suitable model for cytotoxicity evaluating studies [31]. Following 72 h of exposure to both unconjugated and conjugated NPs, cell viability was assessed by MTT assay and IC50 values of free DTX and its formulations were estimated from the results as presented in Figure 8. The IC50 of free DTX, PLGA NPs and PLGA NPs conjugated with HSA were 20.2 ± 0.28, 6.2 ± 0.23 and 5.4 ± 0.21 µg respectively after 72 h incubation with the cell line ($n = 3$). These results may be explained by drug release pattern of various PLGA particulate formulations and their degradation profiles. When DTX is encapsulated in PLGA or PLGA NPs conjugated with HSA a higher DTX concentration may be delivered to the intracellular space which may be the result of the small size of nanoparticles and the passive targeting of macromolecules due to EPR effect. As a result a better efficacy and a lower IC50 is observed for HSA conjugated with PLGA NPs [32].

It should be mentioned that in PLGA NPs conjugated with HSA, the outer layer, HSA, creates a stealth surface which reduces NPs interaction (both interactions between NPs and interaction between cells and NPs) [33].

It is noteworthy that no cellular cytotoxic effect was observed when drug free PLGA NPs and drug free PLGA NPs conjugated with HSA were exposed to HepG2 cell line which confirms these carriers safety.

Conclusions

In this study surface modified PLGA NPs with HSA were developed to prepare a novel drug delivery particulate system which may preferentially target tumor tissues through passive targeting. Specific features of HSA such as its biocompatibility and accumulation in inflamed and tumor tissues make it a good candidate for surface functionalization of carriers. Herein, PLGA NPs conjugated with HSA were developed and fully characterized. The newly developed NPs had an acceptable size and zeta potential and showed promising results in cell culture investigation where a lower IC50 was observed for the conjugated nanoparticles in comparison with free DTX and unconjugated PLGA NPs. It seems that surface modification of PLGA NPs with human serum albumin may represent a promising approach for nanoparticulate delivery system for cytostatic agent delivery.

Competing interests

The authors declare that they have no competing interests.

Authors' contributions

SM conceived the study, carried out the experiments and drafted the manuscript. BD helped with the characterization of the nanoparticles, GK reviewed and revised the manuscript. MA supervised the synthesis and characterization of copolymers, MF assisted in preparation of the manuscript, SNO supervised the MTT assay and cell culture study, FA co-supervised the study, RD designed, coordinated and supervised the study and is the corresponding author of the manuscript. All authors read and approved the final manuscript.

Acknowledgements
This paper is the outcome of a PhD thesis of the first author and was financially supported by Nanotechnology Research Centre, Faculty of Pharmacy, Tehran University of Medical Sciences.

Author details
[1]Department of Pharmaceutics, Faculty of Pharmacy, Tehran University of Medical Sciences, Tehran 1417614411, Iran. [2]Nanotechnology Research Centre, Tehran University of Medical Sciences, Tehran, Iran. [3]Department of Medicinal Chemistry, Faculty of Pharmacy, Tehran University of Medical Sciences, Tehran, Iran. [4]Arash Hospital, Faculty of Medicine, Tehran University of Medical Sciences, Tehran, Iran. [5]Department of Toxicology and Pharmacology, Faculty of Pharmacy, Tehran University of Medical Sciences, Tehran, Iran.

References

1. Dinarvand R, Sepehri N, Manoochehri S, Rouhani H, Atyabi F: **Polylactide-co-glycolide nanoparticles for controlled delivery of anticancer agents.** *Int J Nanomedicine* 2011, **6**:877.
2. Danhier F, Ansorena E, Silva JM, Coco R, Le Breton A, Préat V: **PLGA-based nanoparticles: an overview of biomedical applications.** *J Control Release* 2012, **161**:505–522.
3. Chung YI, Kim JC, Kim YH, Tae G, Lee SY, Kim K, Kwon IC: **The effect of surface functionalization of PLGA nanoparticles by heparin-or chitosan-conjugated Pluronic on tumor targeting.** *J Control Release* 2010, **143**:374–382.
4. Park J, Mattessich T, Jay SM, Agawu A, Saltzman WM, Fahmy TM: **Enhancement of surface ligand display on PLGA nanoparticles with amphiphilic ligand conjugates.** *J Control Release* 2011, **156**:109–115.
5. Kratz F: **Albumin as a drug carrier: design of prodrugs, drug conjugates and nanoparticles.** *J Control Release* 2008, **132**:171–183.
6. Maeda H, Wu J, Sawa T, Matsumura Y, Hori K: **Tumor vascular permeability and the EPR effect in macromolecular therapeutics: a review.** *J Control Release* 2000, **65**:271–284.
7. Taheri A, Atyabi F, Nouri FS, Ahadi F, Derakhshan MA, Amini M, Ghahremani MH, Ostad SN, Mansoori P, Dinarvand R: **Nanoparticles of conjugated methotrexate-human serum albumin: preparation and cytotoxicity evaluations.** *J Nanomaterials* 2011, **2011**:5.
8. Sahoo SK, Labhasetwar V: **Enhanced antiproliferative activity of transferrin-conjugated paclitaxel-loaded nanoparticles is mediated via sustained intracellular drug retention.** *Mol Pharm* 2005, **2**:373–383.
9. Shah N, Chaudhari K, Dantuluri P, Murthy R, Das S: **Paclitaxel-loaded PLGA nanoparticles surface modified with transferrin and Pluronic® P85, an in vitro cell line and in vivo biodistribution studies on rat model.** *J Drug Target* 2009, **17**:533–542.
10. Mo Y, Lim LY: **Paclitaxel-loaded PLGA nanoparticles: potentiation of anticancer activity by surface conjugation with wheat germ agglutinin.** *J Control Release* 2005, **108**:244–262.
11. Bazile D, Ropert C, Huve P, Verrecchia T, Mariard M, Frydman A, Veillard M, Spenlehauer G: **Body distribution of fully biodegradable [^{14}C]-poly (lactic acid) nanoparticles coated with albumin after parenteral administration to rats.** *Biomaterials* 1992, **13**:1093–1102.
12. Esmaeili F, Dinarvand R, Ghahremani MH, Ostad SN, Esmaily H, Atyabi F: **Cellular cytotoxicity and in-vivo biodistribution of docetaxel poly (lactide-co-glycolide) nanoparticles.** *Anticancer Drugs* 2010, **21**:43.
13. Esmaeili F, Hosseini-Nasr M, Rad-Malekshahi M, Samadi N, Atyabi F, Dinarvand R: **Preparation and antibacterial activity evaluation of rifampicin-loaded poly lactide-co-glycolide nanoparticles.** *Nanomedicine* 2007, **3**:161–167.
14. D'Souza SS, DeLuca PP: **Development of a dialysis in vitro release method for biodegradable microspheres.** *AAPS PharmSciTech* 2005, **6**:E323–E328.
15. He C, Hu Y, Yin L, Tang C, Yin C: **Effects of particle size and surface charge on cellular uptake and biodistribution of polymeric nanoparticles.** *Biomaterials* 2010, **31**:3657–3666.
16. Manchanda R, Fernandez-Fernandez A, Nagesetti A, McGoron AJ: **Preparation and characterization of a polymeric (PLGA) nanoparticulate drug delivery system with simultaneous incorporation of chemotherapeutic and thermo-optical agents.** *Colloids Surf B Biointerfaces* 2010, **75**:260–267.
17. Niwa T, Takeuchi H, Hino T, Kunou N, Kawashima Y: **Preparations of biodegradable nanospheres of water-soluble and insoluble drugs with D, L-lactide/glycolide copolymer by a novel spontaneous emulsification solvent diffusion method, and the drug release behavior.** *J Control Release* 1993, **25**:89–98.
18. Feng L, Wu H, Ma P, Mumper RJ, Benhabbour SR: **Development and optimization of oil-filled lipid nanoparticles containing docetaxel conjugates designed to control the drug release rate in vitro and in vivo.** *Int J Nanomedicine* 2011, **6**:2545.
19. Zaske L, Perrin MA, Leveiller F: **Docetaxel: solid state characterization by X-ray powder diffraction and thermogravimetry.** *Le Journal de Physique IV* 2001, **11**:Pr20-221–Pr210-226.
20. Budhian A, Siegel SJ, Winey KI: **Haloperidol-loaded PLGA nanoparticles: systematic study of particle size and drug content.** *Int J Pharm* 2007, **336**:367–375.
21. Song X, Zhao Y, Wu W, Bi Y, Cai Z, Chen Q, Li Y, Hou S: **PLGA nanoparticles simultaneously loaded with vincristine sulfate and verapamil hydrochloride: systematic study of particle size and drug entrapment efficiency.** *Int J Pharm* 2008, **350**:320–329.
22. Mainardes RM, Evangelista RC: **PLGA nanoparticles containing praziquantel: effect of formulation variables on size distribution.** *Int J Pharm* 2005, **290**:137–144.
23. Quintanar-Guerrero D, Fessi H, Allemann E, Doelker E: **Influence of stabilizing agents and preparative variables on the formation of poly (D, L-lactic acid) nanoparticles by an emulsification-diffusion technique.** *Int J Pharm* 1996, **143**:133–141.
24. Chen H, Yang W, Liu L, Gao F, Yang X, Jiang Q, Zhang Q, Wang Y: **Surface modification of mitoxantrone-loaded PLGA nanospheres with chitosan.** *Colloids Surf B Biointerfaces* 2009, **73**:212–218.
25. Misra R, Sahoo SK: **Intracellular trafficking of nuclear localization signal conjugated nanoparticles for cancer therapy.** *Eur J Pharm Sci* 2010, **39**:152–163.
26. Hu Y, Xie J, Tong YW, Wang CH: **Effect of PEG conformation and particle size on the cellular uptake efficiency of nanoparticles with the HepG2 cells.** *J Control Release* 2007, **118**:7–17.
27. Esmaeili F, Ghahremani MH, Esmaeili B, Khoshayand MR, Atyabi F, Dinarvand R: **PLGA nanoparticles of different surface properties: preparation and evaluation of their body distribution.** *Int J Pharm* 2008, **349**:249–255.
28. Musumeci T, Ventura CA, Giannone I, Ruozi B, Montenegro L, Pignatello R, Puglisi G: **PLA/PLGA nanoparticles for sustained release of docetaxel.** *Int J Pharm* 2006, **325**:172–179.
29. Yallapu MM, Gupta BK, Jaggi M, Chauhan SC: **Fabrication of curcumin encapsulated PLGA nanoparticles for improved therapeutic effects in metastatic cancer cells.** *J Colloid Interface Sci* 2010, **351**:19–29.
30. Magenheim B, Levy M, Benita S: **A new in vitro technique for the evaluation of drug release profile from colloidal carriers-ultrafiltration technique at low pressure.** *Int J Pharm* 1993, **94**:115–123.
31. Yoo HS, Oh JE, Lee KH, Park TG: **Biodegradable nanoparticles containing doxorubicin-PLGA conjugate for sustained release.** *Pharm Res* 1999, **16**:1114–1118.
32. Senthilkumar M, Mishra P, Jain NK: **Long circulating PEGylated poly (D, L-lactide-co-glycolide) nanoparticulate delivery of Docetaxel to solid tumors.** *J Drug Target* 2008, **16**:424–435.
33. Panyam J, Labhasetwar V: **Dynamics of endocytosis and exocytosis of poly (D, L-lactide-co-glycolide) nanoparticles in vascular smooth muscle cells.** *Pharm Res* 2003, **20**:212–220.

Protective effects of *Scrophularia striata* in Ovalbumin-induced mice asthma model

Abbas Azadmehr[1,4], Reza Hajiaghaee[2*], Mohammad Ali Zohal[3] and Ghorban Maliji[5]

Abstract

Background: *Scrophularia striata* Boiss. (Scrophulariaceae) is a plant growing in the northeastern part of Iran and being used as a traditional herb for various inflammatory disorders.
This study was designed to investigate the protective effects of the *Scrophularia striata* extract in Ovalbumin (OVA) induced-asthma mice model.

Methods: OVA-sensitized mice were intrapritonealy treated with two doses (100 and 200 mg/kg) of the extract on days 8 to 14 separately. Broncoalveolar lavage fluids (BALF) was collected 48 h after the final OVA challenge and then the number of eosinophils and other inflammatory cells were assessed by direct microscopic counting. In addition, total immunoglubolin (Ig) E and OVA-specific IgE levels in serum, IL-4 and IL-5 cytokines in BALF were determined by Enzyme-Linked Immunosorbent Assay. Moreover, phytochemical assay by thin layer chromatography (TLC) and the 2, 2 diphenyl-1-picrylhydrazyl (DPPH) were used to evaluate the main compounds and the antioxidant capacity of the plant extract, respectively.

Results: The results showed that the main components; including flavonoids, phenolic compounds and phenyl propanoids were presented in the *S. striata* extract. In addition, the treatment with extract significantly reduced the number of inflammatory cells and suppressed T-helper 2 (Th2) cytokines including IL-4 and IL-5 in BALF. Also, total IgE and OVA-specific IgE levels in the serum decreased.

Conclusion: Collectively, it is concluded that the extract has the potential to modulate the Th2 cytokines and could be used as immunomodulatory agent in the treatment of allergic asthma.

Keywords: Asthma, Allergy, Cytokines, Immunoglubolin E, Scrophularia striata

Introduction

Allergic asthma is a chronic inflammatory disease that recognized by airway inflammation and obstruction, mucus hyper secretion and airway hyper responsiveness [1].

The prevalence of inflammatory and allergic airway diseases such as asthma has significantly increased in recent decades. The asthma is associated to T-helper (Th) type 2 cells response, immunoglobulin (Ig) E-mediated mast cell activation, and other inflammatory factors, including eosinophils, B cells, cytokines and chemokines [2].

In addition, Th2 lymphocytes play important role in initiation and progression of allergic diseases such as asthma through their ability to release interleukin (IL)-4 and IL-5 [3].

On the other hand, IL-4 is important to induce of isotype class switching which is required for B cells to express IgE and also, IL-5 is pivotal for growth, differentiation, recruitment and survival of eosinophils [4,5]. Therefore, most efforts are being made to reduce the inappropriate Th2 response to reduce allergic airway diseases. In this regards, Therapeutic concepts include Th2 cytokine inhibitors; neutralizing antibodies directed IgE, histamine and leukotriene blockers, as well as other targets [6,7].

In recent years, many researches have searched to find novel compounds with greater antioxidant activity. In this regard, natural compounds isolated from medicinal plants can be good candidates to study their antioxidant and anti-inflammatory activities. *Scrophularia striata* Boiss. (Scrophulariaceae) is a plant growing in the northeastern part of Iran being used as a traditional herb for

* Correspondence: rhajiaghaee@yahoo.com
[2]Pharmacognosy & Pharmaceutics department of Medicinal Plants Research Center, Institute of Medicinal Plants, ACECR, Karaj, Iran
Full list of author information is available at the end of the article

various purposes. Several species of *Scrophularia* have been used since ancient times as sedative in folk medicine and for treatment of illnesses such as scrophulas, scabies, eczema, psoriasis and tumors [8]. Our previous studies in vitro demonstrated the inhibitory effect of *S. striata* extract on nitric oxide and pro-inflammatory cytokines including TNF-α, IL-1β and PGE2 production by macrophages [9,10]. In addition, the anti-inflammatory and immunomodulatory activity of some species of *Scrophularia* has also been shown by other investigators [11-13]. Moreover, several compounds from various *Scrophularia* species with anti-inflammatory and neuroprotective properties including iridoids and phenyl propanoids have been isolated [13]. In another study, flavonoids, phenolic compound, quercetin and isorhamnetin *3-O*-rutinoside with antioxidant activity were also isolated from *S. striata* [14]. Given these data, we decided to evaluate the anti-asthmatic effect of *S. striata* extract in Ovalbumin-induced mice asthma model.

Materials and methods

Plant material and preparation of the extract

The aerial parts of *S. striata* were collected from Ruin region in northeastern part of Iran, in May 2010 and air dried at room temperature. A sample was authenticated by Dr. Faride Attar, from Tehran University, Faculty of Sciences and a voucher specimen (Herbarium No: 36501) was preserved in the herbarium of the Tehran University Faculty of Sciences, Tehran, Iran. Aerial parts of the plant was dried, powdered (20 g) and macerated with an 80% ethanol solution for 3 days with three changes of the solution. The resulting extract was filtered and evaporated under vacuum into a dried powder extract of *S. striata.* In this study, the extract dissolved in dimethylsulfoxide (DMSO), $(CH_3)_2SO$, (% 0.1 v/v) and then used at appropriate concentrations.

Phytochemical assay

In order to recognize chemical components of extract, thin layer chromatocheraphy (TLC) was used. A variety of indicators including vanillin sulfuric acid; ferric chloride and natural product polyethylene glycol were used in this assay. The indictors were sprayed on prepared thin layers of extract and were observed at 260 and 280 nm wavelengths under UV light.

DPPH assay

The DPPH test was used to evaluate the antioxidant capacity of the plant extract [15]. Briefly, one thousand microlitres of various concentrations (250, 125, 62.5, 31.25, 15.62 and 7.81 μg/ml) of the extract of *S. striata* in ethanol was added to 4 ml of 0.004% methanol solution of DPPH. After a 60 min incubation period at room temperature, the absorbance was read against a blank at 517 nm. Inhibition of free radical by DPPH in percent (I %) was calculated in following way:

$$I\% = [(\text{Ablank}-\text{Asample})/\text{Ablank}]\times 100$$

A blank =Absorbance of the control reaction (containing all reagents except the test compound).

A sample =Absorbance of the test compound. Extract concentration providing 50% inhibition (IC_{50}%) was calculated from the graph plotted inhibition percentage against extract concentration. IC50% values were compared to IC50% value of a "standard" antioxidant, in this case ascorbic acid (AA), obtained by the same procedure.

Determination of total phenolic assay

The total phenolic content of dry herbs was determined by using the Folin-Ciocalteau assay [16]. An aliquot (1 ml) of extract or standard solution of gallic acid (20, 40, 60, 80 and 100 mg/L) was added to 25 ml volumetric flask, containing 9 ml of destilled deionised water (dd H2O). A reagent blank using dd H2O was prepared. One milliliter of Folin-Ciocalteu' sphenol reagent was added to the mixture and shaken. After 5 min, 10 ml of 7% Na2CO3 solution was added to the mixture. The solution was diluted to volume (25 ml) with dd H2O, and mixed. After incubation for 90 min at room temperature, the absorbance against prepared reagent blank was determined at 750 nm. Data of total phenolic contents are expressed as milligrams of gallic acid equivalents (GAE) per gram dry weight (mg $_{GAE}$/g $_{DW}$). All samples were analyzed in duplicates.

Animals

Six- to 7- weeks old male Balb/c mice were purchased from the Pasteur Institute of Iran (Tehran, Iran). In this study, all the animal experiments were approved and performed according to the guidelines of the Ethical Committee of Institute of Medicinal Plant (IMP). All mice had access to standard laboratory rodent chow and water ad libitum. All procedures involving animals were conducted in accordance with the Guidelines for Laboratory Animal Experiments in IMP Animal Research and Care Center.

OVA-sensitization challenge and administration of the extract

OVA sensitization and airway challenge were performed as previously described with minor modification [17]. In brief, mice were sensitization on days 1 and 7 by subcutaneously (SC) injection of 100 μg of ovalbumin (Sigma, USA) emulsified in 1mg of aluminum hydroxide (AL (OH) 3) (Merk, USA) as adjuvant in 200 μl of phosphate buffered saline (PBS). The efficiency of sensitization was assessed by measurement of serum total IgE levels and also eosinophilia and total inflammatory cells count on day 8. Then, mice were challenged with intraperitoneal (IP) injection of 10 μg of ovalbumin in 200 μl of PBS on day 14. The mice were divided into five groups, each containing eight mice. The control group (1) received only PBS (Vehicle). The control group (2) treated with AL (OH) 3. Positive control group (3) was immunized by subcutaneous injection of a suspension containing 100μg of ovalbumin and 1mg AL (OH) 3 in 200 μl of PBS on days 1 and 7. The treatment groups (4 and 5) were sensitized by ovalbumin and then intrapritonealy treated with 100 and 200 mg/kg of extract on days 8 to 14 separately.

Preparation of the bronchoalveolar lavage fluid (BALF) and inflammatory cells count

Lung lavaging was performed 48 h after the last OVA challenge (on day 16) for preparation of bronchoalveolar lavage fluid (BALF). In brief, the thorax cavity of mouse was opened and then sheerd the omohyiod and stylohyoid muscles, then for prevention of lavage reflux, a needle or a fine polyethylene tube was fixed in trachea and 1 ml of PBS was injected to the fixed tube via insulin syrange and then it was aspirated (three time) until 2 ml of BALF was taken. The suspension of BALF was centrifuged and the supernatant collected and stored at −70°C. Inflammatory cell numbers including eosinophil, lymphocyte, neutrophil, macrophage and total cells were determined by direct microscopic counting with a hemocytometer after exclusion of dead cells by trypan blue staining. To determine differential cell counts in BALF, the cells stained using Diff-Quik Stain reagent (B4132-1A; Dade Behring Inc., Deerfield, IL) according to the manufacturer's instructions.

Evaluation of inflammation score by lung histology study

For evaluation of inflammation score, 48 hours after OVA-challenge, the lung tissues removed and fixed in 10% neutral buffered formalin at 4°C for 24 h. Tissues were embedded in paraffin, sectioned at 4 μm thickness, and then stained with hematoxylin and eosin (H&E) to estimate inflammation by light microscopy. The degree of cell inflammation in the lung tissue was scored in a double-blind screen by two independent investigators [18].

Evaluation of total IgE and OVA-specific IgE levels in serum

For evaluation of total IgE and OVA-specific IgE levels, serum samples were collected of the mice on 16 day, respectively. Levels of total mouse IgE and OVA-specific IgE were determined by enzyme-linked immunosorbent assay (ELISA) kits (Serotec, Oxford, UK) according to the manufacturer's instructions. The absorbance was measured at 450 nm by a micro plate ELISA reader.

Table 1 Phytochemical results of *Scrophularia striata* extract

Compounds	Reagents	Standards	Results
Phenylpropanoids and Terpenoids	Vanillin sulfuric acid	Cinamic acid	+
Phenolic compounds	Ferric chloride	Nepitrin	+
Flavonoides	Natural product reagent	Nepitrin	+

Evaluation of Th2 cytokines including IL-4 and IL-5 in BALF

In order to determine Th2 cytokines, the levels of IL-4, IL-5 in BALF were measured by enzyme-linked immunosorbent assay (ELISA) kits (BioSource International, Camarillo,CA) according to the manufacturer's protocol.

Statistical analysis

Data represented as mean ± standard deviation. Statistical analyses were performed by one-way analysis of variance (ANOVA) and a post–hoc Bonferroni's test to express the difference among the groups. All analyses performed using SPSS software16. Data considered statistically significant at $P < 0.05$.

Results

Chemical components of extract

Phytochemical assay by thin layer chromatography showed the main components; including phenyl propanoids, phenolic compounds and flavonoids were presented in the *S. striata* extract (Table 1).

Antioxidant activity and total phenolics compounds

The results of Free radical scavenging capacities of the extract, measured with DPPH assay, and the ratios (IC50%) AA/ (IC50%) extract are shown in Table 2. They represent the ascorbic acid equivalent of the extract antioxidant capacity, i.e. the amount of ascorbic acid in milligrams equivalent to one gram extract. In addition, Phenolic compounds have been recognized as antioxidant agents, which act as free radical terminators [19] and have been known to show medicinal activity as well as exhibiting physiological functions [20]. The total phenolic compounds of dry herb, respectively as shown in Table 2 with gallic acid as standards.

Table 2 Antioxidant capacity and total phenolics compounds of *S. striata* extract

Total Phenolics compounds in dry herb (mg $_{GAE}$/g $_{dw}$)	DPPH radical scavenging activity, $IC_{50\%}$ (mg/l)	Ascorbic acid equivalent of the extract antioxidant capacity (mg/g)
10.96	316.69	29.8

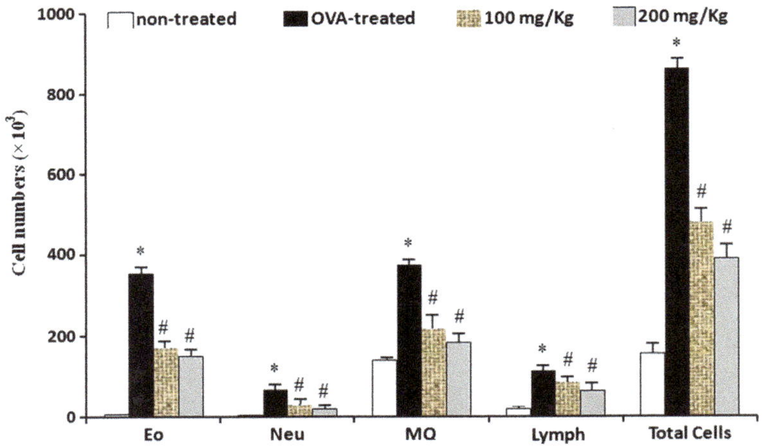

Figure 1 Effect of *S.striata* extract on the recruitment of inflammatory cells in the Broncoalveolar lavage fluid (BALF) of mice. The BALF samples were collected 48 h after the last Ovalbumin (OVA) challenge. The numbers of eosinophils and total inflammatory cells were assessed by direct microscopic counting with a hemocytometer. The results showed that the numbers of eosinophils and total inflammatory cells in BALF were significantly decreased in the *S.striata* extract treated mice. * $P < 0.001$ compared with non-treated OVA (Vehicle), # $P < 0.001$ compared with OVA-treated group.

S. Striata extract reduced the infiltration of eosinophils and other inflammatory cells into BALF and lung tissue

The results of cells number were not shown any significant difference between control groups that received vehicle (1) comparing with control group (2) that received AL (OH) 3. As shown in Figure 1, the numbers of the eosinophils and other inflammatory cells in BALF from the OVA- sensitized or challenged mice were significantly (P<0.05) higher than the negative control mice. However, the infiltration of eosinophils and other inflammatory cells in the BALF

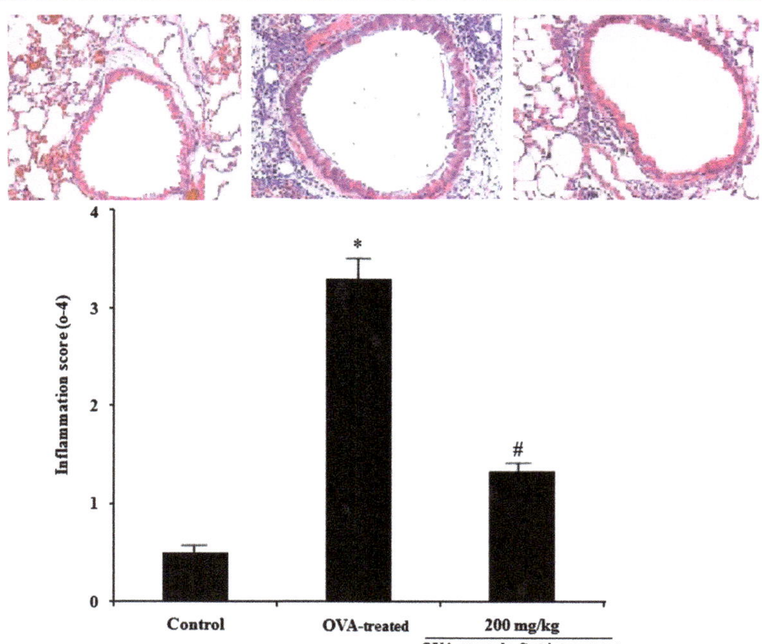

Figure 2 Effect of *S.striata* extract on the inflammation score in lung tissue. Lung tissue from animals of respective groups was stained with hematoxylin and eosin and inflammatory cells were studied by light microscopy. Scoring the scope of inflammation by quantitative analysis of inflammatory cell infiltration in lung sections was performed. Inflammation score significantly (P<0.05) reduced in the extract –treated OVA-challenged groups compared with the control OVA- challenged group. * $P < 0.001$ compared with non-treated OVA (Control), # $P < 0.05$ compared with OVA-treated group.

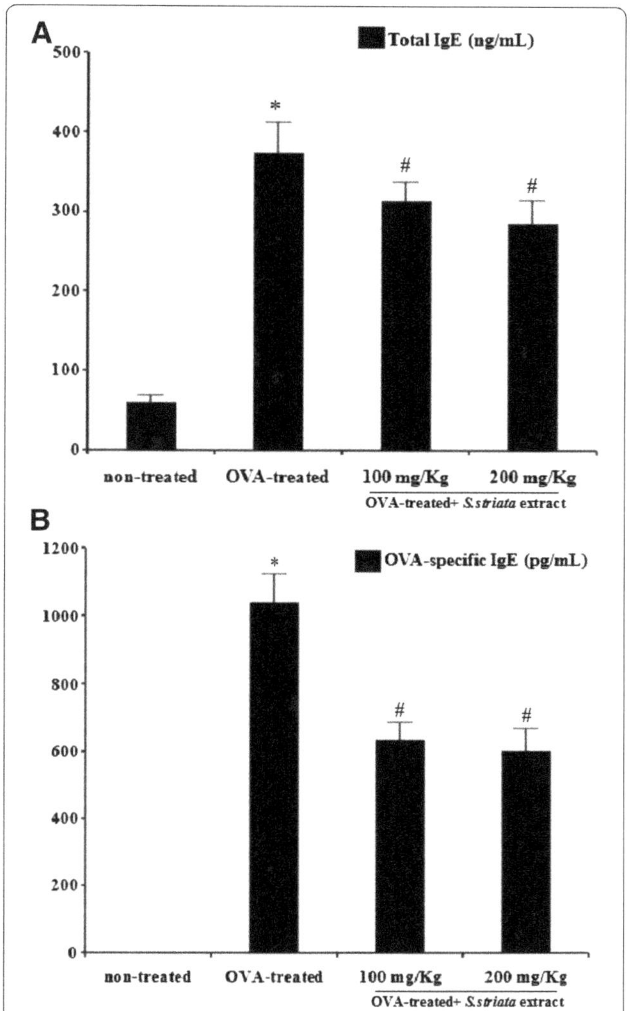

Figure 3 Effect of *S.striata* extract on the total IgE and OVA-specific IgE levels in serum. The serum samples were collected 48 h after the last Ovalbumin (OVA) challenge. **(A)** Total IgE level **(B)** OVA-specific IgE level. The results showed that the total IgE and OVA-specific IgE levels in serum were significantly decreased in the *S.striata* extract treated mice. * $P < 0.001$ compared with non-treated OVA (Vehicle), # $P < 0.001$ compared with OVA-treated group.

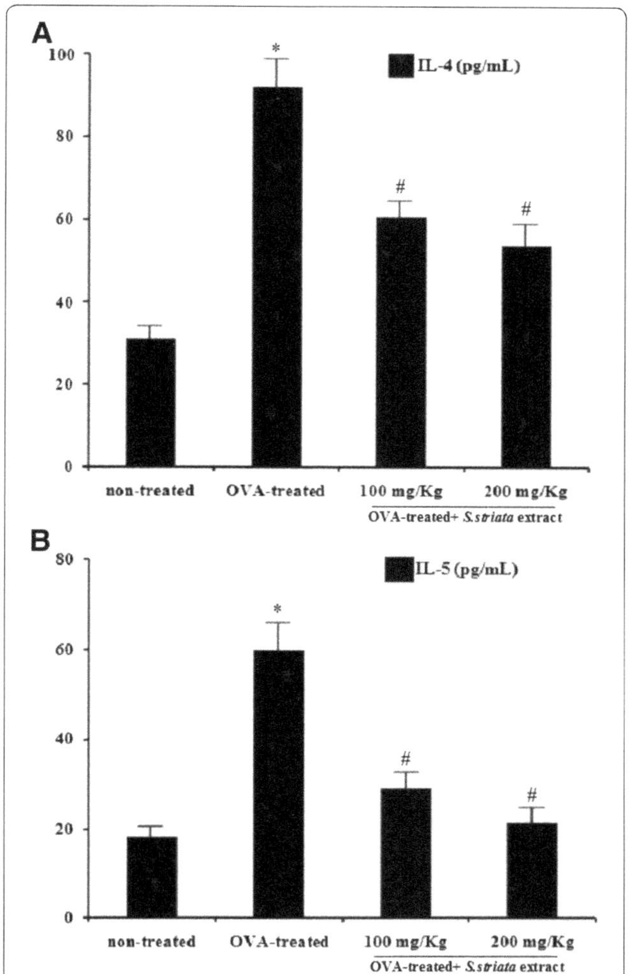

Figure 4 Effect of *S.striata* extract on the levels of IL-4 and IL-5 in BALF. In order to determine of Th2 cytokines, the BALF samples were collected 48 h after the last Ovalbumin (OVA) challenge. IL-4 level **(A)** and IL-5 level **(B)**. The results showed that IL-4 and IL-5 levels in BALF were significantly decreased in the *S. striata* extract treated mice. * $P < 0.001$ compared with non-treated OVA (Vehicle), # $P < 0.001$ compared with OVA-treated group.

significantly decreased in the extract –treated OVA- challenged groups compared with the control OVA- challenged group(P<0.05). Moreover, we determined the suppressive effect of the extract on the infiltration of inflammatory cells in the lung tissue. The results indicated that inflammation score significantly (P<0.05) reduced in the extract –treated OVA- challenged groups compared with the control OVA-challenged group (Figure 2).

S. Striata extract decreased total IgE and OVA-specific IgE in serum

In order to determine the protective effect of *S. striata* extract on the IgE and antigen specific IgE production, the total IgE and OVA-specific IgE levels in serum were evaluated 48 h after the last OVA challenge. The results were not shown any significant difference between the control groups that received vehicle (1) comparing with control group (2) that received AL (OH) 3. As shown in Figure 3A and B; OVA-sensitized or challenged mice showed significantly (P<0.05) higher levels of IgE (total: 382 ng/ml and specific: 1048 pg/ml) compared with negative control mice (total: 65 ng/ml). In addition, treatment with extract significantly decreased the levels of total IgE and OVA-specific IgE antibodies compared with the control OVA- challenged group (P<0.05).

S. striata extract treatment suppressed the Th2 cytokines in BALF

To evaluate the effect of *S. striata* extract on Th2 cytokines in BALF of OVA- sensitized or challenged mice,

IL-4 and IL-5 cytokines were measured by ELISA. The results showed that the levels of IL-4 (94 pg/ml) and IL-5 (60 pg/ml) cytokines in BALF were significantly ($P<0.05$) increased in OVA- sensitized or challenged mice, while the *S. striata* extract treatment with 200 mg/kg significantly ($P<0.05$) decreased the levels of IL-4 to 56 pg/ml and IL-5 to 22 pg/ml compared with the control OVA-challenged group as shown in Figure 4A and B.

Discussion

One of chronic inflammatory disorders is asthma that recognized by airway infiltration of eosinophils and other inflammatory cells, bronchial hyper-responsiveness and airway obstruction [21,22]. On the other hand, in recent decades the prevalence of asthma has significantly increased and extensive efforts have been made to recognize both natural artificial anti-oxidants and anti-asthmatic agents such as medicinal plants. The anti-oxidant, anti-inflammatory and immunomodulatory activity of some species of *Scrophularia* has also been shown by several investigators [9,23-25]. In the present study, we investigated the anti-asthmatic effect of *S. striata extract* in OVA- sensitized /challenged mice asthma model. *S. striata* has been used to treat various inflammatory disorders in animal models. Our previously studies indicated the inhibitory effect of *S. striata* extract on pro-inflammatory mediators production by macrophages including Nitric Oxide (NO), TNF-α, IL-1β and PGE2 and also suppressive effect on matrix metalloproteinases in Wehi-164 tumor cell line in vitro [9,10,25]. The results of this study showed that the treatment with *S. striata* extract (100 and 200 mg/kg) in OVA- sensitized /challenged mice significantly reduced the numbers of eosinophils and total inflammatory cells in the BALF comparing with OVA- sensitized /challenged mice. Th2 cell, a sub-group of lymphocytes, plays an important role in the initiation and progression of allergic asthma by releasing of IL-4 and IL-5 cytokines [26]. Moreover, Th2 response induced airway inflammatory cells infiltration, eosinophil activation, IgE production and mucus secretion [27]. IL-5 cytokine is pivotal for growth, differentiation, recruitment and survival of eosinophils [5]. Our results indicated that *S. striata* extract treatment in OVA-sensitized /challenged mice significantly decreased the levels of IL-4 and IL-5 cytokines in the BALF comparing with OVA- sensitized /challenged mice. The decrease of IL-5 cytokine in the BALF of the mice that had been treated with both extract and OVA may at least in part be responsible for the reduced recruitment of eosinophils. On the other hand, serum IgE level is associated with bronchial asthma and Th2 response [28]. Moreover, IL-4 cytokine is important to the induction of isotype class switching which is required for B cells to express IgE [4]. Our finding in this study showed that treatment with extract significantly decreased total IgE and OVA-specific IgE in the serum of OVA- sensitized /challenged mice that this effect of the extract may at least in part be responsible for the decreased IL-4 cytokine production. In addition, the antioxidant and neuroprotective properties of compounds such as iridoide glycosides and phenylpropanoid esters isolated from *S. buergeriana* have been reported [29-32]. However, in present and previous studies, phenolic compounds, phenyl propanoids and two flavonoids, quercetin and isorhamnetin 3-*O*-rutinoside, were identified from *S. striata* extract [14]. Quercetin is well known dietary antioxidants and phenolic compounds are also an anti-inflammatory and antioxidants that the anti-asthmatic and anti-allergic effects of these compounds have been previously reported [33-36]. Whether these compounds are the main responsible compounds for the anti-asthmatic effects of *S. striata* or other compounds are involved in this activity needs further investigation.

In conclusion, the results of this study showed anti-asthmatic and anti-allergic ability of the *S. striata* extract through reducing the IL-4 and IL-5 cytokines production, total and specific-OVA IgE and also decreasing of eosinophils and total inflammatory cells in the BALF of OVA-sensitized /challenged mice asthma model. Further study needs for identifying the main anti-allergic bioactive compounds of this plant and other anti-asthmatic mechanisms.

Competing interests
The authors declare that they have no competing interests.

Authors' contribution
AA: Project design, conducting and supervising experiment, manuscript preparation. RH: conducting experiment and manuscript preparation. MZ, GhM: supervising project. All authors read and approve the final manuscript.

Acknowledgement
This study was supported by Department of Medicinal Plants Research Center, Institute of Medicinal Plants (IMP), ACECR, Karaj, Iran and Qazvin University of Medical Sciences, Qazvin, Iran. The authors would like to thanks Dr. Saeid Abediankenari from Mazandaran University of Medical Sciences for editing the manuscript.

Author details
[1]Immunology department, Qazvin University of Medical Sciences, Qazvin, Iran. [2]Pharmacognosy & Pharmaceutics department of Medicinal Plants Research Center, Institute of Medicinal Plants, ACECR, Karaj, Iran. [3]Internal medicine department, Qazvin University of Medical Sciences, Qazvin, Iran. [4]Immunology department, Mazandaran University of Medical Sciences, Sari, Iran. [5]Immunology department, Babol University of Medical Sciences, Babol, Iran.

References
1. Buss WW, Rosenwasser LJ: **Mechanisms of asthma.** *J Allergy Clin Immunol* 2003, **111**:s799–804.
2. Herrick CA, Bottomly K: **To respond or not to respond: T cells in allergic asthma.** *Nat Rev Immunol* 2003, **3**:405–412.
3. Brightling CE, Symon FA, Birring SS, Bradding P, Pavord ID, Wardlaw AJ: **TH2 cytokine expression in bronchoalveolar lavage fluid T lymphocytes and bronchial submucosa is a feature of asthma and eosinophilic bronchitis.** *J Allergy Clin Immunol* 2002, **110**:899–905.

4. Steinke JW, Borish L: **Th2 cytokines and asthma. Interleukin-4: its role in the pathogenesis of asthma, and targeting it for asthma treatment with interleukin-4 receptor antagonists.** *Respir Res* 2001, **2**:66–70.
5. Robinson DS: **Th-2 cytokines in allergic disease.** *Br Med Bull* 2000, **56**:956–968.
6. Barnes PJ: **Immunology of asthma and chronic obstructive pulmonary disease.** *Nat Rev Immunol* 2008, **8**:183–192.
7. Holgate ST, Polosa R: **Treatment strategies for allergy and asthma.** *Nat Rev Immunol* 2008, **8**:218–230.
8. Header M, Henderson MRH: **The physicians of myddfai: the Welsh herbal tradition.** *Bot J Scotl* 1994, **46**:623–627.
9. Azadmehr A, Afshari A, Baradaran B, Hajiaghaee R, Rezazadeh S, Monsef-Esfahani H: **Suppression of nitric oxide production in activated murine peritoneal macrophages in vitro and ex vivo by *Scrophularia striata* ethanolic extract.** *J Ethnopharmacol* 2009, **124**:166–169.
10. Azadmehr A, Maliji G, Hajiaghaee R, Shahnazi M, Afaghi A: **Inhibition of pro-inflammatory cytokines by ethyl acetate extract of *Scrophularia striata*.** *Trop J Pharm Res* 2012, **11**(6):893–897.
11. Diaz AM, Abad MJ, Fernandez L, Silván AM, De Santos J, Bermejo P: **Phenylpropanoid glycosides from *Scrophularia scorodonia*: in vitro anti-inflammatory activity.** *Life Sci* 2004, **74**:2515–2526.
12. Bas E, Recio MC, Abdallah M, Máñez S, Giner RM, Cerdá-Nicolás M, Ríos JL: **Inhibition of the pro-inflammatory mediators production and anti-inflammatory effect of the iridoid scrovalentinoside.** *J Ethnopharmacol* 2007, **110**:419–427.
13. Azadmehr A, Hajiaghaee R, Afshari A, Amirghofran Z, Refieian-Kopaei M, yousofi Darani H, Shirzad H: **Evaluation of *in vivo* immune response activity and *in vitro* anti-cancer effect by *Scrophularia megalantha*.** *J Med Plants Res* 2011, **5**:2365–2368.
14. Monsef-Esfahani H, Hajiaghaee R, Shahverdi AR: **Flavonoids, cinnamic acid and phenyl propanoid from aerial parts of *Scrophularia striata*.** *Pharmaceutic Biol* 2010, **48**:333–336.
15. Wojdyło A, Oszmianrski J, Czemerys R: **Antioxidant activity and phenolic compounds in 32 selected herbs.** *Food Chem* 2007, **105**:940–949.
16. Yuan VY, Bone DE, Carrington MF: **Antioxidant activity of dulse (Palmaria palmata) extract evaluated in vitro.** *Food Chem* 2005, **91**:485–494.
17. Ghafourian Boroujerdnia M, Azemi ME, Hemmati AA, Taghian A, Azadmehr A: **Immunomodulatory effects of astragalus gypsicolus hydroalcoholic extract in ovalbumininduced allergic mice model.** *Iran J Allergy Asthma Immunol* 2011, **10**(4):281–288.
18. Myou S, Leff AR, You S, Boetticher E, Tong J, Meliton AY, Liu J, Munoz NM, Zhu X: **Blockade of inflammation and airway hyperresponsiveness in immunesensitized mice by dominant-negative phosphoinositide 3- kinase-TAT.** *J Exp Med* 2003, **198**:1573–1582.
19. Shahidi F, Wanasundara JPD: **Phenolic anioxidants.** *Crit Rev Food Sci Nutr* 1992, **32**:67–103.
20. Sofowora A: *Medicinal plants and traditional medicine in Africa.* Ibadan, Nigeria: Spectrum books Ind; 1993:289.
21. Kay AB: **Asthma and inflammation.** *J Allergy Clin Immunol* 1991, **87**(5):893–910.
22. Djukanović R, Roche WR, Wilson JW, Beasley CR, Twentyman OP, Howarth RH, Holgate ST: **Mucosal inflammation in asthma.** *Am Rev Respir Dis* 1990, **142**(2):434–57.
23. Bas E, Recio MC, Manez S: **New insight into the inhibition of the inflammatory response to experimental delayed-type hypersensitivity reactions in mice by scropolioside A.** *Eur J Pharmacol* 2007, **555**:199–210.
24. Schinella GR, Tournier HA, Prieto JM: **Antioxidant activity of anti-inflammatory plant extracts.** *Life Sci* 2002, **18**:1023–1033.
25. Hajiaghaee R, Monsef-Esfahani HR, Khorramizadeh MR: **Inhibitory effect of aerial parts of *Scrophularia striata* on matrix metalloproteinases expression.** *Phytother Res* 2007, **21**:1127–1129.
26. Barnes PJ: **Efficacy of inhaled corticosteroids in asthma.** *J Allergy Clin Immunol* 1998, **102**(4 Pt 1):531–538.
27. Ngoc PL, Gold DR, Tzianabos AO, Weiss ST, Celedón JC: **Cytokines, allergy, and asthma.** *Curr Opin Allergy Clin Immunol* 2005, **5**(2):161–166.
28. Lin JY, Chen ML, Lin BF: ***Ganoderma tsugae in vivo* modulates Th1/Th2 and macrophage responses in an allergic murine model.** *Food Chem Toxicol* 2006, **44**(12):2025–2032.
29. Jeong EJ, Lee KY, Kim SH: **Cognitive-enhancing and antioxidant activities of iridoid glycosides from *Scrophularia buergeriana* in scopolamine-treated mice.** *Eur J Pharmacol* 2008, **588**:78–84.
30. Kim SR, Lee KY, Koo KA: **Four new neuroprotective iridoid glycosides from *Scrophularia buergeriana* roots.** *J Nat Prod* 2002, **65**:1696–1699.
31. Kim SR, Kim YC: **Neuroprotective phenylpropanoid esters of rhamnose isolated from roots of *Scrophularia buergeriana*.** *Phytochemistry* 2002, **54**:503–509.
32. Kim SR, Koo KA, Sung SH: ***Iridoids from Scrophularia buergeriana* attenuate glutamate induced neurotoxicity in rat cortical cultures.** *J Neurosci Res* 2003, **74**:948–955.
33. Joskova M, Franova S, Sadlonova V: **Acute bronchodilator effect of quercetin in experimental allergic asthma.** *Bratisl Lek Listy* 2011, **112**(1):9–12.
34. Matsuda H, Ando S, Morikawa T, Kataoka S, Yoshikawa M: **Structure-activity relationships of 1′S-1′-acetoxychavicol acetate for inhibitory effect on NO production in lipopolysaccharideactivated mouse peritoneal macrophages.** *Bioorg Med Chem Lett* 2005, **15**(7):1949–1953.
35. Jang YW, Lee JY, Kim CJ: **Anti-asthmatic activity of phenolic compounds from the roots of Gastrodia elata Bl.** *Int Immunopharmacol* 2010, **10**(2):147–154.
36. Medeiros KC, Figueiredo CA, Figueredo TB, Freire KR, Santos FA, Alcantara-Neves NM, Silva TM, Piuvezam MR: **Anti-allergic effect of bee pollen phenolic extract and myricetin in ovalbumin-sensitized mice.** *J Ethnopharmacol* 2008, **119**(1):41–46.

Introduction of a mathematical model for optimizing the drug release in the patient's body

Mohammad Reza Nabatchian[1*], Hamid Shahriari[1] and Mona Shahriari[2]

Abstract

Background: Drug release in a patient's body is of particular interest to the pharmaceutical industry. One of the most essential types of drug release is the gradual release based on a behavior, which is called a profile or modified release. The investigation of the time-oriented quality characteristic is one of the newest topics in the area of product design. There are already several approaches addressing this issue. In this paper, a mathematical model is proposed to find the suitable values of the controllable factors in a drug to achieve the profile of the drug release in the patient's body.

Results: The proposed method has several advantages over the existing methods.

Conclusion: The authors feel that by adjusting the control factors during the production process the drug release profile become closer to the reference profile.

Keywords: Drug release, Time-oriented quality characteristic, Parameter design, Desirability function, Release profile

Introduction

The amount of time it takes a drug to release in a patient's body as well as the time it takes to exert its effects on the target organ are very important factors used to measure the effectiveness of a drug. If this releasing manner is not based on a pre-defined profile, it may cause a reduction of curative properties of the drug and can even have some negative effects on the patient's body. Similarly, in the area of quality engineering, the time-oriented quality characteristics are also assessed. The time-oriented profile of the quality characteristic is specified and the aim of the designer is to find the pre-defined profile with minimum deviation from the target. The quality characteristics are then monitored using the defined profile. In this study, we aim to establish a logical relationship between these two areas and to apply a mathematical modeling approach to investigate the drug release problem in pharmaceutics. In this paper some basic definitions of drug release and quality engineering are presented and then we introduce the four existing approaches for these types of problems and their deficiencies. The proposed method is presented in the next section. Several examples are provided to evaluate the suggested model and in the final section, the conclusions are made.

Definitions

In this section some of the basic terms included in the paper are defined to familiarize the reader with the concepts of the discussion.

Drug release

Drug release is an important stage in the drug life cycle. When the drug is released based on a pre-defined profile, it is more effective on the patient's body. One of the most applicable approaches for measuring the amount of released drugs is to measure the plasma concentration of the drug. The drug is considered effective when the plasma concentration is somewhere between minimum effective concentration (MEC) and minimal toxic concentration (MTC) as is shown in Figure 1 [1-3].

Drugs are usually classified based on the drug release mechanism as follows:

* Correspondence: mrnabatchian@dena.kntu.ac.ir
[1]Department of Industrial Engineering, K.N. Toosi University of Technology, No 7, Pardis St., Mollasadra Ave., Tehran, Iran
Full list of author information is available at the end of the article

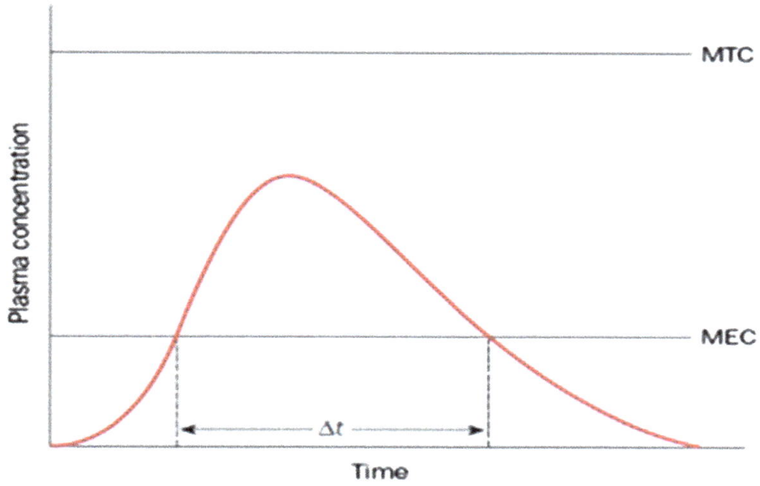

Figure 1 Plasma concentration versus time profile [1].

Immediate release drugs: In this group, the drug is quickly released in the body. This is particularly suitable for drugs that need to take affect rapidly such as pain-killers [1,4].

Modified drug release: In this case by using the pharmaceutical techniques, the time, the amount and the target organ for the drug release is determined. The delayed release and extended release are the methods being used. In the delayed release the drug is released after a pre-determined delay. Figure 2 shows the plasma concentration for this modified release method [1,4].

In the extended release technique, the drug is released gradually over a longer period of time. It is classified into two categories: sustained release and controlled release. In sustained release, the drug is released continuously with a constant rate. In controlled release, the drug is released intelligently so that the concentration remains almost constant in the body. Figure 3 shows the plasma concentration when using this method of drug release [1,5].

Time-oriented quality characteristics

There are several definitions of the quality characteristics in the quality management literature. The most comprehensive of them is the degree of adaptability of the quality characteristic by the user's requirements [6]. Furthermore, the design phase is the principal stage of a product life cycle, because the quality is formed in this stage and control actions at the end of the production process cannot improve the quality of a product with poor quality of design [7].

The Taguchi robust design is a famous design procedure. It is an engineering method for optimizing the product or process condition to minimize the product

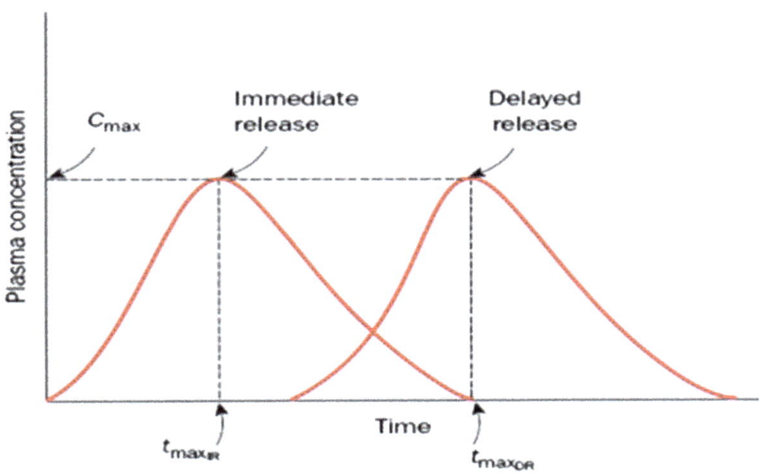

Figure 2 Plasma concentration versus time profile for an immediate release drug and a delayed release drug [1].

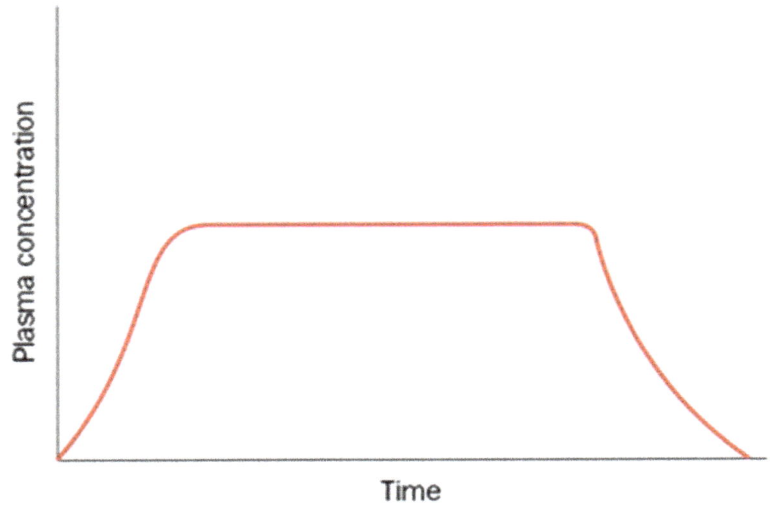

Figure 3 Plasma concentration versus time profile for a controlled release formulation [1].

sensitivity to the noise factors in the environment, such as: ambient temperature, humidity, air pressure and direct sunlight [8]. So, a product with high quality and low cost is being produced. One property of this approach is to investigate the quality characteristics numerically. In this approach the quality characteristics are grouped into three classes as: nominal the best (NTB), larger the better (LTB) and smaller the better (STB). Each of these quality characteristics could be constant or variable over time [9].

The target value and the specification limits for the time-oriented quality characteristics are being changed over time. So, for the design of a product with these quality characteristics, the parameters are designed such that the quality characteristics are being as close to their pre-specified target values as possible.

In this regard, three basic topics need to be introduced.

Design of experiments (DOE)

A collection of statistical methods that are used to find the influenced factors on a quality characteristic and to optimize its conditions. There are several types of DOE techniques including factorial experiments and fractional factorial experiments [10,11].

Response surface methodology (RSM)

A statistical and mathematical method for modeling, analyzing and optimizing the problems with response variables which are directly related to some other independent variables [12].

Desirability function

Is one of the common methods to simultaneously optimize multi response problems. The most applicable method of this type is the Derringer and Suich's which is defined for several types of quality characteristics as follows [13]:

NTB quality characteristic:

$$DF(y) = \begin{cases} \left[\dfrac{y-LSL}{T-LSL}\right]^r, & LSL < y < T \\ \left[\dfrac{y-USL}{T-USL}\right]^s, & T < y < USL \\ 0, & y < LSL; y > USL \end{cases} \tag{1}$$

LTB quality characteristic:

$$DF(y) = \begin{cases} 1, & y > y_i^* \\ \left[\dfrac{y-y_{i_*}}{y_i^*-y_{i_*}}\right]^r, & y_{i_*} < y < y_i^* \\ 0, & y < y_{i_*} \end{cases} \tag{2}$$

STB quality characteristic

$$DF(y) = \begin{cases} 1, & y < y_{i_*} \\ \left[\dfrac{y_i^*-y}{y_i^*-y_{i_*}}\right]^r, & y_{i_*} < y < y_i^* \\ 0, & y > y_i^* \end{cases} \tag{3}$$

In the above equations:

y: value observed for the quality characteristic

T: The target value for quality characteristic applicable for NTB quality characteristic.

USL: Upper specification Limit of NTB quality characteristic

LSL: Lower specification Limit of NTB quality characteristic

y_i^*: optimum point for LTB quality characteristic and highest acceptable value for STB quality characteristic

y_{i*}: Optimum point for STB quality characteristic and lowest acceptable value for LTB quality characteristic

r, s: Weight values, positive constants.

Problem definition

The drugs have a pre-determined profile for release based on the drug's controlled-release mechanism. The aim in any drug laboratory is to find optimum adjustment of the controllable factors, such as material, production machine settings and so on to produce drugs that achieve the pre-determined profile as much as possible. Four methods already exist for parameter design of a drug to achieve its pre-determined profile:

Contour overlay method

This method is applied by Gohel and Amin [14] to find the optimal values to the Diclofenac Sodium formulation. The aim is to determine the suitable values for the three main controllable factors: stirring speed, concentration of $CaCl_2$ and percentage of liquid paraffin, all of which influence the drug efficacy. The pre-determined profile of release is defined in advance. Then, the regression function of the drug release as a response variable and the above-mentioned control factors as independent variables is obtained by the least square method. For each point of time, the response is computed and compared to the pre-specified value. In this method, one variable is kept fixed and a two dimensional plot is used to find the optimal values.

The disadvantage of this method is that when the number of control factors increases, the efficiency of the method to introduce optimal values decreases.

Profile selection

In situations where the profile properties are hard to identify, selection of the best profile is done by using the pre-defined indices. Two of these indices are f_1 and f_2 defined as:

$$f_1 = \frac{\sum_{t=1}^{n} |R_t - T_t|}{\sum_{t=1}^{n} R_t} * 100 \tag{4}$$

$$f_2 = 50 * Log\left\{ \left[1 + \frac{1}{n} \sum_{t=1}^{n} (R_t - T_t)^2 \right]^{-0.5} * 100 \right\} \tag{5}$$

Where:

R_t: Percentage of drug release obtained from the reference formulation

T_t: Percentage of drug release obtained from the test formulation

n: number of observations

The first index, f_1 is defined as the dissimilarity index. As long as its value is small; the profile is close to the reference profile. The second index, f_2 is defined as similarity index and when its value is large; the profile is near to the reference profile [15,16].

MSE minimizing method

This method is applied in three articles. Truong et al. [17] used this method to determine the optimum values for control factors of a regenerative drug based on a profile of seven points.

Park et al. [18] used this method to investigate two quality characteristics separately for six and seven point profiles. Shin et al. [19] used this method to assess two quality characteristics separately for eight and eleven point profiles.

The first step in this method is to gather data and to calculate the basic statistics such as the mean and the variance. Then the RSM for these statistics are computed at each point of time. The optimal values for the control factors are obtained such that the following objective function is minimized.

$$Minimize \sum_{q=1}^{w} \left(\hat{M}(x, t_q) - T_q\right)^2 + \sum_{q=1}^{w} \hat{v}(x, t_q), \ S.t: x \in \Omega \tag{6}$$

Where:

$\hat{M}(x, t_q)$: The mean of the responses at time t_q.

$\hat{v}(x, t_q)$: The variance of the responses at time t_q.

T_q: The pre-specified target value for the response variable for the time q.

w: The number of points in time under study.

Method of minimizing the total cost

This method is used by Goethals and Cho [20] and also the experiment of Gohel and Amin [14] on the Diclufenac Sodium is reassessed. The logic behind this method is to find the optimal values for control factors that minimize the following objective function:

$$Minimize\ E[TC] = \sum_{q=1}^{w} \left[\int_{LSL_q}^{USL_q} L[Y(q)].f[Y(q)].dY(q) + \int_{-\infty}^{LSL_q} NC_{q1}.f[y(q)]dY(q) + \int_{USL_q}^{+\infty} NC_{q2}.f[Y(q)]dY(q) \right] \tag{7}$$

Where:

LSL_q and USL_q: are the lower and the upper specification limits for the quality characteristic, respectively.

f(y(q)): is the probability distribution function for response variable at time q.

NC_{q1} and NC_{q2}: are the costs corresponding to being greater than USL and smaller than LSL, respectively.

L(y (q)): is the quality loss function for the quality characteristic within the acceptable region, but not on the target.

w: is the number of time points under study.

The proposed method

The proposed method is a systematic and straightforward technique for determining the optimum values for the control factors for a drug. So that in a specified time interval, the drug release follows its premeditated profile. This method requires the following steps:

1. Determination of the drug release profile: Considering the kind of drug and its mechanism of release, the pharmaceutics design of the release profile of a drug by consulting the specialist physicians. To facilitate the comparison between the standard profile and the drug profile function, some points on time are considered and the experiments are run in these points. At each time point, the target value and the upper and the lower specification limits are determined. Selection of the number of points under study is based on the type of the drug and its life cycle in the patient's body.
2. Determination of the experiment templates: In this stage, many controllable factors such as raw material and production factors for the drug under study are determined. Several combinations of these controllable factors are being tested by running the experiments. One important logic of the DOE is to find as much as information possible from the minimum number of experiments. For each combination of the factor levels at each time point some data is collected. Then, the data are organized based on the Table 1. The primary statistics such as the mean, the variance and the coefficient of variation for each time point and the covariance between observations in different time points are calculated. The computational formulas used to compute these statistics are as follows:

$$\bar{y}_{qr} = \frac{\sum_{w=1}^{m} y_{qrw}}{m} \tag{8}$$

$$s_{qr}^2 = \frac{\sum_{w=1}^{m} \left(y_{qrw} - \bar{y}_{qr}\right)^2}{m-1} \tag{9}$$

$$\left(\frac{s}{m}\right)_{qr} = \frac{s_{qr}}{\bar{y}_{qr}} \tag{10}$$

$$s_{i,j} = \frac{\sum_{r=1}^{m} \left(y_{ipr} - \bar{y}_{ip}\right)\left(y_{jpr} - \bar{y}_{jp}\right)}{m-1} \tag{11}$$

3. Determination of the relationships among the statistics and the control factors: By using RSM technique, the relationships are defined. For the sake of simplicity and prevention of using data with several scales, the control factors are coded by linear relationships.

$$\hat{\mu}_q(x) = x\hat{\beta}_{\mu q}\ ,\ \hat{\beta}_{\mu q} = \left(x'x\right)^{-1} x'\bar{y}_q\ ,\ x = \begin{bmatrix} 1 & \cdots & x_{1,k-1} \\ \vdots & \ddots & \vdots \\ 1 & \cdots & x_{n,k-1} \end{bmatrix}$$
$$\bar{y}_q = \left[\bar{y}_{q1}, \bar{y}_{q2}, \ldots, \bar{y}_{qn}\right]' \tag{12}$$

$$\hat{s}_q^2(x) = x\hat{\beta}_{s^2 q}\ ,\ \hat{\beta}_{s^2 q} = \left(x'x\right)^{-1} x's_q^2\ ,\ x = \begin{bmatrix} 1 & \cdots & x_{1,k-1} \\ \vdots & \ddots & \vdots \\ 1 & \cdots & x_{n,k-1} \end{bmatrix}$$
$$s_q^2 = \left[s_{q1}^2, s_{q2}^2, \ldots, s_{qn}^2\right]' \tag{13}$$

$$\left(\left(\frac{\hat{s}}{m}\right)\right)_q(x) = x\hat{\beta}_{(s/m)}q\ ,\ \hat{\beta}_{(s/m)}q = \left(x'x\right)^{(-1)} x'(s/m)_q,$$
$$x = \begin{bmatrix} 1 & \cdots & x_{1,k-1} \\ \vdots & \ddots & \vdots \\ 1 & \cdots & x_{n,k-1} \end{bmatrix} \tag{14}$$
$$\left(\frac{s}{m}\right)_q = \left[\left(\frac{s}{m}\right)_{q1}, \left(\frac{s}{m}\right)_{q2}, \ldots, \left(\frac{s}{m}\right)_{qn}\right]'$$

Table 1 Experimental format [20]

Run	*x*	*Y(1)*	$\bar{y}_1$	s_1^2	...	*Y(w)*	$\bar{y}_w$	s_w^2
1	Control factor settings	$y_{111}\ldots y_{11m}$	$\bar{y}_{11}$	s_{11}^2	...	$y_{w11}\ldots y_{w1m}$	$\bar{y}_{w1}$	s_{w1}^2
2		$y_{121}\ldots y_{12m}$	$\bar{y}_{12}$	s_{12}^2	...	$y_{w21}\ldots y_{w2m}$	$\bar{y}_{w2}$	s_{w2}^2
.		...	...	...	...	...	...	...
r		$y_{1r1}\ldots y_{1rm}$	$\bar{y}_{1r}$	s_{1r}^2	...	$y_{wr1}\ldots y_{wrm}$	$\bar{y}_{wr}$	s_{wr}^2
.		...	...	...	...	...	...	...
n		$y_{1n1}\ldots y_{1nm}$	$\bar{y}_{1n}$	s_{1n}^2	...	$y_{wn1}\ldots y_{wnm}$	$\bar{y}_{wn}$	s_{wn}^2

$$\hat{s}_{i,j}(x) = x\hat{\beta}_{s_{i,j}}, \hat{\beta}_{s_{i,j}} = (x'x)^{-1}x's_{i,j}, \; x = \begin{bmatrix} 1 & \cdots & x_{1,k-1} \\ \vdots & \ddots & \vdots \\ 1 & \cdots & x_{n,k-1} \end{bmatrix}$$
$$s_{i,j} = [s_{i,j,1}, s_{i,j,2}, \ldots, s_{i,j,n}]' \quad (15)$$

In the interest of time and cost, the number of control factors is reduced before running the experiments by using any technique such as screening experiments, as well as the forward, backward and stepwise regression.

4 Model optimization: Using the desirability function method, the optimal values for control factors are determined based on the type of quality characteristics and their specification limits such that their values come as close to the target values as possible. The desirability function of interest is:

$$Maximize D_{total} = \left\{ \left[\prod_{i=1}^{n} D(\mu_i)^{w_i}\right] \cdot \left[\prod_{i=1}^{n} D(s_i^2)^{w_i'}\right] \cdot \left[\prod_{i=1}^{n} D\left(\frac{s_i}{m_i}\right)^{w_i''}\right] \cdot \left[\prod_{i=1}^{n} D(s_{i,j})^{w_i'''}\right] \right\} \times \left(\frac{1}{\sum_{i=1}^{n}\left(w_i + w_i' + w_i''\right) + \sum_{i=1}^{\binom{n}{2}} w_i'''} \right) \quad (16)$$

The results are robust as long as the covariances between the observations for each pair of points are close to zero. So, when there is a deviation in some time intervals, they would not be transmitted to the other points.

The other advantage of the proposed method is its ability to be used for any part of the desirability function. For instance when we don't have access to the entire data and only the mean and the variance of the observations are available, the covariance part of the model may be eliminated. Or if the mean of the observations at each point of time for different combinations is in hand, only the mean part of the model is being used. Also, by using the desirability function and its weighted values, one may use any indices in some points under study. For the sake of simplicity, in the examples provided in Section 5, equal weights are assigned to all statistical indices in all time periods.

Numerical examples

To illustrate the applications of the proposed method, seven examples for different drugs are presented in this section adapted from credible pharmaceutical papers. These examples are solved by the proposed method to find the optimum values for the control factors of the drugs. The required material, the methods of pharmaceutical experiments and the data for each example are presented in the stated indicated references.

Example 1

Diclufenac Sodium

The release profile of this drug is investigated by Gohel [14] and Goethals [20]. The contour overlay and the minimization of quality loss function methods are introduced in their papers, respectively. This drug has three main control factors given in Table 2.

The first step is to code the control factors using the following relationships:

$$x_{1(\text{new})} = \frac{x_1 - 1000}{500}, x_{2(\text{new})} = \frac{x_2 - 10}{5}, x_{3(\text{new})} = \frac{x_3 - 25}{25}$$

In this research, three points of time for the drug release profile are being investigated with properties shown in Table 3.

The response surface relationships for the mean, the variance, the coefficient of variation and the covariance between each pair of points under study are presented in the Appendix 1. Optimum values are shown in Table 4.

Example 2

Terazosin HCl dehydrate

The release profile for this drug is investigated by Shin [19] and the problem is solved by the MSE minimization method. This experiment has ten control factors as shown in Table 5.

Noticing the large number of control factors in this example, five control factors x_1, x_3, x_7, x_8 and x_{10} are identified as significant control factors by using the stepwise regression method. The control factors are coded by the following relationships:

$$x_{i-new} = \begin{cases} \dfrac{x_i - 93.71}{7.03}, i = 1 \\ \dfrac{x_i}{7.03}, i = 2, 3, \ldots, 10 \end{cases}$$

In this research, 11 points of time of drug release profile are being investigated as presented in Table 6.

Table 2 Main control factors influencing Diclufenac Sodium release

Variable	Control factor	Level 1	Level 2	Level 3
x_1	Stirring speed (RPM)	500	1000	1500
x_2	Concentration of calcium chloride	5%	10%	15%
x_3	Percentage of liquid paraffin	0%	25%	50%

Table 3 The target values and lower and upper values for example 1

Response	Delay after usage	LSL	Target	USL
y_1	1 hour	20%	30%	40%
y_2	6 hour	50%	60%	70%
y_3	8 hour	65%	72.5%	80%

The response surface relationships for the mean and the variance of the underlying data are presented in Appendix 2. Optimum values for this example are shown in Table 7.

Example 3

Verapamil HCl

The release profile of this drug is investigated by Siva [21]. The three main control factors for this drug are presented in Table 8.

The control factors are coded by the following relationships:

$$x_{1(\text{new})} = \frac{x_1-11}{3}, x_{2(\text{new})} = \frac{x_2-36}{12}, x_{3(\text{new})} = \frac{x_3-90}{30}$$

In this research, five points of time are investigated from release profile as shown in Table 9.

The RSM relationships for the mean, the variance and the coefficient of variation for the points in Table 8 are presented in Appendix 3. By using the desirability function method the optimum values obtained for control factors are shown in Table 10.

Example 4

Metformin

The release profile for this drug is investigated by Nagrava [22]. The three main control factors are defined for this drug release as shown in Table 11.

The values of the control factors are coded using the following relationships:

$$x_{1(\text{new})} = \frac{x_1-1.758}{1.25}, x_{2(\text{new})} = \frac{x_2-0.25}{0.25}, x_{3(\text{new})} = \frac{x_3-3.75}{1.25}$$

The three points of time for the release profile are investigated in this research have the properties provided in Table 12.

The RSM relationships for the mean, the variance and the coefficient of variation for the data are presented in Appendix 4. By using the desirability function method the optimum values obtained for control factors are shown in Table 13.

Table 4 Optimum values for example 1

Variable	Control factor	Coded value	Uncoded value
x_1	Stirring speed (RPM)	−0.7576	621.2 rpm
x_2	Concentration of calcium chloride	−0.3939	8.0305%
x_3	Percentage of liquid paraffin	1	50%

Table 5 Control factors influencing Terazosin HCl dehydrate release

Variable	Control factor	Level 1	Level 2	Level 3	Level 4	Level 5
x_1	PEO	93.71	100.77	107.77	171.04	234.31
x_2	LH-11	0	7.03	14.06	77.33	140.6
x_3	Syloid	0	7.03	14.06	77.33	140.6
x_4	Ac-Di-Sol	0	7.03	14.06	77.33	140.6
x_5	Na-CMC	0	7.03	14.06	77.33	140.6
x_6	HEC	0	7.03	14.06	77.33	140.6
x_7	NaH_2PO_4	0	7.03	14.06	77.33	140.6
x_8	Citric acid	0	7.03	14.06	77.33	140.6
x_9	Pharma coat 603	0	7.03	14.06	77.33	140.6
x_{10}	Polyox N10	0	7.03	14.06	77.33	140.6

Example 5

Rhinetedin

The release profile of this drug is investigated by Patel [23]. The two main control factors for this drug are presented in Table 14.

The control factors are coded by the following relationships:

$$x_{1(\text{new})} = \frac{x_1-672}{168}, x_{2(\text{new})} = \frac{x_2-168}{84}$$

In this research three time points are investigated from release profile are shown in Table 15.

In this example, the index f_2 is the measure of similarity between the drug release profile and the target profile. The RSM relationships are presented in Appendix 5 and the optimum values are shown in Table 16.

Example 6

Metoprolol

The release profile for this drug is investigated by Gohel [24]. The two main control factors defined for this drug are shown in Table 17.

The control factor values are coded by using the following relationships:

$$x_{1(\text{new})} = \frac{x_1-30}{10}, x_{2(\text{new})} = \frac{x_2-20}{10}$$

The three points of time for the drug release profile are presented in Table 18.

In the study of this drug, f_2, t_{50} (the time required for 50% of drug to be released) and mean dissolution time (MDT) are the measures of the similarity factor between

Table 6 The target values and lower and upper values for example 2

	y_1	y_2	y_3	y_4	y_5	y_6	y_7	y_8	y_9	y_{10}	y_{11}
Time	0.5 h	1 h	1.5 h	2 h	3 h	4 h	6 h	8 h	10 h	12 h	24 h
LSL	4.8	8.8	10.24	12.88	18.08	23.84	34.8	41.12	48.24	54.8	65.84
Target	6	11	12.8	16.1	22.6	29.8	43.5	51.4	60.3	68.5	82.3
USL	7.2	13.2	15.36	19.32	27.12	35.76	52.2	61.68	72.36	82.2	98.76

release profile and the predefined profile, the time required to dissolve half of the drug and the mean dissolution time, respectively. The RSM relationships for the means and these measures are presented in Appendix 6. By using the proposed method, the optimum values are obtained as shown in Table 19.

Comparison of the proposed method and the existing ones

The disadvantages of the existing methods are:

Contour overlay method:

This method has a limited application and when the number of variables exceeds from two, the model may not be optimized unless the additional variables are being fixed at a constant level.

Profile selection method:

In this method, the number of test profiles is adjusted based on the experimenter point of view and the best profile is selected among the existing ones. It is possible that the optimum values for the control factors may not be included in these profiles.

MSE minimizing method:

In this method, there is no attention paid to the specification limits, while in the real world, passing these limits has substantial penalties.

Minimizing the total cost method:

In this method all deviations from the target values are evaluated by means of money terms, while in human problems, e.g. pharmaceutical studies, adverse events may have human fallout which cannot be measured by money terms.

The proposed method overcomes all the above disadvantages.

Conclusions

Investigation of the pharmaceutics problems in an industrial engineering framework is very constructive. The key point here is the problem presentation by the engineering terms. In this research, the drug release problem which is an important subject of pharmaceutics is being studied. In this area, applying the complex formulas is avoided. So, the experts with minimum knowledge of mathematics and statistics may apply this approach to solve the pharmaceutics problems. The results of the examples show the ability of the proposed model for solving the controlled release problems and to assure that the intended drug is resolved as its predefined profile. The simultaneous optimization of drugs with multi time-oriented quality characteristics is a topic for the future research.

Table 7 Optimum values for control factors for example 2

Variable	Control factor	Coded value	Uncoded value
x_1	PEO	15.556	203.069
x_3	Syloid	0.691	4.858
x_7	NaH_2PO_4	14.748	103.675
X_8	Citric acid	0	0
X_{10}	Polyox N10	20	140.6

Appendix 1

$$\begin{aligned}\mu_{1(1h)} = {} & 39.929 + 2.365x_1 - 2.206x_2 - 1.959x_3 \\ & + 0.202x_1^2 + 1.971x_2^2 - 0.912x_3^2 - 1.389x_1x_2 \\ & + 0.797x_1x_3 + 0.079x_2x_3\end{aligned}$$

$$\begin{aligned}\mu_{2(6h)} = {} & 73.368 + 4.388x_1 - 5.031x_2 - 2.379x_3 \\ & + 0.399x_1^2 + 0.579x_2^2 - 0.127x_3^2 - 1.525x_1x_2 \\ & - 0.062x_1x_3 - 0.359x_2x_3\end{aligned}$$

$$\begin{aligned}\mu_{3(8h)} = {} & 83.203 + 4.165x_1 - 4.562x_2 - 2.498x_3 \\ & - 0.624x_1^2 - 0.907x_2^2 + 1.176x_3^2 - 2.37x_1x_2 \\ & + 0.151x_1x_3 - 1.632x_2x_3\end{aligned}$$

$$\begin{aligned}V_{1(1h)} = {} & 7.31 - 0.642x_1 + 0.032x_2 + 2.799x_3 \\ & + 1.698x_1^2 + 5.377x_2^2 + 4.895x_3^2 + 5.543x_1x_2 \\ & + 1.893x_1x_3 - 0.686x_2x_3\end{aligned}$$

$$\begin{aligned}V_{2(6h)} = {} & 5.74 - 1.195x_1 + 1.609x_2 - 5.458x_3 \\ & + 7.112x_1^2 + 0.037x_2^2 + 9.608x_3^2 + 11.9x_1x_2 \\ & - 4.042x_1x_3 + 0.98x_2x_3\end{aligned}$$

$$\begin{aligned}V_{3(8h)} = {} & 11.548 - 6.216x_1 + 3.632x_2 - 0.354x_3 \\ & + 2.053x_1^2 + 2.293x_2^2 + 2.581x_3^2 - 5.282x_1x_2 \\ & + 2.575x_1x_3 - 5.902x_2x_3\end{aligned}$$

Table 8 Main control factors influencing Verapamil HCl release

Variable	Control factor	Level 1	Level 2	Level 3
x_1	Coating weigh gain	8%	11%	14%
x_2	Duration of coating	24 h	36 h	48 h
x_3	Amount of plasticizer	60%	90%	120%

Table 9 The target values and lower and upper values for example 3

	y_1	y_2	y_3	y_4	y_5
Time	2 h	4 h	6 h	9 h	12 h
LSL	13.36%	26.64%	40%	50%	80%
Target	16.7%	33.3%	50%	75%	100%
USL	20.04%	39.96%	60%	90%	120%

$$\left(\frac{s}{m}\right)_{1(1h)} = 0.063–0.005x_1–0.001x_2 + 0.012x_3 + 0.007x_1^2 + 0.008x_2^2 + 0.014x_3^2 + 0.021x_1x_2 + 0.008x_1x_3–0.003x_2x_3$$

$$\left(\frac{s}{m}\right)_{2(6h)} = 0.04–0.002x_1 + 0.007x_2–0.003x_3 + 0.006x_1^2–0.004x_2^2 + 0.009x_3^2 + 0.013x_1x_2–0.008x_1x_3 + 0.004x_2x_3$$

$$\left(\frac{s}{m}\right)_{3(8h)} = 0.039–0.009x_1 + 0.008x_2 + 0.002x_3 –0.0002x_1^2 + 0.004x_2^2 + 0.006x_3^2–0.007x_1x_2 +0.002x_1x_3–0.006x_2x_3$$

$$(s_{12})_{(1h–6h)} = 1.89 + 2.507x_1–0.799x_2 + 0.299x_3 + 0.677x_1^2–2.227x_2^2–4.571x_3^2–2.594x_1x_2 –0.655x_1x_3–2.289x_2x_3$$

$$(s_{13})_{(1h–8h)}= 1.091 + 1.603x_1 1.572x_2 + 3.023x_3 –3.872x_1^2–3.299x_2^2 + 3.353x_3^2–1.879x_1x_2 +0.966x_1x_3 + 2.559x_2x_3$$

$$(s_{23})_{(6h–8h)} = –2.945–1.711x_1–1.729x_2–3.296x_3 + 2.541x_1^2 + 2.411x_2^2–2.738x_3^2–0.22x_1x_2 + 3.237x_1x_3 + 3.732x_2x_3$$

Appendix 2

$$\mu_{1(0.5h)} = 4.844–0.039x_1 + 0.023x_3–0.006x_7–0.005x_8 –0.001x_{10} + 0.0001x_1^2–0.00007x_3^2 + 0.00006x_7^2 +0.00002x_8^2 + 0.00003x_{10}^2 + 0.0006x_1x_3$$

$$V_{1(0.5h)} = 0.71–0.008x_1 + 0.0001x_3–0.00078x_7 + 0.006x_8–0.006x_{10} + 0.00003x_1^2 + 0.000006x_3^2 + 0.00003x_7^2–0.00002x_8^2 + 0.00004x_{10}^2–0.00003x_1x_3$$

Table 10 Optimum values for control factors for example 3

Variable	Control factor	Coded value	Uncoded value
x_1	Coating weigh gain	–0.6566	9.0302
x_2	Duration of coating	0.5152	29.8176
x_3	Amount of plasticizer	1	120

Table 11 Main control factors for example 3

Variable	Control factor	Level 1	Level 2	Level 3
x_1	Concentration of sodium alginate	1.25%	1.75%	2.25%
x_2	Concentration of gellan gum	0%	0.25%	0.5%
x_3	Concentration of metformin	2.5%	3.75%	5%

$$\mu_{2(1h)} = 7.644–0.027x_1 + 0.015x_3–0.01x_7 + 0.017x_8 –0.014x_{10} + 0.0001x_1^2 + 0.000001x_3^2 + 0.0001x_7^2 +0.0002x_8^2 + 0.0001x_{10}^2 + 0.0004x_1x_3$$

$$V_{2(1h)} = 1.103–0.041x_1–0.027x_3–0.002x_7 +0.021x_8 + 0.006x_{10} + 0.0001x_1^2 +0.00008x_3^2 + 0.00002x_7^2–0.00007x_8^2 –0.00002x_{10}^2 + 0.0009x_1x_3$$

$$\mu_{3(1.5h)} = 7.228 + 0.109x_1 + 0.018x_3–0.029x_7 + 0.033x_8 –0.035x_{10}–0.0003x_1^2–0.0005x_3^2 + 0.0003x_7^2 +0.0003x_8^2 + 0.0002x_{10}^2–0.0044x_1x_3$$

$$V_{3(1.5h)} = 0.292 + 0.021x_1 + 0.035x_3–0.031x_7 +0.033x_8–0.004x_{10}–0.00005x_1^2–0.000009x_3^2 +0.0002x_7^2–0.0001x_8^2 + 0.00003x_{10}^2–0.0009x_1x_3$$

$$\mu_{4(2h)} = 8.611 + 0.165x_1 + 0.248x_3–0.074x_7 +0.074x_8–0.05x_{10}–0.0005x_1^2–0.0007x_3^2 +0.0006x_7^2 + 0.0002x_8^2 + 0.0003x_{10}^2–0.006x_1x_3$$

$$V_{4(2h)} = 1.582–0.082x_1–0.05x_3–0.033x_7 + 0.058x_8 + 0.027x_{10} + 0.0003x_1^2 + 0.0002x_3^2 +0.0002x_7^2–0.0002x_8^2–0.0001x_{10}^2 + 0.002x_1x_3$$

$$\mu_{5(3h)} = 12.428 + 0.207x_1 + 0.309x_3–0.09x_7 + 0.089x_8–0.049x_{10}–0.0006x_1^2–0.0008x_3^2 +0.0007x_7^2 +0.0003x_8^2 +0.0004x_{10}^2–0.008x_1x_3$$

$$V_{5(3h)} = 1.69–0.078x_1–0.033x_3–0.021x_7 + 0.052x_8 + 0.033x_{10} + 0.0003x_1^2 + 0.0001x_3^2 +0.0001x_7^2–0.0002x_8^2–0.0001x_{10}^2+ 0.001x_1x_3$$

$$\mu_{6(4h)} = 16.417 + 0.287x_1 + 0.388x_3–0.11x_7 + 0.126x_8–0.07x_{10}–0.0008x_1^2–0.001x_3^2 +0.0009x_7^2+ 0.0003x_8^2+ 0.0005x_{10}^2–0.011x_1x_3$$

Table 12 The target values and lower and upper values for example 4

Response	Delay after usage	LSL	Target	USL
y_1	0.5 hour	21%	23.5%	26%
y_2	3.5 hours	62%	63.5%	65%
y_3	8 hours	91%	92.5%	94%

Table 13 Optimum values of control factors for example 4

Variable	Control factor	Coded value	Uncoded value
x_1	Concentration of sodium alginate	1	2.25%
x_2	Concentration of gellan gum	−0.9192	0.0202%
x_3	Concentration of metformin	−1	2.5%

$$V_{6(4h)} = 3.123-0.134x_1-0.074x_3-0.035x_7 + 0.061x_8 + 0.053x_{10} + 0.0005x_1^2 + 0.0002x_3^2 + 0.0002x_7^2-0.0002x_8^2-0.0002x_{10}^2 + 0.003x_1x_3$$

$$\mu_{7(6h)} = 21.874 + 0.563x_1 + 0.691x_3-0.174x_7 + 0.109x_8-0.084x_{10}-0.002x_1^2-0.002x_3^2 + 0.001x_7^2 + 0.0006x_8^2 + 0.0007x_{10}^2-0.02x_1x_3$$

$$V_{7(6h)} = 4.719-0.22x_1-0.104x_3-0.056x_7 + 0.073x_8 + 0.105x_{10} + 0.0008x_1^2 + 0.0003x_3^2 + 0.0003x_7^2-0.0002x_8^2-0.0004x_{10}^2 + 0.005x_1x_3$$

$$\mu_{8(8h)} = 28.588 + 0.811x_1 + 0.963x_3-0.221x_7 + 0.073x_8-0.11x_{10}-0.002x_1^2-0.003x_3^2 + 0.001x_7^2 + 0.0007x_8^2 + 0.001x_{10}^2-0.03x_1x_3$$

$$V_{8(8h)} = 5.417-0.226x_1-0.064x_3-0.072x_7 + 0.061x_8 + 0.158x_{10} + 0.0008x_1^2 + 0.0001x_3^2 + 0.0004x_7^2-0.0002x_8^2-0.0006x_{10}^2 + 0.004x_1x_3$$

$$\mu_{9(10h)} = 37.1 + 0.886x_1 + 1.086x_3-0.249x_7 + 0.058x_8-0.094x_{10}-0.003x_1^2-0.003x_3^2 + 0.002x_7^2 + 0.001x_8^2 + 0.001x_{10}^2-0.032x_1x_3$$

$$V_{9(10h)} = 7.351-0.28x_1-0.085x_3-0.088x_7 + 0.046x_8 + 0.201x_{10} + 0.001x_1^2 + 0.0002x_3^2 + 0.0005x_7^2-0.0002x_8^2-0.0008x_{10}^2 + 0.005x_1x_3$$

$$\mu_{10(12h)} = 44.362 + 1.017x_1 + 1.237x_3-0.229x_7 + 0.055x_8-0.144x_{10}-0.003x_1^2-0.004x_3^2 + 0.001x_7^2 + 0.0006x_8^2 + 0.001x_{10}^2-0.036x_1x_3$$

$$V_{10(12h)} = 7.482-0.267x_1-0.049x_3-0.095x_7 + 0.055x_8 + 0.217x_{10} + 0.001x_1^2 + 0.00001x_3^2 + 0.0005x_7^2-0.0002x_8^2-0.001x_{10}^2 + 0.004x_1x_3$$

$$\mu_{11(24h)} = 82.688 + 0.577x_1 + 0.705x_3-0.056x_7 + 0.06x_8 + 0.044x_{10}-0.002x_1^2-0.002x_3^2 + 0.004x_7^2-0.00004x_8^2 + 0.0001x_{10}^2-0.02x_1x_3$$

Table 14 Main control factors for example 5

Variable	Control factor	Level 1	Level 2	Level 3
x_1	Amount of gelucire 43/01	504	672	840
x_2	Amount of ethylcellulose	84	168	252

Table 15 The target values and lower and upper specifications for example 5

Response	Delay after usage	LSL	Target	USL
y_1	1 hour	26%	32.5%	39%
y_2	5 hours	54%	67.5%	81%
y_3	10 hours	68%	85%	102%

$$V_{11(24h)} = 7.503-0.104x_1-0.025x_3-0.097x_7-0.005x_8 -0.004x_{10} + 0.0005x_1^2 + 0.00004x_3^2 + 0.0006x_7^2-0.0001x_8^2-0.0001x_{10}^2 + 0.001x_1x_3$$

Appendix 3

$$\mu_{1(2h)} = 12.986-2.16x_1-x_2 + 0.68x_3 + 0.121x_1^2-0.279x_2^2 + 0.221x_3^2 + 0.038x_1x_2 + 0.038x_1x_3 + 0.163x_2x_3$$

$$\nu_{1(2h)} = 1.274 + 0.057x_1 + 0.33x_2-0.235x_3-0.064x_1^2 + 0.056x_2^2-0.298x_3^2-0.002x_1x_2 + 0.426x_1x_3 + 0.292x_2x_3$$

$$\left(\frac{s}{m}\right)_{1(2h)} = 0.082 + 0.013x_1 + 0.017x_2-0.015x_3 -0.006x_1^2 + 0.011x_2^2-0.016x_3^2 + 0.002x_1x_2 + 0.014x_1x_3 + 0.015x_2x_3$$

$$\mu_{2(4h)} = 25.121-5.2x_1-2x_2 + 1.43x_3 + 0.47x_1^2-0.331x_2^2 + 0.619x_3^2 + 0.163x_1x_2 + 0.063x_1x_3 + 0.338x_2x_3$$

$$\nu_{2(4h)} = 1.747 + 0.112x_1 + 0.004x_2-0.564x_3-1.017x_1^2 + 1.813x_2^2-0.732x_3^2-0.442x_1x_2 + 0.185x_1x_3-0.185x_2x_3$$

$$\left(\frac{s}{m}\right)_{2(4h)} = 0.046 + 0.01x_1 + 0.002x_2-0.011x_3 -0.013x_1^2 + 0.025x_2^2-0.009x_3^2-0.004x_1x_2 + 0.0004x_1x_3-0.004x_2x_3$$

$$\mu_{3(6h)} = 42.938-7.27x_1-2.87x_2 + 2.31x_3-0.257x_1^2 -0.257x_2^2-0.057x_3^2 + 0.913x_1x_2 + 0.463x_1x_3 -0.688x_2x_3$$

$$\nu_{3(6h)} = 3.412 + 0.072x_1 + 0.965x_2 + 0.052x_3 + 3.869x_1^2-1.106x_2^2-1.351x_3^2-1.126x_1x_2 + 0.936x_1x_3-0.049x_2x_3$$

$$\left(\frac{s}{m}\right)_{3(6h)} = 0.042 + 0.009x_1 + 0.008x_2-0.002x_3 -0.023x_1^2-0.005x_2^2-0.007x_3^2-0.006x_1x_2 + 0.004x_1x_3 + 0.001x_2x_3$$

Table 16 Optimum values for example 5

Variable	Control factor	Coded value	Uncoded value
x_1	Amount of gelucire 43/01	−0.909	657.7288
x_2	Amount of ethylcellulose	1	252

Table 17 Main control factors for example 7

Variable	Control factor	Level 1	Level 2	Level 3
x_1	% of xanthan gum	20%	30%	40%
x_2	% of Methocel	10%	20%	30%

$$\mu_{4(9h)} = 67.278-11.37x_1-3.02x_2+3.27x_3-2.541x_1^2 + 3.709x_2^2-3.841x_3^2+0.125x_1x_2+0.825x_1x_3 + 0.05x_2x_3$$

$$v_{4(9h)} = 3.563+0.311x_1-0.064x_2+0.085x_3-0.895x_1^2 +0.32x_2^2+0.425x_3^2+0.523x_1x_2-0.208x_1x_3 -0.09x_2x_3$$

$$\left(\frac{s}{m}\right)_{4(9h)} = 0.027+0.007x_1+0.002x_2-0.002x_3-0.001x_1^2 +0.001x_2^2+0.003x_3^2+0.003x_1x_2 -0.002x_1x_3-0.001x_2x_3$$

$$\mu_{5(12h)} = 82.395-12.84x_1-5.25x_2+3.8x_3-0.567x_1^2 -0.417x_2^2+0.333x_3^2-0.675x_1x_2+0.625x_1x_3 +0.125x_2x_3$$

$$v_{5(12h)} = 3.944-0.428x_1+0.038x_2-0.142x_3+1.018x_1^2 -1.592x_2^2-0.662x_3^2+0.705x_1x_2-0.065x_1x_3 +0.643x_2x_3$$

$$\left(\frac{s}{m}\right)_{5(12h)} = 0.024+0.002x_1+0.002x_2-0.002x_3 +0.004x_1^2-0.006x_2^2-0.002x_3^2+0.003x_1x_2 -0.001x_1x_3+0.003x_2x_3$$

Appendix 4

$$\mu_{1(0.5h)} = 31.153-3.546x_1-3.884x_2+3.243x_3 + 0.667x_1^2+1.874x_2^2-3.391x_3^2 + 2.897x_1x_2-0.767x_1x_3+1.175x_2x_3$$

$$v_{1(0.5h)} = 0.669-0.456x_1-0.45x_2-0.839x_3+1.542x_1^2 -1.429x_2^2+2.026x_3^2-1.309x_1x_2-1.167x_1x_3 +0.649x_2x_3$$

$$\left(\frac{s}{m}\right)_{1(0.5h)} = 0.028+0.002x_1+0.0004x_2-0.016x_3 +0.01x_1^2-0.01x_2^2+0.022x_3^2-0.016x_1x_2 -0.01x_1x_3+0.002x_2x_3$$

Table 18 The target values and lower and upper specification limits for example 7

Response	Delay after usage	LSL	Target	USL
y_1	1 hour	15%	17.5%	20%
y_2	4 hours	20%	30%	40%
y_3	12 hours	60%	65%	70%
t_{50}	-	6 h	7 h	8 h
MDT	-	8 h	9 h	10 h

Table 19 Optimum values for example 7

Variable	Control factor	Coded value	Uncoded value
x_1	% of xanthan gum	0.0458	30.458
x_2	% of Methocel	0.6726	26.726

$$\mu_{2(3.5h)} = 64.474-6.603x_1-4.648x_2+3.1x_3-0.977x_1^2 +4.658x_2^2+1.287x_3^2-1.168x_1x_2-0.65x_1x_3 -0.705x_2x_3$$

$$v_{2(3.5h)} = 0.841-0.063x_1+0.215x_2+0.12x_3-0.173x_1^2 +0.765x_2^2+0.048x_3^2-0.084x_1x_2-0.56x_1x_3 -0.371x_2x_3$$

$$\left(\frac{s}{m}\right)_{2(3.5h)} = 0.011+0.001x_1+0.003x_2-0.001x_3 -0.001x_1^2+0.007x_2^2-0.0003x_3^2-0.00003x_1x_2 -0.004x_1x_3-0.002x_2x_3$$

$$\mu_{3(8h)} = 92.466-4.383x_1-2.878x_2+1.811x_3-1.242x_1^2 + 2.206x_2^2-0.987x_3^2-1.1x_1x_2+0.168x_1x_3 + 2.018x_2x_3$$

$$v_{3(8h)} = 0.895-0.192x_1+0.213x_2-0.302x_3 + 0.029x_1^2-0.564x_2^2+0.786x_3^2-0.135x_1x_2 + 0.088x_1x_3-0.284x_2x_3$$

$$\left(\frac{s}{m}\right)_{3(8h)} = 0.01-0.001x_1+0.001x_2-0.001x_3 +0.0001x_1^2-0.004x_2^2+0.004x_3^2-0.001x_1x_2 +0.001x_1x_3-0.001x_2x_3$$

Appendix 5

$$\mu_{1(1h)} = 37.191-7.918x_1-3.955x_2+1.148x_1^2-1.432x_2^2 -0.558x_1x_2$$

$$v_{1(1h)} = 1.957+0.862x_1-0.693x_2-0.105x_1^2-0.04x_2^2 -1.32x_1x_2$$

$$\left(\frac{s}{m}\right)_{1(1h)} = 0.038+0.015x_1-0.003x_2-0.002x_1^2-0.001x_2^2 -0.012x_1x_2$$

$$\mu_{2(5h)} = 75.29-6.358x_1-8.795x_2+1.035x_1^2-1.345x_2^2 + 0.745x_1x_2$$

$$v_{2(5h)} = 5.129+0.25x_1+0.915x_2-2.223x_1^2-0.583x_2^2 -1.18x_1x_2$$

$$\left(\frac{s}{m}\right)_{2(5h)} = 0.031+0.003x_1+0.006x_2-0.009x_1^2 -0.002x_2^2-0.005x_1x_2$$

$$\mu_{3(10h)} = 89.216-8.49x_1-7.528x_2+3.797x_1^2-1.728x_2^2 -3.195x_1x_2$$

$$v_{3(10h)} = 3.026-0.145x_1-1.292x_2+2.372x_1^2-1.968x_2^2 + 0.75x_1x_2$$

$$\left(\frac{s}{m}\right)_{3(10h)} = 0.017 + 0.002x_1 - 0.003x_2 + 0.007x_1^2 - 0.004x_2^2 - 0.003x_1x_2$$

$$f_2value = 50.157 + 7.52x_1 + 9.473x_2 - 5.26x_1^2 - 1.49x_2^2 - 0.66x_1x_2$$

Appendix 6

$$\mu_{1(1h)} = 20.778 - 3.317x_1 - 4.017x_2 + 0.183x_1^2 - 0.917x_2^2 - 0.325x_1x_2$$

$$\mu_{2(4h)} = 38.678 - 4.5x_1 - 5.7x_2 + 1.583x_1^2 - 1.467x_2^2 - 1.425x_1x_2$$

$$\mu_{3(12h)} = 68.822 - 5.483x_1 - 5.5x_2 + 2.317x_1^2 - 1.333x_2^2 + 0.15x_1x_2$$

$$\mu_{4(t_{50})} = 6.222 + x_1 + 1.167x_2 - 0.333x_1^2 + 0.167x_2^2$$

$$\mu_{5(MDT)} = 8.222 + 0.767x_1 + 0.933x_2 - 0.333x_1^2 + 0.267x_2^2 - 0.1x_1x_2$$

$$\mu_{6(f2)} = 68.556 + 11.183x_1 + 11.45x_2 - 2.483x_1^2 - 3.583x_2^2 - 1.525x_1x_2$$

Abbreviations
MEC: Minimum effective concentration; MTC: Minimal toxic concentration; NTB: Nominal the best; LTB: Larger the better; STB: Smaller the better; DOE: Design of experiments; RSM: Response surface methodology; LSL: Lower specification limit; USL: Upper specification limit; MDT: Mean dissolution time.

Competing interests
The authors declare that they have no competing interests.

Authors' contributions
Authors contributed to the manuscript according to their responsibility. MRN designed and carried out the study. HS was the dissertation supervisor. MS validated the findings and proofread the final version. All authors read and approved the final manuscript.

Acknowledgements
This research was part of Mohammad Reza Nabatchian PhD Dissertation.

Author details
[1]Department of Industrial Engineering, K.N. Toosi University of Technology, No 7, Pardis St., Mollasadra Ave., Tehran, Iran. [2]Department of Dermatology, University of Connecticut Health Center, Farmington, CT, USA.

References
1. Perrie Y, Rades T: *Pharmaceutics-drug delivery and targeting.* UK: Pharmaceutical press; 2012:7–14.
2. Hillery A, Loyd A, Swarbrick J: *Drug delivery and targeting.* USA: Taylor and Francis; 2005:20–42.
3. Li X, Jasti B: *Design of controlled release drug delivery systems.* USA: McGraw-Hill; 2006:10–35.
4. Wen H, Park K: *Oral Controlled Release formulation design and drug delivery.* USA: John Wiley & Sons; 2010:21–46.
5. Rathbone M, Hadgraft J: *Modified-release drug delivery technology.* USA: Marcel Dekker, Inc; 2003:1–20.
6. Juran J, Godrey A: *Juran's quality handbook.* 5th edition. USA: McGraw-Hill; 1999:5–20.
7. Taguchi G, Chowdhury S, Taguchi S: *Taguchi's quality engineering handbook.* USA: John Wiley & Sons; 2005:20–60.
8. Phadke M: *Quality engineering using robust design.* USA: Prentice-hall international; 1989:5–40.
9. Park S, Antony J: *Robust design for quality engineering and six sigma.* USA: World Scientific; 2008:25–60.
10. Montgomery DC: *Design and analysis of experiments.* 5th edition. USA: John Wiley & Sons; 2001:21–60.
11. Dean A, Lewis S: *Screening: methods for experimentation in industry, drug discovery and genetics.* USA: Springer; 2006:1–45.
12. Myers R, Montgomery DC: *Response surface methodology.* 2nd edition. USA: John Wiley & Sons; 2002:20–50.
13. Derringer G, Suich R: **Simultaneous optimization of several response variables.** *J Qual Technol* 1980, **12**(4):214–219.
14. Gohel A, Amin A: **Formulation optimization if controlled release diclofenac sodium microspheres using factorial design.** *J Control Release* 1998, **51**:115–122.
15. Moore J, Flanner H: **Mathematical comparison of curves with an emphasis on in-vitro dissolution profiles.** *J Pharm Technol* 1996, **20**(6):67–74.
16. Freitag G: **Guidelines on dissolution profile comparison.** *Drug Inf J* 2001, **35**:865–874.
17. Truong N, Shin S, Choi Y, Jeong S, Cho B: **Robust design with time-oriented responses for regenerative medicine industry.** In *Proceeding of the 3rd International Conference on the Development of biomedical engineering: 11-14 January 2010.* Edited by Toi V, Khoa T. Vietnam: Springer; 2010:67–70.
18. Park J, Shin J, Truong N, Shin S, Choi Y, Lee J, Yoon J, Jeong S: **A pharma robust design method to investigate the effect of PEGand PEO on matrix tablets.** *Int J Pharm* 2010, **393**:79–87.
19. Shin S, Choi D, Truong N, Kim N, Chu K, Jeong S: **Time-oriented experimental design method to optimize hydrophilic matrix formulations with gelatin kinetics and drug release profiles.** *Int J Pharm* 2011, **407**:53–62.
20. Goethals P, Cho B: **The development of a robust design methodology for time-oriented dynamic quality characteristics with a target profile.** *Qual Reliability Eng Int* 2011, **27**:403–414.
21. Vaithiyalingam S, Khan M: **Optimization and characterization of controlled release multi-particulate beads formulated with a customized cellulose acetate butyrate dispersion.** *Int J Pharm* 2002, **234**:179–193.
22. Nagarwal R, Srinatha A, Pandit J: **In situ forming formulation: development, evaluation, and optimization using 3^3 factorial design.** *AAPS pharm sci tech* 2009, **10**(3):977–983.
23. Patel D, Patel N, Patel V, Bhatt D: **Floating granules of ranitidine hydrochloride-gelucire 43/01: formulation optimization using factorial design.** *AAPS pharm sci tech* 2007, **8**(2):1–7.
24. Gohel M, Parikh R, Nagori S, Jena D: **Fabrication of modified release tablet formulation of metoprolol succinate using hydroxypropyl methylcellulose and xanthan gum.** *AAPS pharm sci tech* 2009, **10**(1):62–68.

Permissions

All chapters in this book were first published in DARU-JPS, by BioMed Central; hereby published with permission under the Creative Commons Attribution License or equivalent. Every chapter published in this book has been scrutinized by our experts. Their significance has been extensively debated. The topics covered herein carry significant findings which will fuel the growth of the discipline. They may even be implemented as practical applications or may be referred to as a beginning point for another development.

The contributors of this book come from diverse backgrounds, making this book a truly international effort. This book will bring forth new frontiers with its revolutionizing research information and detailed analysis of the nascent developments around the world.

We would like to thank all the contributing authors for lending their expertise to make the book truly unique. They have played a crucial role in the development of this book. Without their invaluable contributions this book wouldn't have been possible. They have made vital efforts to compile up to date information on the varied aspects of this subject to make this book a valuable addition to the collection of many professionals and students.

This book was conceptualized with the vision of imparting up-to-date information and advanced data in this field. To ensure the same, a matchless editorial board was set up. Every individual on the board went through rigorous rounds of assessment to prove their worth. After which they invested a large part of their time researching and compiling the most relevant data for our readers.

The editorial board has been involved in producing this book since its inception. They have spent rigorous hours researching and exploring the diverse topics which have resulted in the successful publishing of this book. They have passed on their knowledge of decades through this book. To expedite this challenging task, the publisher supported the team at every step. A small team of assistant editors was also appointed to further simplify the editing procedure and attain best results for the readers.

Apart from the editorial board, the designing team has also invested a significant amount of their time in understanding the subject and creating the most relevant covers. They scrutinized every image to scout for the most suitable representation of the subject and create an appropriate cover for the book.

The publishing team has been an ardent support to the editorial, designing and production team. Their endless efforts to recruit the best for this project, has resulted in the accomplishment of this book. They are a veteran in the field of academics and their pool of knowledge is as vast as their experience in printing. Their expertise and guidance has proved useful at every step. Their uncompromising quality standards have made this book an exceptional effort. Their encouragement from time to time has been an inspiration for everyone.

The publisher and the editorial board hope that this book will prove to be a valuable piece of knowledge for researchers, students, practitioners and scholars across the globe.

List of Contributors

Khosrou Abdi
Department of Medicinal Chemistry, Tehran, Iran
Department of Nuclear Pharmacy, Tehran, Iran

Ali Khalaj
Department of Medicinal Chemistry, Tehran, Iran
Department of Nuclear Pharmacy, Tehran, Iran

Syeed-Naser Ostad
Department of Pharmacology & toxicology, Tehran, Iran

Mohammad Reza Khoshayand
Department of Drug and Food Control, Faculty of Pharmacy, Tehran University of Medical Sciences, Tehran, Iran

Maryam Ehsani
Department of Endodontics, Dental Material Research Center, Faculty of Dentistry, Babol University of Medical Sciences, Babol, Iran

Ali-Akbar Moghadamnia
Department of Pharmacology, Faculty of Medicine, Babol University of Medical Sciences, Babol, Iran

Samir Zahedpasha
Department of Endodontics, Dental Material Research Center, Faculty of Dentistry, Babol University of Medical Sciences, Babol, Iran

Ghorban Maliji
Cellular and Molecular Biology Research Center, Babol University of Medical Sciences, Babol, Iran

Sina Haghanifar
Department of Oral and Maxillofacial Radiology, Faculty of Dentistry, Babol University of Medical Sciences, Babol, Iran

Seyyed Mohsen Aghajanpour Mir
Cellular and Molecular Biology Research Center, Babol University of Medical Sciences, Babol, Iran

Narges Mousavi Kani
Cellular and Molecular Biology Research Center, Babol University of Medical Sciences, Babol, Iran

Kaveh Eslami
Faculty of Pharmacy and Pharmaceutical Sciences Research Centre, Tehran University of Medical Sciences, Tehran, IranFaculty of Pharmacy, Ahvaz Jondishapour University of Medical Sciences, Ahvaz, Iran

Ata Mahmoodpoor
Department of Anesthesiology and Critical Care Medicine, Faculty of Medicine, Tabriz University of Medical Sciences, Tabriz, Iran

Arezoo Ahmadi
Department of Anesthesiology and Critical Care Medicine, Sina Hospital, Faculty of Medicine, Tehran

Mohammad Abdollahi
Faculty of Pharmacy and Pharmaceutical Sciences Research Centre, Tehran University of Medical Sciences, Tehran, Iran

Koorosh Kamali
Department of Public Health, School of Public Health, Zanjan University of Medical Sciences, Zanjan, Iran

Sarah Mousavi
Clinical Pharmacy Department, Faculty of Pharmacy and Research Center for Rational Use of Drugs, Tehran University of Medical Sciences, Tehran, Iran

Atabak Najafi
Department of Anesthesiology and Critical Care Medicine, Sina Hospital, Faculty of Medicine, Tehran
University of Medical Sciences, Tehran, Iran

Maryam Baeeri
Faculty of Pharmacy and Pharmaceutical Sciences Research Centre, Tehran University of Medical Sciences, Tehran, Iran

Hadi Hamishehkar
Clinical Pharmacy Department, Faculty of Pharmacy, Tabriz University of Medical Sciences, Tabriz, Iran

Leila Kouti
Faculty of Pharmacy, Ahvaz Jondishapour University of Medical Sciences, Ahvaz, Iran

Mohammad Reza Javadi
Faculty of Pharmacy and Pharmaceutical Sciences Research Centre, Tehran University of Medical Sciences, Tehran, Iran

Mojtaba Mojtahedzadeh
Faculty of Pharmacy and Pharmaceutical Sciences Research Centre, Tehran University of Medical Sciences, Tehran, Iran
Department of Anesthesiology and Critical Care Medicine, Sina Hospital, Faculty of Medicine, Tehran
University of Medical Sciences, Tehran, Iran

Negar Mohammadhosseini
Department of Chemistry, North Tehran Branch, Islamic Azad University, Tehran, Iran
Department of Medicinal Chemistry, Faculty of Pharmacy and Pharmaceutical Sciences Research Center, Tehran University of Medical Sciences, Tehran, Iran

Zahra Alipanahi
Department of Chemistry, North Tehran Branch, Islamic Azad University, Tehran, Iran

Eskandar Alipour
Department of Chemistry, North Tehran Branch, Islamic Azad University, Tehran, Iran

Saeed Emami
Department of Medicinal Chemistry and Pharmaceutical Sciences Research Center, Faculty of Pharmacy, Mazandaran University of Medical Sciences, Sari, Iran

Mohammad Ali Faramarzi
Department of Pharmaceutical Biotechnology, Faculty of Pharmacy, Tehran University of Medical Sciences, Tehran, Iran

Nasrin Samadi
Department of Pharmaceutical Biotechnology, Faculty of Pharmacy, Tehran University of Medical Sciences, Tehran, Iran

Nika Khoshnevis
Department of Pharmaceutical Biotechnology, Faculty of Pharmacy, Tehran University of Medical Sciences, Tehran, Iran

Abbass Shafiee
Department of Medicinal Chemistry, Faculty of Pharmacy and Pharmaceutical Sciences Research Center, Tehran University of Medical Sciences, Tehran, Iran

Alireza Foroumadi
Department of Medicinal Chemistry, Faculty of Pharmacy and Pharmaceutical Sciences Research Center, Tehran University of Medical Sciences, Tehran, Iran

Parisa Azerang
Drug Design and Bioinformatics Unit, Medical Biotechnology Department, Biotechnology Research Center, Pasteur Institute, Tehran, Iran13164

Ali Hossein Rezayan
Department of Life Science Engineering, Faculty of New Science and Technology, University of Tehran, Tehran, Iran

Soroush Sardari
Drug Design and Bioinformatics Unit, Medical Biotechnology Department, Biotechnology Research Center, Pasteur Institute, Tehran, Iran13164

Farzad Kobarfard
Department of Medicinal Chemistry, School of Pharmacy, Shahid Beheshti University of Medical Sciences, Tehran, Iran
Phytochemistry Research Centre, Shahid Beheshti University of Medical Sciences, Tehran, Iran

Mitra Bayat
Phytochemistry Research Centre, Shahid Beheshti University of Medical Sciences, Tehran, Iran

Kimia Tabib
Department of Medicinal Chemistry, School of Pharmacy, Shahid Beheshti University of Medical Sciences, Tehran, Iran

Narges Khaghanzadeh
Shiraz Institute for Cancer Research, Shiraz University of Medical Sciences, School of Medicine, Shiraz, Iran
Department of Immunology, Shiraz University of Medical Sciences, School of Medicine, Shiraz, Iran

Zahra Mojtahedi
Shiraz Institute for Cancer Research, Shiraz University of Medical Sciences, School of Medicine, Shiraz, Iran

Mohammad Ramezani
Pharmaceutical Research Center, School of Pharmacy, Mashhad University of Medical Sciences, Mashhad, Iran

Nasrollah Erfani
Shiraz Institute for Cancer Research, Shiraz University of Medical Sciences, School of Medicine, Shiraz, Iran

Abbas Ghaderi
Shiraz Institute for Cancer Research, Shiraz University of Medical Sciences, School of Medicine, Shiraz, Iran
Department of Immunology, Shiraz University of Medical Sciences, School of Medicine, Shiraz, Iran

Adile Ayati
Department of Medicinal Chemistry and Pharmaceutical Sciences Research Center, Faculty of Pharmacy, Mazandaran University of Medical Sciences, Sari, Iran

Mehraban Falahati
Department of Parasitology, Faculty of Medicine, Tehran University of Medical Sciences, Tehran, Iran

Hamid Irannejad
Department of Medicinal Chemistry and Pharmaceutical Sciences Research Center, Faculty of Pharmacy, Mazandaran University of Medical Sciences, Sari, Iran

Saeed Emami
Department of Medicinal Chemistry and Pharmaceutical Sciences Research Center, Faculty of Pharmacy, Mazandaran University of Medical Sciences, Sari, Iran

Amir Gharib
Department of Laboratory Sciences, Borujerd Branch, Islamic Azad University, Borujerd, Iran

Zohreh Faezizadeh
Department of Laboratory Sciences, Borujerd Branch, Islamic Azad University, Borujerd, Iran

Masoud Godarzee
Department of Biology, Borujerd Branch, Islamic Azad University, Borujerd, Iran

Mona Noori Koopaei
Novel Drug Delivery Lab, Faculty of Pharmacy, Tehran University of Medical Sciences, Tehran 1417614411, Iran

Mohamad Shahab Maghazei
Novel Drug Delivery Lab, Faculty of Pharmacy, Tehran University of Medical Sciences, Tehran 1417614411, Iran

Seyed Hossein Mostafavi
Nanotechnology Research Centre, Faculty of Pharmacy, Tehran University of Medical Sciences, Tehran, Iran

Hossein Jamalifar
Department of Drug and Food Control, Faculty of Pharmacy, Tehran University of Medical Sciences, Tehran, Iran

Nasrin Samadi
Department of Drug and Food Control, Faculty of Pharmacy, Tehran University of Medical Sciences, Tehran, Iran

Mohsen Amini
Department of Medicinal Chemistry, Faculty of Pharmacy, Tehran University of Medical Sciences, Tehran, Iran

Soheyl Jafari Malek
Novel Drug Delivery Lab, Faculty of Pharmacy, Tehran University of Medical Sciences, Tehran 1417614411, Iran

Behrad Darvishi
Novel Drug Delivery Lab, Faculty of Pharmacy, Tehran University of Medical Sciences, Tehran 1417614411, Iran

Fatemeh Atyabi
Novel Drug Delivery Lab, Faculty of Pharmacy, Tehran University of Medical Sciences, Tehran 1417614411, Iran
Nanotechnology Research Centre, Faculty of Pharmacy, Tehran University of Medical Sciences, Tehran, Iran

Rassoul Dinarvand
Novel Drug Delivery Lab, Faculty of Pharmacy, Tehran University of Medical Sciences, Tehran 1417614411, Iran
Nanotechnology Research Centre, Faculty of Pharmacy, Tehran University of Medical Sciences, Tehran, Iran

Shirin Hasani-Ranjbar
Endocrinology and Metabolism Research Institute, Tehran University of Medical Sciences, Tehran, Iran

Zahra Jouyandeh
Endocrinology and Metabolism Research Institute, Tehran University of Medical Sciences, Tehran, Iran

Mostafa Qorbani
Endocrinology and Metabolism Research Institute, Tehran University of Medical Sciences, Tehran, Iran

Mahbubeh Hemmatabadi
Endocrinology and Metabolism Research Institute, Tehran University of Medical Sciences, Tehran, Iran

Bagher Larijan
Endocrinology and Metabolism Research Institute, Tehran University of Medical Sciences, Tehran, Iran

Fowad Khurshid
Faculty of Pharmacy, Jamia Hamdard (Hamdard University), New Delhi 110062, India
Pharmacoeconomics and Outcomes Research Unit; Department of Clinical Pharmacy, College of Pharmacy, King Saud University, P.O Box: 2457, Riyadh 11451, Saudi Arabia

Mohammed Aqil
Faculty of Pharmacy, Jamia Hamdard (Hamdard University), New Delhi 110062, India

Mohammad Shamshir Alam
Faculty of Pharmacy, Jamia Hamdard (Hamdard University), New Delhi 110062, India

Prem Kapur
Majeedia Hospital, Jamia Hamdard (Hamdard University), New Delhi 110062, India

Krishna K Pillai
Faculty of Pharmacy, Jamia Hamdard (Hamdard University), New Delhi 110062, India

Negar Mohammadhosseini
Department of Medicinal Chemistry, Faculty of Pharmacy and Pharmaceutical Sciences Research Center, Tehran University of Medical Sciences, Tehran 14176, Iran

Parastoo Saniee
Department of Microbiology, Faculty of Sciences, University of Tehran, P.O. Box: 14155-6455, Tehran, Iran

Ameneh Ghamaripour
Department of Biology, Faculty of Science, Golestan University, Gorgan, Iran

Hassan Aryapour
Department of Biology, Faculty of Science, Golestan University, Gorgan, Iran

Farzaneh Afshar
Department of Chemistry, Science and Research Branch, Islamic Azad University, Arak, Iran

Najmeh Edraki
Department of Medicinal Chemistry, Faculty of Pharmacy and Pharmaceutical Sciences Research Center, Tehran University of Medical Sciences, Tehran 14176, Iran

Farideh Siavoshi
Department of Microbiology, Faculty of Sciences, University of Tehran, P.O. Box: 14155-6455, Tehran, Iran

Alireza Foroumadi
Department of Medicinal Chemistry, Faculty of Pharmacy and Pharmaceutical Sciences Research Center, Tehran University of Medical Sciences, Tehran 14176, Iran

Abbas Shafiee
Department of Medicinal Chemistry, Faculty of Pharmacy and Pharmaceutical Sciences Research Center, Tehran University of Medical Sciences, Tehran 14176, Iran

Ali Mandegary
Department of Pharmacology & Toxicology, School of Pharmacy and Pharmaceutics Research Center, Kerman University of Medical Sciences, Kerman, Iran

Arastoo Saeedi
Physiology Research Center, Kerman University of Medical Sciences, Kerman, Iran

Aziz Eftekhari
Department of Pharmacology & Toxicology, School of Pharmacy and Pharmaceutics Research Center, Kerman University of Medical Sciences, Kerman, Iran

Vahideh Montazeri
Department of Pharmacology & Toxicology, School of Pharmacy and Pharmaceutics Research Center, Kerman University of Medical Sciences, Kerman, Iran

Elham Sharif
Herbal and Traditional Medicines Research Center, Kerman University of Medical Sciences, Kerman, Iran

Ali Rafinejad
Department of Medicinal Chemistry, Faculty of Pharmacy and Drug Design & Development Research Center, Tehran University of Medical Sciences, Tehran, Iran

Asal Fallah-Tafti
Department of Medicinal Chemistry, Faculty of Pharmacy and Drug Design & Development Research Center, Tehran University of Medical Sciences, Tehran, Iran

Rakesh Tiwari
Department of Biomedical and Pharmaceutical Sciences, College of Pharmacy, The University of Rhode Island, Kingston, RI, USA

Amir Nasrolahi Shirazi
Department of Biomedical and Pharmaceutical Sciences, College of Pharmacy, The University of Rhode Island, Kingston, RI, USA

Deendayal Mandal
Department of Biomedical and Pharmaceutical Sciences, College of Pharmacy, The University of Rhode Island, Kingston, RI, USA

Abbas Shafiee
Department of Medicinal Chemistry, Faculty of Pharmacy and Drug Design & Development Research Center, Tehran University of Medical Sciences, Tehran, Iran

Keykavous Parang
Department of Biomedical and Pharmaceutical Sciences, College of Pharmacy, The University of Rhode Island, Kingston, RI, USA

Alireza Foroumadi
Department of Medicinal Chemistry, Faculty of Pharmacy and Drug Design & Development Research Center, Tehran University of Medical Sciences, Tehran, Iran

Tahmineh Akbarzadeh
Department of Medicinal Chemistry, Faculty of Pharmacy and Drug Design & Development Research Center, Tehran University of Medical Sciences, Tehran, Iran

Ahmad Mohammadi-Farani
Department of Pharmacology, Toxicology and Medical Services, Faculty of Pharmacy, Kermanshah University of Medical Sciences, Kermanshah, Iran

Aram Ahmadi
Students Research Committee, Kermanshah University of Medical Sciences, Kermanshah, Iran
Department of Medicinal Chemistry, Faculty of Pharmacy, Kermanshah University of Medical Sciences, Kermanshah, Iran

Hamid Nadri
Neurobiomedical Research Center, Shahid Sadoughi University of Medical Sciences, Yazd, Iran

Alireza Aliabadi
Department of Medicinal Chemistry, Faculty of Pharmacy, Kermanshah University of Medical Sciences, Kermanshah, Iran

MH Yazdi
Department of Pharmaceutical Biotechnology and Biotechnology Research Center, Faculty of Pharmacy, Tehran University of Medical Sciences, Tehran, Iran

Z Niazzadeh Najafi
Department of Pharmaceutical Biotechnology and Biotechnology Research Center, Faculty of Pharmacy, Tehran University of Medical Sciences, Tehran, Iran

MR Khorramizadeh
Department of Medical Biotechnology, School of Advanced Medical Technologies, Tehran University of Medical Sciences, Tehran, Iran

M Amini
Drug Design and Development Research Center, Faculty of Pharmacy, Tehran University of Medical Sciences, Tehran, Iran

AR Shahverdi
Department of Pharmaceutical Biotechnology and Biotechnology Research Center, Faculty of Pharmacy, Tehran University of Medical Sciences, Tehran, Iran

Khosrou Abdi
Department Radiopharmacy, Tehran University of Medical Sciences, Tehran 14174, Iran
Department of Medicinal Chemistry, Tehran University of Medical Sciences, Tehran 14174, Iran

Ali Khalaj
Department of Medicinal Chemistry, Tehran University of Medical Sciences, Tehran 14174, Iran
Drug Design & Development Research Center, Tehran University of Medical Sciences, Tehran 14174, Iran

Seyed Nasser Ostad
Department of Toxicology & Pharmacology, Tehran University of Medical Sciences, Tehran 14174, Iran

Navid Lamei
Drug Design & Development Research Center, Tehran University of Medical Sciences, Tehran 14174, Iran

Mohammad Reza Khoshayand
Department of Drug and Food Control, Faculty of Pharmacy, Tehran University of Medical Sciences, Tehran 14174, Iran

Ali Almasirad
Department of Medicinal Chemistry, Pharmaceutical Sciences Branch, Islamic Azad University, Tehran, Iran

Zahra Mousavi
Department of Toxicology and Pharmacology, Pharmaceutical Sciences Branch, Islamic Azad University, Tehran, Iran

Mohammad Tajik
Department of Medicinal Chemistry, Faculty of Pharmacy and Pharmaceutical Sciences Research Center, Tehran University of Medical Sciences, Tehran, Iran

Mohammad Javad Assarzadeh
Department of Medicinal Chemistry, Pharmaceutical Sciences Branch, Islamic Azad University, Tehran, Iran

Abbas Shafiee
Department of Medicinal Chemistry, Faculty of Pharmacy and Pharmaceutical Sciences Research Center, Tehran University of Medical Sciences, Tehran, Iran

Eskandar Alipour
Department of Chemistry, Islamic Azad University, Tehran-North Branch, Zafar St, Tehran, Iran

Zinatsadat Mousavi
Department of Chemistry, Islamic Azad University, Tehran-North Branch, Zafar St, Tehran, Iran

Zahra Safaei
Department of Chemistry, Islamic Azad University, Tehran-North Branch, Zafar St, Tehran, Iran

Mahboobeh Pordeli
Department of Biochemistry, Institute of Biochemistry and Biophysics, University of Tehran, Tehran, Iran

Maliheh Safavi
Biotechnology Department, Iranian Research Organization for Science and Technology, Tehran, Iran

Loghman Firoozpour
Drug Design and Development Research Center, Tehran University of Medicinal Sciences, Tehran, Iran

Negar Mohammadhosseini
Department of Medicinal Chemistry, Faculty of Pharmacy and Pharmaceutical Sciences Research Center, Tehran University of Medical Sciences, Tehran, Iran

Mina Saeedi
Department of Medicinal Chemistry, Faculty of Pharmacy and Pharmaceutical Sciences Research Center, Tehran University of Medical Sciences, Tehran, Iran

Sussan Kabudanian Ardestani
Department of Biochemistry, Institute of Biochemistry and Biophysics, University of Tehran, Tehran, Iran

Abbas Shafiee
Department of Medicinal Chemistry, Faculty of Pharmacy and Pharmaceutical Sciences Research Center, Tehran University of Medical Sciences, Tehran, Iran

Alireza Foroumadi
Department of Medicinal Chemistry, Faculty of Pharmacy and Pharmaceutical Sciences Research Center, Tehran University of Medical Sciences, Tehran, Iran

Jinho Lee
Department of Chemistry, Keimyung University, Daegu 704-701, Korea

Jina Kim
Department of Chemistry, Keimyung University, Daegu 704-701, Korea

Victor Sukbong Hong
Department of Chemistry, Keimyung University, Daegu 704-701, Korea

Jong-Wook Park
Department of Immunology, Keimyung University School of Medicine, Daegu 704-701, Korea

Tatiane Teixeira Oliveira
Instituto de Ciências da Saúde, Universidade Federal da Bahia, Salvador, Bahia, Brazil

Keina Maciele Campos
Instituto de Ciências da Saúde, Universidade Federal da Bahia, Salvador, Bahia, Brazil

Ana Tereza Cerqueira-Lima
Instituto de Ciências da Saúde, Universidade Federal da Bahia, Salvador, Bahia, Brazil

Tamires Cana Brasil Carneiro
Instituto de Ciências da Saúde, Universidade Federal da Bahia, Salvador, Bahia, Brazil

Eudes da Silva Velozo
Faculdade de Farmácia, Universidade Federal da Bahia, Salvador, Bahia, Brazil

Ingrid Christie Alexandrino Ribeiro Melo
Centro de Biotecnologia, Universidade Federal da Paraíba, João Pessoa, Paraíba, Brazil

Eugênia Abrantes Figueiredo
Centro de Biotecnologia, Universidade Federal da Paraíba, João Pessoa, Paraíba, Brazil

Eduardo de Jesus Oliveira
Centro de Biotecnologia, Universidade Federal da Paraíba, João Pessoa, Paraíba, Brazil

Darizy Flávia Silva Amorim de Vasconcelos
Instituto de Ciências da Saúde, Universidade Federal da Bahia, Salvador, Bahia, Brazil

Lain Carlos Pontes-de-Carvalho
Centro de Pesquisas Gonçalo Moniz, Fundação Oswaldo Cruz, Salvador, Bahia, Brazil

Neuza Maria Alcântara-Neves
Instituto de Ciências da Saúde, Universidade Federal da Bahia, Salvador, Bahia, Brazil

Camila Alexandrina Figueiredo
Instituto de Ciências da Saúde, Universidade Federal da Bahia, Salvador, Bahia, Brazil

Arash Khorrami
Department of Pharmacology and Toxicology, Faculty of Pharmacy, Tabriz University of Medical Sciences, Tabriz, Iran
Student Research Committee, Tabriz University of Medical Sciences, Tabriz, Iran

Mojtaba Hammami
Student Research Committee, Tabriz University of Medical Sciences, Tabriz, Iran

Mehraveh Garjani
Student Research Committee, Tabriz University of Medical Sciences, Tabriz, Iran

Nasrin Maleki-Dizaji
Department of Pharmacology and Toxicology, Faculty of Pharmacy, Tabriz University of Medical Sciences, Tabriz, Iran

Alireza Garjani
Department of Pharmacology and Toxicology, Faculty of Pharmacy, Tabriz University of Medical Sciences, Tabriz, Iran

Atabak Najafi
Department of Anesthesiology and Critical Care Medicine, Sina Hospital, Faculty of Medicine, Tehran University of Medical Sciences, Tehran, Iran

Mojtaba Mojtahedzadeh
Department of Anesthesiology and Critical Care Medicine, Sina Hospital, Faculty of Medicine, Tehran University of Medical Sciences, Tehran, Iran
Department of Clinical Pharmacy, Faculty of Pharmacy, Tehran University of Medical Sciences, Tehran, Iran
Faculty of Pharmacy and Pharmaceutical Sciences Research Center, Tehran University of Medical Sciences, Tehran, Iran

Keyvan Haji Ahmadi
Department of Clinical Pharmacy, Faculty of Pharmacy, Tehran University of Medical Sciences, Tehran, Iran

Mohammad Abdollahi
Faculty of Pharmacy and Pharmaceutical Sciences Research Center, Tehran University of Medical Sciences, Tehran, Iran

Maryam Mousavi
Department of Clinical Pharmacy, Faculty of Pharmacy, Mashhad University of Medical sciences, Mashhad, Iran

Legese Chelkeba
Department of Clinical Pharmacy, Faculty of Pharmacy, Tehran University of Medical Sciences, Tehran, Iran
Faculty of Pharmacy and Pharmaceutical Sciences Research Center, Tehran University of Medical Sciences, Tehran, Iran

Farhad Najmeddin
Department of Clinical Pharmacy, Faculty of Pharmacy, Tehran University of Medical Sciences, Tehran, Iran

Arezoo Ahmadi
Department of Anesthesiology and Critical Care Medicine, Sina Hospital, Faculty of Medicine, Tehran University of Medical Sciences, Tehran, Iran

Zahra Daman
Aerosol Research Laboratory, Department of Pharmaceutics, School of Pharmacy, Tehran University of Medical Sciences, Tehran, Iran

Kambiz Gilani
Aerosol Research Laboratory, Department of Pharmaceutics, School of Pharmacy, Tehran University of Medical Sciences, Tehran, Iran
Medicinal Plants Research Center, Tehran University of Medical Sciences, Tehran, Iran

Abdolhossein Rouholamini Najafabadi
Aerosol Research Laboratory, Department of Pharmaceutics, School of Pharmacy, Tehran University of Medical Sciences, Tehran, Iran

Hamid Reza Eftekhari
Aerosol Research Laboratory, Department of Pharmaceutics, School of Pharmacy, Tehran University of Medical Sciences, Tehran, Iran

Mohammad Ali Barghi
XRD Research Laboratory, School of Sciences, Tehran University, Tehran, Iran

Bagher Alinejad
Department of Pharmacology, School of Medicine, Mashhad University of Medical Sciences, Mashhad, Iran

Reza Shafiee-Nick
Department of Pharmacology, School of Medicine, Mashhad University of Medical Sciences, Mashhad, Iran
Pharmacological Research Center of Medicinal Plants, School of Medicine, Mashhad University of Medical Sciences, Mashhad, Iran

Hamid Sadeghian
Department of laboratory Sciences, School of Paramedical Sciences, Mashhad University of Medical Sciences, Mashhad, Iran

Ahmad Ghorbani
Pharmacological Research Center of Medicinal Plants, School of Medicine, Mashhad University of Medical Sciences, Mashhad, Iran

Mohsen Vosooghi
Department of Medicinal Chemistry, Faculty of Pharmacy, Tehran University of Medical Sciences, Tehran, Iran

Loghman Firoozpour
Drug Design and Development Research Center, Tehran University of Medical Sciences, Tehran, Iran

Abolfazl Rodaki
Drug Design and Development Research Center, Tehran University of Medical Sciences, Tehran, Iran

Mahboobeh Pordeli
Institute of Biochemistry and Biophysics, University of Tehran, PO Box 13145–1384, Tehran, Iran

Maliheh Safavi
Department of Biotechnology, Iranian Research Organization for Science and Technology, Tehran, Iran

Sussan K Ardestani
Institute of Biochemistry and Biophysics, University of Tehran, PO Box 13145–1384, Tehran, Iran

Armin Dadgar
Department of Medicinal Chemistry, Faculty of Pharmacy, Tehran University of Medical Sciences, Tehran, Iran

Ali Asadipour
Neuroscience Research Center, Institute of Neuropharmacology, Kerman University of Medicinal Sciences, Kerman, Iran

Mohammad Hassan Moshafi
Neuroscience Research Center, Institute of Neuropharmacology, Kerman University of Medicinal Sciences, Kerman, Iran

Alireza Foroumadi
Neuroscience Research Center, Institute of Neuropharmacology, Kerman University of Medicinal Sciences, Kerman, Iran
Pharmaceutical Sciences Research Center, Tehran University of Medical Sciences, Tehran, Iran

Nahid Kabiri
Department of Physiology, Faculty of Veterinary Medicine, Shahid Chamran University of Ahvaz, Ahvaz, Iran

Mohammad Reza Tabandeh
Department of Biochemistry and Molecular Biology, Faculty of Veterinary Medicine, Shahid Chamran University of Ahvaz, Ahvaz, Iran

Seyed Reza Fatemi Tabatabaie
Department of Physiology, Faculty of Veterinary Medicine, Shahid Chamran University of Ahvaz, Ahvaz, Iran

Hasan Fallah Huseini
Medicinal Plants Research Center, Institute of Medicinal Plants, ACECR, Karaj, Iran

Maryam Sotoudeh Anvari
Clinical and Surgical Pathology Department Tehran Heart Center, Tehran University of Medical Sciences, Tehran, Iran

Yaser Tajallizadeh khoob
Endocrinology and Metabolism Research Center, Endocrinology and Metabolism Clinical Sciences Institute, Tehran University of Medical Sciences, Tehran, Iran

Shahram Rabbani
Experimental Research Center, Tehran Heart Center, Tehran University of Medical Sciences, Tehran, Iran

Farshad Sharifi
Elderly Health Research Center, Endocrinology and Metabolism Population Sciences Institute, Tehran University of Medical Sciences, 4th floor, No 4, Ostad Nejatollahi Street, Engelab Avenue, Tehran, Iran

Seyed Masoud Arzaghi
Elderly Health Research Center, Endocrinology and Metabolism Population Sciences Institute, Tehran University of Medical Sciences, 4th floor, No 4, Ostad Nejatollahi Street, Engelab Avenue, Tehran, Iran

Hossein Fakhrzadeh
Elderly Health Research Center, Endocrinology and Metabolism Population Sciences Institute, Tehran University of Medical Sciences, 4th floor, No 4, Ostad Nejatollahi Street, Engelab Avenue, Tehran, Iran

Alireza Aliabadi
Pharmaceutical Sciences Research Center, School of Pharmacy, Kermanshah University of Medical Sciences, Kermanshah, Iran
Department of Medicinal Chemistry, Faculty of Pharmacy, Kermanshah University of Medical Sciences, Kermanshah, Iran

Ahmad Mohammadi-Farani
Pharmaceutical Sciences Research Center, School of Pharmacy, Kermanshah University of Medical Sciences, Kermanshah, Iran
Department of Pharmacology, Toxicology and Medical Services, Faculty of Pharmacy, Kermanshah University of Kermanshah, Iran

Zeinab Hosseinzadeh
Department of Medicinal Chemistry, Faculty of Pharmacy, Kermanshah University of Medical Sciences, Kermanshah, Iran
Students Research Committee, Kermanshah University of Medical Sciences, Kermanshah, Iran

Hamid Nadri
Neurobiomedical Research Center, Yazd Shahid Sadoughi University of Medical Sciences, Yazd, Iran

Alireza Moradi
Neurobiomedical Research Center, Yazd Shahid Sadoughi University of Medical Sciences, Yazd, Iran

Farahnaz Ahmadi
Pharmaceutical Sciences Research Center, School of Pharmacy, Kermanshah University of Medical Sciences, Kermanshah, Iran
Department of Pharmacology, Toxicology and Medical Services, Faculty of Pharmacy, Kermanshah University of Medical Sciences, Kermanshah, Iran

Amol S Shete
Department of Pharmaceutics, Shree Santkrupa College of Pharmacy, Ghogaon, Tal. Karad Dist, Satara, MS, India

Adhikrao V Yadav
Gourishankar Institute of Pharmaceutical Education and Research, Limb, Satara 415002, India

Srinivasa M Murthy
Vignan Institute of Pharmaceutical sciences, Deshmukhi, 508284, Nalgonda Dist, India

Maliheh Barazandeh Tehrani, Melika Namadchian and Effat Souri
Department of Medicinal Chemistry, Faculty of Pharmacy and Pharmaceutical Sciences Research Center, Tehran University of Medical Sciences, Tehran, Iran

Sedigheh Fadaye Vatan
R & D Department, Kish Medipharm Company, No. 64, Kish free zone island, Iran

Effat Souri, Abbas Kaboodari and Massoud Amanlou
Department of Medicinal Chemistry, Faculty of Pharmacy and Drug Design and Development Research Center, Tehran University of Medical Sciences, Tehran 14155-6451, Iran

Noushin Adib
Department of Pharmaceutics, Food and Drug Laboratory Research Center, Ministry of Health, Tehran, Iran

Saeed Manoochehri and Behrad Darvishi
Department of Pharmaceutics, Faculty of Pharmacy, Tehran University of Medical Sciences, Tehran 1417614411, Iran

Golnaz Kamalinia
Nanotechnology Research Centre, Tehran University of Medical Sciences, Tehran, Iran

Mohsen Amini
Department of Medicinal Chemistry, Faculty of Pharmacy, Tehran University of Medical Sciences, Tehran, Iran

Mahdieh Fallah
Arash Hospital, Faculty of Medicine, Tehran University of Medical Sciences, Tehran, Iran

Seyed Naser Ostad
Department of Toxicology and Pharmacology, Faculty of Pharmacy, Tehran University of Medical Sciences, Tehran, Iran

Fatemeh Atyabi and Rassoul Dinarvand
Department of Pharmaceutics, Faculty of Pharmacy, Tehran University of Medical Sciences, Tehran 1417614411, Iran
Nanotechnology Research Centre, Tehran University of Medical Sciences, Tehran, Iran

Abbas Azadmehr
Immunology department, Qazvin University of Medical Sciences, Qazvin, Iran
Immunology department, Mazandaran University of Medical Sciences, Sari, Iran

Reza Hajiaghaee
Pharmacognosy & Pharmaceutics department of Medicinal Plants Research Center, Institute of Medicinal Plants, ACECR, Karaj, Iran

Mohammad Ali Zohal
Internal medicine department, Qazvin University of Medical Sciences, Qazvin, Iran

Ghorban Maliji
Immunology department, Babol University of Medical Sciences, Babol, Iran

Mohammad Reza Nabatchian and Hamid Shahriari
Department of Industrial Engineering, K.N. Toosi University of Technology, No 7, Pardis St., Mollasadra Ave., Tehran, Iran

Mona Shahriari
Department of Dermatology, University of Connecticut Health Center, Farmington, CT, USA